PREVENTION PRACTICE

Strategies for
Physical Therapy
and
Occupational Therapy

Jeffrey Rothman, EdD, PT

Director of Health Sciences
The College of Staten Island of
The City University of New York
Staten Island, New York

Ruth Levine, OTR/L, FAOTA, EdD

Professor and Chairman
Department of Occupational Therapy
College of Allied Health Sciences
Thomas Jefferson University
Philadelphia, Pennsylvania

PREVENTION PRACTICE

Strategies for Physical Therapy and Occupational Therapy

W. B. SAUNDERS COMPANY

Harcourt Brace Jovanovich, Inc.

Philadelphia   London   Toronto   Montreal   Sydney   Tokyo

W. B. SAUNDERS COMPANY
Harcourt Brace Jovanovich, Inc.

The Curtis Center
Independence Square West
Philadelphia, Pennsylvania 19106

Library of Congress Cataloging-in-Publication Data

Prevention practice: Strategies for physical therapy and
occupational therapy
/ edited by Jeffrey Rothman, Ruth Ellen Levine.

p. cm.

ISBN 0–7216–3261–0

1. Health promotion.   2. Medicine,
    Preventive.   I. Rothman, Jeffrey, Ed. D.
    II. Levine, Ruth Ellen.

[DNLM: 1. Health Promotion.
2. Preventive Medicine.   WA 108 P94224]

RA427.8.P75   1992

DNLM/DLC   91-26441

Editor: Margaret M. Biblis
Developmental Editor: Rosanne Hallowell
Designer: Terri Siegel
Cover Designer: Megan Costello Connell
Production Manager: Bill Preston
Manuscript Editors: Marjory I. Fraser and Mary Day McCoy
Illustration Specialist: Cecelia Roberts
Indexer: Ann Cassar

Prevention Practice: Strategies for Physical Therapy
and Occupational Therapy   ISBN 0–7216–3261–0

Printed in the United States of America.

Last digit is the print number: 9   8   7   6   5   4   3   2   1

This book is dedicated to those seeking healthier and more productive lives.

CONTRIBUTORS

John M. Barbis, M.A., P.T., O.C.S. □ Assistant Professor, Department of Physical Therapy, College of Allied Health Sciences, Thomas Jefferson University, Philadelphia, Pennsylvania. □ *Chapter 4: Prevention and Management of Low Back Pain*

Robert D. Bazley, P.T., M.A.T. □ Private Practice, Atlantic Rehabilitation Services, Manasquan, New Jersey. □ *Chapter 3: Promoting Health Through Exercise*

Julie Belkin, O.T.R./L., C.O. □ Director, Occupational Therapy, Mercy Medical Center, Baltimore, Maryland. □ *Chapter 8: Injury Prevention Through Splinting*

Sally H. Bennett, M.S.L.S., O.T.R./L. □ Adjunct Clinical Instructor—Thomas Jefferson University, College of Allied Health Sciences, Philadelphia, Pennsylvania; Staff Occupational Therapist, Institute of Pennsylvania Hospital, Philadelphia, Pennsylvania. □ *Chapter 14: Low Vision: Clinical Aspects and Interventions*

Susan M. Blackmore, M.S., O.T.R., C.H.T. □ Assistant Chief of Occupational Therapy, The New York Hospital, Cornell Medical Center, New York, New York. □ *Chapter 8: Injury Prevention Through Splinting*

Caroline Robinson Brayley, Ph.D., O.T.R./L., F.A.O.T.A. □ Chair and Associate Professor, Department of Occupational Therapy, School of Health Related Professions, University of Pittsburgh, Pittsburgh, Pennsylvania. □ *Chapter 6: Prevention and Management of Chronic Pain*

Ernest A. Burch, Jr., P.T. □ Chief Executive Officer, Burch, Rhoads, and Loomis, P.A., Baltimore, Maryland. □ *Chapter 30: Marketing, Health Promotion, and Injury Prevention Programs*

Theresa Cappelli Calibey, A.T.C., O.T.R. □ Chief of Occupational Therapy, St. Francis Hospital, Wilmington, Delaware. □ *Chapter 7: Prevention, Treatment, and Rehabilitation of Sports Injuries*

Pascale Carayon, Ph.D. □ Assistant Professor, Department of Industrial Engineering, University of Wisconsin-Madison, Madison, Wisconsin. □ *Chapter 23: Physical and Mental Strain in Computerized Workplaces: Causes and Remedies*

Cheryl A. Cott, B.P.T., Dip. Geront, M.Sc. □ Lecturer, Division of Physical Therapy, Faculty of Medicine, University of Toronto, Toronto, Ontario, Canada; Geriatric Consultant, Physiotherapy Department, Sunnybrook Health Science Centre, Toronto, Ontario, Canada. □ *Chapter 13: Preventing Accidental Falls by the Elderly*

Quinten M. Davis, M.B.A. □ Vice President for Operations, B.I.M.C., Baltimore, Maryland. □ *Chapter 30: Marketing, Health Promotion, and Injury Prevention Programs*

Wendy S. Davis, M.Ed., O.T.R./L. □ Clinical Associate Professor, Thomas Jefferson University, Philadelphia, Pennsylvania; Clinical Coordinator of Occupational Therapy, Children's Rehabilitation Hospital, Philadelphia, Pennsylvania. □ *Chapter 15: Promoting Health and Wellness in the Pediatric Disabled and "At Risk" Population*

Elizabeth DePoy, O.T.R./L., M.S.W., Ph.D. □ Assistant Professor, University of Maine, Orono, Maine. □ *Chapter 29: Program Evaluation*

Phil Dunphy, B.S., P.T. □ Private Practice, New Jersey. □ *Chapter 28: Assessment of Exercise and Fitness Equipment*

Laura N. Gitlin, Ph.D. □ Assistant Professor, Department of Occupational Therapy, Research Coordinator, College of Allied Health Sciences, Thomas Jefferson University, Philadelphia, Pennsylvania. □ *Chapter 20: Use of the Environment for Promoting Optimal Function in the Chronically Disabled*

Pamela J. Holliday, B.Sc.(P.T.), M.Sc. □ Research Associate, Department of Surgery and Division of Physical Therapy, University of Toronto, Toronto, Ontario, Canada; Research Associate, Centre for Studies in Aging, Sunnybrook Health Science Centre, Toronto, Ontario, Canada. □ *Chapter 13: Preventing Accidental Falls by the Elderly*

Susan J. Isernhagen, B.S., P.T. □ Clinical Instructor, Program in Physical Therapy, University of Minnesota; President, Isernhagen & Associates, Inc., Duluth, Minnesota. □ *Chapter 21: Corporate Fitness and Prevention of Industrial Injuries*

Caryn R. Johnson, M.S., O.T.R./L. □ Clinical Assistant Professor, Thomas Jefferson University, Philadelphia, Pennsylvania. □ *Chapter 17: Aquatics for Promoting Health in People with Physical Disabilities*

Julie Moyer Knowles, E.D.D., A.T.C., P.T. □ Adjunct Professor, University of Delaware, Newark, Delaware; Adjunct Professor, Delaware Technical and Community College, Wilmington, Delaware; Clinical Assistant Professor, Thomas Jefferson University, Philadelphia, Pennsylvania; Director of Rehabilitation, Pike Creek Sports Medicine Center, Wilmington, Delaware. □ *Chapter 7: Prevention, Treatment, and Rehabilitation of Sports Injuries*

Elissa Krasnopolsky-Levine, M.S., R.D., C.N.S.D. ☐ Chief, Quality Management and Staff Development Section, Dietetic Service, Department of Veterans Affairs, Brooklyn, New York. ☐ *Chapter 18: Nutrition in Health and Wellness: Planning for Services*

Ruth E. Levine, O.T.R./L., F.A.O.T.A., Ed.D. ☐ Professor and Chairman, Department of Occupational Therapy, College of Allied Health Sciences, Thomas Jefferson University, Philadelphia, Pennsylvania. ☐ *Chapter 20: Use of the Environment for Promoting Optimal Function in the Chronically Disabled*

Susan Johnson Lieber, B.S., O.T.R./L. ☐ Formerly Coordinator of Work Performance Assessment Rehabilitation Program, University of Pittsburgh Medical Center, Pain Evaluation and Treatment Institute, Pittsburgh, Pennsylvania. ☐ *Chapter 6: Prevention and Management of Chronic Pain*

Edmund J. McTernan, Sr., M.P.H., Ed.D., Sc.D. ☐ Professor of Health Sciences, School of Allied Health Professions, Health Sciences Center, State University of New York, Stony Brook, New York. ☐ *Chapter 1: Promoting Health Through Public Policy*

Susan Morrill, P.T., M.A. ☐ District Manager, Rehabilitation People, Inc., Langhorne, Pennsylvania; Private Practice Consultant Specializing in Holistic Health, Ardmore, Pennsylvania. ☐ *Chapter 19: Holistic Stress Management*

Julie Mount, M.A., P.T. ☐ Assistant Professor, Department of Physical Therapy, College of Allied Health Sciences, Thomas Jefferson University, Philadelphia, Pennsylvania. ☐ *Chapter 12: Designing Exercise Programs for the Elderly*

David L. Nelson, Ph.D., O.T.R., F.A.O.T.A. ☐ Professor, Department of Occupational Therapy, Western Michigan University, Kalamazoo, Michigan. ☐ *Chapter 2: The Roles of Occupational Therapy in Preventing Further Disability of Elderly Persons in Long-Term Care Facilities*

Jane O'Callaghan, B.Sc. Rehabilitation Med., M.Ed., O.T.(C.) P.T. ☐ Partner, TOC Consulting Inc., Toronto, Ontario, Canada. ☐ *Chapter 22: Primary Prevention and Ergonomics: The Role of Rehabilitation Specialists in Preventing Occupational Injury*

Lynda Olender-Russo, B.S.N., M.A., C.N.S.N. ☐ Adjunct Faculty Member, New York University, New York, New York; Nutrition Support Clinician, Brooklyn VA Medical Center, Nursing Service Designee for Nutrition Committee, Brooklyn, New York. ☐ *Chapter 18: Nutrition in Health and Wellness: Planning for Services*

Jean Duffy Rath, P.T., Dip. Mech., D.T. ☐ Director, Spine Center of New Jersey, Raritan, New Jersey; Faculty Member, McKenzie Institute, U.S.A. ☐ *Chapter 5: Prevention of Musculoskeletal Injury*

Wayne W. Rath, P.T., Dip. Mech., D.T. ☐ Clinical Assistant Professor, Department of Physical Therapy, Thomas Jefferson University, Philadelphia, Pennsylvania; Director, Spine Center of New Jersey, Raritan, New Jersey; Faculty Member, McKenzie Institute, U.S.A. ☐ *Chapter 5: Prevention of Musculoskeletal Injury*

Margaret E. Rinehart, M.S., P.T. ☐ Assistant Professor, Department of Physical Therapy, College of Allied Health Sciences, Thomas Jefferson University, Philadelphia, Pennsylvania. Contract Physical Therapist, Thomas Jefferson University Home Health Services and Prime Physical Therapy Group, Inc., Philadelphia, Pennsylvania. ☐ *Chapter 9: Prevention of Spinal Cord Injury*

Jeffrey Rothman, Ed.D., P.T. ☐ Director of Health Sciences, The College of Staten Island of The City University of New York, Staten Island, New York. ☐ *Chapter 27: Problem-Solving Approach to Health and Wellness: An Educational-Model*

Robert L. Rubinstein, Ph.D. ☐ Associate Director of Research, Philadelphia Geriatric Center, Philadelphia, Pennsylvania. ☐ *Chapter 25: How to Find Meaning in Client Interaction*

Roseann C. Schaaf, M.Ed., O.T.R./L. ☐ Instructor, Department of Occupational Therapy, Thomas Jefferson University, Philadelphia, Pennsylvania. ☐ *Chapter 15: Promoting Health and Wellness in the Pediatric Disabled and "At Risk" Population*

Kieron Sheehy, B.A.(Hons.), M.Ed., Cert. Ed., C. Psychol. ☐ Lecturer in Behavioural Science, St. Loyes School of Occupational Therapy, Exeter, Devon, England. ☐ *Chapter 16: Preventing Disabilities in Children: Active Intervention in the Developmental Process*

Roger O. Smith, M.O.T., O.T.R. ☐ Associate Researcher and Lecturer, Department of Therapeutic Science and Trace Research and Development Center, University of Wisconsin-Madison; Computer Access and Interface Specialist, Communications Aids and Systems Clinic, University of Wisconsin Hospitals and Clinics, Madison, Wisconsin. ☐ *Chapter 23: Physical and Mental Strain in Computerized Workplaces: Causes and Remedies*

Clint Stucky, B.A. ☐ Department of Occupational Therapy, Hutchinson Hospital, Hutchinson, Kansas. ☐ *Chapter 2: The Roles of Occupational Therapy in Preventing Further Disability of Elderly Persons in Long-Term Care Facilities*

Rodney S. Taylor, B.Sc.(Hons), Ph.D. ☐ Senior Lecturer, Department of Biological Sciences, St. Loyes School of Occupational Therapy, Exeter, England; Research Fellow, Department of Postgraduate Medicine, University of Exeter, Exeter, Devon, England. ☐ *Chapter 11: Prevention for Cardiac Patients*

Wendy D. Torresin, Dip. P.&O.T., M.H.Sc. □ Assistant Professor, School of Occupational and Physiotherapy, McMaster University, Hamilton, Ontario, Canada; Director, Physiotherapy, Chedoke-McMaster Hospitals, Hamilton, Ontario, Canada. □ *Chapter 13: Preventing Accidental Falls by the Elderly*

Mary Winegardner Voth, B.S. □ Owner and Clinic Director, Myofascial & Manual Therapy Institute, Richardson, Texas. □ *Chapter 10: Prevention and Management of Temporomandibular Joint Dysfunction*

Katherine LeGuin White, Ph.D., P.T. □ Associate Professor and Program Director, UMDNJ—School of Health Related Professions, Wenonah, New Jersey. □ *Chapter 26: Ethical Considerations in the Prevention and Rehabilitation of Injuries*

Karen A. Williams, O.T.R. □ Director, Michigan Hand Rehab Center, Inc., Warren, Michigan. □ *Chapter 24: Consultative Work Programs for Cumulative Trauma Disorders*

Debra S. Zelnick, M.S., O.T.R./L. □ Adjunct Instructor, College of Allied Health Sciences, Thomas Jefferson University, Philadelphia, Pennsylvania; Regional Manager, Therapy Care Systems, Blue Bell, Pennsylvania. □ *Chapter 9: Prevention of Spinal Cord Injury*

FOREWORD

The editors of this book, *Prevention Practice: Strategies for Physical Therapy and Occupational Therapy*, have chosen a timely topic that provides a comprehensive perspective of the role that prevention may have in concert with traditional treatment and rehabilitation provided by occupational and physical therapists. To ignore the contributions associated with prevention after injury occurs is to be self-serving, because no one who has treated patients and clients after an accident can be more aware of the need for prevention: prevention to prevent accidents and trauma and prevention to reduce and, when possible, avoid the sequelae that may follow an injury.

To provide a context for prevention, before and after accidents, one need only examine the consequences of one diagnostic category—traumatic head injury—to understand the consequences and costs that may be associated with injuries. Head injury is the major cause of disability in young adults: 63% of its victims are under 25 years of age, and males outnumber females by two to one (Committee on Trauma Research, 1985).

The prevalence of head injuries in the United States is estimated to be between 1,000,000 and 1,800,000 cases per year, of which 50,000 to 90,000 individuals will sustain injuries that preclude a return to normal lifestyles. It is estimated that the survivors will incur hospitalization and treatment costs averaging 4 billion dollars as a result of their injuries. In addition to this direct cost, it is further estimated that their injuries will cost the United States an estimated additional 75 to 100 billion dollars in lost economic activity and productivity (National Head Injury Foundation, 1984). The survivors of head injuries generally have a normal life expectancy of 35 to 60 years postinjury (Klein, cited in Moore and Bartlow, 1900), resulting in persistent economic, social, and personal costs (Cope, cited in Berry, 1985).

One additional factor not considered in these figures is that it is not unusual for one or more family members to give up productive employment to provide care for a family member with traumatic head injury. These figures are staggering, and yet they reveal little about the personal consequences experienced by survivors and their families, many of whose lives may be permanently changed. However, even though these survivors may not regain normal lifestyles, it is still possible for them to experience health, in its broadest sense.

To their credit, the editors have included many of the preventive considerations that contribute to or affect health and that must be addressed by occupational and physical therapists who provide treatment services to persons with acute injuries as well as to persons with chronic conditions: cultural differences, nutrition, public policy, ethical considerations, the use of activity to promote health, and the contributions of exercise to health. By implication, health is thus defined as more than return to employment. It becomes a quality of life that is accessible to those with chronic conditions and to individuals who may never return to school or work but who can have a meaningful life. Health thus becomes an important factor in reducing or preventing secondary problems, such as depression, low energy, or contractures, that arise from inactivity, inadequate nutrition, and poor positioning. Involvement in meaningful activities that give one a sense of purpose, fulfillment, and participation may also contribute to health.

This book, whose purpose is to address pragmatic concerns of treatment, will be a valuable contribution to the professional literature and should broaden the domains of professional practice and responsibility to include prevention, thus reducing secondary health care costs. The ultimate consequence, however, is that the lives and health of many persons with disabilities and their families will be enriched.

JERRY A. JOHNSON, ED.D., O.T.R./L, F.A.O.T.A.
Professor and Graduate Coordinator
Thomas Jefferson University
Past President, American Occupational Therapy Association, Inc.

References

Berry S: Rehabilitation planning for the severely head injured. J Appl Rehab Counselling 16:46–48, 1985

Committee on Trauma Research: Head injury in America. Washington, National Academy Press, 1985.

Moore RL and Bartlow CL: Vocational limitations and assessment of the client who is traumatically brain injured. J Appl Rehab Counselling 21(1):3–8, 1990.

National Head Injury Foundation, Inc: The Silent Epidemic. Framingham, MA, National Head Injury Foundation, 1984.

FOREWORD

The notion of prevention and preventive care is not new. It enjoys its origins in many ancient cultures of the world that placed great value on physical well-being and health. The ancient societies of China focused on the balance of Yin and Yang in promoting health; Rome, Greece, and the Scandinavian countries valued the importance of health and physical culture; and the earliest Hebrew societies documented the importance of certain dietary restrictions to promote health and to avoid illness or disease.

Throughout this century public health professionals have advocated the importance of preventive care as an integral element of the quality of health and medical care. Those professionals have also developed an extensive literature relating to prevention.

For many years, the Physical and Occupational Therapy professions have been among those considered as "rehabilitation" professions. In the perspective of many, particularly with the Physical Medicine and Rehabilitation (PM&R) residency development following World War II, our professions were providers of services that came after all other life-saving measures. To some extent that may still be a valid perspective. However, this book presents an expanded view of the roles of Physical and Occupational Therapists in multiple aspects to preventive care.

I urge readers to direct specific attention to the authors' definitions of the levels of prevention and preventive care. Note that prevention in its narrow sense means health promotion and specific disease prevention. However, in its broader interpretation, it means prevention of further sequelae at any point along the primary, secondary, or tertiary level of prevention.

There is an additional point I wish to make regarding definitions, and it is critically important to Physical Therapists, Occupational Therapists, and to students enrolled in our preprofessional education programs. In the late 19th and early 20th centuries, it was comparatively easy and comfortable to identify preventive care measures in terms of the control of communicable diseases such as malaria or influenza. However, our contemporary society is laden with the incidence and prevalance of chronic diseases. Those of us practicing in the so-called "rehabilitation" professions interact with clients who are experiencing multichronicity. For example, we may develop a plan of care related specifically to a pathologic condition such as a hip fracture or a cerebrovascular accident. However, that same client may also have a history of coronary heart failure, chronic obstructive pulmonary disease, and diabetes. In effect, the presence of multichronicity obligates us to be alert to make preventive interventions at any point along the health service spectrum.

In our practices of Physical and Occupational Therapy, we enjoy the challenging opportunities of facilitating functional outcomes for our clients.

This book, consisting of 30 chapters, provides us with many efficacious directions in that regard.

I commend the authors on the timeliness of this book which, in my opinion, has the potential of becoming a major text for practitioners and for students. Most important, this book may reap its greatest value in expanding the horizons of other health care professionals with regard to their understanding and expectations of our professional contributions to health care.

JANE S. MATHEWS
Past President, American Physical Therapy Association,
and Rehabilitation Team Leader, Visiting Nurse Association of North Shore,
Gloucester, Massachusetts

PREFACE

Prevention Practice: Strategies for Physical Therapy and Occupational Therapy is a guide for physical and occupational therapists in the United States, United Kingdom, and Canada who want to incorporate the concept of prevention of disability into their daily practices. Although the idea of prevention in therapy is not new, the authors who took the effort and time to share their programs here are modern-day pioneers, because our present health care system remains focused on acute or tertiary care. Recently, as health care consumes more and more of our national income, the concept of prevention is once again gaining attention.

The recent interest in prevention began in 1979 when the Surgeon General issued a report delineating goals for a healthier population. Dr. Koop urged Americans to quit smoking and to change their eating habits and sexual practices, stating that these changes could have a positive impact on health and happiness. The Department of Health and Human Services announced a prevention program on September 6, 1990, when Secretary of Health Louis W. Sullivan released a report entitled *Healthy People 2000,* a culmination of 3 years of effort by the U.S. Public Health Service. The agency is committed to achieving health promotion and disease prevention objectives by setting up priority areas. (The report can be obtained from the Superintendent of Documents, Government Printing Office, Washington, D.C. 20402-9325 [Telephone 202-783-3238], Stock No. 017-001-00473-1.) As health professionals, therapists will have to

---

Injury Prevention and Rehabilitation: Definition of Terms

Health Promotion—focuses on maintaining or improving the general health of individuals, families, and communities. Interventions by physical therapists and occupational therapists are directed toward developing the resources of persons to maintain or enhance their well-being.

Primary Prevention—includes generalized health promotion as well as specific protection against disease, precedes disease or dysfunction and is applied to a population generally considered both physically and emotionally healthy. It is not therapeutic, does not use therapeutic treatments, and does not involve symptom identification. The purpose is to decrease the vulnerability of the individual or population to illness or dysfunction.

Secondary Prevention—emphasizes early diagnosis and prompt treatment to halt the pathologic process, thus shortening its duration and severity and enabling the individual to return to a former state of health at the earliest time possible. Ranges from providing screening techniques and treating early stages of disease to limiting disability by averting or delaying the consequences of advanced disease. Screening and health teaching are important aspects.

Tertiary Prevention—not only stops at the disease process but also prevents complete disability. The objective is to return the affected individual to a useful place in society within the constraints of the disability. It occurs when a defect or disability is permanent and irreversible.

Prevention—in a narrow sense means averting the development of disease. In a broad sense it consists of the measures that limit the progression of disease at any point along its course.

---

define their roles in this new arena, develop strategies to achieve their goals, and obtain appropriate levels of fiscal support.

Today, most therapists work in tertiary care to stop the progression of a disease. We also use secondary prevention when we teach patients how to prevent disease and encourage them to seek help early in the disease process. This is not enough, though, since we have little time to promote healthy lifestyles and encourage prevention of disability. Although many of the programs explained in this book focus on secondary and tertiary prevention, you will find a wealth of information on new areas of practice in which prevention and health promotion are central aspects of care.

Because of their knowledge and skills, therapists are uniquely qualified to work with individuals and to encourage health and wellness. Physical therapists have a thorough understanding of the musculoskeletal, cardiopulmonary, and neuromuscular systems and are skilled in biomechanics, kinesiology, and therapeutic exercise. Occupational therapists have a thorough understanding of the relationship between functional performance and motor, sensory-perceptual, cognitive, emotional, cultural, and social aspects of behavior. Skilled in promoting competence, occupational therapists try to actively engage the person in a "just-right challenge."

The authors contributing to this book were selected because of their reputation as creators of successful programs that promoted prevention and wellness. They were asked to consider the individual as the center of a model of concentric circles in which family and social groups, institutions, and the environment exerted influence on health. Thus, many of the authors address the needs of the person in relation to the immediate family, the community, and larger groups such as institutions. This was not always easy to describe, since the opportunities to direct prevention programs have to be created by the therapists.

There are 30 chapters in the book organized in four parts.

I. Promoting a Health Lifestyle. This part has three chapters that describe programs that promote health by influencing public policy through activity and through exercise.

II. Prevention and Treatment Strategies for Specific Problems. In the second part specific problems are addressed through chapters that focus on clinical issues. These chapters include specific information on the goals, population, treatment, equipment, and setting for the program. Case study material and charts and illustrations reinforce the program ideas.

III. Workplace and Environment. In the third part, programs for the workplace and environment are described. Some chapters offer specific program ideas, but others are designed to encourage creative thinking about progressive treatment.

IV. Issues for the Therapist and Educator. In the final section, the authors offer ideas for improving clinical intervention.

Two leaders in prevention, Jerry Johnson and Jane Matthews, wrote the Forewords for the book. Both have extensive international and national experience with academic and clinical occupational and physical therapy programs in prevention. We are glad that they offered their invaluable guidance and support for the book.

We hope that you, the reader, will find the authors' ideas useful and that you can design new programs with the help of these clinicians and educators, whose hard-won experience is often the best teacher. The chapters are concrete and practical, with information formatted for easy incorporation into clinical practice. We hope to hear of many new programs that were started as a result of this book.

We are delighted with the opportunity to encourage new directions for patient care. The high cost of and limited access to the health care system, as well as the growing illness of segments of our society, are worrisome to all of us. In some small way we hope that you will feel supported in your desire to start a new program that improves health care for patients.

JEFFREY ROTHMAN, ED.D., P.T.
RUTH E. LEVINE, O.T.R./L., F.A.O.T.A., ED.D.

ACKNOWLEDGMENTS

The strength of this text lies in its authors' commitment to improving health care services. We are grateful to the contributors to *Prevention Practice: Strategies for Physical Therapy and Occupational Therapy* who agreed to share their visionary ideas with you, the reader. Many of these authors contributed material in subject areas in which there are few models to follow. We would like to thank them and to acknowledge their dedication to improving client services.

We would also like to acknowledge the staff of the W.B. Saunders Company, in particular our editor, Margaret Biblis, as well as other members of the Saunders staff, including Rosanne Hallowell, Marjory I. Fraser, Bill Preston, Cecelia Roberts, Karen O'Keefe, and David Nazaruk—a dedicated and thoroughly professional group of individuals whose goal is to improve the quality of health care texts. We also extend appreciation to our colleagues, clients, staff, and students who have expressed interest in this book and encouraged our efforts.

Finally, on a personal level, we would like to extend a special note of gratitude to our families and friends for the patience and understanding that they expressed throughout the planning, writing, and editing process. Elise, Erica, and Blair Rothman and Richard Schemm—a big thank you for your support.

CONTENTS

13
Preventing Accidental Falls by the Elderly 234

Pamela J. Holliday
Cheryl A. Cott
Wendy D. Torresin

14
Low Vision: Clinical Aspects and Interventions 258

Sally H. Bennett

15
Promoting Health and Wellness in the Pediatric Disabled and "At Risk" Population 270

Roseann C. Schaaf
Wendy S. Davis

16
Preventing Disabilities in Children: Active Intervention in the Developmental Process 284

Kieron Sheehy

PART III Workplace and Environment

20
Use of the Environment for Promoting Optimal Function in the Chronically Disabled 347

Ruth E. Levine
Laura N. Gitlin

21
Corporate Fitness and Prevention of Industrial Injuries 356

Susan J. Isernhagen

22
Primary Prevention and Ergonomics: The Role of Rehabilitation Specialists in Preventing Occupational Injury 370

Jane O'Callaghan

PREVENTION PRACTICE

Strategies for
Physical Therapy
and
Occupational Therapy

Promoting a Healthy Lifestyle

1

Edmund J. McTernan, Sr.

Promoting Health Through Public Policy

The primary purpose of this chapter is to focus on how public policy is developed and maintained in the contemporary American society, especially in the context of policies that promote health or prevent illness and disability. Public policy includes all those actions adopted by a government to promote public welfare.

PRIMER ON PUBLIC POLICY: DEFINING THE WILL OF THE PEOPLE

The usual measure of any recommended addition to public policy may be summed up by asking, "Is this for the public good and will it serve the best interests of at least a majority of the community at large?" The path from a good idea into the public policy of the community is likely to be lengthy and arduous.

Whereas an individual or a group may support a concept or policy that they believe is beneficial to the total society, that concept must be adopted into the legislative structure of the total community before it can be considered public policy. This is often a very difficult objective to achieve. According to Alger (1990), it is much easier to defeat a bill than to enact one. Since 1974, fewer than 5% of all bills introduced in Congress have been enacted.

AMERICAN FEDERAL SYSTEM

The American system of government affects and ultimately controls policy development in the health field as it does with all public policy. The checks and balances, which result from the tensions between the executive, legislative, and judicial branches will frequently modify a policy suggested by any of the three, whereas the different levels of government (national, state, and local) may similarly stimulate, attenuate, or impede the incorporation of a well-intentioned health proposal into the law of the land (Fig. 1–1).

Executive Branch

The executive branch of our federal government reaches its apogee in the office of the president. The penultimate level is that of the several federal departments, each headed by a secretary. From these levels, a command chain of federal officials extends downward to the lowest grade clerk earning a living in some obscure regional office many miles from the national capital.

Obviously, the president is not alone in discharging the many duties of the office. He or she has a large staff of assistants and aides, many of them familiar because of their frequent exposure in the media; others are unknown and unrecog-

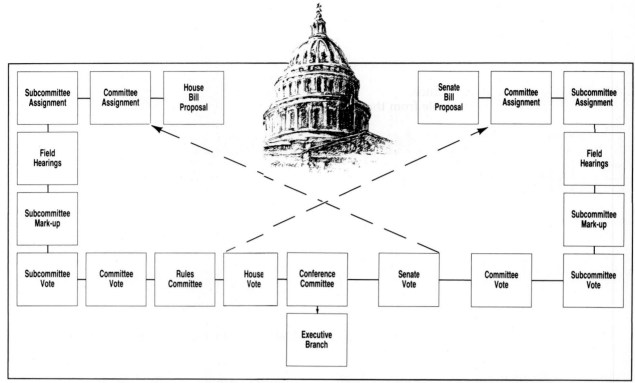

Figure 1–1. A schematic representation of the system by which the U.S. Congress works. (From the *Educational Record* 71(3):22–23, 1990. Reprinted by permission of the publisher, American Council on Education.)

nized outside the precincts of the White House or of the Executive Office Building. Along this chain are countless individuals who may be in a position to help along legislation they see as desirable or to impede the progress of other proposals intended for adoption as public policy, which they may view as unnecessary or undesirable.

Interacting with the "Feds"

In the arena of health promotion/disease prevention (HP/DP) efforts, the most important federal agency to contact and seek support from is the Public Health Service (PHS). PHS's Office of Disease Prevention and Health Promotion is, of course, the key contact agency, but there are countless other federal agencies that have an interest, role, and voice on this topic. These were detailed in a special supplement to the September–October 1983 issue of *Public Health Reports*, the official journal of the PHS.

That supplement, entitled "Implementation Plans for Attaining the Objectives for the Nation" (U.S. Department of Health and Human Services, Office of Disease Prevention/Health Promotion (USDHHS: ODPHP), 1983) used 176 quarto-sized pages of reduced type, setting forth the many plans and programs toward the achievement of the 1980 *Objectives for the Nation* (USDHHS: ODPHP, 1980), which had been developed by every agency and subdivision of the PHS.

Although in most cases the PHS or other divisions of the DHHS are likely to be most frequently contacted by proponents or opponents of health promotion legislation, one must also be alert to the interests and influence of other federal agencies, wherein the responsibilities of those agencies overlap into the area of health concerns. For example, the U.S. Department of Transportation is a major player in one area of health promotion (accident prevention) and parenthetically in setting standards for the training of emergency medical technicians.

The first step in approaching federal employees of the executive branch on issues relating to health is to identify one key official who can and might be helpful. In the HP/DP arena, the ODPHP is frequently a good place to start. Staff of this office are also very helpful about suggesting other officials who might be contacted for additional information or assistance.

Two useful documents available from the U.S. Government Printing Office are the *U.S. Government Manual* and the *Congressional Directory, One Hundred First Congress.* Updated editions of these books are published frequently, and they list essentially all the federal officials and all departments that one might wish to contact.

Impact of the Executive Branch on National Legislation

In our national system, laws are of course made by the Congress. However, those laws are subject to presidential approval or veto, so the executive branch certainly exercises considerable influence over the form that a proposed piece of legislation eventually takes.

All laws must be implemented and enforced if they are to be meaningful. This requires the adoption of administrative regulations that interpret and define the law. The development of these regulations occurs within the executive branch.

There are, within Congress, legislators who are from the same political party as the president. Although these lawmakers may not always agree with the chief executive, it is almost beyond imagination that the president could not prevail on at least a few members of both houses to introduce a bill that he or she supports.

Finally, the office of president carries with it immense persuasive power, particularly when the incumbent is a forceful and respected personality. For all these reasons, it is a bit simplistic to say that Congress makes the laws. Indeed, Congress must pass the legislation, but the president must accept it (unless a presidential veto is overridden), and it is the executive branch that will shape the implementation of the legislation through the administrative policies that it will adopt.

Legislative Branch

Conversely, the ultimate decision concerning proposed legislation that will be voted on in the House of Representatives and in the Senate is clearly a congressional decision. Any proposed legislation can be stopped or expedited at a number of points as it makes its way toward incorporation into the law of the land.

Proponents of new laws must first enlist at least one member of either House to introduce a bill that addresses the subject in which they are interested. Generally with the help of their primary sponsor, proponents must then obtain a sponsor in the other House. Developing a list of several cosponsors in both the House and the Senate is a very helpful step.

Proposed laws, once introduced, are then referred to the appropriate committees. Here again, the sympathy and support of members of these important committees, including bipartisan support if possible, are great advantages. Once released by the committee, a bill passed in both Houses will go to a conference committee for resolution of any differences between the Senate and House versions.

Countless laws have been passed by the Congress, with significant authorizations (a sum of money recommended for dedication to that legislation), which were then seriously diluted or even hamstrung by a lack of sufficient appropriations (the sum of monies actually released for the purpose of that bill). The latter decision comes in the first instance from an appropriations committee in each House, which divides the total available pot of funding across all the legislation for which funding is required. The appropriations recommended by the two Houses are often at different levels; the difference is then resolved by a House–Senate Joint Conference Committee, which must agree on the amount to be provided for the purposes of each act or law.

The allied health provisions of the Public Health Act Section 796(a), Title 7, provide a useful case in point of this process. The provision of federal funds in support of allied health education per se ended in 1981. Over the next several years, effective lobbying by the American Society of Allied Health Professions and others culminated in the passage of new authorizing legislation at a level of 2.5 million dollars in 1988. However, no funds were provided in support of the act in 1989. Because of increased lobbying efforts, $750,000 was appropriated in fiscal year 1990, and the first allied health education grants were approved and funded in that year. In fiscal year 1991 1.3 million dollars were appropriated for allied health education.

Judicial Branch

The judicial branch can of course affect legislation and, consequently, federal funding as it exercises its responsibility to rule on the constitutionality of new laws and on the ways in which those laws are interpreted. For example, judicial endorsement of public health laws requiring child immunizations has supported the cause of public health and preventive care on many occasions. However, because interventions by the judiciary are a much less common path toward the development of public policy regarding health promotion, judicial influence will not be discussed in depth here.

AFFECTING NATIONAL LEGISLATION AND ADMINISTRATION

Health professionals interested in the adoption of a particular program into official public policy typically interact with the process of legislation and regulation through either the executive or legislative branches of the federal government. Although it is conceivable that an issue could be brought to the judicial review of the Supreme Court by a series of lawsuits and appeals through the system, this would be an unusual and extraordinary occurrence.

Informing, Testifying, and Lobbying

What does happen frequently, probably daily, is that we attempt to affect legislation, or to foster or modify federal policy, through lobbying efforts directed to members of either House of Congress or officials of the executive branch of government. Lobbying is properly used only in reference to efforts directed at members of a legislative body. The term is used here in a somewhat broader context.

The simplest example of lobbying is when citizens write to a legislator, giving their views on a particular law, proposed law, or problem in need of legislative attention. Most commonly, these letters are addressed to the legislators elected to represent the district in which the writers live and vote. The next escalation of the effort is when the communication takes the form of a telegram or a telephone call. A third level of expressing interest or concern is a personal visit to the legislator in his or her Washington office or home district office. Most legislators maintain two offices: one in the national capital (or in the state capital in the case of state legislators), and the other in their home district. In large districts there may also be subsidiary offices. Each office has one or more staff members to meet and respond to constituents in the absence of the legislator.

Professional Lobbyists

Because few practicing health-care professionals could afford more than an occasional visit to lobby a legislator, organized groups of practitioners with continuing interest in an issue or a field of issues may employ a professional lobbyist. The national capital and most if not all state capitals are the operation ground of a number of professional lobbyists, some who lobby full time and some of them lawyers who engage in lobbying on a part-time basis.

Large organizations often employ one or more full-time lobbyists who devote their entire effort to the interests of that organization. Other lobbyists accept clients on a part-time basis, representing such clients on a regular or as-needed basis, charging a retainer and often a unit-of-time fee as agreed on by contract. Typically, the employing group must also underwrite any expenses incurred by the lobbyist working on its behalf.

The principal advantage of the professional lobbyist is that of access to key personnel within the legislative or executive system. If lobbyists are effective, they know the right person to reach, how to do it, and when. They are usually respected and well liked by those with whom they deal and therefore have fairly ready access to the halls of government.

Key Players: Administrative and Legislative Staff Members

Whether lobbying on their own or using a lobbyist, proponents or opponents of a particular issue must recognize that the entire business of government does not take place under the aegis of the elected official alone. Every legislator and every administrative officer of government has a staff. Much of the study of an issue, and the determination of a position on that issue, is performed by these staff members. Senior legislators often have specialists on their staff who concern themselves with specific types of issues and legislation that relate to their specialty area such as health, aging, and so on.

Responsiveness of Legislators

In most cases, staff decide when an issue merits serious attention. They study all aspects of the issue and report a recommended stand to the elected or appointed official for whom they work. Thus, major progress on a proposed policy may occur before the legislator or appointed official even hears of it.

Most people are surprised at the level of responsiveness that they encounter when they first make contact with one of their legislators. Constituents who request an appointment to visit their legislator's office will rarely be discouraged or dismissed. If legislators are unavailable, or even if they are on hand, an appropriate staff member will often be asked to sit in and to follow up on the concern, suggestion, or need that is discussed. Similarly, mail to elected legislators rarely goes unanswered! Not infrequently, the letter is acknowledged, with a promise of follow-up; in due course, the results of that follow-up are reported in a letter.

What is not surprising is that the most solicitous attention is reserved for the people in a position to re-elect or defeat the legislator: home-district constituents. However, it is a rare office holder who does not treat all visitors with courtesy and attention.

Much of the effective work of legislative bodies occurs through a committee structure. In bicameral systems such as our federal and state systems—except for Nevada, which has a unicameral legislature—there are committees in each House, often with different titles, that carry on the work of developing, passing, or modifying laws. Each develops a program that is then presented to the full body. Differences that emerge between the programs adopted by the two Houses are then resolved by a joint conference committee, which has equal membership from both Houses.

Committees, too, have their own staff who carry on much of the work. At this level, staff members tend to be even more specialized than those who serve an individual legislator. For example, the Committee on Health and the Environment in the U.S. Senate has in recent years had a full-time physician as chief member of its staff.

Therapists interested in encouraging legislation in the area of HP/DP should certainly inform their legislator of their support. This information might be conveyed in a letter, in a mailgram, or by a personal visit to the legislator's office. Often, a letter followed up by a personal visit has added power in communicating interests and concerns. Group visits by constituents and members of an affinity group (such as American Occupational Therapy Association) are especially effective. Beyond a visit to the home-district legislators, however, it is important to get the message to the relevant committees. A list of members of the appropriate committees should be obtained and, whenever possible, colleagues who share your viewpoint and who reside in the districts of the members should be enlisted in the campaign. A letter from "your constituent" followed by an office visit by that individual, alone or with a small group able to articulate the concern effectively, including one or more constituents, if possible, is an excellent course of action.

If there is an issue of great importance to the affinity group, a visit by delegates from that group to the chairpeople of the appropriate committees in both Houses of the legislative body is another important step.

Some Tips on Lobbying

John DiBiaggio, President of Michigan State University, suggested some useful tips on effective lobbying in an article published in *Educational Record* (DiBiaggio, 1990). President DiBiaggio presented a list of 10 tips developed from the perspective of the university president. Several of these suggestions are just as relevant for the health professional interested in furthering the cause of a health issue such as increased federal emphasis on HP/DP. In abbreviated form, DiBiaggio's recommendations include the following:

1. Know the senators and representative; don't just know about them.
2. Be as considerate of a representative's office time as you [would] want people to be of yours. Have data and other support materials readily available in your mind and in your briefcase. Be clear and concise in your presentation. . . . Above all, do your homework on the issues.
3. Do your homework on members of Congress, as

well. Know the legislative and personal interests of those you visit.

4. Be prepared to promptly assist congressional member needs, inquiries, and requests for expertise.

5. Recognize that . . . members of Congress enjoy capable, hard-working staff support. . . . Know exactly to what issues the individual staff members are assigned.

6. Work closely . . . with [your professional] associations . . . that effectively represent you in Washington. . . . Staff members at these organizations are up-to-date on issues and are invaluable resources on Federal relations. In order for the staff members to help you on [Capitol] Hill, notify the associations well in advance of your visit; don't just drop in.

7. [Do not make] a practice of dropping in unannounced on members of Congress.

8. Appreciate your folks on the Hill. Members of Congress, on the whole, are doing the best they can under pressure . . . serving the unrelenting demands and needs of diverse constituencies with limited funding, minimal staff, and only 24-hour days.

The value of organized lobbying to the allied health professions was lucidly presented in an article that first appeared in *Advance for Physical Therapists* (Pronsati, 1990a) and later reprinted, in modified form, in *Advance for Occupational Therapists* (Pronsati, 1990b). The later article is reprinted in the Appendix.

Realities of Partisan Politics: Caveat Emptor

Although, on the whole, the American system of government works remarkably well in serving the interests of the American people, it would be a bit too naive to imply that suggestions relative to legislation encouraging HP/DP will always be received with full approbation or that the best person will always win. Politics is, in the last analysis, the science of the possible and the persistent! Elected and appointed officials carry on a great deal of their work through negotiation. Even though federal representatives from a tobacco-growing district might be personally convinced that smoking is deleterious to one's health, the overwhelming resistance of their constituents to tobacco-control legislation may remove those legislators as a potential source of antismoking support. The dictates of party policy may impede support of a particular issue. The costs of being re-elected may give a political action committee a louder voice than is

possessed by a pro-health group. (A political action committee is supported by an interest group that makes financial contributions to support the campaigns of politicians perceived as friendly to the goals of that interest group.)

What is certainly true is that one's viewpoint will not be considered or weighed if it is never placed before the attention of the legislator. The first steps are to communicate, to encourage, and to maintain enthusiasm.

Recognizing Special Health-Related Interests of Specific Legislators and Other Public Officials

As noted in President DiBiaggio's recommendations, certain legislators have particular interests in the health arena; therefore, they have a special interest in keeping well informed on matters that relate to those interests. Perhaps the best example of that kind of interest was the late Representative Claude Pepper of Florida, who came to symbolize the national concern for the elderly. Senator Edward F. Kennedy's concern for the well-being of less privileged Americans, especially in terms of their health care, is another illustration.

Allied health professionals interested in promoting policies supportive of improved HP/DP policies would do well to determine where the special interests of legislators to whom they have access intersect with the cause they are promoting. A visit to those legislators to discuss this mutuality of interest, preferably by a colleague who is a constituent of the legislator, is another very effective measure.

ENCOURAGING LEGISLATION AT THE STATE LEVEL

Influencing Policy

Not all legislation relating to HP/DP occurs at the federal level. A significant amount of activity also occurs within the legislative and executive branches of the governments of the several states. Sometimes this activity is a precursor to later, comparable federal action. At other times, it may supplement or extend federal health policies.

There is, of course, a good deal of variation among the legislative structures of the 50 states and of the Commonwealth of Puerto Rico. However, to a significant extent, many of these reflect the federal system, with the same three divisions of government—executive, legislative, and judicial—and with a process in the development of legislation that approximately parallels that used in the federal system. All the principles and recommendations for lobbying or informing the federal government apply in general to most of the states. Members of the state executive branch, state legislators, staff members of legislative committees, officials of state departments of health and education, and staff members assisting individual legislators (where they exist) are typically very receptive to visits, information, and recommendations from constituents, especially when those contacts appear to be intended for the public good.

Summaries of Health-Related Legislation in All States

Although interested health practitioners will usually be concerned primarily with the actions of the particular state in which they practice, there are also a number of reasons why there may be an interest in monitoring relevant legislative activity all across the nation. The legislatures of every state and of Puerto Rico participate in the National Conference of State Legislatures. Each year for the past 7 years that conference has "tracked" health-legislation activities in all states.

Annually, a summary is published of all state-level health-care legislation that has occurred in the preceding year. This summary is indexed, and one category of the index is health promotion. A review of this index shows only limited activity in health promotion. A review of the summaries for the past 3 years showed eight entries in 1986, six from California and one each from Delaware and Florida (King and Francis, 1987). In 1987, there were only four entries, one each from Michigan, Ohio, Tennessee, and Washington State (Landes, 1988). The 1988 summary listed 45 entries (Hooker et al, 1989). Of these, Arizona was the source of two, as were Michigan, Nebraska, and Pennsylvania. Three entries each were included for Hawaii, Indiana, Maryland, and New York. Actions in Illinois accounted for four entries, and Louisiana led the list with six new acts relating to health promotion.

Of course, nothing says that numerous acts,

each possibly quite limited, are more effective than one act that may be fairly comprehensive. To truly examine the commitment of each state to the principles of HP/DP, it would be necessary to examine each piece of legislation in some detail. Unfortunately, space limitations do not permit the luxury of that exercise. What this brief tabulation does show, however, is that as of 1988 there was still strong interest in HP/DP in many parts of the nation. It is quite likely that this activity will be reinforced as a follow-up to the publication of the new PHS document: *Healthy People: 2000* (USDHHS:ODPHP, 1990).

The California Example

The potential importance of state legislation for support of HP/DP activities is illustrated by experience in California. Several actions by the state legislature have permitted the continuance of several strong and unique HP/DP initiatives under the aegis of allied health interests, despite the termination of much of the federal support that was previously available for such activities. Notable was California State Senate Bill No. 143 (1985), which established state-funded health-education contract programs for California institutions. Funds from this program have enabled one California institution, the College of Allied Health at Charles R. Drew University of Medicine and Science, to mount a spectrum of unique and important health-promotion programs aimed at the community in which the school is located. These programs could not have been developed if the special funding provided by California under this program had not been available (HE Douglas, personal communication, September 1990).

PUBLIC POLICY FOR HEALTH PROMOTION AT THE LOCAL LEVEL

In some local jurisdictions (county, city, town, village), there is also potential to implement HP/DP policies through statutes adopted by the elected legislative body of such jurisdictions. For example, in Suffolk County, New York, the county legislature mandated separate smoking and nonsmoking dining areas in most places of public accommodation long before the state turned its attention to this issue. The same legislative body, acting on the recommendation of the Suffolk County Health Commissioner David Harris, MD, also proposed to limit severely the access of youthful purchasers to cigarette vending machines.

These are, of course, only a small sampling of examples of local action that could be cited. The point, of course, is that both local appointed and elected officials are potential allies in an effort to gain the adoption of HP/DP goals into public policy.

PROMOTION OF PUBLIC POLICY DEVELOPMENTS BY CORPORATE SUPPORT AND PRIVATE PHILANTHROPY

Corporate Sector

Although only legislative agencies of government have the power to enact laws, and only the executive branches have authority to draft regulations that govern the application of those laws, the activities of charitable organizations and corporations frequently create trends or pressures that may eventually be adopted and incorporated into public policy. Corporate actions especially may be taken that defuse or frustrate efforts to promote health legislation that may be in the public interest, but that may contravene the fiscal interests of segments of the business community.

In the area of HP/DP, one can readily find both inspiring and appalling intervention by the business community. The Wellness Councils of America (WELCOA) is sponsored by the Health Insurance Association of America and the American Council of Life Insurance, and is actively supported by executives of several major corporations such as Johnson and Johnson, Metropolitan Life, Berkshire Hathaway, AT&T, and the Union Pacific Railroad (the AFL-CIO is also represented on WELCOA's Board of Directors).

The Kimberly Clark Corporation and many other corporate entities both large and small have moved ahead with effective and innovative HP/DP programs without federal funds because of their own conviction that these efforts are in both the corporate and public interest. Certainly, legislators and other policy makers, seeing the value of these demonstration projects, are disposed to actions that extend similar benefits to all.

At the other end of the spectrum, the tobacco industry is perhaps the most notable for its resistance to a beneficial health behavior that would clearly improve the status of the public health; that is, the cessation of cigarette smoking. Both individual tobacco companies and the Tobacco Council that they formed have resisted antismoking legislation and have sought any apparent evidence that would deflect the conviction that "smoking [is the] single most important preventable cause of death and disease . . . associated with heart and blood vessel disease, chronic bronchitis and emphysema, cancers of the lung, larynx, pharynx, oral cavity, esophagus, pancreas and bladder, and with other problems such as respiratory infections and stomach ulcers" (USDHHS:ODPHP, 1980).

Philanthropy

The Robert Wood Johnson Foundation and the W. K. Kellogg Foundation are notable, among others, for their efforts to encourage new departures in the health-care system that will improve the quality of care and cost effectiveness of the way in which care is delivered.

Terrance Keenan, Special Program Consultant to the Robert Wood Johnson Foundation, recently wrote:

> Foundations are specifically prohibited from attempting to influence specific legislation under the provisions of the Tax Reform Act of 1969. On the other hand, the purpose of foundation giving is to advance the public good. Very often this involves the shaping and development of public policy regarding the areas in which the foundation works. Two major ways this is accomplished are: (1) objective, fact-finding studies of critical problems affecting the public welfare; (2) demonstrations of new approaches to solving such problems, which, if successful, are likely to be adopted by government bodies." (T Keenan, personal communication, 1990)

Johnson's Teaching Nursing Home program was an innovative departure in extending the understanding of care of older Americans and thereby reducing morbidity and perhaps avoiding institutionalization of later generations of senior citizens.

In the 1980s, Kellogg redirected its grant-making policies. A major priority would be health promotion and public health (e.g., disease prevention) efforts "judged to be of highest consequence to the public" (DeVries, 1983). These demonstration grants, when effective, are also noted by both federal and state legislators and may represent the blueprint of legislation that is later developed.

Role of Voluntary Health Agencies

Already cast as allies in the effort to improve positive health behaviors are voluntary health agencies, many of which operate at national, state, and local levels. The American Heart Association and the American Lung Association are only two of many examples of agencies with organ-system or disease-specific interests in HP/DP. The National Easter Seal Society deserves special merit because of its recognition of allied health professionals in its advisory groups. Planned Parenthood does great work in the area of prevention of sexually transmitted diseases despite constant harassment from pro-life advocates.

Many allied health professionals interested in HP/DP find that their common cause with these voluntary agencies makes the act of reaching out to them worthwhile. Giving support and expecting support in return is a very realistic policy.

Health-Profession Organizations

Our own professional organizations may also serve as bellwethers of good HP/DP practice and may in time encourage positive legislation and the development of positive public policy. One of the early allied health groups to make a strong public commitment to HP/DP was the American Association for Respiratory Therapy (now known as the American Association for Respiratory Care).

In 1985, the American Association for Respiratory Therapy (1985) adopted a position paper that "identifies . . . the involvement of the respiratory care practitioner in the promotion of health and the prevention of disease." This document encourages the "instill[ation of] awareness for the opportunity to improve the patient's quality and longevity of life" and

"recognizes the respiratory care practitioners' *responsibility* [emphasis added] to participate in pulmonary disease teaching, smoking cessation programs, pulmonary function studies for the public, air pollution alerts, allergy warnings, and sulfite warnings . . . as well as in research in those and other areas where

efforts could promote improved health and disease prevention."

(American Association for Respiratory Therapy, 1985.)

Similarly, the American Academy of Physician Assistants has included concerns for patient wellness in its list of responsibilities of physician assistants (P Lombardo, personal communication, September 1990).

These policies are notable in that they identify the responsibility of the individual allied health practitioner to serve as a role model for HP/DP. In an age when many health-care practitioners take a "Do as I say, not as I do" attitude, this recognition of personal responsibility by the practitioner is especially effective and direct.

Health Credentialing Agencies

As noted during the 1984 PHS workshops (see later discussion), actions by licensing, certification, registration, and accrediting bodies to require HP/DP content in professional education would dramatically and quickly raise practitioner interest in these issues. Unfortunately, response by these agencies to recommendations that HP/DP be mandated in their requirements has been limited (USDHHS: Bureau of Health Professionals, 1984).

HEALTH PROMOTION AS A MODEL FOR PUBLIC POLICY

An individual or group, committed to some special cause or idea, may promote that cause and recruit others by virtue of pronouncements, writings, or example. However, to integrate such efforts into the fabric and philosophy of the population, those advocates must achieve the adoption of their cause into the public policy of their community or nation.

The importance of HP/DP to the public health provides an excellent case in point for proof of the foregoing statement. Almost every significant, large-scale advance in the health status of the American population can be attributed to public health efforts that have led to changes in community health behavior. Changing behavior in a more positive direction is the ultimate goal of health promotion.

Whereas dramatic pharmacologic or surgical breakthroughs may reduce morbidity or mortality for small numbers of individuals, it has been the advances achieved on a community-wide scope that have led to massive improvements in the health status of whole communities. Some examples of this include the provision and use of clean water supplies, safe disposal of sewage, and mass vaccination programs.

Neglect of Prevention by the American Health-Care System

With the advent of scientific medicine (notably in the period between World Wars I and II and thereafter), the recognized importance of and support for public health initiatives fell into decline. Ceaseless media exposure of one medical miracle after another assured us that no one had to die or limit his or her behavioral patterns for health reasons. There would always be a new wonder drug or other medical intervention to restore us to shining good health.

Before the 1970s, neglect of public health and health promotion had proceeded to a point where only about 4% of all the states' expenditure on health, and a similar portion of the total federal expenditure, was devoted to preventive purposes (USDHHS: HCF, 1989). Clearly, support for health promotion was a very low priority item of public policy.

One effect of the explosion of medical knowledge and technology was that the nature of the most frequent causes of illness and death had changed dramatically. Whereas one was most likely to die from an infectious disease during the first part of the 20th century, by the latter years of that century the principal causes of death and disability were due to lifestyle behaviors (or, minimally, secondary to nonhealthful lifestyles). Five leading causes of death among adults in the United States in 1989 were related to negative lifestyle behaviors (USDHHS: Centers for Disease Control, National Center for Health Statistics, 1990). Our bodies succumb largely because of what we ourselves do to them, not because of the predations of some foreign infectious agent.

New Emphasis on Prevention

Voices in the wilderness began to be heard. Thoughtful, insightful, and concerned people (or occasionally actuaries who were tracking the payment of medical care costs) suggested that the

abandonment of some of the most damaging lifestyle behaviors, by at least a majority of the population, might contribute to reduced chronic and other lifestyle-related diseases, just as the advent of antibiotics had contributed to the reduction of the infectious illnesses of an earlier day.

The breakthrough of these concerns into the arena of public policy occurred with the publication in 1979 of *Healthy People*. In his foreword to this report, Secretary Joseph A. Califano, Jr., Surgeon General of the PHS, wrote:

> [The purpose of] . . . the first Surgeon General's Report on Health Promotion and Disease Prevention . . . is to encourage a second public health revolution in the history of the United States. . . . It represents an emerging consensus among scientists and the health community that the nation's health strategy must be dramatically recast to emphasize the prevention of disease. (U.S. Department of Health, Education, and Welfare, Office of Surgeon General, 1979, p. vii)

One year later (1980), a companion report, *Promoting Health/Preventing Disease: Objectives for the Nation* (USDHHS: ODPHP, 1980), was released. Beginning with the goals set forth in *Healthy People*, these objectives presented a series of measurable improvements in the nation's health status to be attained by the year 1990.

In 1984, the PHS sponsored a series of six workshops on HP/DP, five of which focused on the integration of prevention into different divisions of health-profession education. The sixth workshop summarized and compared the others (USDHHS: BHP, 1984). One of these workshops specifically addressed the role, potentials, and obstacles to optimal participation of the allied health disciplines in HP/DP practice (USDHHS: BHP, 1984). All six workshops called for modifications in restrictive legislation, accreditation, and credentialing designed to empower all the nonphysician health disciplines to play a much larger role in prevention and promotion interventions.

Within the PHS, the ODPHP was established directly within the Office of the Secretary of Health and Human Services. These actions clearly heralded a strong, new commitment of the federal health establishment to preventive efforts and, it was hoped, a trend toward reemphasis on pro-active care throughout our health-care system.

Eleven years after the publication of *Healthy People*, a new set of health objectives for the year

2000 was announced. The new objectives were published in a report entitled *Healthy People, 2000* (USDHHS: ODPHP, 1990).

Impact of the Objectives

The 1990 Health Objectives for the Nation: A Midcourse Review (USDHHS: ODPHP, 1986), which assessed the 226 measurable targets presented in the 1980 publication mentioned earlier, showed that about half the objectives were either already achieved or were on track to be achieved by the end of the decade; 26% were unlikely to be achieved, and data were insufficient to perceive trends for another 26%.

Nevertheless, in the opinion of many, the sweeping redirection of emphasis toward preventive interventions that had been projected has fallen far short of what was projected in 1979. For allied health professionals especially, the emphasis and attention given to preventive efforts has been disappointing.

Because preventive interventions had not previously been stressed in any but a few of the allied health disciplines, there was a need for an organized and vigorous effort to modify curriculum, credentialing requirements, attitudes, and modes of practice. For a 3-year period (1983 to 1986), the federal government provided funds for demonstration projects to introduce the concept of prevention and health promotion to the allied health disciplines. Then the restrictions on social programming enforced under the Reagan administration removed the modest funds being provided for these pump-priming activities, and most of the demonstration projects ended because of a lack of financial support. Little progress has been made toward major involvement of the allied health disciplines in the HP/DP effort for the past decade.

Contemporary American Commitment to HP/DP

The optimistic view in 1979 was that many decades of neglect of public health and its separation from the mainstream of American health care and commitment were ending. Sadly, the time for this was not quite right, and the goal of real and widespread commitment to HP/DP continued to be elusive.

However, many observers of the health-care

system now believe that major new technical breakthroughs, which will significantly improve the status of the public health, are likely to be few and far between in the future. Certainly, as has been cited, today's most common causes of morbidity and mortality are lifestyle-related, and are unlikely to be amenable to a magic-bullet approach or to any solution other than changes in how we live and act.

Secretary Califano was very emphatic in his assessment of the objectives set forth in *Healthy People.* In his foreword, he stated:

> We are killing ourselves by our own careless habits. We are killing ourselves by carelessly polluting the environment. We are killing ourselves by permitting harmful social conditions to persist—conditions like poverty, hunger, and ignorance—which destroy health." (p. viii)

The PHS has continued its commitment to HP/DP. On September 6, 1990, DHHS Secretary Louis W. Sullivan released a new report that had been in preparation with wide participation for 3 years. This document, *Healthy People, 2000,* provides new goals and objectives for the nation for the new decade of the 1990s. It is hoped that this decade will witness policy trends at all levels of government, accompanied by necessary fund appropriations to permit the public health revolution that Secretary Califano called for in 1980 to become a reality by the year 2000.

It is hoped that the nation's immense and rich resource of non-physician/non-nurse health professionals (i.e., the allied health professions), including rehabilitation therapists, will be major participants in this health-care revolution. In fact, the current congressional definition of an allied health professional includes the practice of HP/DP.

RESPONSIBILITIES OF THE PROFESSIONAL

All these efforts start with the involvement and determination of a single individual, and then of groups of individuals of increasing number who encourage their colleagues, associations, and employers to take the lead in promoting better health practices and in placing greater emphasis on the prevention of disease. Some allied health professionals, by virtue of established relationships with officials of philanthropic foundations, may also be in a position to encourage increased attention by those foundations to HP/DP demonstration projects, especially ones that involve or integrate the allied health disciplines.

As noted by the National Committee for Injury Prevention and Control, "one person *can* make a difference. To date, advances in injury prevention can be credited more to individual leadership than to agency initiative" (USDHHS: Education Development Center, National Committee for Injury Prevention and Control, 1989, p. 21).

PROFESSIONAL AND PERSONAL COMMITMENT OF REHABILITATION THERAPISTS TO INVOLVEMENT IN HP/DP ACTIVITIES

Every health professional inevitably assumes three personas, among which they alternate as they go about their daily lives. The first is the private citizen. It is hoped that the individual who is intelligent and committed enough to gain professional status will also be an informed and concerned citizen and voter, taking the kind of active interest in public policy that educated citizens in a democracy should.

The second persona is one that the local community in which the individual health professional lives will inevitably endow them: that of a neighborhood authority on health issues. It does not seem to make much difference to which discipline one belongs; when information is needed the man next door and the woman across the street are very likely to turn to a health professional known to them in their community for advice on health-care decisions.

The third and final persona is the professional. This role in turn has two faces; that of the practitioner, caring for and advising patients, and that of the involved member of a discipline participating in decisions of the organized profession. In all of these roles, the activities of the individual professional allow considerable latitude as to how one's profession may be practiced and how one spends energies as a neighbor, a leader, and a citizen.

Empowerment for the Nonphysician to Practice HP/DP

Rehabilitation therapists cannot ethically perform services beyond their legal scope of practice or ethically contradict the clients' diagnoses and treatment plans of the primary care giver. How-

ever, there are a number of areas in which they have great latitude.

In their professional role, rehabilitation therapists should certainly be aware of the latest intelligence about HP/DP, health behaviors, and about how observance of those behaviors can reduce morbidity and mortality. They have a responsibility to be a teacher to their clients and a model of health behavior for clients to emulate. As leaders in their professions, they can and should promote positive HP/DP positions and activities by their professional group and join with other professionals in promoting constructive public policy in the HP/DP realm.

In their role as a health authority in the community, rehabilitation therapists may be able to add a positive health voice in community organizations such as school boards, parent–teacher associations, and other groups. Again, by virtue of possession of current knowledge concerning HP/DP, they should be able to offer good advice and guidance to their neighbors and friends.

As citizens and as professionals, rehabilitation therapists can and should add their personal prestige to those of other allied health disciplines, supporting and, when necessary, arguing for the adoption into the public policy of health-positive laws, activities, and concepts.

Levels of Intervention in HP/DP

HP/DP takes many forms. Smoking cessation and other interventions and behavioral changes targeted in the objectives cited earlier have received the most attention in recent years, but there are countless other efforts that could be made to improve the health status of the American public.

Although the partial achievement, that of identification of the objectives, represents an enormous stride toward health improvement, those objectives only scratched the surface. Developed principally by people with public health backgrounds, they were focused exclusively on the arena of primary prevention or on efforts intended to prevent the occurrence of disease or injury in the first instance. Certainly, allied health practitioners can and should support and participate in primary prevention.

Some allied health disciplines in fact devote all or most of their professional efforts within the realm of primary prevention. As an obvious example, the primary activities of dental hygienists are dedicated to the prevention of dental disease. Other disciplines, however, engage in forms of professional practice that offer at best only limited opportunities for involvement in primary prevention. Many will have greater opportunity to engage in secondary or tertiary prevention efforts. Rehabilitation therapists are perhaps obvious examples of the second group. Prevention is any intervention that reduces the likelihood that a disease or disorder will affect an individual or that interrupts or slows the progress of the disorder. *Primary* prevention reduces the likelihood that a particular disease or disorder will develop in a person. *Secondary* prevention interrupts or minimizes the progress of a disease or irreversible damage from a disease by early detection and treatment. *Tertiary* prevention slows the progress of the disease and reduces the resultant disability through treatment (Spitzer, 1990).

ECONOMICS: WHO PAYS?

HP/DP practice requires not only the constant updating of knowledge on prevention issues but also the expenditure of professional time in effective health-education interventions. Because time is money to the practitioner, the question arises, "Who will pay for this time and service?" Unfortunately, few third-party payors have yet to become enlightened about HP/DP to the point where they provide coverage for health-education service.

Perhaps this important health-policy issue will become a major goal of the nation's allied health professionals in the years ahead. Meanwhile, the conscientious professional will somehow find ways to carry on a reasonable amount of client education, even in the absence of reimbursement for the time used in this effort.

CONCLUSION: OBLIGATIONS OF THE ALLIED HEALTH PROFESSIONAL TO FUNCTION PRO BONO PUBLICO

It is the responsibility of the professional to support improved health. The effective, long-term incorporation of a strong commitment to HP/DP as a plank of the nation's public health policy must eventually be in the form of legislation. Effective demonstration programs implemented by foundations, voluntary agencies, or professional groups can be powerful ammunition

in lobbying efforts to obtain HP/DP legislation, but the struggle to achieve such legislation requires vigorous, logical, and continuing effort by professionals and others committed to this goal: pro bono publico . . . in the interests of the public. The old adage that the longest journey starts with a single step is certainly true in the promotion of public policy supporting prevention. One can say with conviction that the incorporation of effective HP/DP into the national public health policy must begin with individual and concerned health-care professionals.

Acknowledgments

I gratefully acknowledge the assistance of Mrs. Michele L. McTernan, who contributed many hours of her expertise to editing and to the technical preparation of the text, and to Robert O. Hawkins, Ph.D, and Nanci C. Rice, Ph.D, of State University of New York at Stony Brook allied health faculty, each of whom offered numerous and useful suggestions.

References

Alger KR: A layman's guide to Congress. Educ Rec 71(3):22–23, 1990.

American Association of Respiratory Therapy: Health Promotion and Disease Prevention. Dallas, TX, American Association of Respiratory Therapy, 1985.

California State Senate Bill No. 143: An act to add Article 3 to Part 1.95 of Division of the Health and Safety Code relating to health (chap. 832). Approved September 19, 1985.

DeVries, R: Editorial. Health considerations for improving human well-being in the 1980's. J Health Admin Educ 1(3):222, 1983.

DiBiaggio J: Ten tips for higher education leaders. Educ Rec 71(3):17, 1990.

Douglas HE: Dean, College of Allied Health, Drew University of Medicine and Science. Personal Communication, September 1990.

Editorial. J Health Admin Educ 1(3):219, 1983.

Hooker TA, Harden SL, and Landes D: 1988 Health Care Legislation. Denver, CO, National Conference of State Legislatures, 1989.

King MP and Francis D: 1986 Health Care Legislation. Denver, CO, National Conference of State Legislatures, 1987.

Landes D: 1987 Health Care Legislation. Denver, CO, National Conference of State Legislatures, 1988.

Pronsati MP: Here's how we get it: PTs urged to tap lobbying potential. Adv Phys Ther 1(4):7, 1990a.

Pronsati MP: Organized lobbying pays dividends. Adv Occup Ther G(23):12, 1990b.

Spitzer WO: The scientific admissibility of evidence on the effectiveness of preventive intervention. In Goldbloom RB and Lawrence RS (eds): Preventing Disease: Beyond the Rhetoric. New York, Springer-Verlag, 1990.

Sullivan LW: Viewpoint: Healthy people, 2000: Promoting health and building a culture of character. Am J Health Promotion 5(1):5–6, 1990.

U.S. Department of Health and Human Services, Bureau of Health Professionals. Proceedings from the Workshop on Health Promotion/Disease Prevention: Impact on Health Professions Education—Allied Health. Silver Springs, MD, Applied Management Science Inc, 1984a.

U.S. Department of Health and Human Services, Bureau of Health Professionals: Proceedings from the Workshop on Health Promotion/Disease Prevention: Impact on Health Professions Education—Summary Conference. Silver Springs, MD, Applied Management Science Inc, 1984b.

U.S. Department of Health and Human Services, Centers for Disease Control, National Center for Health Statistics: Health–United States, 1989, and Prevention Profile. Hyattsville, MD, U.S. Government Printing Office, 1990.

U.S. Department of Health and Human Services, Education Development Center, National Committee for Injury Prevention and Control. Injury prevention: Meeting the challenge. Am J Prevent Med, Spring 1989, p. 21.

U.S. Department of Health and Human Services, Office of Disease Prevention/Health Promotion: Healthy People 2000 (publication no. 017-001-00474-0). Washington, DC, U.S. Government Printing Office, 1990.

U.S. Department of Health and Human Services, Office of Disease Prevention/Health Promotion: Implementation Plans for Attaining the Objectives for the Nation (Supplement to Public Health Rep). Washington, DC, U.S. Government Printing Office, 1983.

U.S. Department of Health and Human Services, Office of Disease Prevention/Health Promotion: Promoting Health/Preventive Objectives for the Nation. Washington, DC, U.S. Government Printing Office, 1980.

U.S. Department of Health and Human Services, Office of Disease Prevention/Health Promotion: The 1990 Health Objectives for the Nation: A Midcourse Review. Washington, DC, U.S. Government Printing Office, 1986.

U.S. Department of Health, Education, and Welfare, Office of Surgeon General: Healthy People: Surgeon General's Report on Health Promotion/Disease Prevention (publication No. 79-55071). Washington, DC, U.S. Government Printing Office, 1979.

Bibliography

Goldbloom RB and Lawrence RS (eds): Preventing Disease: Beyond the Rhetoric. New York, Springer-Verlag, 1990.

Health Affairs (special issue): Promoting Health 9(2), 1990.

Joint Committee on Printing of the Congress of the United States, 1989–90 Congressional Directory, One Hundred First Congress. Washington, DC, U.S. Government Printing Office, 1989.

National Archives and Records Administration, Office of the Federal Register: U.S. Government Manual, 1989–90. Washington, DC, U.S. Government Printing Office, 1989.

U.S. Department of Health, Education, and Welfare, Office of Surgeon General: Healthy People: Surgeon General's Report on Health Promotion/Disease Prevention (publication no. 79-55071). Washington, DC, U.S. Government Printing Office, 1979.

U.S. Department of Health, Education, and Welfare, Office of Surgeon General: Surgeon General's Report on Smoking and Health. Washington, DC, U.S. Government Printing Office, 1979.

U.S. Department of Health and Human Services, Bureau of Health Professions. Proceedings from the Workshop on

Health Promotion/Disease Prevention: Impact on Health Professions Education–Allied Health. Silver Springs, MD, Applied Management Science Inc, 1984.

U.S. Department of Health and Human Services, Bureau of Health Professions: Proceedings from the Workshop on Health Promotion/Disease Prevention: Impact on Health Professions Education–Summary Conference. Silver Springs, MD, Applied Management Science Inc, 1984.

U.S. Department of Health and Human Services, Centers for Disease Control, National Center for Health Statistics: Health–United States, 1989, and Prevention Profile. Hyattsville, MD, U.S. Government Printing Office, 1990.

U.S. Department of Health and Human Services, Health Care Finance Administration, Office of Research and Demonstration: National health expenditures. Health Care Rev 10(4):1–36, 1989.

U.S. Department of Health and Human Services, Office of Disease Prevention/Health Promotion: The 1990 Health Objectives for the Nation: A Midcourse Review. Washington, DC, U.S. Government Printing Office, 1986.

U.S. Department of Health and Human Services, Office of Disease Prevention/Health Promotion: Disease Prevention/Health Promotion: The Facts. Palo Alto, CA, Bull Publishing, 1987.

U.S. Department of Health and Human Services, Office of Disease Prevention/Health Promotion: Healthy People, 2000 (publication no. 017-001-00474-0). Washington, DC, U.S. Government Printing Office, 1990.

U.S. Department of Health and Human Services, Office of Disease Prevention/Health Promotion: Promoting Health/Preventing Disease: Objectives for the Nation. Washington, DC, U.S. Government Printing Office, 1980.

U.S. Department of Health and Human Services, Office of Disease Prevention/Health Promotion: Promoting Health/Preventing Disease. Implementation Plans for Attaining the Objectives for the Nation (supplement to Public Health Rep). Washington, DC, U.S. Government Printing Office, 1983.

APPENDIX I: ORGANIZED LOBBYING PAYS DIVIDENDS*

With the right blend of legislative knowledge, confidence, and homework, occupational therapists can make impressions on state and federal lawmakers that could persuade them to support causes important to the health care professions.

Research, establishing contacts, lobbying and personal meetings with lawmakers or aides all have big parts in bringing vital issues to the attention of those with legislative power.

"One of the most important things to keep in mind is that you are a constituent. These lawmakers really are interested in hearing from you, because you put them in office," explained Pamela Phillips, associate director of an allied

---

*From Pronsati MP: Organized lobbying pays dividends. Adv Occup Ther 6(23):12, 1990. Reprinted with permission of the publishers, Merion Publications, Inc.

Promoting Health Through Public Policy ☐ **17**

health association's department of government affairs.

Speaking recently at a government affairs forum here, Ms. Phillips said allied health professionals across the country can make a difference in the state and federal lawmaking process, once a good knowledge base is established and societies organize to present a unified, articulate front.

During a presentation titled "The Legislative Process and You," Ms. Phillips briefed allied health care personnel on the workings of the legislative branch and the intricacies of bill passage, and provided tips on how to stage a successful meeting with a legislator or congressional representative.

A key to any successful lobbying effort is a good understanding of how a bill becomes law.

The process is often lengthy and confusing, although the premise appears simple on paper.

In Congress, 65% of bills originate in the House, including all revenue bills, which, under the Constitution, must start there.

After a bill is filed, it is referred to a committee, which assigns it to a subcommittee. The subcommittee does most of the work on the legislation, researching it and fine-tuning the provisions and language.

During this period, most of the lobbying is done in the form of phone calls, meetings, and letters from constituents or other lawmakers. The subcommittee usually holds one or more hearings on the bill and eventually votes to recommend or reject it.

The bill then moves on to the full committee, which usually follows the subcommittee recommendation. If it is a House bill, the House Rules Committee then dictates how the legislation will be handled on the floor, setting conditions for debate and deciding whether amendments will be permitted. In the Senate, bills proceed directly from full committee to the floor with no conditions on floor activity.

The procedure in state legislatures is markedly different. The committee's role is paramount there, because most legislatures do not have subcommittees. In addition most states do not use their rules committees to set conditions for floor action, and the only limits imposed on debate are those contained in the state constitution, or those agreed on by vote of the membership.

Another difference between state legislatures and Congress is the importance of hearings. On the state level, testimony and input received at a hearing may well influence a legislator's vote.

"I've testified at the state level, and I think in some cases we were able to turn legislators around right at that point," Ms. Phillips said.

Congressional hearings have a different purpose, however, because most representatives and senators have already made up their minds by the time the hearing begins.

"Hearings in Congress have much less of an impact than at the state level," Ms. Phillips continued. "By the time a Congressional hearing starts, everything is more or less decided. The work has already been done, and usually there will be only one to three members of Congress present. Basically they will just thank you for your time."

Ms. Phillips also noted several other differences between the state and federal governments.

"Obviously, the federal government is much larger, more complicated, and more bureaucratic," Ms. Phillips said. "In Congress, aides are very important. In fact, legislative assistants are often the key."

Health legislative assistants, known on Capitol Hill as health LAs, assume much of the responsibility for development and research of health-related bills, and lawmakers have only a small role in the process.

"You should not be disappointed if you do not meet with a member of Congress," Ms. Phillips related. "It is a big help for you to talk to the legislative assistants."

Aides and legislative assistants are not as prevalent in the state legislatures, and administrative assistants or secretaries are valuable sources to cultivate as allies. State representatives and senators tend to be more accessible to the public than members of Congress, and the activities of state legislatures are more closely reported by local newspapers.

Another fact about Congress is that it passes fewer bills than state legislatures.

The numbers are a little misleading, however, because although fewer bills are passed, many small bills end up in large, multifaceted pieces of legislation called omnibus bills.

Amendments are also more abundant in Congress, as lawmakers attempt to add programs, provisions and funds that will help their district. The well-known term for this is "pork barreling."

Ready to tackle a legislative issue? The first thing you should do is reach a consensus on the issue, or the bill in which it is addressed.

Gather all relevant facts and develop a succinct

written and oral presentation about the situation. Statistics are particularly effective. Ask chapter members to write letters to the state legislator or member of Congress who is, or could be, amenable to supporting legislation on the issue.

After these mailings begin, contact the lawmaker's office, ask to speak to the health LA (if you are working with Congress) and request a meeting. Speak to the administrative assistant or secretary if you are lobbying a state senator or representative.

Send a follow-up letter to confirm the time and date. On the assigned day, arrive early so that you can begin the meeting on time. Elected officials, particularly those in Congress, maintain very detailed schedules.

"Try not to be intimidated," Ms. Phillips advised. "You are the expert. Unfortunately, many lawmakers do not even know what an occupational therapist is, but the health LA will."

Begin the meeting by introducing yourself and stating where you live and work. Be sure to point out that you live in the district the legislator represents.

"Emphasize that you are a constituent," she said. "You may have to tell the legislator what an OT is. You should also let the legislator know how many OTs reside and practice in your state.

Next, ask the legislator if rehabilitation issues are familiar topics, and whether his or her office has received correspondence from OTs. Identify the major features of the bill for which you are lobbying, or the issue you hope he or she will support. Explain the personal impact the bill would have on you and your colleagues and present copies of position statements from your regional or state organization.

After discussing the bill, follow up by questioning the lawmaker about chances for passage and whether you can expect support for the legislation.

"If the legislator is opposed to it, you can try again to convince him or her but do not be argumentative," Ms. Phillips said. "That is one of the worst things you can do; it does nothing but turn the staff totally off. You do not want to burn bridges."

You may want to question the lawmaker politely about the reasons for the opposition so you can address those concerns in the future.

If the legislator supports your issue, ask him or her to sponsor or cosponsor a bill, and also ask what your organization can do to help.

Offer to send supplemental information, reports, or studies to assist lawmakers in reaching their decision.

Let the lawmaker know how you plan to follow up on the issue to ensure his or her continued attention and support.

Also ask which staff member you should contact for updates on pertinent legislative activity.

"One of the most important things to do after the meeting is to send a letter thanking the legislator for their time, whether they're for or against the bill," Ms. Phillips said.

It is also a good idea to contact the lawmaker's district or home office by letter, summarizing the meeting and the points covered.

If you can, set up an appointment with an aide in the local office to reinforce your position on the issue.

Congressional Information

To determine the status of legislation.
House Bill Status Office
3669 House Office Building
Annex #2
Washington, DC 20515
(202) 225-1772

Senate Bill Status Office
Senate Library
The Capitol, S332
Washington, DC 20510
(202) 224-2971

To obtain copies of House or Senate bills and documents:
House Documents Room
The Capitol, H226
Washington, DC 20515
(202) 225-3456

Senate Documents Room
The Capitol, S325
Washington, DC 20510
(202) 224-4321

To find out where in the government you need to go for information:
Federal Information Center
General Services Administration
7th and D Streets, SW
Washington, DC 20407
(202) 755-8660

CHAPTER

2

David L. Nelson
Clint Stucky

The Roles of Occupational Therapy in Preventing Further Disability of Elderly Persons in Long-Term Care Facilities

Readers of this book might assume that all of today's health-care professionals place a high value on health promotion and disease prevention, particularly in relation to vulnerable populations such as the elderly. Such an assumption would be wrong: We have much work to do.

The literature suggests that concepts of preventive medicine are frequently rejected or ignored. In the *Journal of the American Geriatrics Society*, physicians Black and Kapoor (1990) reported on a recent survey of physicians' attitudes regarding health promotion and disease prevention in the elderly. They found that 73% of attending physicians slightly or strongly agreed with the statement, "Lifestyle changes made after the age of 65 do not have a significant impact on health." Only 27% strongly disagreed that lifestyle changes do not have a significant impact on health. A majority of those surveyed (56%) strongly disagreed with this statement: "Adopting a healthy lifestyle is an important way of reducing one's risk of disease." In addition, only 24% strongly agreed that "I feel a

strong personal commitment to promoting healthy lifestyle changes in all my clients."

Black and Kapoor confirmed what Woo and associates (1985) reported earlier: Many physicians are less likely to conduct prevention-oriented tests and examinations on elderly individuals than on younger persons. The prevention of disease in elderly people is often a low priority in American health care. In an editorial for the *Journal of the American Medical Association*, Wetle (1987) argued that age is a significant risk factor for inadequate treatment.

Bortz (1982, 1989) has been a consistent champion of the potential of older persons to influence the state of their own health. He has also been a critic of the ageism frequently demonstrated by adherents of the medical model who confuse disease with aging and who harbor negative attitudes as to the value of disease prevention among the elderly.

As Bortz (1982) stated, "Disuse [of the body] expands morbidity." The active promotion of "using" the self in meaningful, purposeful oc-

19

cupation—an important health-promotion idea—is the method of disease prevention discussed in this chapter. Here we maintain that occupation is a vital force in disease prevention and health promotion, especially in regard to the elderly who reside in long-term care facilities.

LONG-TERM CARE FACILITIES FOR THE ELDERLY

This chapter specifically focuses on occupation and occupational therapy. Lewis (1987) discussed many of these issues from a physical therapist's point of view. The first point to make is that the vast majority of elderly people do not need and do not live in nursing homes. Most elderly people are best off in their own homes with family members or in special residences for the elderly that have no special tie to nursing or medical care (Kane et al, 1984). Indeed, it sometimes is an excellent treatment goal for the person residing in a nursing home to be discharged to a community residence. However, the long-term care facility is sometimes the only viable option for a minority of elderly persons.

According to a report of the Institute of Medicine (1986), there are 15,000 Medicare- or Medicaid-certified nursing homes in the United States, and these nursing homes provide 1.5 million beds. Larson and associates (1989) reported that the annual cost of U.S. nursing homes exceeds $20 billion and will continue to rise as the population ages.

Most nursing homes are large and structured like hospitals, with corridors leading from nursing stations to hospital-like rooms. Physicians' orders usually receive the highest priorities for institutional action, with emphasis on the correct dispensation of medicines and other treatments. Well described by Gillick (1989), uniformity, orderliness, and cleanliness are prized. Frequently, these values are associated with promoting docility and passivity in residents. These values can clash with the individual's inherent need for autonomy and a sense of control over the environment. Individually meaningful and purposeful occupation frequently creates conflicts in orderly, medically oriented institutions.

TYPICAL IMPAIRMENTS, DISABILITIES, AND PERFORMANCE DEFICITS

Residents of nursing homes may have a variety of impairments and disabilities. One way of in-

troducing some of these problems is reference to the uniform terminology categories used by the American Occupational Therapy Association Uniform Terminology Task Force (1989). These categories are: sensory motor performance components, cognitive performance components, and psychosocial performance components.

In the sensory motor performance component, elderly nursing-home residents often have visual or auditory deficits. Ambulation is frequently impaired; pain and joint limitations resulting from arthritis are common. Common clinical conditions, such as stroke or Parkinson's disease, result in characteristic patterns of motor deficits. Pulmonary, cardiovascular, and neoplastic diseases reduce physical capacity. Lower extremity amputations secondary to diabetes are frequently seen.

As for the cognitive performance component, the U.S. Department of Health and Human Services (1981) estimated that 55% of nursing-home residents have cognitive impairments. In many cases of dementia, including Alzheimer's disease, remote long-term memory is often superior to short-term memory. Judgment and orientation to present person, time, or place may be impaired. Alternatively, it is important to note that many nursing-home residents have no major cognitive deficit and are fully capable of problem solving and other intellectual functions.

In the psychosocial component, Rovner and colleagues (1986) found that 94% of nursing-home patients surveyed had diagnosable psychiatric conditions. These conditions include, but are not limited to, the dementias just mentioned in reference to the cognitive component. Dementia results in affective and social disorders as well as in cognitive disabilities. Less severe psychosocial disorders commonly seen in nursing-home residents include exaggerations of previous personality patterns; depression; and reactive disorders following physical losses and disease.

The American Occupational Therapy Association uniform terminology also recognizes the importance of three occupational performance areas: activities of daily living (ADL), work, and play/leisure. In terms of ADL, the National Nursing Home Survey by the U.S. Department of Health and Human Services (1981) revealed that 80% of residents need help with bathing; 69% need help with dressing; and 53% need assistance with toileting. A person who is truly independent in self-care and instrumental ADL should not be in a nursing home. In terms of the area of work, nursing-home life rarely if ever involves paid employment; moreover, there are few opportunities for residents to be socially productive as volunteers. As for leisure, structured activity programs are mandated by law; however, nursing-home residents often spend too much time in passive or escapist types of occupations.

EMPHASIS ON ABILITY AND LATENT CAPACITY

Hasselkus (1989) is among the leading occupational therapists in gerontology who urged a "focus on function" as opposed to an orientation toward disease processes. All nursing-home residents have disabilities; however, what is more important is the fact that nursing-home residents also have many functional abilities that can be tapped in comprehensive programs of health promotion and disease prevention. The concept of latent capacity is particularly relevant to nursing-home residents (Baltes et al, 1986). Provision of an environment that is sensitive to the individuality of the residents can lead to competent performance that surprises those who know the residents only in the context of insensitive environments. For example, given the right kind of music and setting, the individual with dementia might be a competent pianist or dancer. Alternatively, in a relaxed social setting, the depressed resident might show a sophisticated sense of humor and insight.

Disability in the sensory or motor areas can often be compensated for so that individuals can fully exercise their intact cognitive functions. Even if higher level cognition is irreversibly lost, the environment (or what some occupational therapists call the occupational form) can be restructured so as to ensure that individuals function successfully at tasks (or occupations) within their capacity. Psychosocial abilities are especially amenable to adaptation; social isolation and depression are frequently reversible if residents see that their efforts can have beneficial results. A focus on the nursing-home residents' strengths reinforces their sense of personal efficacy and becomes the best way to treat or compensate for disabilities.

Naturally, the best therapist is skilled at recognizing the clients' strengths and weaknesses. However, if we were nursing-home residents and had to choose between a therapist who was

highly skilled at identifying clinically relevant disabilities but insensitive to remaining capacities and a therapist with the opposite characteristics, we would unhesitatingly choose the one who could relate to our abilities. The choice might be different in an acute-care setting. However, occupational therapy in a long-term care facility requires a special focus on function, because activation of function (occupation) is a main method of health promotion and disease prevention.

A final introductory point is that the importance of health promotion and disease prevention does not diminish just because the individual already suffers from a disease process. The individual with one type of disease is usually especially vulnerable to the development of other disease processes. For example, the individual whose first disease impedes mobility tends to become especially vulnerable to cardiovascular disease. For another example, infectious pulmonary diseases tend to be likely following supposedly unrelated clinical conditions restricting mobility. In addition, psychiatric disorders frequently follow the experience of functional losses as a result of neuromuscular disorders. In other words, primary prevention and secondary prevention of new disease processes are especially important for individuals who are already experiencing an impairment. This idea is particularly relevant to nursing-home elderly. The fact that some disabling condition makes residential treatment a necessity only underscores the need for an overall strategy oriented to prevention.

PREVENTIVE OCCUPATION: PRINCIPLES AND PRACTICE

Healthy and Unhealthy Patterns of Occupation

Occupation is a powerful force in human life. One person's pattern of daily occupations might provide sufficient challenges that sustain and promote sensory motor, cognitive, and psychosocial capabilities. For example, an elderly woman residing in a nursing home might move through her daily occupations in such a way that she feels stimulated, competent, autonomous, appreciated for her uniqueness, and valued as a community member. Despite present or threatened disabilities, she routinely encounters situations that make sense to her, interest her, are compatible with her way of looking at herself and her world, elicit a sense of purpose in her, give her choices within her capabilities, give her the chance to see that she can still have an impact on the world around her, help her compensate for any incorrectable impairments, and help her to help herself through her own actions. For such a person, occupational situations (occupational forms) are health promoting and disease preventing. Personal dignity and integrity are promoted as well.

However, just as one's occupational pattern can be a powerful force for the good, so can it be a powerfully negative force. The daily occupational situations of the individual might sometimes provide challenges that simply cannot be met given the person's current state of health. Also unfortunately, the environment might provide little or no challenge at all. Any combination of failure because of inordinate challenges and boredom through the lack of challenges can weaken the sensory motor, cognitive, and psychosocial capabilities of the person (Lawton, 1982). For example, the elderly woman who encounters overly demanding situations cannot make sense of what is going on, cannot relate it to her past remembered experience, feels only a desire to escape the situation one way or another, feels trapped if physical escape is impossible, anticipates failure and humiliation, and learns lessons of personal helplessness. She literally might wish that she were dead. As another example, an elderly woman might encounter unstimulating, antiseptic situations promoting passivity and demanding little but compliance. Either way, the result is a progressive deterioration in functional ability. Muscles and joints that do not move atrophy and stiffen. Cognitive abilities that are not used become dull. Psychosocial skills unused in daily life are forgotten.

As Fidler and Fidler (1978) said, as we do, so we become. Through our occupations, we adapt in healthy ways, or, through our occupations, we maladapt in unhealthy ways.

Occupation Defined

The potency of occupation in promoting health has long been recognized; this recognition is the basis for the existence of the profession of occupational therapy. However, concise, internally consistent, and useful definitions of occupation and related terms such as meaning, purpose, performance, impact, and adaptation have been lacking until the past few years (Christiansen, 1990). Here these terms are defined in accordance with a previous publication (Nelson, 1988). Examples are given that are particularly relevant to the use of occupation as a preventive measure for elderly persons living in nursing homes.

An occupation is the relationship between an occupational form and an occupational performance (Fig. 2–1). In other words, occupation is something—the form—that is done—the performance.

To illustrate the concepts defined in this section, let us use some typical occupations in nursing homes. Eating dinner in the community dining hall is an occupation, as is an exercise class and as is a visit with one's family. In the case of the dinner, the occupational form is made up of the food, the dishes, and tableware, other physical objects such as tables and chairs, and the presence of other people. In the case of the exercise class, the occupational form consists of the group leader's instructions and demonstrations, the exercise equipment, and the actions of fellow exercisers. As for the family visit, the family members and the step-by-step flow of their words are the most important aspects of the occupational form, but other aspects include the room, its decorations, and the visual or auditory presence of staff or fellow residents.

In all cases, the occupational form has not only a physical nature but also a sociocultural nature. Culture permeates environments (Levine and Merrill, 1987). In our culture, we all understand what a community dining hall is all about: It is an eating and socializing situation. Any acculturated person can immediately identify and distinguish typical and atypical features within the context of a community dining hall. Similarly, most of us know what is generally expected in our culture when we see an exercise situation.

Although many occupational forms are interpretable to almost everyone within a culture or

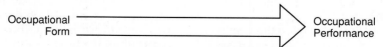

Figure 2–1. An occupation is the relationship between an occupational form and an occupational performance. (Redrawn from Nelson DL: Occupation: Form and performance. Am J Occup Ther 42:633–641, 1988.)

even cross-culturally, some occupational forms are interpretable only within smaller social units. For example, the gestures made by family members during a visit might be easily interpretable within one ethnic group and perplexing within a different ethnic group. Holiday decorations in a nursing home might be specific to members of a certain religion or cultural background. Even family units have their own agreed-upon ways of interpreting signs and symbols. The same words that represent warm, friendly kidding within one family could be considered rude in another. An individual must be a social insider to interpret many occupational forms correctly.

Occupational performance is the carrying out of the occupational form. If all goes well in the dining hall, the typical occupational performance of the individual is to manipulate the utensils, eat the food, and engage in conversation. The predictable occupational performance in the exercise class is to engage in voluntary movements (these can be analyzed kinesiologically). The occupational performance in the family visit includes talking, gesturing, and otherwise communicating with family members.

Occupational performance is the voluntary doing of the individual. Occupational form is the environmental context (physical as well as sociocultural) that elicits the individual's doing.

An especially human characteristic is that different individuals emit different occupational performances in relation to the same occupational forms. For example, in the same exercise class, one elderly man might move vigorously, whereas another dozes off. Figure 2–2 accounts for the importance of individual differences in occupational performances. The meaning assigned to an occupational form always depends on the unique developmental structure of the individual. "Meaning" is the entire interpretive process. The man dozing off in the exercise class might not find the occupational form meaningful because he cannot interpret the instructor's words. Another possibility is that he can interpret the instructions but does not see the value of exercising; indeed, he might see exercise as either dangerous to his health or as something that he did enough of when he was younger (Mobily, 1982; Nelson and Peterson, 1989). A lack of meaning leads to a lack of purpose or motivation.

In contrast, the man who is exercising vigorously finds definite meanings in the exercise situation; the situation makes sense to him. The meaningfulness of the occupational form leads to a sense of purpose. Perhaps, indeed, he has several purposes at once (i.e., to feel healthier, win the praise of the exercise instructor, and experience the joy of moving for its own sake).

As Figure 2–2 depicts, the individual's sense of purpose (or lack of it) leads to occupational performance (or its lack). The individual's unique developmental structure explains the meaningfulness of the occupational form and the purposefulness of the occupational performance.

Figure 2–2 also depicts occupational dynamics. Through occupational performance, the individual has an impact on subsequent occupational forms in the environment. For example, the diner cleans his or her plate. The exerciser elicits praise by the instructor and influences others in the group. The person who is visited by family members has an impact on those visitors. This impact can serve as feedback to the individual.

Besides having an impact on the environment, occupational performance and having a sense of purpose can also result in adaptations to the individual's own developmental structure. An

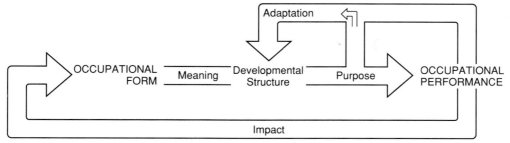

Figure 2–2. Each individual interacts in a unique way with the occupational form, depending on the individual's *developmental structure*. The form takes on *meaning*, which can result in a sense of *purpose*. Occupational dynamics include *impact* as well as *adaptation*. (Redrawn from Nelson DL: Occupation: Form and performance. Am J Occup Ther 42:633–641, 1988.)

adaptation is any change in the developmental structure from what would have otherwise occurred without the occupational performance. Thus the exerciser might have enhanced flexibility, endurance, strength, or self-esteem because of the occupational performance. An adaptation of the person dining might be to maintain self-feeding skills (if the person did not regularly feed oneself, the skills would decay). In addition, adaptations of the elderly person who conversed with family members might include renewed orientation to time, place, and person as well as enhanced functional memory.

Whereas Figure 2–2 depicts occupation in general, Figure 2–3 includes the role of the occupational therapist, which is to collaborate in synthesizing occupational forms that lead to meaningful, purposeful occupational performance. In synthesizing a therapeutic occupational form, the occupational therapist considers physical as well as sociocultural factors and makes a match between these factors and the client's unique developmental structure. Therapeutic occupational performance, in turn, leads to individuals having an effect on the environment (impact) as well as to changes in their own developmental structure (adaptation).

Occupational synthesis is a collaborative process between the occupational therapist and the resident of the long-term care facility. Some residents are able to have considerable impacts on their occupational synthesis; some are not. For example, some residents enjoy having a menu in advance so that they can plan their meals. Others, for various reasons (e.g., cognitive, sensory, and so on) might be perplexed by the options. The guideline is for the resident to synthesize as many naturalistic (socioculturally

typical) options as possible. Indeed, an increase in self-determination (more personally satisfying and appropriate impact) is often a treatment goal.

The occupational therapist's motive is always to construct an occupational form that elicits meaning, purpose, and full-fledged performance on the resident's part. This occupational performance might (a) provide evaluative data, (b) serve as a compensation for performances that are no longer possible, or (c) result in adaptations to the developmental structure. As an example of an occupational synthesis for the goal of providing evaluative data, provision of certain foods can reveal information to the occupational therapist about the residents' fine motor and oral-motor functions. An example of occupational synthesis for the goal of compensation is to provide assistive equipment (e.g., plateguard, nonslip plate, built-up handles on utensils) to enable successful occupational performance. An example of occupational synthesis for the goal of adaptation is to provide the tactile input recommended by neuromotor therapies to encourage changes in oral-motor abilities.

THERAPEUTIC OCCUPATION AND LEVELS OF PREVENTION

Tertiary Prevention Through Occupation

Occupational therapists are often most familiar with tertiary prevention: measures taken to minimize disabilities following disease. Historically, occupational therapists have used occupation to minimize sensory motor, cognitive, or psychosocial disabilities following any of the many disease processes that might strike elderly residents

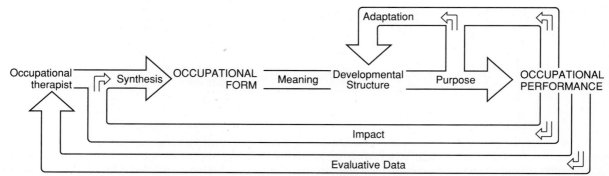

Figure 2–3. The role of the occupational therapist is to collaborate in synthesizing occupational forms that lead to meaningful, purposeful occupational performance.

of long-term care facilities. Here occupational therapists might synthesize occupational forms designed to elicit performances that increase motor control or decrease hemineglect in a stroke patient. Alternatively, an occupational therapist might encourage occupations involving range of motion or graded strengthening in clients with arthritis.

It is important to note that the occupational therapist is not always physically present when therapeutic occupation occurs. After proper positioning in a wheelchair, therapeutic occupations involving mobility can occur whether or not the therapist is present. The same holds for assistive devices, architectural modifications, and orientation aids. Frequently, the role of the therapist involves supervision or consultation with nursing staff and others to ensure that devices and aids are used properly.

Secondary Prevention Through Occupation

Therapists also have an important role in terms of screening for incipient impairments and alerting medical staff so that early diagnosis is possible. For example, therapists providing direct service might well recognize the symptoms of transient ischemic attacks. Communication with medical staff can lead to the prevention of more serious cerebrovascular accidents through appropriate medical intervention. Similarly, at the secondary level of prevention, therapists can frequently identify postures that might be associated with the beginnings of decubital or skeletal deformities.

Another role is the monitoring of the observable effects of psychotropic medications (Rogers, 1986). Intended as well as unintended effects should be monitored. Larson and colleagues (1989) argued that psychotropic medications are frequently overused in nursing homes and may lead to lethargy and unnecessarily low levels of function. Another common result of high-dosage psychotropic medications is tardive dyskinesia. The best context in which to observe dyskinesia is everyday, naturalistic occupation.

Through indirect service and staff training, therapists can instill an attitude of watchfulness among staff so that small problems do not lead to larger ones. Examples include a wariness toward evidence of visual or auditory loss and ensuring that residents regularly wear their prescribed eyeglasses or hearing aids. Yet another example involves some dementia-like conditions related to nutrition that can be successfully treated, especially if identified early.

Primary Prevention Through Occupation

Perhaps one of the most important and yet least fulfilled roles for therapists in long-term care facilities is primary prevention. An important example of primary prevention is systematic programming against falls, an important cause of morbidity and mortality among the elderly. Occupational therapists can assist by identifying at-risk clients and by developing training programs targeted for them. Mayo and co-workers (1989) identified variables that predict falling for the first time in rehabilitation clients. Statistically significant predictors were (a) stroke, (b) incontinence, (c) anticonvulsant medications, and (d) topical eye preparations. Other factors cited in the literature include (a) previous falls, (b) postural sway, (c) muscle weakness and limitation of movement, (d) feet abnormalities, (e) cardiovascular abnormalities, (f) visual disorders, and (g) improperly fitting canes or walkers (Tideiksaar, 1989). Targeted programs oriented to those at risk for falling can include assistive devices (e.g., elevated toilet seats, grab bars, shower seats), architectural modifications (e.g., nonslip floor surfaces, good lighting, and elimination of lighting glare), patient training, and staff training.

Exercise programs are also important in terms of primary prevention. Shephard (1990) reviewed the scientific basis for prescribing exercise for the very old and concluded that exercise reduces cardiovascular risks; lowers blood pressure; slows the rate of osteoporosis; corrects constipation; helps to ensure adequate nutrition and to control obesity; enhances sleep; increases cerebral arousal; enhances body image and self-esteem; increases strength and flexibility; fosters overall functional capacity; and decreases anxiety, depression, and anger. Morgan (1989, p. 125) theorized that "institutionalized elderly people with some degree of cognitive impairment appear to be a particularly appropriate target group" for demonstrating the psychologic benefits of physical activity.

Primary prevention of psychosocial disabilities is programmable in many ways also. For example, much depression is reactive to circumstances and can be prevented, especially when it is associated with feelings of loss and lack of control. In these cases, depression can often be prevented through occupation. Nursing-home residents need to see that they can impact their environments through their own occupations. Their living space can be personalized so that individual identity is respected. Staff can also demonstrate that the individual is a respected and productive member of the residential community. An institutional focus on individually meaningful and purposeful occupation is an excellent method for preventing depression.

PROGRAMMING PREVENTIVE OCCUPATIONS IN TEN SPECIFIC WAYS

Orientation Aids/Sensory Compensations

Given the sensory and perceptual problems of many residents, special care must be taken in designing the living space (the enduring occupational forms) in long-term care facilities. Koncelik (1976, 1982) analyzed the orientation needs of elderly persons from an architect's point of view, and Christenson (1989) conducted similar analyses from an occupational therapist's point of view.

To compensate for problems of visual acuity, bright localized lighting, elimination of glare (e.g., through carpeted hallways as opposed to shiny linoleum), and extra-large signs are recommended. Because the pupillary response to changes in lighting tends to be slow in elders, major differences in lighting levels from room to room should be avoided. Each community area, especially hallways, should have clear, unique landmarks facilitating orientation and direction (even healthy adults can become disoriented in labyrinths of unmarked corridors). Landmarks with textural, touchable features (e.g., large plants and wall-hangings) are especially valuable for elders. Music is another possibility. A general principle is to provide redundant, multisensory information by stimulating vision, audition, and touch in natural ways. A special caution is to avoid sound-distorting echoes; this can be done through the use of acoustical materials.

Assistive Devices/Motor Compensations

As with sensory compensations, the purpose of assistive devices is to promote compensatory occupation. Rogers (1981) stated that compensations can be just as important in gerontic occupational therapy as restoration or adaptation. Kiernat (1987) and Hasselkus (1989) argued that it is often more therapeutic to focus on changing the environment than changing the person. The fitting of assistive equipment to promote occupational performance is a major role for occupational therapy; here we focus on the role of assistive equipment in the prevention of injury and helplessness.

Bed rails, other strategically located handrails, and grab bars can promote safe transfers. Bathrooms can be equipped with shower seats and raised toilet seats if necessary. Nonslip surfaces are critical for safety. Different types of equipment designed to facilitate hygiene, feeding, communication, and dressing are readily available from several suppliers. The mobile arm support is an example of a multipurpose device that compensates for shoulder and elbow weakness (Wells et al, 1986). This device can be mounted to a wheelchair. Dynamic splints and universal cuffs can sometimes substitute for hand and finger weakness; of course, dynamic splints also have a role in restoration of motor ability.

Seating, Positioning, and Mobility

This section deals with intimate, touchable aspects of the occupational form. Until recently, there has been very little research into innovative seating systems for elderly patients. The technological breakthroughs that are routinely applied in pediatrics (the customized fitting of space-age metals, plastics, and electronics) are seldom applied in geriatrics. This is another example of ageism that runs counter to the philosophy of health promotion and disease prevention.

Olin (1987) described some of the problems that can be created by a standard wheelchair when used by a typical elderly person. These preventable problems include slouched posture, kyphosis, neck hyperextension, excessive pressure on the coccyx and sacrum, low back pain, skin deterioration, a narrow base of support with knees together, difficulty with foot-propelled mobility, difficulty with hand propulsion because of both posture and the weight of the chair, a lack of arm support at appropriate height, and even difficulty in transport by others (family members might not take the resident for day visits outside the nursing home because of the wheelchair's size, weight, maneuverability, and storage capacity). Occupational therapists and physical therapists can prevent these problems (Plautz & Timen, 1989; Epstein and Sadownick, 1989; Gromak and Gessert, 1989; Zacharkow, 1988). However, funding is often not available.

Sometimes relatively inexpensive modifications can enhance the daily occupational performance of nursing-home residents. Wheelchairs in some facilities can often be improved by simple repairs or by elementary adjustments (e.g., foot plates or armrests). Extended handles on wheelchair locks can facilitate safe transfers, and hand-rim projections can sometimes mean the difference between personal mobility and immobility. Firm seat inserts or back inserts can reverse the damage done by vinyl sling seats and sling backs, and gel cushions can provide comfort and reduce the likelihood of skin breakdown. Lateral trunk supports can correct for excessive chair width.

Sometimes inexpensive solutions work well. However, staff training and staff cooperation are essential because inexpensive accessories are not built into the design of the product and are easy to misplace or ignore.

Other critical issues in relation to mobility involve the provision and adjustment of canes and walkers. In a nursing home, it is one thing for an elderly person to be able to walk, for example, in a gait-training session. It is an entirely different matter to ensure that the individual actually gets up out of the bed, the chair, or the wheelchair and walks in the performance of everyday, naturalistic occupation. The first guideline here is to provide an occupational form that has meaning and purpose for the individual so that walking has personal value.

Activities (Occupations) of Daily Living

Performance of basic self-care occupations is a matter of personal integrity and self-esteem. Eating, dressing, washing, and hygiene take much more time and effort in elders than they do in younger people. One reason why occupational therapists should concentrate on ADL is that these occupations are so important within the daily occupational configuration of most nursing-home residents.

As with all preventive occupations, the occupational therapist focusing on ADL makes a therapeutic match between a synthesized occupational form and the individual's developmental structure. Rogers (1989) hypothesized that ADL performance depends as much on "task and environmental variables" (i.e., the occupational form) as on the client's developmental structure. Hasselkus (1989) argued that long-term chronic care requires a focus on the removal of environmental barriers and disincentives as opposed to the acute-care assumption that the problem is within the individual.

Dining occupations are often the most important in the nursing-home resident's day, and this is particularly true of residents with relatively severe impairments. The community dining hall calls for all the occupational therapist's expertise in analyzing occupations on sensory motor, cognitive, and psychosocial dimensions. Positioning, assistive devices, orientation aids, and group process all come into play in synthesizing therapeutic occupational forms. For example, table heights should vary depending on type of chair or wheelchair used; the spacing of tables influences wheelchair accessibility (frequently there is not enough space); and the size of the table influences resident-to-resident communication (smaller tables with individuals at homogeneous levels of function tend to elicit more mealtime satisfaction). A small matter such as the provision of chairs with arms can make the difference between occupational success and occupational failure.

As with the tables and chairs, the plates and flatware should be individually selected for residents with motor disabilities. For example, some flatware is too heavy for many residents, but certain individuals, such as those with tremor secondary to Parkinson's disease, might benefit from weighted flatware. Built-up handles are frequently the most useful assistive devices in our equipment inventory.

Individuals with cognitive disabilities require a different type of occupational synthesis. For example, a man with advanced Alzheimer's disease can suddenly forget that he is in an eating situation, or he can become confused by having several different types of food and several different types of utensils. Such an individual is often fed by staff. However, the dining occupation might be the person's last remaining area in which to exercise personal control. Staff can promote maximal performance by simplifying the situation (providing small amounts of one type of food at a time to be eaten with a single utensil).

Although nonverbal cuing is particularly valuable, staff verbalizations can also assist in orienting the individual to the occupation at hand. Sometimes staff can initiate and stimulate conversations between residents by referring to immediate stimuli (e.g., flowers or weather outside the window) in naturalistic ways. Generally speaking, the community dining hall should not be a training area (systematically restoring self-feeding skills could take place on a one-to-one basis elsewhere). To the greatest extent possible, residents should not have to endure the inappropriate behavior of peers or the corrections of staff. Overall, staff need to internalize the values of independence and naturalism. Just because some individuals might need help in cutting meat does not mean that they have to be fed forkful by forkful.

The same principles of using the physical as well as the human features of the occupational form apply to other ADL tasks. Is the sink accessible by wheelchair within the person's room? Is the mirror at the right height? Can assistive devices (e.g., elongated handles or stocking assists) promote function? For residents with cognitive deficits, will pictures of clothes on the dresser help them to participate in dressing, or will a picture of a toilet on the bathroom door cue them to avoid incontinence and discomfort? Frequently, a small change in the occupational form will make a major difference. In addition, even individuals who are unable to move well enough to dress themselves might enjoy making a choice as to what is worn.

Promoting Privacy, Promoting Community

Institutional settings are known for depriving their residents of privacy and autonomy (Kiernat, 1987) and for discouraging a sense of community empowerment (Moos and Lemke, 1984). In promoting passivity, residences designed to provide health care sometimes inadvertently promote clinical depression and a gap between what residents are able to do and what they actually do on a day-to-day basis.

The inadvertent encouragement of passive dependency is often deeply embedded in institutional policy and in the attitudes of staff. Perhaps the most important role for long-term care therapists is as advocates for the power of self-directed occupational choice as a health promoter

and disease preventer. Attitudes that promote occupational dysfunction must be constantly challenged. For example, there is the attitude that it does not matter whether residents contribute to their own self-care occupations as long as the job gets done. Then there is the attitude that the presence of personally meaningful objects in the residents' room and community space interferes with the orderliness of the institution. Another destructive attitude is that all residents should be treated alike and should adhere to the same schedule without options regardless of individual interest, background, or ability level. Most destructive of all, the attitude exists that it makes little difference whether residents become ill and incapacitated this week or in a month from now because they are thought to be on a progressively deteriorating course of disease toward death anyhow. All of these attitudes have no place in a health-care facility, and all can be combated by advocacy of meaningful, purposeful occupation.

A specific strategy to begin empowering nursing-home residents is to conduct institutional evaluations designed for this purpose. The Multiphasic Environmental Assessment Procedure (Moos & Lemke, 1984) assesses policy choice (options that residents have in choosing daily occupations); policy clarity; resident control (resident influence in running the facility); privacy; self-exploration (the extent to which residents are urged to express their feelings and concerns); and any gaps between what is available in the facility and what is actually used. Another instrument that initiates dialogue at the institutional level is the Situational Control of Daily Activities Scale (Chang, 1978).

An example of encouraging personal control is to provide residents with locked drawers in their rooms and activity areas. Keys can be built up with paddle handles, and therapists or nurses can help residents devise a plan for safeguarding keys, if necessary. Some residents can safely lock their doors at night. Each resident should be encouraged or assisted in personalizing his or her room with photographs and mementos as well as new decorations. An institutional priority should be to provide peace and security to residents who might be disturbed by disruptive behavior or vocalizations of other residents. Even apparently minor choices (types of music, entertainment, snacks) can be important in giving residents a sense of control.

Leisure and Productivity

The role of occupational therapists in relation to "activities programs" in long-term care facilities is not always clear. As Crepeau (1986) wrote, trained as well as untrained individuals may direct the activity programs at various facilities. If trained, the individual might be an occupational therapist or might be from a different discipline (e.g., recreational therapy, music therapy, dance therapy, art therapy, social work). Occupational therapists are also involved as consultants, program planners, administrators, or supervisors (Crepeau, 1986).

Regardless of role, occupational therapists are vitally concerned with leisure and productivity. To the greatest extent possible, nursing-home residents should be encouraged to have high levels of meaning and purpose in all they do. According to the definition of occupation presented in an earlier section, all occupations have some level of meaning and purpose; otherwise they would not be done. However, different occupations are not equal in terms of meaning and purpose. Unfortunately, too many occupations in the daily life of many nursing-home residents are escapist, diversional, or performed for minimal or extrinsic purposes (e.g., to get something over with or to please others). Lacking are occupations in which the individual is totally, vitally involved; occupations that are done for their own sake; and occupations that offer the experience of challenge and, eventually, mastery.

Helping residents to find deeply involving occupations is very much an individual matter. In some cases, the occupation might be identified through an occupational (activity) history, but in other cases residents might become involved in a novel occupation little valued until old age. Lifelong gardeners might shun plants because of unpleasant associations, but these individuals might take on a special passion for photography.

Although individualized programming is essential, general programming is also characteristic of most healthy communities. There should be a balance in occupational forms offered: (a) group and individual; (b) parallel, reciprocal, and project; (c) product-oriented and product-free; (d) spectator-oriented and participative; and (e) long-term/multisession and short-term/single session. Most important, opportunities should be provided on weekends, holidays, and evenings for those residents able to participate. One tool occupational therapists can use in raising institutional consciousness about the quality of programming is the activity (occupational) configuration (Cynkin and Robinson, 1990). Is there a balance of occupations throughout the week? Who takes part? What needs are met by occupation?

A special need for many elderly people is a sense of productivity. After a long life of work, many elderly people continue to need to make socially recognized contributions. For some people, avocational pursuits fulfill this need. Others take a special interest in helping to care for fellow residents in appropriate ways. Riessman (1965) described the helper-therapy principle: the placing of service recipients into the helper/volunteer role. Therapeutic benefits are potentially reciprocal for the helped and the helper. Altruistically motivated occupations can be structured in a variety of ways. Hatter and Nelson (1987) found experimentally that elderly subjects were significantly more likely to attend a scheduled activity if their work products (impact of performance) were to be given to others in need as opposed to being kept. In a follow-up study, Getz (1987) demonstrated that elderly women residing in a nursing home made significantly more stationery and engaged longer in the occupation when the stationery was to be given to abused children as opposed to being kept. The making of valued products for others is a way of fulfilling the need for productivity in individuals lacking the necessary interpersonal skills for face-to-face helping.

Exercise for General Fitness

A previous section of this chapter summarized the many physical and psychologic benefits of exercise in the very old. For more on the scientific basis for prescribing exercise in the very old, see Shephard (1990). The focus in this section is on programming exercise in nursing homes, with a special focus on residents' motivation.

Currently in our society, aerobics and various types of group fitness programs are common. However, they were not so common in the cultural milieu in which elderly people, especially women, grew to maturity. This change in social values can explain in part the reluctance of some nursing-home residents to participate in exercise groups. For those who refuse to participate in typical exercise classes, programming is still possible, however. For example, the best exercise for many people, elderly or not, is walking. Use of walkers involves some upper extremity exercise as well. Walking can be embedded into naturalistic, everyday occupation if residents who are able to walk have somewhere to walk to with purpose and if the use of wheelchairs is discouraged. Each resident should have a clear treatment plan in regard to personal mobility and its relation to exercise.

Kemp (1988) and Mobily (1982) argued that motivation in geriatric rehabilitation is a two-sided phenomenon: The elderly person might have motives not to exercise as well as motives to exercise. Possible motives to avoid exercise include (a) avoidance of expected pain or fatigue; (b) fear of failure and appearance of weakness in the eyes of peers or staff; (c) the idea that exercise is dangerous to health; (d) the belief that enough exercise was done earlier in life; (e) fear of instability and falling; and (f) a generalized sense of learned helplessness. Alternatively, possible motives for exercise include (a) desire for enhanced health; (b) avoidance of future disability; (c) relaxation and release of stress; (d) desire for a sense of autonomy; (e) wanting to please the therapist; and (f) pursuit of added purposes in such a way that the exercise is embedded within a meaningful occupation (Nelson and Peterson, 1989).

One of the problems in initiating an exercise program is that many of the motives for exercise are not experienced until after a regular exercise program is well established; hence the importance of initial motivation. Recent research demonstrates the effects of various types of occupational forms on exercise motivation in nursing-home residents. For example, Yoder, Nelson, and Smith (1989) found experimentally that elderly women engaged in significantly more exercise repetitions when the exercise was embedded in a food-preparation occupation than in a controlled–for rote exercise condition. Another experiment by Riccio, Nelson, and Bush (1990) demonstrated that the use of imagery (verbal cues referring to materials not immediately present) elicited more exercise repetitions than a rote exercise (control) condition. Music and aspects of group process are also possible motivators. One of the earliest ideas within the profession of occupational therapy was the embedding of exercise within meaningful, purposeful occupations. Occupational therapists should assert their heritage in programming health-promoting exercise.

Restorative Adaptations (Rehabilitation)

It has been argued that the rehabilitation model with its emphasis on restoration of abilities within the individual applies more to the aftermath of the acute phase of a disease process than to a chronic disability (Hasselkus, 1989; Kiernat, 1987). The fact is that elderly people in nursing homes do experience disease processes (including psychiatric disorders) at a rate much higher than the general population and that placement in rehabilitation hospitals is frequently impossible in the aftermath of disease. Therefore, a rehabilitation approach with structured occupational therapy and physical therapy to restore specific performance components is appropriate. Indeed, failure to provide rehabilitation is another example of the medically common ageism discussed at the beginning of this chapter.

Occupational therapists can advocate that the nursing home recognize that certain residents are clients within a rehabilitation model, whereas others are residents within a community living model. Although the two models have many things in common (e.g., holistic conception of the individual, concern for integration of skills into everyday life), the two models have differences that should be clear to staff. In rehabilitation, formal assessments are frequent, therapists' expectations of client performance are explicit, and instructions are often quite directive. There is the attempt to establish an atmosphere in which therapists and clients are working vigorously together on targeted goals. There is also the assumption that intensive treatment will come to an end after the maximum restoration is achieved. In contrast, the community living model uses a less directive approach, and the focus is on compensatory alterations of the environment (occupational form) instead of on changes (adaptations) within the person's developmental structure.

There is no reason that the two models cannot be in operation within the same facility. Residents with acute impairments whose abilities can be restored deserve rehabilitation. Residents with stable conditions deserve a less directive approach.

Community Integration

Total institutions, such as many nursing homes, are noted for being isolated from the communities around them (Gillick, 1989). There are many negative consequences of this isolation. To some degree, everyday occupation depends on environmental expectations (the human context of the occupational form). In most community life, there is an expectation of productivity, responsibility, responsiveness, and alertness. Isolation from the hustle and bustle of everyday life can lead to low expectations of occupational performance, and low expectations can be self-fulfilling. The norm for behavior should be "a robust person" not "a person who causes no trouble."

Therapists can combat the negative effects of isolation in two basic ways: Bring more of the community into the nursing home, and take more of the nursing home out into the community. Most nursing homes encourage family members and friends to visit. The problems are that hours of visitation are often restricted artificially and that the environment (occupational form) of the visit is seldom ideal. Family members deserve privacy and freedom from the potential distractions provided by other residents. Even more so, family members and friends need environments in which they can do things with residents.

Conversation is a good occupation for some elderly persons in nursing homes, but many residents function better when involved in structured occupations involving materials. A given family might enjoy a game of cards. My grandmother Esther used to play a game called "Seven-Up" with my sister and me when we were children, and we enjoyed playing this game with her later in life when she had trouble engaging in conversation without the support provided by materials. Playing our old game, she got a twinkle in her eye and talked easily and meaningfully. Craft areas and materials should be made available to residents with visitors. Food preparation and dining are excellent family-involving occupations that often encourage reminiscence and shared meanings.

Other members of the community have much to offer. Many nursing-home residents have active spiritual and religious lives. Clergy and lay people make great contributions to nursing-home life. Many nursing homes have entertainment programs. Spectator-oriented entertainers are helpful, but most helpful are those entertainers who are able to elicit active participation by residents in singing, dancing, the theatre, and so on. Students and volunteers of all ages should be encouraged to develop one-to-one relation-

ships with residents. Intergenerational exchanges between children and elderly residents can be powerfully therapeutic.

The other side of community integration is the movement of residents outside the walls of the building. That begins with access to the facility's grounds and immediate surround. The problem with most institutions is that ingress and egress are tightly controlled because a small minority of residents tend to wander and become lost. Their safety can be ensured without restricting the freedom of others, and each facility should have a clear plan of how to do this. Even those who might wander off should have access in good weather to an outside patio with architectural features that are secure yet not prison-like.

Visits to family member's houses should be encouraged as much as visits in the opposite direction. To facilitate this, family members often need specific guidance from staff in terms of wheelchair management, architectural barriers, medication, transfers, and ADL, including toileting. Frequently, people hesitate to bring a family member home for a holiday because they are afraid to ask practical questions (they might feel that staff expect them to know everything without asking).

Staff-accompanied trips and visits to community facilities should also be a valued occupation. Once again, spectator-oriented events are fine, but participative situations are usually better. It is remarkable to see how an elderly person can perk up and appear to change personality when taken to a shopping mall or a supermarket! It is good for nursing-home residents to experience naturalistic everyday occupational forms, and it is good for community members to experience the presence of all their fellow citizens.

Employee Wellness

Staff training has been mentioned several times in this chapter, and it is mentioned again because it is a vital role in nursing homes. However, staff training and ultimately staff performance depend on employees' abilities to handle the stresses associated with the job (Benjamin and Spector, 1990).

Factors potentially contributing to excessive stress and burnout involve the workplace, the organization, and personality (Schuster et al, 1984). Workplace factors include excessive caseload and residents who are difficult to work with.

Organizational factors include insensitive or unfair supervision and inability to contribute to policy-making. Personality factors include perfectionism and low self-concept. Many employees of nursing homes feel that they are poorly paid and that they have low status in the community. Whatever the problems of the community, they find their way into the informal organizational structure of the nursing home.

The consequences of excessive stress and burnout can be devastating because residents are so dependent on day-to-day interactions with staff. Staff might actively resist training and sabotage the best-laid plans for ADL. Inadvertently, staff might encourage passivity and dependence. Verbal or physical abuse is possible, especially in relation to demanding, unresponsive, or defiant behavior by residents.

Occupational therapists have a role in health promotion among staff as a method to achieve the health of residents. The lines of communication between staff and their supervisors should be tested in both directions. Staff should not feel isolated at night, on weekends, or on holidays. Employee-recognition programs are appropriate. Formal employee-wellness programs with provisions for physical and mental health are desirable.

ROLES AND FUNDING

As the architect Koncelik (1976, p. 46) said, "Much of the general activity found in nursing homes is directly related to occupational therapy even though it may not be prescribed." Indeed, a visionary approach to long-term care facilities for the aged would be to aim toward developing what would be called "nursing and occupational homes" or even "occupational and nursing homes!" Nurses and occupational therapists would team up to direct the facility. Both professions have a holistic philosophy and complementary skills.

In addition to a management role in long-term care facilities, occupational therapists have several other valuable roles to play. Primary, secondary, and tertiary levels of prevention are involved depending on the role. Primary prevention is usually accomplished through consultancy, staff training, supervision, and advocacy. Most nursing homes actively seek occupational therapists as consultants and staff educators. However, funds are seldom adequate for developing comprehensive programs built on a philosophy of meaningful, purposeful occupation. Consultancy is often related to orientation aids, assistive devices, positioning, and ADL rather than to an overall emphasis on occupational performance.

Funding from Medicare, Medicaid, and insurance companies tends to be most straightforward when the resident is a clear candidate for rehabilitation (the tertiary level of prevention). Direct service seems to be more attractive to many occupational therapists than the indirect service of consultancy or management. Rogers (1981) stated that this preference for direct service might be due to the emphasis in basic educational preparation on direct service functions. She argued that many occupational therapists might see indirect service roles as "unattractive, ambiguous, and threatening" because they received little formal instruction about these roles.

An especially neglected area is the treatment of psychiatric disorders in long-term care facilities. Larson and associates (1989) pointed out that many psychiatric disorders that would merit well-funded intervention if presented by younger people are simply ignored if presented by the elderly. As with roles in consultancy, many of today's occupational therapists avoid psychiatrically related practice. Psychogeriatric practice is unfortunately not a popular area of practice, despite the outstanding potential of occupational therapy in this practice area.

Service provision and funding can be problematic in other areas of practice also. Gromak and Gessert (1989) described difficulties in obtaining equipment reimbursement and strategies for doing so. Olin (1987) wrote specifically about custom-ordered wheelchairs, which often cost twice as much as standard wheelchairs but which prevent the development of multiple impairments. Olin (1987, p. 45) stated that "Medicare . . . appears reluctant to fund this new technology and routinely limits or denies coverage." Strategies recommended by Olin include appeals to Medicare if funding is denied; careful justification of the functional importance of the equipment to insurance carriers; and presentation of the value of the product to the patient and, in some cases, to family members so that a personal spending decision can be made. Epstein and Sadownick (1989) reported that funds for inexpensive fabrications can sometimes be supported by nursing budgets, and they urged the use of photographs to supplement narrative in obtaining funds for larger items.

New roles for occupational therapists are emerging. Positioning equipment manufacturing companies are being developed by occupational therapists. Occupational therapists are also consulting or collaborating with architects to design visionary residential facilities. The problem here again is funding. Funding issues have not improved since Koncelik (1976) described the dilemma he faced after carefully designing a model room for the elderly person in a nursing home. According to Koncelik, $1,000 was allotted for each room, but an acceptable bed cost $650. That left little money for basic furnishings and no money for innovative design. Once again, however, some individuals might be able to afford a supportive environment.

Another role for occupational therapists is research. As in many areas of practice, gerontologic occupational therapy is not a regular recipient of research funds. This creates a vicious circle, of course. The less research we have demonstrating the therapeutic power of occupation, the less likely we are to receive clinical funding for many of our preventive interventions. In turn, however, it is difficult to justify research funding without a well-recognized clinical base and without a strong prior record of research. This problem can be addressed if not solved by clinical–academic partnerships supported by the American Occupational Therapy Association and the American Occupational Therapy Foundation.

Acknowledgments

We gratefully acknowledge the support, encouragement, and persistence of editors Rothman and Levine; the invaluable input of clinician/administrator Diane S. Stern, OTR, currently with Visiting Nurse Association, Kalamazoo, Michigan; the helpful suggestions and bibliographic assistance of Anne L. Morris, MPA, OTR, of the American Occupational Therapy Association; and the example of a meaningful, purposeful occupation (playing "Seven-Up") provided by my grandmother Esther Nelson and cited in this chapter.

References

American Occupational Therapy Association Uniform Terminology Task Force: Uniform Terminology for Occupational Therapy, 2nd ed. Am J Occup Ther 43:808–815, 1989.

Baltes PB, Dittman-Kohli C, and Kliegel R: Reserve capacity of the elderly in aging—seventeen tests of true intelligence. Psychol Aging 1:172–177, 1986.

Benjamin LC and Spector J: The relationship of staff, resident and environmental characteristics to stress experienced by staff caring for the dementing. Int J Geriatr Psychiatry 5:25–31, 1990.

Black JS and Kapoor W: Health promotion and disease prevention in older people: Our current state of ignorance. J Am Geriatr Soc 38:168–172, 1990.

Bortz WM: Disuse and aging. JAMA 248:1203–1208, 1982.

Bortz WM: Redefining human aging. J Am Geriatr Soc 37:1092–1096, 1989.

Chang B: Perceived situational control of daily activities: A new tool. Res Nurs Health 1:181–188, 1978.

Christenson M: Rehabilitation of the elderly: Adaptations that compensate for sensory changes. Source Program Guide: The American Occupational Therapy Association Practice Symposium. Rockville, MD, American Occupational Therapy Association, 1989.

Christiansen C: The perils of plurality. Occup Ther J Res 10:259–265, 1990.

Crepeau EL: Activity programming. In Davis LJ and Kirkland M (eds): The Role of Occupational Therapy with the Elderly. Rockville, MD, American Occupational Therapy Association, 1986.

Cynkin S and Robinson AM: Occupational Therapy and Activities Health: Toward Health Through Activities. Boston, Little, Brown, 1990.

Epstein CE and Sadownick PM: Specialized seating for the institutionalized elderly: Prescription, fabrication, funding. In Technology Review, 1989: Perspectives on Occupational Therapy Practice. Rockville, MD, American Occupational Therapy Association, 1989, pp 13–16.

Fidler GS and Fidler SW: Doing and becoming: Purposeful action and self-actualization. Am J Occup Ther 32:305–310, 1978.

Getz CJ: The Effects of Altruism on Activity Productivity in Elderly Women in Skilled-Care Nursing Facilities. Unpublished master's thesis, Western Michigan University, 1987.

Gillick MR: Long-term care options for the frail elderly. J Am Geriatr Soc 37:1198–1203, 1989.

Gromak PA and Gessert V: Working "smarter": A systems approach to meeting government regulations for restorative care in long-term care facilities. Healthy Aging, Creighton Regional Geriatric Newsletter 2(1):3–4, 8–9, 1989.

Hasselkus BR: Occupational and physical therapy in geriatric rehabilitation. Phys Occup Ther Geriatr 7(3):3–20, 1989.

Hatter JK and Nelson DL: Altruism and task participation in the elderly. Am J Occup Ther 41:379–381, 1987.

Institute of Medicine: Improving the Quality of Care in Nursing Homes. Washington, DC, National Academy Press, 1986.

Kane R, Ouslander J, and Abrass, I: Essentials of Clinical Geriatrics. New York, McGraw-Hill, 1984.

Kemp BJ: Motivation, rehabilitation, and aging: A conceptual model. Top Geriatr Rehabil 3(3):41–51, 1988.

Kiernat JM: Promoting independence and autonomy through environmental approaches. Top Geriatr Rehabil 3(1):1–6, 1987.

Koncelik JA: Aging and the Product Environment. Stroudsburg, PA, Hutchinson Ross, 1982.

Koncelik JA: Designing the Open Nursing Home. Stroudsburg, PA, Dowden, Hutchinson and Ross, 1976.

Larson DB, Lyons JS, Hohmann AA, et al: A systematic review of nursing home research in three psychiatric journals: 1966–1985. Int J Geriatr Psychiatr 4:129–134, 1989.

Lawton MP: Competence, environmental press, and the adaptation of older people. In Lawton MP, Windley PG, and Byers TO (eds): Aging and the Environment: Theoretical Approaches. New York, Springer, 1982.

Levine RE and Merrill SC: Psychosocial aspects of the environment. Top Geriatr Rehabil 3(1):27–34, 1987.

Lewis BC (speaker): Dismobility in the Elderly: Evaluation and Treatment (Video conference). Pittsburgh, American Rehabilitation Educational Network, 1987.

Mayo NE, Korner-Bitensky N, Becker R, and Georges P: Predicting falls among patients in a rehabilitation hospital. Am J Phys Med Rehabil 68:139–146, 1989.

Mobily KE: Motivational aspects of exercise for the elderly: Barriers and solutions. Phys Occup Ther Geriatr 1(4):43–53, 1982.

Moos RH and Lemke S: Multiphasic environmental assessment procedure (MEAP). Stanford, CA, University Medical Center, 1984.

Morgan K: Trial and error: Evaluating the psychological benefits of physical activity. Int J Geriatr Psychiatr 4:125–127, 1989.

Nelson DL: Occupation: Form and performance. Am J Occup Ther 42:633–641, 1988.

Nelson DL and Peterson CQ: Enhancing therapeutic exercise through purposeful activity: A theoretic analysis. Top Geriatr Rehabil 4(4):12–22, 1989.

Olin DW: The therapist's role in improving the person-environment fit. Top Geriatr Rehabil 3(1):43–47, 1987.

Plautz RE and Timen BM: Seating/positioning of the institutionalized elderly. In Technology Review, 1989: Perspectives on Occupational Therapy Practice. Rockville, MD, American Occupational Therapy Association, 1989.

Riccio CM, Nelson DL, and Bush MA: Adding purpose to the repetitive exercise of elderly women through imagery. Am J Occup Ther 44:714–719, 1990.

Riessman F: The helper therapy principle. Soc Work 10:27–32, 1965.

Rogers JC: Gerontic occupational therapy. Am J Occup Ther 35:633–666, 1981.

Rogers JC: Occupational therapy services for Alzheimer's disease and related disorders (position paper). Am J Occup Ther 40:822–824, 1986.

Rogers JC: Therapeutic activity and health status. Top Geriatr Rehabil 4(4):1–11, 1989.

Rovner B, Kafonek S, Fillipp L, et al: Prevalence of mental illness in a community nursing home. Am J Psychiatr 143:1446–1449, 1986.

Schuster ND, Nelson DL, and Quisling C: Burnout among physical therapists. Physical Therapy 64:299–303, 1984.

Shephard RJ: The scientific basis of exercise prescribing for the very old. J Am Geriatr Soc 38:62–70, 1990.

Skolaski-Pellitteri T: Environmental intervention for the demented person. Phys Occup Ther Geriatr 3:55–59, 1984.

Tideiksaar R: Geriatric falls: Assessing the cause, preventing recurrence. Geriatrics 44:57–64, 1989.

U.S. Department of Health and Human Services. Characteristics of nursing home residents, health status and care received. National Nursing Home survey. PHS 81–1712. Vital and Health Statistics, Series 13, No. 51, 1981.

Wells MA, Chew TA, Lars B, and Campbell BA: Therapeutic adaptations. In Davis LJ and Kirkland M (eds): The Role of Occupational Therapy with the Elderly. Rockville, MD, American Occupational Therapy Association, 1986.

Wetle T: Age as a risk factor for inadequate treatment. JAMA 258:516, 1987.

Woo B, Woo B, Cook EF, et al: Screening procedures in the asymptomatic adult: Comparison of physicians' recommendations, patients' desires, published guidelines, and actual practice. JAMA 254:1480, 1985.

Yoder RM, Nelson DL, and Smith DA: Added-purpose versus rote exercise in female nursing home residents. Am J Occup Ther 43:581–586, 1989.

Zacharkow D: Posture: Sitting, Standing, Chair Design and Exercise. Springfield, IL, Charles C Thomas, 1988.

APPENDIX I: ORGANIZATION RESOURCES

Administration on Aging
Department of Health and Human Services
330 Independence Avenue, SW
Washington, DC 20201
(202) 245-2158

The Alzheimer's Disease and Related Disorders Association
70 East Lake Street
Chicago, IL 60601
(301) 853-3060

American Occupational Therapy Association
1383 Piccard Drive
Rockville, MD 20850
(301) 948-9626

American College of Health Care Administrators
(formerly American College of Nursing Home Administrators)
4650 East-West Highway
Bethesda, MD 20014
(301) 652-8384

American Geriatrics Society
10 Columbus Circle
New York, NY 10019

Association of Long Term Care Gerontology Centers, Inc.
℅ Eric A. Pfeiffer, MD, President
Suncoast Gerontology Center
USF, 12901 North 30th Street
Tampa, FL 33612

Asociacion Nacional Pro Personas Mayores
National Association for Hispanic Elderly
1730 West Olympic Boulevard
Suite 401
Los Angeles, CA 90015

Federal Council on Aging
330 Independence Avenue, SW
Room 4620, North Building
Washington, DC 20201
(202) 245-0441

Gerontology Standing Committee
% Practice Division
American Occupational Therapy Association
1383 Piccard Drive
Rockville, MD 20850
(301) 948-9626
(Note: Most state organizations of occupational therapy have gerontology special interest sections.)

The Gerontological Society of America
1835 K Street, NW
Suite 305
Washington, DC 20006

Jewish Association for Services for the Aged
222 Park Avenue, South
New York, NY 10003
(212) 677-2530

National Alliance of Senior Citizens
2525 Wilson Boulevard
Arlington, VA 22201
(703) 528-4380

National Association of Senior Living
  Industries
The Directory of Senior Living Industries
Annapolis, MD 21401

National Center on Arts and the Aging
600 Maryland Avenue, SW
West Wing 100
Washington, DC 20024
(202) 479-1200

National Center on Ministry with the Aging
1000 West 42nd Street
Indianapolis, IN 46208
(317) 924-1331

National Center on the Black Aged
1424 K Street, NW
Suite 500
Washington, DC 20005
(202) 637-8400

National Citizens Coalition for Nursing
  Home Reform
1309 L Street, NW
Suite 300
Washington, DC 20005
(201) 393-7979

National Clearinghouse on Aging
Department of Health and Human Services
330 Independence Avenue, SW
Washington, DC 20201

National Council on the Aging, Inc.
600 Maryland Avenue, SW
Washington, DC 20024

National Council on Senior Citizens
1511 K Street, NW
Washington, DC 20005

National Council for Therapy and
  Rehabilitation Through Horticulture
701 North St. Asaph Street
Alexandria, VA 22314
(703) 836-4609

National Institutes of Health
National Institute on Aging
Building 31, Room 5C-12
9000 Rockville Pike
Bethesda, MD 20205

Western Gerontological Society
833 Market Street, Room 516
San Francisco, CA 94103

CHAPTER

3

Robert D. Bazley

Promoting Health Through Exercise

The United States has become a nation of spectators. It is not unusual to see millions of Americans watching a football game on a Sunday afternoon, and yet only a small percentage of those viewers actually participate in any type of regular exercise or activity themselves. It is more than coincidence that the leading cause of death in the United States is coronary heart disease, a condition prevalent in wealthy, sedentary societies. Although it has been speculated for centuries that regular exercise has a positive effect on health, only recently has research shown that regular exercise can help prevent not only heart disease but also many of the other degenerative diseases. Today, a great deal has been written in the popular literature about the benefits of exercise. We are told that through regular exercise we will lose weight, look better in our clothes, and even look and feel younger. More important, if we are active on a regular basis our hearts are healthier, our blood pressures are lower, and we are more resistant to stroke and diabetes. We feel more "positive" and may even ward off certain types of cancer.

Over the past decade, "fitness" has grown into a billion dollar per year industry. Health clubs have sprung up across the entire United States. High-tech clothing, shoes, and computerized exercise equipment are commonplace. Despite the seemingly complex nature of fitness, the principles of exercise are simple and the benefits can

be enjoyed by everyone. It is not necessary to join an expensive club or wear the latest exercise fashion to achieve fitness and health. All you need is the desire to be healthier and a little knowledge of how to begin. On the following pages the benefits of exercise will be discussed and a simple yet effective fitness program, aimed at promoting good health, will be outlined.

Why have most Americans remained spectators rather than participants in sport and exercise? According to de Vries (1980), the American system of physical education may be to blame for this phenomenon. It has emphasized the development of a relatively small group of scholastic athletes for sports such as football, basketball, and baseball, rather than teaching the larger population about fitness activities that can be pursued and enjoyed over a lifetime.

Will a regular regimen of physical activity actually help to prevent disease? Empirically, exercise, or more specifically, the physical fitness achieved via regular exercise, seems to produce a healthier human body that is more resistant to disease. Over the years, however, the skeptics in the medical world have pointed to the paucity of good research as their reason for not encouraging their patients to exercise. The debate over exercise and health may be as old as medicine itself, but only recently has science, backed by sound research, concluded that there is a direct relationship between regular physical exercise and good health.

HISTORICAL PERSPECTIVE

The notion that exercise can promote good health is not new. Hippocrates (4th century B.C.) wrote that moderate exercise can make the body healthier and slow the aging process. Conversely, a sedentary lifestyle leads to illness and to a shorter life span. He actually prescribed walking and other forms of exercise to treat various ailments. The ancient Greek ideal was "a sound mind in a sound body." This philosophy was so vital in daily Greek life that exercise and sport became the focal point of their religious festivals, the most famous being the Olympic Games.

Although the emphasis on sport and exercise declined during the Middle Ages, it was embraced heartily by the Teutonic tribes of Northern Europe, the Vikings, and the English (Nixon and Jewett, 1969). Survival in a world dominated by constant warfare between tribes depended on fitness and health. These cultures would later influence the development of physical education and physical therapy in 20th century America. Through the Renaissance (14th and 15th centuries) and Enlightenment (18th century), the "fitness-health" connection was strengthened, first by the "rebirth" of the classical ideal and, later, by the belief in the power of human reason (Nixon and Jewett, 1969).

The Industrial Revolution in America, during the 19th and early 20th centuries, further reinforced the idea that health was related to exercise and activity. America experienced a shift in demographics from the farm to the city. People were thrust into a world of pollution, noise, new mechanical inventions, and a faster-paced lifestyle. Lovett, an orthopedist, stated in his "presidential address" to the American Association for the Advancement of Physical Education in 1901:

The tremendous pressure of American Life, the rush, the tension, the steadily increasing demands of life, are pauperizing the community in a physical way. (pp. 300–302.)

Physical education was becoming part of the curricula of American schools. This was the great era of immigration, and the Germans and Scandinavians brought with them their love of sport and exercise. German, Swedish, and Danish systems of "gymnastics" were soon introduced into the American physical educational programs. Also related to this European influence was the realization that exercise could be used to treat victims of injury and disease. During this time

the physical therapy profession had its beginnings, working with patients stricken with "infantile paralysis" and soldiers injured during World War I (Pinkston, 1989).

Exercise for Health. During the first half of the 20th century, there was an ever-growing awareness of the "exercise-health" connection. The rise of organizations like the Boy Scouts and Girl Scouts; the YMCAs and YWCAs; the American Red Cross swimming programs; and the building of playgrounds, pools, and athletic facilities in the 1930s by the Work Projects Administration (WPA) and Public Works Administration (PWA) is evidence that there was a growing consensus that physical activity was important (Nixon and Jewett, 1969).

Interest in exercise and health grew even faster after World War II. There are many reasons for this rise in interest. Now, Americans had more leisure time and a higher standard of living. More people had free weekends and vacation time. The sporting goods industry was born. Television brought live coverage of sports events like baseball, football, and Olympic Games into the home. And, probably most important, President Eisenhower established the President's Council on Youth Fitness (1956). Exercise was recognized officially by the U.S. Government as being important. However, the medical critics were still not convinced, and only a small portion of the American public actually was physically active on a regular basis.

During the 1950s and 1960s there was an ever-growing body of knowledge and awareness of physical fitness, but the proponents of exercise were at the very least considered eccentric and at the worst, fanatical, or even mad. Even with the advances of science, no one could prove that exercise could promote good health or prolong life. One of the fitness "gurus" of this era was Cerutty, the Australian track coach/philosopher whose athletes won Olympic medals. He was considered radical even by his colleagues. He wrote in his book *Be Fit! or Be Damned!* (Published by Pelham Books, 1967):

It is this marked alteration in man's living habits—food, exercise, sedentary work, that are the factors that have reduced his capacity to live healthily and survive reasonably. Could it be that his very security: his freedom from want: ample food, and the substitution of natural stresses by the artificial stresses associated with business and ambition, his urban life, even the air he breathes, that these are the contributing factors to his ill-health, and the customary physical decline after middle-age and often, before! (pp. 32–33.)

Cerutty's formula for fitness, "walking 2 miles per day in 30 minutes," does not seem radical in today's world of hi-tech exercise. Cerutty most certainly had an impact on the rise of physical fitness "down under" and, due to the success of his athletes in international competition, worldwide. Hailing from exercise-oriented cultures, Maitland (from Australia) and Paris and McKenzie (from New Zealand) were certainly influenced by this phenomenon. In turn, these practitioners have greatly influenced the practice of physical therapy throughout the world today.

Exercise and Preventive Medicine. Cooper (1982) stated that in the late 1960s there was little interest in the medical world in preventive medicine. Medicine at that time was concerned with treating existing conditions. Cooper had developed a fitness program for the U.S. Air Force Astronaut program and later for the entire Air Force. This program was based on research that included 27,000 subjects. His first book, *Aerobics* (1968), was the first well-documented fitness program that suggested exercise would promote good health. Cooper even coined a new term in the English language, "aerobics" (i.e., any of the various sustained exercises, such as jogging, rowing, swimming, or cycling, that stimulates and strengthens the heart and lungs, thus improving the body's utilization of oxygen). After leaving the military, Cooper established the Institute for Aerobics Research, Dallas, Texas, where he continues to study the impact of exercise on health. The book *Aerobics* (1968) and the televised win of American Frank Shorter in the 1972 Olympic Marathon have been cited as two major events that started the "fitness revolution" of the 1970s in the United States.

Throughout history many of the giants of medicine—Hippocrates, Osler (1958), Joslin (1985), and White (1937)—had extolled the value of exercise, but there had not been conclusive proof that physical activity prevented disease. Although, by the 1980s, many members of the medical community agreed that regular physical activity promoted fitness, the dissenters doubted the claims of prophylaxis and longevity. At the end of the decade, however, two landmark studies, one by Paffenbarger and associates (1986), the other by Blair and associates (1989), concluded that regular aerobic exercise reduces the risk of disease and death in healthy individuals.

The first study, carried out by Paffenbarger and colleagues (1986), examined the relationship between mortality rates and physical activity (defined as walking, stair climbing, and sports played) of 16,936 Harvard alumni. This population consisted of men who entered college from 1916 to 1950. Personal and lifestyle characteristics of their college days (including medical histories) were obtained via questionnaires. More than 75% of the known surviving alumni responded, and information such as causes of death was obtained through the Harvard Alumni Office. Fewer than 1% of the alumni were lost to follow-up without death notification.

During the 12 to 16 years of follow-up (1962 to 1978) 1,413 alumni died (8%). Cardiovascular disease accounted for 45% of these deaths; cancer claimed 32%; other natural causes 13%, and trauma 10%. An inverse relationship was found between exercise and total mortality. Furthermore, a decline in death rates was seen as the intensity of exercise increased. Paffenbarger used energy expended in kilocalories (kcal) per week to express the intensity of exercise. Walking seven city blocks required the expenditure of 56 kcal, climbing 70 stairs equaled 28 kcal. Sports were rated as light (5 kcal/min), vigorous (10 kcal/min), or mixed (7.5 kcal/min). Thus, death rates declined as energy expended per week from less than 500 to 3500 kcal per week. Those alumni who expended 2000 kcal or more per week had a one quarter to one third lower death rate than their less active classmates. Even considering factors such as hypertension, cigarette smoking, obesity, or family history, the physically active alumni had lower death rates. The group with the highest death rate were men who were smokers, had hypertension, and were sedentary.

The second study conducted by Blair and Associates (1989) examined the relationship between physical fitness and all-cause mortality. Unlike Paffenbarger, Blair examined the relationship between physical fitness, rather than physical activity, and all-cause mortality. Physical activity is a determinant of physical fitness; therefore, fitness can be viewed as a measure of habitual physical activity. Blair believes that physical fitness, because it can be quantified easier than physical activity, is a more objective factor to examine in relation to all-cause mortality.

Data were collected for 20 years at Cooper's Institute for Aerobics Research, Dallas, Texas. 10,224 men and 3,120 women were studied with an average follow-up of 8 years. Each subject received a complete preventive medical evaluation that included the following: a personal and family health history, physical examinations, questionnaire on demographic characteristics and health habits, anthropometry, resting electrocardiogram (ECG), blood chemistry test, blood pressures, and a maximal treadmill exercise test. Subjects who were free of known chronic disease (i.e., no personal history of heart attack, hypertension, stroke, or diabetes; no resting ECG abnormalities; no abnormal responses on the exercise ECG) were selected for the study.

Physical fitness was measured by the treadmill exercise test. Subjects were assigned to fitness categories based on their age, sex, and results of the treadmill test. Five categories (1 = lowest fitness to 5 = highest fitness level) were established for each age and sex group.

The results showed a consistent inverse relationship between high level of physical fitness and all-cause mortality rates in both men and women. This favorable result was seen even after adjustments were made for age, smoking habits, cholesterol level, systolic blood pressure, fasting blood glucose level, parental history of coronary heart disease, and follow-up interval. Furthermore, decreased mortality rates due to cardiovascular disease and cancer were seen in the subjects of the higher fitness categories. The major decrease in death rate occurred between the first and second fitness levels. A decline in mortality rates, especially among the women, was seen in the middle fitness groups and only a slight continued reduction was evident in the most fit subjects. This important result indicates that even a modest improvement of physical fitness can yield significant protection against the degenerative diseases.

In 1989 the U.S. Preventive Services Task Force (USPSTF), concluded that physical inactivity is a risk factor for degenerative diseases and that physicians should counsel their patients on the benefits of exercise. Finally, after 2,500 years of debate, exercise has become recognized as an effective treatment.

DEGENERATIVE DISEASES: THE "DISEASES OF CIVILIZATION"

Fisher and Worth (1986) showed that the major cause of death in the United States at the turn of the century was infectious diseases such as influenza, pneumonia, tuberculosis, diphtheria, and poliomyelitis. These diseases were responsible for more than 500 deaths in 100,000 persons. By 1983, only 25 of 100,000 died of infectious disease. As medical cures were found for these diseases, and as people lived longer and more sedentary lives, the leading causes of death have become the degenerative diseases such as coronary heart disease (CHD), cancer, and cerebrovascular accident (Powell et al, 1989).

Eaton and associates (1988) called these degenerative processes the "diseases of civilization" and stated that they accounted for 75% of all deaths in the western world. Eaton believed that modern Homo sapiens are genetically identical to their Stone Age ancestors. What has changed drastically, especially since the Industrial Revolution, is man's way of life. This "mismatch" of genetics and lifestyle has given rise to the diseases of civilization. (Interestingly, these diseases are rare in the primitive societies that still exist today.)

The ancient hunter-gatherers lived very physical lives in order to survive. Transportation was by foot (either walking or running). The men tracked wild game for miles, sometimes for several days, while the women gathered fruits and vegetables and tended to the children. These small bands of ancient humans were usually nomadic, following the migrations of the animals they depended on for food and clothing.

How different our world is today! Because of the automobile, humans no longer need to walk. Modern appliances have taken the physical effort out of most of our daily chores. Jobs have become very specialized and stressful. The human body is exposed constantly to man-made toxins in our environment.

Nixon (1980), a British cardiologist, considered that degenerative disease may be a result of the demands placed on man by his "hard and urbanized society." He developed the human function curve (HFC) (Fig. 3–1), which illustrates that ill health and ultimate breakdown may be a result of the tension that develops between a person's actual performance and the level that he or she thinks is expected of him or her. Nixon defined arousal as a continuum from "unconsciousness and drowsiness" through "normal levels of alertness" to heightened states of emotion such as "rage, terror, and revulsion." Performance relates to "accomplishment of action and work" and the "skill of coping." "P" represents the "breakdown" point.

In order to stay healthy, Nixon considered that

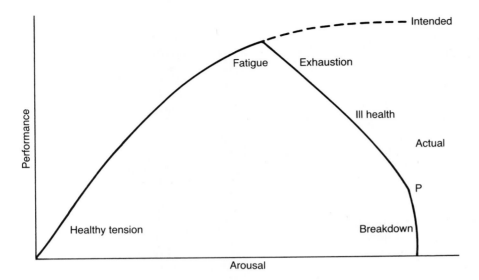

Figure 3–1. The human function curve illustrates the gap between a human's actual performance and what that person thinks is expected of him or her. (Adapted from Nixon PGF: Human functions and the heart. *In* Seedhouse D and Cribb A [eds]: Changing Ideas in Health Care. New York, John Wiley, 1989.)

individuals must live their lives in a "homeostasis." The individual must therefore increase performance when demanded by the challenges of self or environment and reduce the effort when demands are fewer. If a person can live on the up side of the curve, he or she will be successful; however, if a person falls to the down side, he or she will eventually have ill health and an ultimate breakdown. In terms of primary prevention, the HFC must be kept high enough to support one's chosen lifestyle without going to the point of exhaustion and breakdown. When counseling clients about their goals and behaviors, Nixon tells his clients to ask themselves:

1. Is this what I want?
2. Should I make myself fit enough and tough enough to endure?
3. Should I "off-load" until I can succeed?

He suggests the following behaviors to help shift the HFC in a healthier direction:

1. Adequate rest (not imprisonment in inactivity)
2. Adequate sleep
3. Reduced arousal states permitting tolerable levels of sympatho-adrenomedullary (S-AM) and pituitary-adrenocortical (P-AC) activity and enhancing the parasympathetic influence
4. Physical training to promote long-distance stamina

PHYSICAL FITNESS IN THE UNITED STATES

Despite the wealth of information that exists today supporting the health benefits of exercise, relatively few people in the U.S. exercise regularly or intensely enough to receive any health benefit (Stephens et al, 1985) (Fig. 3–2). A review of the literature (Wenger and Bell, 1986) suggested that aerobic exercise (i.e., low-intensity, long-duration exercise such as walking, running, cycling, and swimming) will improve cardiorespiratory fitness. The exercise must be performed for at least 20 to 30 minutes, 3 to 4 times per week. The intensity must be at least 50% of V_{O_2} max. Stephens (1988) and associates reported that only 20% of the population of the United States and Canada exercise at a level high enough to gain cardiorespiratory fitness. Forty per cent exercise at levels below the recommended level and the remaining 40% are described as being completely sedentary. The 40% who exercise below the recommended level may be receiving some health benefit, but there is so much variation of frequency, duration, and intensity in this group that fitness is difficult to quantify. The persons most likely to exercise regularly are the young (teenagers and younger) and those from higher socioeconomic status (white-collar workers are more likely to exercise than blue-collar workers). Men and women are equally likely to exercise, although men tend to exercise more intensely and frequently. At this point, no stud-

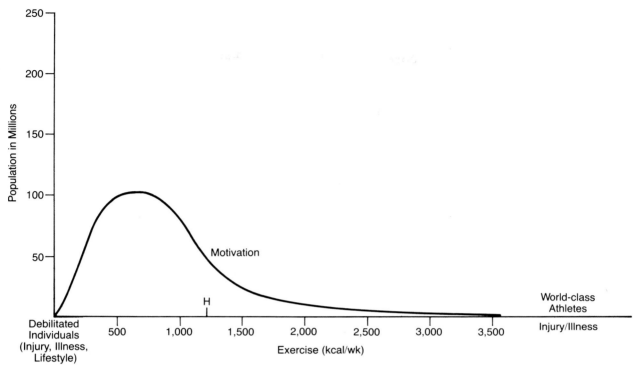

Figure 3–2. *The Exercise Distribution Curve (EDC)* illustrates the state of physical fitness in the United States today. The population is viewed as a continuum from the debilitated individual who is completely sedentary (due to injury, illness, or lifestyle) to the world-class athlete who may exercise in excess of 10,000 kcal/wk. Ironically, the specter of "Injury/Illness" appears again at the far left of the curve, due to overuse syndromes. *H* is the "health benefit" point (1,000–1,200 kcal/wk) for most individuals. Unfortunately, most Americans do not reach this level of fitness. Motivation refers to the reasons or incentives for exercising, which may include factors such as job demands, health/fitness, relaxation, and enjoyment. Motivation is the key to shifting the EDC to the right, thus reducing the risk of degenerative disease in the U.S. population.

ies indicate difference in exercise habits among races. Furthermore, the proportion of the population defined as active declines with age, the steepest decline seen during adolescence and early adulthood. This is alarming especially because most of the degenerative diseases, although they may begin insidiously, are not usually diagnosed until later in life.

The Target Population. The United States Preventive Services Task Force (Harris et al, 1989) recommended that all patients be counseled to engage in a regular physical exercise program with the goal of disease prevention. This program is aimed at healthy adults. A healthy individual is someone with no personal history of heart attack, stroke, hypertension, diabetes, resting ECG abnormalities, or abnormal responses on exercise ECG (Blair et al, 1989).

EXERCISE AND THE PREVENTION OF DISEASE

A sedentary lifestyle has been recognized as an important risk factor in CHD, hypertension, non–insulin-dependent diabetes mellitus (NIDDM), osteoporosis, obesity, depression and anxiety, and colon cancer. Several studies show that exercise can be used as a primary preventive intervention for these degenerative disease processes (Blair et al, 1984; Harris et al, 1989; Haskell et al, 1985; Siscovick et al, 1985).

Coronary Heart Disease (CHD). Paffenbarger and Hale demonstrated the relationship between physical activity and reduced risk of CHD in studies of San Francisco longshoreman (1975) and Harvard College alumni (1986). The risk of CHD was lower for those who engaged in higher levels of physical activity. Morris and associates (1980) studied the leisure time habits of civil servants in Great Britain. They found that subjects who did not partake in vigorous activity had a higher risk of CHD than their more active counterparts. Many other studies also show the relationship between vigorous physical activity and prevention of CHD (Garcia-Palmieri et al, 1982; Salonen et al, 1982; Siscovick et al, 1982).

Exercise protects individuals from CHD in two ways: (1) improved cardiovascular fitness and (2) improved metabolic fitness (Table 3–1). Paffenbarger stated that exercise also helps to protect against CHD indirectly by decreasing the cigarette habit, improving the weight-to-height ratio, and minimizing certain adverse familial tendencies (Rippe et al, 1987).

Hypertension. Several studies show a relationship between regular exercise and lower blood pressure. Hicky (1975) and Cooper and associates (1976) showed that on the average subjects who were regularly active had diastolic blood pressures 2 to 5 mm Hg less than the inactive subjects, even after statistical corrections were made for age, weight, and percentage of body fat. Paffenbarger and associates (1983) discovered that Harvard college alumni who did not currently engage in vigorous sports were at 35% greater risk of hypertension than those who were active. This finding was independent of other risk factors, such as higher body mass index, weight gain since college, and family history. A study by Blair and colleagues (1984) showed that persons who had low physical fitness had 52% greater risk of hypertension than their highly fit counterparts. Bjorntorp (1982) suggested that exercise may reduce sympathetic nervous system activity, thus lowering blood pressure, although the biochemical mechanism responsible for this remains unclear.

Non–Insulin-Dependent Diabetes Mellitus (NIDDM). A number of important studies have examined the effect of physical activity on individuals with NIDDM. Exercise acts to reduce blood glucose levels and to increase insulin sensitivity (Richter and Schneider, 1981). It is thought that because of these effects, regular physical exercise may have a prophylactic effect against NIDDM. Two cross-sectional studies of natives of the South Pacific (King et al, 1984; Zimmet et al, 1981) showed that the sedentary groups had higher incidences of NIDDM than their active counterparts. It has been observed clinically that vigorous physical activity improves glucose control in diabetic children and inactivity seems to worsen it (Siscovick et al, 1985). Physical activity seems to have a role in the prevention of NIDDM, but more research needs to be conducted before exercise can be prescribed safely to those with NIDDM.

Osteoporosis. Physical activity, especially weight-bearing exercise, has been shown to decrease the risk of osteoporosis and fracture (Chalmers and Ho, 1970). Patients confined to bed and astronauts in weightless environments lose approximately 1% of trabecular bone mass per week; however, this trend is reversed upon resuming weight-bearing exercise (Mazess and Wheedon, 1983). Studies (Alois et al, 1978; Dalen and Olsson, 1974) on distance runners have shown that runners have greater bone densities than nonrunners. Furthermore, osteoporosis may be postponed in postmenopausal women who engage in weight-bearing physical exercise 30 to 60 minutes three times per week (Alois et al, 1978). There has been some evidence (Chalmers and Ho, 1970; Paganini-Hill et al, 1981) that the risk of hip fracture is reduced by regular exercise, but, because of the increased potential of falling, exercise must be carefully prescribed and monitored in the older population. Ironically, too much aerobic exercise such as marathon running may have a negative effect on bone

Table 3–1. How Exercise Can Prevent Coronary Heart Disease

Improved Cardiovascular Fitness
Increased collateral circulation
Slower heart rate at rest and during any specific workload
Improved peripheral circulation via increased capillary-to-fiber ratio
Lower blood pressure
Increased stroke volume
Larger coronary vessels
Increased cardiac output
Increased physical work capacity
Improved aerobic capacity (VO_2 max)

Improved Metabolic Fitness (i.e., improved lipid profile and reduced blood glucose levels)
Lower blood concentrations of low-density lipoprotein cholesterol (LDL-C)
Lower concentrations of very low density lipoprotein cholesterol (VLDL-C)
Reduced levels of serum triglycerides
Increased levels of high-density lipoprotein cholesterol (HDL-C)
Decreased fibrinolytic activity at rest via reduced circulating catecholamines
Increased insulin sensitivity
Increased blood volume

density in women. Chronic long-distance training is known to cause amenorrhea in female distance runners. This condition has been associated with lowered bone density and stress fractures (Drinkwater et al, 1984).

Obesity. Obesity has been identified as a risk factor for hypertension, hyperlipidemia, diabetes, CHD, decreased self-esteem, and several other conditions (Harris et al, 1989). Epstein and Wing (1980) have demonstrated the effect of aerobic exercise on weight control. As long as caloric intake is controlled, weight loss is achieved via the calories burned during exercise and the appetite suppression that occurs (in some individuals) after exercise. Aerobic exercise, 30 to 40 minutes per session, 3 to 4 times per week, can be effective in controlling weight.

Depression and Anxiety. Although several studies have shown a positive association between regular physical activity and affect (defined as mood, depression, and anxiety), there is little evidence that exercise has a significant impact on actual clinically recognized disorders (Folkins and Sime, 1981; Stephens, 1988). Taylor and associates (1985) stated that regular exercise can be effective in alleviating some symptoms associated with mild to moderate depression as well as improving self-image, social skills, and cognitive functioning. It can also reduce the symptoms of anxiety and help alter type A behavior. More research is needed to determine the impact on clinically diagnosed mental disorders.

Colon Cancer. Paffenbarger (1984) and associates have shown that those persons who regularly exercise have lower incidences of all cancers than those who are sedentary. A number of studies (Powell et al, 1989) have shown an inverse relationship between regular physical activity and the occurrence of colon cancer. Cordain and colleagues (1986) believed that physical activity may help to prevent colon cancer because it reduces intestinal transit time, thus reducing the exposure of the bowel mucosa to potential carcinogens. Although a positive relationship has been identified between physical activity and colon cancer, other risk factors (except increasing age) are poorly understood. Further, it is difficult to control for family history, alcohol and vitamin A ingestion, dietary fat, fiber, and other factors associated with colon cancer (Powell et al, 1989). Further study is indicated in order to shed more light on the relationship of physical exercise and the decreased incidence of cancer.

EXERCISE AND CHRONIC ILLNESS

The role of regular physical exercise in preventing disease has been established; however, its place in the treatment of those diagnosed with chronic disease is less clear (and not in the scope of this chapter). Haskell and associates stated that a high level of physical fitness does not necessarily increase resistance to disease. He cited the examples of patients with emphysema or schizophrenia, who may become more fit by exercising regularly but who will not change the disease itself or the prognosis (Haskell et al, 1985).

Fitness and health are not synonymous, but they are related. Exercise may yield both fitness and health benefits, but the biologic changes responsible for improvement in health may differ from those causing improved fitness. Regular aerobic exercise will improve fitness levels and also reduce the risk of CHD, but the biologic changes responsible for these two phenomena are different. The increased fitness is a result of improved oxygen transport and utilization capacity, whereas the decreased risk of CHD is probably due to metabolic changes such as a more favorable lipoprotein profile and decreased fibrinolytic activity (Haskell et al, 1985).

Sheehan (1989) made a distinction between "disease" and "illness." He called "disease" a biologic event that affects an organ (e.g., heart, lungs, liver, kidney). It can be diagnosed by various investigative procedures (e.g., x-ray, computed tomography [CT] scan, biopsies). Illness, on the other hand, is a physical event that is defined by the impact that the disease has on the patient's performance. Disease has an effect on longevity whereas illness is related to life expectancy or to what the patient expects out of a particular day or every day. The quality of the patient's life is due more to the level of his or her fitness than to the disease.

Sheehan cites the example of the patient with CHD who can choose to become completely sedentary and suffer the consequences of inactivity or who can exercise regularly, lose weight, stop smoking, and eventually outperform his or her presumably healthy neighbor.

Can regular exercise change the disease itself? Sheehan (1987) said:

What exercise *may* do is cause regression of a disease process. This is still problematical once structural changes occur in the heart, lung, kidneys, and other organs and systems . . . it seems unlikely that exercise will reverse them. Nevertheless, regression of coronary artery disease has been reported, as has improvement in osteoporosis; and clearing of clinical non-insulin dependent diabetes and hypertension. At present, we should be content with the many good things that exercise will do for the patient, rather than demand that it do even more.

Fitness Program for Healthy Individuals

The Center for Chronic Disease Prevention and Health Promotion (a branch of the Centers for Disease Control [CDC]) strongly urges all health professionals to encourage their clients to exercise regularly (Koplan et al, 1989). Physical and occupational therapists are in a unique position to develop exercise and activity programs for their clients. Perhaps a team approach utilizing the physical and occupational therapists, the nurse, physician, social worker, dietitian, and family members would be in the client's best interest. Most patients seen by physical and occupational therapists are in a state of decreased physical fitness, resulting from a sedentary lifestyle that is due either to an injury or illness or to premorbid habits. An exercise program aimed at promoting good health should be developed for the client sometime during the course of his or her treatment. Exercise and a return to the activities of daily living can often be started during acute care and should continue to be monitored through the client's discharge from outpatient services.

The author usually includes some form of aerobic training in each client's therapy program. Because fewer insurance companies today are reimbursing for prevention programs, exercise geared at long-term health promotion must be uniquely integrated into each patient's program. For example, a patient being treated for a torn ACL may begin cycling with the immediate goal of improving range of motion and strength in the knee, the intermediate goal of regaining cardiovascular fitness for the return to sports, and the long-term goal of lifelong fitness and health. Similarly, a patient with cerebrovascular accident (CVA) with hemiparesis may begin walking on a treadmill initially as a means of improving quality of gait, but eventually to improve physical work capacity to allow for independence in activities of daily living. As patients are eventually weaned from physical therapy they are well versed in aerobic exercise, they know how to monitor themselves, and they continue independently on individualized home programs geared toward lifelong health. Examples of these programs can be seen in the case studies included in this chapter.

The exercise programs outlined in the following section can be administered by any health professional who has an interest and background in exercise physiology. Traditionally, it has been the physical therapist who has developed the exercise programs, but the patient might benefit more if the other members of the rehabilitation team are involved. The occupational therapist may see the fitness program as a way in which a patient can improve physical work capacity, enabling him or her to resume normal activities of daily living. Those involved regularly in daily activities, such as mowing the lawn, walking to work, and gardening, have been shown to have fewer signs of CHD than those who are sedentary (Monahan, 1987). Thus, the physical and occupational therapists can work together in developing a program uniquely tailored to a patient's interests, aimed at preventing disease.

EXERCISE PROGRAMS

Client Goals

As a result of participating in a lifelong, regular exercise program, the client will:

1. Improve his or her physical work capacity
2. Improve his or her functioning (e.g., for activities of daily living, hobbies, sports, work)
3. Reduce his or her risk of specific diseases or conditions
4. Improve his or her sense of well-being
5. Improve his or her quality of life

Screening

Health care professionals are more likely to counsel their patients about physical exercise if the following three conditions are met: (1) low-level screening techniques are used, (2) the program can be integrated into a patient's treatment session, (3) the patient can be easily monitored (Harris et al, 1989). There has been much debate about whether patients should be screened via exercise ECG before they embark on an exercise program, but exercise ECGs have two limitations: (1) They produce many false-positive results (estimated at as high as 80%) in asymptomatic persons (Shepard, 1984). Therefore, it does not make sense economically to look for occult disease in asymptomatic clients or to subject them unnecessarily to the discomfort or even risk of mortality from this test. (2) Even if CHD is detected, the client will probably be placed on an exercise program as part of his or her treatment.

The Physical Activity Readiness Questionnaire is a simple and reliable pre-exercise screening tool (Harris et al, 1989). The questionnaire consists of seven questions designed to give the health care professional information regarding the client's medical history. If the client answers "yes" to any of the questions, he or she should return to the referring physician for a medical examination before commencing with the exercise program.

Physical Activity Readiness Questionnaire
(Chisholm et al, 1975)

1. Has your doctor ever said that you had heart trouble?
2. Do you frequently have pains in your heart and chest?
3. Do you often feel faint or have spells of severe dizziness?
4. Has a doctor ever said your blood pressure was too high?
5. Has your doctor ever told you that you have a bone or joint problem such as arthritis that has been aggravated by exercise or that might be made worse by exercise?
6. Is there a good physical reason not mentioned here why you should not follow an activity program even if you wanted to?
7. Are you over 65 years of age and are you unaccustomed to doing vigorous exercise?

The American College of Sports Medicine (ACSM) has also established guidelines for pre-exercise screening (American College of Sports Medicine, 1986). If the patient is under 35 years of age and has no history of CHD or known CHD risk factors, it is safe to start him or her on an exercise program. However, all persons over 35 years of age and those under 35 years of age with a history of symptoms are advised to have a complete medical examination prior to participation in an exercise program.

The Programs

Four aerobic exercise programs are outlined in Tables 3–1 to 3–4. Walking, jogging, swimming, and cycling have been chosen because they are simple activities to do and, except for swimming, require no special facilities and can be performed independently at home. Swimming has been included because many people enjoy it. Also, it is an ideal activity for persons with arthritis or musculoskeletal deficiency. The goal of the therapist is to have the patient perform one activity or a combination of activities independently 3 to 4 times per week for 30 to 40 minutes each session. The prescription of "3 to 4 times per week, 30 to 40 minutes per session" has become known as the "fitness formula" and is the frequency and duration of exercise needed to stimulate an aerobic effect and help prevent disease. It will take approximately 11 to 12 weeks to reach the desired aerobic level, and exercise must be maintained over a lifetime in order to continue to maintain the aerobic and protective benefit (Wenger and Bell, 1986) (Tables 3–2 to 3–5).

Borg's Perceived Exertion Scale

Unlike many programs that specify how far and fast to walk or run, the protocols outlined in Tables 3–1 to 3–4 are based on minutes of exercise and rate of perceived exertion (RPE). The swimming program is the only exception, because it is easier to count laps than to keep track of time in the pool. RPE is also used to determine the intensity of the swimming workout.

In the late 1960s, Borg (1967) developed a scale of perceived exertion that related subjective feel-

	Table 3–2. Walking Program		
Week	Time (min)	Frequency/wk	RPE (Rate of Perceived Exertion)
1	10	4	9
2	15	4	9
3	20	4	9–10
4	20	4	9–11
5	25	4	11
6	25	4	11–12
7	30	4	12
8	35	4	12
9	35	4	12
10	40	4	12
11	45	4	12–13
12	45–50	4	12–13

Week		Time (min)	Frequency/wk	RPE†
1	Walking:	Begin with 40 min, work up to 50 min by week's end.	4	11–12
2	Walking:	50–60 min (as above)	4	12
3		a. Walk 10 min	4	11
		b. Alternate 1 min of jogging with 1 min of walking for 20 min		12
		c. Walk 10 min		10–11
4		a. Walk 10 min	4	11
		b. Alternate 2 min of jogging with 1 min of walking for 20 min		12
		c. Walk 10 min		10–11
5		a. Walk 10 min	4	11
		b. Alternate 4 min of jogging with 1 min of walking for 20 min		12
		c. Walk 10 min		10–11
6		a. Walk 10 min	4	12
		b. Alternate 6 min of jogging with 1 min of walking for 20 min		12
		c. Walk 10 min		10–11
7		a. Walk 5 min	4	11
		b. Alternate 8 min of jogging with 1 min of walking for 26 min		12
		c. Walk 5–10 min		10–11
8		a. Walk 5 min	4	11
		b. Alternate 10 min of jogging with 1 min of walking for 22 min		11–12
		c. Walk 5–10 min		10–11
9		a. Walk 5 min	4	11
		b. Jog 20 min nonstop		11–12
		c. Walk 5–10 min		10–11
10		a. Walk 5 min	4	11
		b. Jog 25 min		12
		c. Walk 5 min		10–11
11		a. Walk 5 min	4	11
		b. Jog 30 min		12
		c. Walk 5 min		10–11
12		a. Walk 5 min	4	11
		b. Jog 30 min		12–13
		c. Walk 5 min		10–11

Table 3–3. Jogging Program*

*Must be able to walk 60 min at RPE 12 to 13.
†RPE = rate of perceived exertion.

ings of exertion with objective measures such as heart rate. After studying thousands of healthy subjects, he found that RPE was directly related to heart rate and that RPE rises in a linear fashion. Borg assigned numeric values for ratings of perceived exertion followed by subjective descriptions of the effort (Table 3–6). The numeric value multiplied by 10 is equal to the heart rate. Thus, if a healthy individual is exercising at an RPE of "11," which is described as "fairly light," his or her heart rate is approximately 110 BPM.

Morgan and Borg (1976) found that RPE was consistently reliable (reliability coefficient 0.90) in estimating exercise work load. Pollack and associates (1986) concurred and found that RPE was applicable not only to exercise but also to activities of daily living. RPE can be learned quickly, usually in two to three workout sessions. Clients can be placed on a stationary bicycle or treadmill and exercised at gradually increasing loads (up to RPE 13). Periodically (every 3 to 4 minutes), heart rate can be measured and the client should

Table 3–4. Swimming Program

Week		Distance		Frequency/wk	RPE*
1 Mon.	5 × 25 yd	Full recovery after each swim		4	9–10
Wed.	7 × 25 yd	Full recovery after each swim			9–10
Fri.	9 × 25 yd	Full recovery after each swim			9–10
Sat. or Sun.	12 × 25 yd	Full recovery after each swim			9–10
2 Mon.	5 × 25 yd	1 min recovery after each		4	10–11
	2 × 50 yd	Full recovery after each			10–11
Wed.	4 × 25 yd	1 min recovery after each			10–11
	3 × 50 yd	Full recovery after each			10–11
Fri.	3 × 25 yd	1 min recovery after each			10–11
	4 × 50 yd	Full recovery after each			10–11
Sat. or Sun.	2 × 25 yd	1 min recovery after each			10–11
	5 × 50 yd	Full recovery after each			10–11
3 Mon.	6 × 50 yd	1 min recovery		4	11
Wed.	6 × 50 yd	30 sec recovery			11
Fri.	7 × 50 yd	30 sec recovery			11
Sat. or Sun.	8 × 50 yd	30 sec recovery			11
4 Mon.	4 × 100 yd	1 min recovery		4	11–12
Wed.	4 × 100 yd	1 min recovery			11–12
Fri.	4 × 100 yd	30 sec recovery			11–12
Sat. or Sun.	2 × 200 yd	1 min recovery			11–12
5 Mon.	2 × 250 yd	1 min recovery		4	11–12
Wed.	2 × 250 yd	45 sec recovery			11–12
Fri.	2 × 250 yd	30 sec recovery			11–12
Sat. or Sun.	2 × 250 yd	15 sec recovery			11–12
6 Mon.	1 × 500 yd	Rest at 250 10–15 sec only if needed		4	11–12
Wed.	500 yd	Rest at 250 10–15 sec only if needed			11–12
Fri.	500 yd	Rest at 250 10–15 sec only if needed			11–12
Sat. or Sun.	500 yd	Rest at 250 10–15 sec only if needed			11–12
7 Mon.	500 yd	Nonstop		4	11–12
Wed.	550 yd	Nonstop			11–12
Fri.	600 yd	Rest at 300 yd 10–15 sec if needed			11–12
Sat. or Sun.	600 yd	Rest at 300 yd 10–15 sec if needed			11–12
8 Mon.	600 yd	Nonstop		4	12
Wed.	600 yd	Nonstop			12
Fri.	600 yd	Nonstop			12
Sat. or Sun.	600 yd	Nonstop			12
9 Mon.	650 yd	Nonstop		4	12
Wed.	650 yd	Nonstop			12
Fri.	700 yd	Nonstop			12
Sat. or Sun.	700 yd	Nonstop			12
10 Mon.	700 yd	Nonstop		4	12
Wed.	700 yd	Nonstop			12
Fri.	750 yd	Nonstop			12
Sat. or Sun.	750 yd	Nonstop			12
11 Mon.	800 yd	Nonstop		4	12
Wed.	800 yd	Nonstop			12
Fri.	800 yd	Nonstop			12
Sat. or Sun.	800 yd	Nonstop			12
12 Repeat week 11				4	12–13

*RPE = rate of perceived exertion.

be asked to rate his or her RPE. RPEs of 12 to 13 correspond well with 60 to 70% of VO_2 max (Pollack), which is the intensity goal of most aerobic exercise programs. Thus, clients, without constantly stopping their activity to take a pulse, will be able to sense a safe and efficient level of exercise or activity.

The exercise programs outlined in Tables 3–2

Table 3–5. Cycling Program

Week	Time	Frequency/wk	RPE*
1	20 min (alternate periods of 4 min of cycling with 2 min of coasting)	4	9–10
2	24 min (alternate periods of 6 min of cycling with 2 min of coasting)	4	9–10
3	28 min (alternate periods of 8 min cycling with 2 min of coasting or cycling at easier rate)	4	10–11
4	33 min (alternate periods of 10 min cycling with 1 min of coasting or cycling at easier rate)	4	11
5	32 min (alternate periods of 15 min cycling and 1 min of coasting or cycling at easier rate)	4	11–12
6	30 min of continuous cycling (coasting only for turns or safety)	4	11–12
7	30 min of continuous cycling (coasting only for turns or safety)	4	12
8	35 min of continuous cycling (coasting only for turns or safety)	4	12
9	40 min of continuous cycling (coasting only for turns or safety)	4	12
10	30–40 min of continuous cycling (coasting only for turns or safety)	4	12–13
11	35–40 min of continuous cycling (coasting only for turns or safety)	4	12–13
12	40 min of continuous cycling (coasting only for turns or safety)	4	12–13

*RPE = rate of perceived exertion.

to 3–5 are broken down on a weekly basis for 12 weeks. They are guidelines and are not meant to be "cookbooks" on exercise. Each program will probably have to be modified for each individual. Each program assumes that the client has no exercise background and is essentially beginning in a deconditioned state. Those who are in better physical condition may begin at a higher level or may advance through the program faster. However, the initial weeks of each program are designed to be easy in order to allow the specific muscle groups used in the exercise to become accustomed to the activity and avoid injury.

Table 3–6. Borg's Scale of Perceived Exertion*

Rating of Perceived Exertion	Description of Exertion	Heart Rate (RPE × 10) BPM†
6		60
7	Very, very light	70
8		80
9	Very light	90
10		100
11	Fairly light	110
12		120
13	Somewhat hard	130
14		140
15	Hard	150
16		160
17	Very hard	170
18		180
19	Very, very hard	190
20		200

*Adapted from Borg GAV and Linderholm H: Perceived exertion and pulse rate during graded exercise in various age groups. Acta Med Scand 472:194–206, 1967. In Monahan T: Perceived exertion: An old exercise tool finds new applications. Physician Sports Med 16(10):174–179, 1988.
†BPM = beats per minute; RPE = rate of perceived exertion.

Furthermore, if a client is struggling during a particular week he or she can drop back 1 week until he or she feels ready to advance.

Each workout should consist of three phases: (1) the warm-up; (2) the exercise itself; and (3) the cool-down. The warm-up should consist of light activity, such as submaximal walking, cycling, or swimming, and stretching. Walking is a sufficient warm-up for the jogging program. The goal is to bring the heart rate up to the exercise level. The therapist should design a general stretching program that addresses the major muscle groups and, especially, the specific muscles used in the activity. The warm-up period usually takes 10 to 15 minutes.

The exercise phase consists of the activity itself for the specified time and RPE. By week 12 the client should be able to tolerate 30 to 40 minutes of continuous exercise at an RPE of 12 to 13. For individuals who tend to underestimate their RPE (the overaggressive types), they should be instructed to exercise at a level at which they can talk to someone. If they are too out of breath to talk, they are probably working too hard.

The cool-down consists of light activity such as walking and stretching. The goal of this phase is to gradually allow the body to return to its resting level and to help remove lactic and other metabolites from the muscles.

Walking and Jogging

The walking exercise program is aimed primarily at "healthy" (see definition earlier) but unfit individuals as a means of promoting fitness and preventing illness. It can also be used to prevent the recurrence of disease, as is seen in case studies 1 and 3.

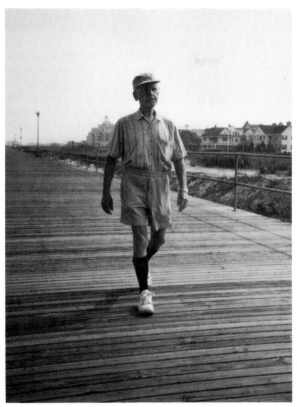

Figure 3–3. Walking is a simple, enjoyable yet effective means of achieving fitness and health.

The walking program is straightforward, and because most healthy individuals walk as part of their activities of daily living, they should have no problem with advancing through the program. The beauty of the walking program is its simplicity. Walking can be done any time and anywhere, with a partner or alone (Fig. 3–3). It can even be incorporated into the workday. Walk at lunchtime, or park 1 mile from work and walk from the car to work and back to the car at the end of the day. Those who wish to begin a jogging program should complete the walking program first in order to adapt the musculoskeletal system to the stresses that will be encountered during jogging (Fig. 3–4). Ask the client to invest in a good pair of running shoes. Progress from one level to the next only when the previous level begins to feel easy.

A discussion of running shoes could take a chapter in itself. It is difficult to recommend a particular brand or model because people's feet vary so greatly. A sports-oriented health professional should be able to suggest to the patient the type of shoe that he or she will need, based on the foot type and on the level of running. It may be wise to purchase shoes from a specialty shop (where the employees actually use the equipment) rather than a department store.

Swimming

The swimming program is somewhat different from the other programs in that work bouts alternated with rest intervals are used in the initial weeks (Fig. 3–5). Assuming that the client has been sedentary, the muscles used in swimming will probably be deconditioned and unable to tolerate extended periods of activity. Thus, the distances swum become longer and the rest intervals become shorter throughout the 12-week period until the client can swim 800 yards continuously at an RPE of 12 to 13. The client may use any stroke (most favor the crawl) or a combination of strokes. Enrollment in an instructional program is encouraged to learn proper swim mechanics. Swimming is much more enjoyable and efficient if a good technique is mastered.

Cycling

The cycling program is designed for cycling on a standard bicycle outside (Fig. 3–6). Bicycles

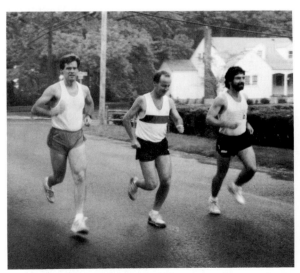

Figure 3–4. For the more ambitious, running can be an invigorating and challenging way to stay fit.

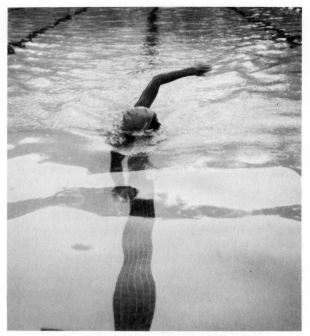

Figure 3–5. Swimming is an excellent means of achieving fitness, especially for people with orthopedic problems.

should be in a good state of repair, and seats and handlebars should be adjusted at the appropriate levels. It might be wise to have your bicycle checked out at the local bike shop to ensure that it is in good repair and properly adjusted. Clients should be instructed to pedal in the mid-gear range at an RPM of 60 to 90. Continuous pedaling is difficult to maintain while outside because there is a tendency to coast and "sightsee" while cycling. Although enjoying the outdoors is the advantage of outdoor cycling, continuous pedaling must be maintained in order to achieve the aerobic benefits. Like the swimming program, the initial stages of the cycling protocol have work bouts and rest intervals. The goal of the program is to cycle for 40 minutes continuously by week 12. The same program can be used with an indoor stationary bicycle or a wind trainer. Substitute coasting or easier cycling with full rest or cycling at a lower RPM (e.g., if you are cycling at a rate of 90 RPM, drop down to 30 RPM during the rest interval).

Cross Training

There has been a growing interest in the concept of "cross training," popularized by those training for the triathlon, in recent years. Cross training is simply the alternating use of two or more forms of exercise to achieve fitness. Cross training has three major advantages over single exercise training: (1) By alternating exercise types (e.g., jogging 1 day followed by swimming the next day), the individual can avoid overuse injuries that are often associated with the chronic use of the same musculoskeletal structures. (2) The variety of physical activity provides for more flexibility in the training program. The individual can adapt his or her program to weather, work schedule, family, and personal responsibilities. (3) The variety of activity also helps the individual to avoid boredom, a factor that often leads to dropping out of exercise programs.

The individual should become proficient in at least one program before attempting cross training. An example of cross training is:

Mon: Walking 45 min
Wed: Cycling 40 min
Fri: Jogging 30 min
Sat or Sun: Swimming 800 yd

For the sedentary older patient who may not be receptive to a standard exercise program, the following "cross training" regimen might apply:

Mon: Walking 30 to 40 min
Wed: Gardening
Fri: Walking 30 to 40 min
Sat or Sun: Mowing lawn (pushing the mower)

Patient Compliance

The combinations of activities are infinite, limited only by the individual's imagination. The key to adherence is enjoyment. Rather than focusing on the benefits of regular exercise, help the client to find an activity that he or she loves to do. If the client looks forward to going out for a walk, a bicycle ride, or gardening, he or she will make it a priority. The health benefits will be "icing on the cake."

It has been the author's experience that working with a client on a one-on-one basis helps the individual discover the type of exercise best suited for him or her. The author has been known to exercise with the client, letting him or her set the pace while observing and correcting technique. It should be something readily available to the client (e.g., he or she may enjoy swimming but may not have access to a pool).

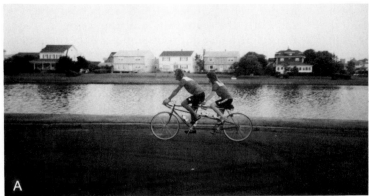
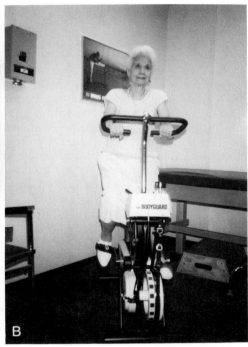

Figure 3–6. *A*, Enjoy the pleasure of the outdoors and the benefits of fitness through cycling. *B*, When the weather does not permit or when you cannot get out of the house, try cycling indoors.

Each client's program should be individualized for his or her own interests and special situation. The therapist can set a good example by becoming involved in a variety of activities. If the therapist can speak about exercise from personal experience, it helps to motivate the client to begin and to stay with a program. If the client has difficulty in staying motivated, help him or her to find an appropriate club, group of friends or family member to exercise with the client. Sometimes the social interaction is all the incentive that a client needs to continue exercising.

Studies on compliance are mixed. Research on cardiac rehabilitation programs show that 50% of clients drop out of programs during the first 6 months (Harris et al, 1989). However, 75% of those who began fitness programs at the Cooper Clinic were still exercising 3.5 years later (Blair, 1985). Harris (1989) stated that compliance with an exercise program is greater if a fitness program is offered at work. Johnson and Johnson's "Live for Life Program," in addition to exercise, has other health-related goals such as weight control and smoking cessation. They report that 55% of their employees exercise at the Live for Life facility. Seventy-five to 85% of the employees participate in some component of the program. This has been termed a "total immersion" ap-

proach, and it is hoped that the constant reinforcement at work will encourage Johnson and Johnson employees to adopt a healthier lifestyle (Bly et al, 1986).

Financial Implications

With the ever-increasing cost of health care in the United States, the federal government has become more interested in the concept of disease prevention. Several government agencies within the Department of Health and Human Services oversee the development and implementation of preventive health programs in the United States. These include the CDC, the National Institutes of Health (NIH), the Office of Disease Prevention and Health Promotion (ODPHP), and the President's Council on Physical Fitness and Sports (PCPFS). The federal government has set an example for the private sector to follow by establishing fitness programs for its 3 million employees (Simmons, 1987). There are more than 50 federally sponsored fitness programs in Washington, D.C., and several more established throughout the United States. Federal employees contribute a fee for participation, which is deducted from their paychecks.

The CDC has developed physical fitness and exercise objectives for 1990, but a mid-course review in 1985 revealed that these goals will probably not be met (Centers for Disease Control, 1989). Recommendations for the year 2000 have shifted from those who are already active, to encouraging the sedentary population to begin lower-level programs such as walking. This may be a more realistic approach, because there is evidence that health benefits may be achieved at lower intensities of exercise than what was originally thought (Blair et al, 1989). Morgan (Rippe et al, 1987) believed that the emphasis should be placed on the children who normally are active but who at some point are encouraged to become sedentary. He thought that the schools should ensure that the youth of the United States should remain active and should retain their love of play and exercise. In 1987, the federal government urged state governments to mandate daily physical education classes for all children, from kindergarten through twelfth grade; however, as of now, this has not happened. Ironically, in many school districts throughout the United States, physical education classes have been cut back rather than increased (Iverson et al, 1985).

In the private sector, while some businesses have initiated exercise programs, only 25% of employers offer such programs to their employees (Nice perk . . . , 1990). Most of these corporate fitness programs are only open to executives of the company. Johnson and Johnson's Live for Life program is an exception in that all employees are encouraged to participate. Usually employees contribute some portion of their salaries to join such programs.

Iverson and associates (1985) reported that the greatest number and variety of fitness programs exist at the community level. These include the YMCAs, YWCAs, Jewish Community Centers, running clubs, cycling clubs, ski clubs, softball leagues, and county and local programs. Although these programs seem to affect the public awareness of exercise, they have not yet changed the statistics of participation.

Ultimately, the cost for participation in an exercise program will be borne by the individual. Even though a preparticipation physical examination and the health professional's counseling time can be expensive, the money saved through a program of prevention will easily justify the initial screening costs (Harris et al, 1989). Fortunately, extensive, sophisticated pre-exercise testing is not indicated for the majority of the population. The USPSTF (1990) sees a changing role for both the clinician and the patient in the future. The health professional will become more of a counselor and teacher, advising the patient on how to prevent disease. Patients, on the other hand, will have to take a more active role in taking care of themselves. Together, they will form a partnership to improve the status of health care in the United States.

CASE STUDIES

The following three case studies illustrate how an aerobic exercise program can be integrated into a patient's physical therapy program. As mentioned earlier, the four tables are only guidelines; they must be modified for each patient's goals and medical condition. The case studies presented here depict three vastly different clients, but they all benefited from aerobic training. The following criteria must be kept in mind when developing aerobic programs for all clients.

1. The effects of aerobic conditioning are long term. The patient, who is referred to P.T. for an injury or medical condition, may not show great aerobic progress while he or she is under your care for the primary condition. Therefore, use aerobic exercises that will initially help to treat the primary problem. After discharge, this program will not only maintain the health of the injured body part but will also play a role in the prevention of certain diseases. For example, if your client was referred for an orthopedic problem in the knee, bicycling may be a good way to improve range of motion and strength, and, at the same time, begin aerobic conditioning.
2. Always consider the contraindications of exercise. Will the aerobic program that you are designing for your client be safe orthopedically? Does your client have a pre-existing condition, such as heart disease? These questions must be kept in mind when designing an aerobic program for your client. The author uses the Physical Activity Readiness Questionnaire (see text) to help determine the appropriateness of an exercise program aimed at health promotion.
3. Set realistic goals with your client. A client who has never been athletic prior to an injury is unlikely to run a 4-minute mile or win Wimbledon afterwards. Appropriate goals such as restoring full range of motion and strength and returning to prior activities are more realistic. Sometimes a client may have to give up one sport due to his or her limita-

tions after an injury but may make a successful transition to another sport, as in Case Study 2. Of course, the long-range goal of the aerobic exercise is the prevention of disease and the promotion of good health.

4. Build a program around activities that your client enjoys and/or will need to achieve his or her goals (see Case Studies 1 and 3). Patients are more likely to continue with a program if they enjoy what they are doing and see a reason for doing it.
5. Begin at an easy level and progress only when a present level of exercise is no longer challenging. Usually the author wants clients to exercise in the comfortable range, RPE "11 to 12." If a patient's RPE drops to "8–9," it may be time to advance the program.
6. Move the client toward an independent home program. In order to gain the disease prevention benefits of aerobic exercise, the client must continue the program on a lifelong basis. Ultimately, the client must take the responsibility to exercise on his or her own. Let the client work the program into his or her daily routine. In this way, exercise will become a vital part of the client's daily schedule.
7. After discharge, follow up on the client's progress periodically. This can be done by telephone or in writing. The author has found that a telephone call helps to motivate former clients. During these calls, any problems the client may be having with his or her program are discussed. Often exercise programs are modified and new goals are set. Even though the client is working independently, he or she knows that help is only a telephone call away.

Case Study 1: Betty is a 74-year-old white female who suffered a right CVA 3 years ago that resulted in a left-sided hemiparesis. By the time that we examined her in the clinic her hemiparesis had resolved; however, due to her sedentary lifestyle her left lower extremity weakness remained. Betty lives alone in a small house and is assisted by a neighbor who helps her with cleaning, shopping, and coming to physical therapy. The neighbor reports that Betty is often "depressed" and is resistant to the idea of exercise.

Betty's past medical history included hypertension, which fluctuated due to her inconsistency in taking medication. It ranged from 120/80 to 150/95. She was also obese (5'4", 185 lb). The initial evaluation revealed a pleasant, alert, and oriented × 3 elderly woman with residual weakness in the left lower extremity. The left gluteus medius, hamstrings, quadriceps, and anterior tibialis were especially weak (fair -). No abnormal

muscle tone was found, and deep tendon reflexes were normal. At this point, her left lower extremity weakness was probably due more to her sedentary lifestyle than to her CVA. She could ambulate 200' independently with a walker before tiring (actually, she did not need her walker, but she relied on it for "security"). Betty was a moderately heavy smoker, consuming "at least 1 pack per day." Betty's general physician referred her to physical therapy for "general strengthening," and it was determined that she was a good candidate for the disease prevention exercise program. This program would integrate well with a program aimed at strengthening her left lower extremity and improving her overall strength and endurance.

Betty began a program of physical therapy three times per week for 2 months. Each session began with proprioceptive neuromuscular facilitation (PNF) activities to increase strength, proprioception, and coordination in her trunk, pelvis, and left lower extremity. Next, she performed general flexibility exercises for the cervical, thoracic, and lumbar spines, both upper extremities and lower extremities (focusing on the quadriceps, hamstrings, and gastrocsoleus group). Then, Betty performed the following progressive resistance exercise (PRE) program for both lower extremities:

1. Terminal knee extension (TKE)
2. Straight leg raise (SLR)
3. Hip abduction/adduction
4. Hip flexion/extension
5. Knee flexion/extension

She began with one set of ten repetitions with no weight and progressed to three sets of ten with 2½ lb by the end of 6 weeks. Betty was also encouraged to begin a program to stop smoking. Betty began a stationary bicycling program during the second physical therapy session. She had not performed any aerobic exercise in many years, so she began her program at a lower level than outlined in Table 3–4. Betty's first workout consisted of three sets of 4-minute work bouts with no resistance and full recovery after each. She was shown Borg's Scale of perceived exertion (see Table 3–5) during the workout and was told to keep the effort at "6 to 7" or "very, very light."

Betty was able to complete the workout but said that the effort was more like "11 to 12." Her pulse remained at 88 to 90 bpm. However, because she was taking propranolol hydrochloride (Inderal) (a beta-blocker), heart rate would not be a valid means of monitoring effort. RPE would prove to be a better method. Betty stayed at this work level for three sessions and by the end of the first week stated that her RPE for the entire workout was "7 to 8."

During the second week a fourth 4-minute work bout was added and rest intervals were limited to 4 minutes. She was asked to pedal between 40 and 50 rpm. Still, no resistance was applied. She reported RPE of "8 to 9" for this level. By the third week of physical therapy, Betty was able to tolerate the program listed under week no. 1 in Table 3–4. She no longer used her walker and progressed to using a straight cane. During the next 3 weeks, she followed a modified version of the program outlined in Table 3–4. This was her sixth week of physical therapy and she was cycling two work bouts of 10 minutes, resistance of 150 kpm (60 rpm), with 2-minute rest intervals between bouts. Her RPE for this level of work was "11." Betty's RPE was telling us when to increase the duration of the work bout or decrease the rest interval. Our goal for her was to cycle 20 to 30 minutes, three times a week, at an RPE of 11 to 12. Once her RPE dropped to a lower number, it was time to increase the duration of the cycling, decrease the rest interval, or increase the resistance on the ergometer (or a combination of these variables).

By week 8 of therapy, Betty was able to cycle for 25 minutes continuously at a resistance of 150 kpm (60 rpm), at an RPE of "11 to 12."

At this point, Betty was ready for discharge and was given a home program that included:

1. Continuation of her general flexibility exercises
2. Stationary cycling 20 to 30 minutes 3 to 4 times per week at an RPE of 11 to 12
3. Walking program (modified version of Table 3–1). Goal: 30 minutes on noncycling days

Betty began walking with her neighbor and reported to us that she was cycling 3 days and walking (with a cane) 2 days per week.

Results: Betty was re-evaluated at the end of 3 months. She kept track of her exercise by simply recording on a wall calendar how many minutes of cycling or walking was performed and the RPE. At the end of 12 weeks, Betty had:

1. Lost 20 lb
2. Resting heart rate 72 bpm
3. Resting blood pressure consistently at 130/80 (she also reported better compliance with her medication while she was on the exercise program)
4. Left lower extremity strength at "good" or 4/5 level
5. Reported that she was sleeping better
6. "A more positive attitude"
7. Stopped smoking

Case Study 2: When the author first treated Geoff, he was a 17-year-old white male who tore the anterior cruciate ligament (ACL) in his right knee while he was playing in a high school football game. Arthroscopic surgery revealed a complete tear of the right ACL, but no damage to either meniscus or to other ligaments. Geoff, his parents, and his physician discussed the possibility of ACL reconstruction, but it was decided that he would receive physical therapy first and re-evaluate the knee after 3 months. If Geoff was having instability problems at that time, an ACL reconstruction would be reconsidered.

Although he was an outstanding player, Geoff did not wish to pursue football after high school. His physician felt that if he was no longer planning on participating in contact sports, his knee might function well without reconstructive surgery. If rehabilitation went well, Geoff hoped to run spring track.

Past Medical History: Geoff is a well-developed young male with no history of serious medical problems. Orthopedically, he had a history of a grade II sprain of the right ankle caused by playing football.

Geoff began physical therapy 1 day after having arthroscopic surgery. He presented to us with significant swelling and ecchymosis around the right knee joint. Active range of motion of the right knee was 30 to 110 degrees. Strength could not be determined at this time due to his inability to move comfortably through the full range of motion. He was ambulating on crutches and non–weight bearing on the right lower extremity.

Our initial goals were to:

1. Reduce pain in the right knee
2. Reduce swelling
3. Restore full range of motion
4. Ambulate partial weight bearing on the right lower extremity
5. Enhance proprioceptive awareness in the right knee
6. Improve strength
7. Prevent aerobic deconditioning

Geoff began a physical therapy program three times a week. He progressed well for the first month. Pain and swelling resolved, and active range of motion improved to 0 to 120 degrees in the right knee. By the end of 4 weeks he was full weight bearing on the right lower extremity without an assistive device. Geoff's knee rehabilitation program included traditional modalities to decrease his pain and swelling, PNF techniques, and PREs to improve range of motion, strength, and proprioceptive awareness in the right lower extremity. He began a program of light stationary cycling during the second week of P.T., initially to increase range of motion at the knee and eventually to begin an aerobic conditioning program. By week 4, Geoff was performing a modified version of cycling program week 1 (see Table 3–4). He was cycling four bouts of 4 minutes at 60 RPM, 750 kpm, RPE of 11. Geoff was in very good physical condition prior to his injury and was able to make rapid progress. Although his cardiovascular system was ready for harder work, he held back on intensity until I knew that his knee could tolerate increased workloads.

During week 5, Geoff began the swimming program (see Table 3–3). Again, due to his prior conditioning, he was able to begin at a relatively high level. He started with 10 sets of 50 yards with a 1-minute rest interval after each. His RPE was "10 to 11," and he performed this program 3 days per week (nontherapy days). He was also encouraged to walk as much as possible emphasizing proper gait mechanics. Thus, instead of riding the bus to school, Geoff walked 1 mile to and from school each day.

At week 6, we introduced isokinetic velocity spectrum training for the right hip, knee, and ankle. Our goal was to maximize strength and endurance in the right lower extremity, especially in the hamstrings that would act as secondary restraints in the right knee during running/walking and lateral/rotatory movements. At the same time his cycling program had progressed to three sets of 10 minutes, 90 RPM, 1,000 kpm, with 1-minute rest intervals. RPE was "11 to 12."

At 8 weeks the isokinetic program continued, emphasizing high-velocity work. Proprioceptive facilitation continued by means of PNF, balance beams, and wobble boards. There had been no signs of instability at the right knee since physical therapy commenced. Geoff's swimming program progressed to eight sets of 100 yards with 30-second rest intervals and an RPE of 12. His cycling progressed to 30 minutes of continuous cycling, 90 RPM, 1,200 kpm, RPE "12 to 13." Consistent with Borg's Scale (see Table 3–5), Geoff's pulse was consistently in the 120 to 130 bpm range during his cycling. He continued walking to and from school (1 mile each way) at a brisk pace. Geoff was essentially on a program of cross training (see text).

By 12 weeks, isokinetic testing revealed that Geoff's right quadriceps were essentially equal in power and speed to the left. His right hamstrings were now 20% stronger than the left hamstrings. Proprioceptive re-education continued, emphasizing weight-bearing activities. No incidents of instability were observed or reported. Geoff's swimming program progressed to 3×400 yards with a 30-second rest interval

after each set and an RPE of "12 to 13." Swimming was performed three times each week. The cycling program progressed to 30 minutes three times per week, 90 RPM, 1,500 kpm, with an RPE of "12 to 13."

Based on Geoff's desire to run spring track (team practice was to begin in 2 weeks) and his progress in strength and function in the right knee, it was determined that a running program could be introduced (see Table 3–2). Geoff had been walking 2 miles/day all winter, so he could begin running immediately, without the 2-week walking period advocated in Table 3–2. We began running on a nearby beach. We ran at low tide, when the sand was flat and firm. The first workout consisted of 10 repetitions of 300 yards (approximately 1 minute of running) with a 300-yard walk/rest after each set. Emphasis was placed on proper running mechanics. RPE was reported as "11 to 12." This program was repeated on Monday, Wednesday, and Friday of the first week. On Saturday, Geoff ran for 20 minutes continuously on the boardwalk with an RPE of "11 to 12." Geoff was able to begin his running program at a relatively high level because of his progressive aerobic program during the preceding 3 months. If Geoff was going to be competitive in track, we would have to gear his program to the stresses that he would encounter in competition. Our goals for this phase of his rehabilitation were:

1. Protect the right knee (by continuing strengthening and proprioceptive re-education program)
2. Maximize aerobic conditioning
3. Begin anaerobic training to prepare for the 800-meter run.

Geoff was encouraged to run on soft, firm, and even surfaces such as hard packed sand, golf course fairways, or the boardwalk. This would reduce the impact and stresses on the right knee. It was important to remember that, although his cardiovascular conditioning was improving satisfactorily, we had to make sure that we were not overtaxing his skeletoarticular system (i.e., his right knee).

At this point in the physical therapy program we began to shift emphasis from rehabilitation of the injury to preparation for athletic competition. Geoff was scheduled to run his first 800-meter race against a rival high school in 5 weeks. He already had a good aerobic base of conditioning and had begun some submaximal anaerobic conditioning. The 800-meter run is basically an anaerobic event, lasting for about 2 minutes; thus we began introducing faster interval work at distances of 200, 400, and 600 meters. A typical workout would be 8 to 10×200 meters, 6 to

8 × 400 meters, or 4 to 5 × 600 meters, eventually working down to race pace.

To determine the pace to begin this type of training, we used the "Oregon System" developed by Bowerman (1982), former track and field coach at the University of Oregon. Geoff was asked to run an 800-meter time trial at 75% effort, or RPE of "12." He was able to run 2:14.0 (which works out to be two 400 meters in 67 seconds each). We decided to begin interval training at a slightly faster pace (i.e., 65 seconds for the 400 meters, 32 for the 200 meters, and 1:37.0 for the 600 meters). During the previous year Geoff had recorded a personal best of 2:02.0 for the 800 meters, so we set a goal for 5 weeks of matching that time. This meant that the interval training pace would drop approximately 1 second for the 400 meters per week (a 2:02.0 800 meters requires back-to-back 400s at 61 seconds). Geoff's training program was:

Sunday:
Progress from 20 minutes continuous running to 45–50 minutes. RPE "11."
Monday:
Warm-up: 10 minutes jogging followed by general flexibility exercises.
6 × 400 meters or 3 to 4 × 600 meters progressively working down to 61 seconds pace (RPE 15 to 16).
Rest interval 200 meters—jog/walk between each.
Cool-down: 10 minutes jogging.
Tuesday:
30 minutes continuous running RPE "11"
OR
Swimming 800–1,000 yards RPE "11"
Wednesday:
Same warm-up and cool-down as Monday.
8 × 200 meters beginning at 32–33 seconds and, over 5 weeks, progress to 29–30 seconds.
RPE 15–16, 200-meter jog/walk rest interval.
Thursday:
Rest
Friday:
Race (*or* 30–40 minutes running RPE 11–12)
Saturday:
Swimming or rest

On April 1, Geoff ran his first race and won it, recording a personal record of 2:00.0 for the 800 meters. He eventually progressed to 1:56.0 by the end of the spring track season, finishing second in his division of the state championship.

Isokinetic re-evaluation halfway through the season showed equal power and speed in both quadriceps and a 20% increase in the right hamstrings. No reports of knee instability were noted.

During a 6-year follow-up, Geoff went on to compete as a middle distance runner in college, recording a personal best of 1:51.0 for the 800 meters. He was also able to participate in informal basketball games and tennis without any reports of knee dysfunction. In the 2 years since he graduated from college, Geoff has run 4 days per week, 40 to 60 minutes per session, and competes occasionally in a road race. He presents a good example of how an aerobic fitness program can be integrated into a physical therapy program. Geoff's program was uniquely modified to prepare him for competition, and then, after college, his program was modified once more with the goal of maintaining lifelong fitness and health. Geoff is one of the new generation of people who have started fitness programs in their youth and are committed to lifelong fitness and health.

Case Study 3: Al is a Lutheran minister who had myocardial infarction (MI) when he was 39 years old. Prior to his MI he routinely put in 60 to 80 hours per week attending to the needs of his congregation. Weddings, baptisms, funerals, support groups, visiting the ill at home and in the hospital, and preparing sermons for Sunday's service are all part of his responsibility. He is truly devoted to his work, and before the MI he made himself available at any hour of the day or night. In addition he is married with two children, and he often says that he was "on the go" 24 hours a day.

Early on a Friday morning in 1987, just before an especially busy weekend, Al awoke with chest pains and diaphoresis. His wife, an R.N., immediately recognized the symptoms and rushed him to the hospital. Serum enzyme levels and ECG changes confirmed that he had an inferior wall MI. He was placed on a Lidocaine drip, valium, lopressor, and aspirin. Orders for phase I cardiac rehabilitation were written by his attending physician.

Ironically, Al's previous medical history was unremarkable. He did have three risk factors, however. He had a family history of heart disease (his father had an MI at 49 years of age), he was 15 to 20 lb over his ideal weight, and he had a great amount of stress in his work. Al exercised regularly: He swam between a half-mile and a mile three to four times a week and walked 30 to 40 minutes three times a week.

Phase I cardiac rehabilitation began on the second day of his hospital stay. The author introduced the program to Al and explained that our goal was to get him back to work and exercise. Al was eager to begin exercise and was already knowledgeable about the benefits of exercise and proper diet. He stated that he was well aware of the fact that he was working too many hours and that it had been "catching up to him." His plan was to take some time off from work to recover from the MI and go through phase II (outpatient) cardiac rehabilitation. The Lutheran Church would provide a substitute minister until he could return. Upon returning to work, Al made up his mind to limit his work hours to 40 hours per week and to delegate some responsibility.

Phase I began with general active range-of-motion exercises for the entire body and a progressive walking program within the hospital. Fortunately, Al's MI was uncomplicated and he rapidly progressed through his 10-day hospital stay to the point at which he was walking 5 minutes continuously three times a day. Upon discharge he was referred to the phase II program.

On the following Monday, Al reported to the hospital to begin outpatient cardiac rehabilitation. He had a submaximal stress test prior to discharge and target heart rate (THR) was established at 110 bpm. Due to the lopressor (a beta-blocker) he could not elevate his heart rate above 110 during the stress test. Two other stress tests would be administered during the 3-month program: one at 6 weeks and a final one at 12 weeks to monitor progress and document cardiac status.

Al was placed on a cardiac monitor during the first month of exercise and heart rate and blood pressures were recorded before and after each bout of exercise. Al began his outpatient program with general range-of-motion exercises for both upper and lower extremities and the spine. In Al's case we focused on the hamstrings, gastrocsoleus group, and lumbar spine, because these were the areas where he was least flexible. Next, he performed 4-minute work bouts on each of the following pieces of equipment: stationary bicycle, upper extremity ergometer (UE Ergometer), treadmill, and rowing machine. He was instructed to work at a "comfortable" pace (RPE "11") and was given a full rest interval after each exercise. He performed light stretching at the end of the session, waited for the heart rate and blood pressure to return to resting levels, and was sent home. He was given a home walking program (see Table 3–1) that he would perform on days that he did not attend phase II rehabilitation (patients attend phase II 3 days per week—usually on Monday, Wednesday, and Friday).

During the first week, Al was introduced to Borg's Scale of Perceived Exertion (see Table 3–5). Because he was on beta-blocking medication, his pulse was not an accurate indication of his exertion. Therefore, RPE would be a more reliable indicator. Al was able to pick up the "Perceived Exertion" concept quickly, possibly be-

cause he had a background of regular exercise prior to his MI.

By the end of 4 weeks, Al was performing 10 minutes of walking on the treadmill at 3.5 mph (0% elevation), two sets of 5 minutes on the stationary bicycle with 1 minute of easy cycling as a rest interval (60 RPM, 900 kpm), 5 minutes on the upper extremity ergometer (30 RPM), and 5 minutes of rowing. All exercises were performed at an RPE of "11 to 12" or "comfortable," and rest breaks were limited to 1 minute between exercise stations. He was taken off the ECG monitor and would now monitor his effort based solely on RPE. We continued random pulse checks and blood pressures as needed.

Al continued to progress well over the next 4 weeks. His second stress test revealed a stable cardiac status. By week 8, Al was walking on the treadmill for 10 minutes at 4 mph (5% grade), cycling for 10 minutes (90 RPM, 1,000 kpm), upper extremity ergometer 5 minutes 40 RPM, and rowing for 5 minutes. The goal for the final 4 weeks was to have Al exercise continuously for 30 to 40 minutes at an RPE of "12" and to prepare him for discharge by designing a home program.

Al continued his home walking program and was walking 30 to 35 minutes, four times a week, at an RPE of "11 to 12." He voiced interest in returning to swimming and possibly beginning jogging, so we geared his phase 2 program toward those goals over the next 4 weeks. We began alternate minutes of jogging and walking on the treadmill. Al would walk for 5 minutes at 4 mph (0% grade), then alternate minute intervals of jogging and walking over the next 5 minutes (jogging at 6 mph). Then he would walk 5 minutes more at 4 mph. Next, we upped the U.E. ergometer program to three sets of 3 minutes (50 RPM) with 1-minute rest intervals to prepare his upper extremities for swimming. Rowing continued at 5 minutes and cycling 10 minutes at 90 RPM (1,200 kpm). RPE remained at "12." By week 12, Al was alternating 10 minutes of jogging and walking (6 mph and 4 mph), doing three sets of 4 minutes on the upper extremity ergometer at 40 RPM, cycling 10 minutes at 90 RPM (1,200 kpm), and rowing for 5 minutes. In addition, he was walking 50 minutes to 1 hour at an RPE of 12, 3 to 4 days per week. He was ready to be discharged. Al was placed on the swimming program (see Table 3–3) and essentially progressed week by week on the identical program. He also continued his walking program three to four times per week.

On a 3-year follow-up, Al continues regular exercise. He states that his "day is not complete without swimming or walking." His medication has been modified to atenolol (Tenormin) (a beta-blocker) 12.5 mg/qd, Lopid (which decreases serum lipids) 600 mg bid, dipyridamole (Persantine) 25 mg tid, and one aspirin qd. His exercise regime is as follows:

SUMMER
Walking: 4 × week 45 minutes–1 hour (covers 3 to 4 miles)
Swimming: 3 × week 30–35 minutes (⅔ mile)

WINTER
Walking: 4 × week 45 minutes to 1 hour (3 to 4 miles)
Swimming: 2 × week 30 to 35 minutes (⅔ mile)
Rowing: 1-2 × week 10 minutes

Al has dropped 20 lb since his MI 3 years ago, and all follow-up examinations have been excellent. Al states that he has not been ill since he started the aerobic exercise program after his MI. In addition, he has been counseling cardiac patients in his congregation.

References

Alois JF, Cohn SH, Ostuni JA, et al: Prevention of involutional bone loss by exercise. Ann Intern Med 89(3): 356–358, 1978.
American College of Sports Medicine: Guidelines for Graded Exercise Testing and Prescription, 3rd ed. Philadelphia, Lea & Febiger, 1986.
Blair SN: Physical activity leads to fitness and pays off. Physician Sports Med 13(3): 153–157, 1985.
Blair SN, Goodyear NN, Gibbons LW, and Cooper KH: Physical fitness and incidence of hypertension in healthy normotensive men and women. JAMA 252(4): 487–490, 1984.
Blair SN, Kohl HW, Paffenbarger RS, et al: Physical fitness and all-cause mortality: A prospective study of healthy men and women. JAMA 262(17): 2395–2401, 1989.
Bjorntorp P: Hypertension and exercise. Hypertension 4(III):56–59, 1982.
Bly JL, Jones RC, and Richardson JE: Impact of worksite health promotion on health care costs and utilization: Evaluation of Johnson & Johnson's live for life program. JAMA 256(23): 3235–3240, 1986.
Borg GAV and Linderholm H: Perceived exertion and pulse rate during graded exercise in various age groups. Acta Med Scand 472:194–206, 1967.
Bowerman, W.J. Returning to running after injury. In the American Academy of Orthopedic Surgeons Symposium on: The foot and leg in running sports. C.V. Mosby Co. 1982. pp 162–166.
Centers for Disease Control: Progress toward achieving the 1990 national objectives for physical fitness and exercise. JAMA 262(6):746–753, 1989.
Cerutty P: Be Fit or Be Damned! London, Pelham, 1967.
Chalmers J and Ho KC: Geographical variations in senile osteoporosis: The association of physical activity. J Bone Joint Surg 52: 667–675, 1970.
Chisholm DM, Collis ML, and Kulak LL: Physical activity readiness. Br Columbia Med J 17: 375–378, 1975.
Cooper KH: Aerobics. New York, M. Evans, 1968.
Cooper KH: The Aerobics Program of Total Well-Being. New York, Bantam Books, 1982.
Cooper KH, Pollock ML, Martin RP, et al: Physical fitness levels vs selected coronary risk factors: A cross-sectional study. JAMA 236(2): 166–169, 1976.
Cordain L, Latin RW, and Behnke JJ: The effect of an aerobic running program on bowel transit time. J Sports Med Phys Fitness 26(1): 101–104, 1986.
Dalen N and Olsson KE: Bone mineral content and physical activity. Acta Scandinavica 45:170–174, 1974.
de Vries HA: Physiology of Exercise for Physical Education and Athletics, 3rd ed. Dubuque, IA, Wm. C. Brown, 1980.
Drinkwater BL, Nilson K, Chestnut CH, et al: Bone mineral content of amenorrhic and eumenorrheic athletes. N Engl J Med 311(5): 277–281, 1984.
Eaton BS, Konner M, and Shostak M: Stone agers in the fast lane: chronic degenerative diseases in evolutionary perspective. Am J Med 84(4): 739–749, 1988.
Epstein LH and Wing RR: Aerobic exercise and weight. Addict Behav 52:667–675, 1980.
Fisher AC and Worth W: America's health in the 20th century. ACSH News & Views 7: 1–7, 1986.
Folkins CH and Sime WE: Physical fitness training and mental health. Am Psychol 36(4): 373–389, 1981.
Garcia-Palmieri MR, Costas R, Cruz-Vidal M, et al: Increased physical activity: A protective factor against heart attacks in Puerto Rico. Am J Cardiol 50(4): 749–755, 1982.
Harris SS, Caspersen CJ, DeFriese GH, and Estes EH: Physical activity counseling for healthy adults as a primary preventive intervention in the clinical setting: Report for the U.S. preventive services task force. JAMA 261(24): 3588–3598, 1989.
Haskell WL, Montoye HJ, and Orenstein D: Physical activity and exercise to achieve health-related physical fitness components. Public Health Rep 100(2): 202–212, 1985.
Hicky N: Study of coronary risk factors related to physical activity in 15,171 men. Br Med J 5982(3): 507–509, 1975.
Iverson DC, Fielding JE, Crow RS, and Christenson GM: The promotion of physical activity in the United States population: The status of programs in medical, worksite, community, and school settings. Public Health Rep 100(2): 212–224, 1985.
Jones WHS (ed and trans): Hippocrates: Regimen I, Vol. 4. Cambridge, Harvard University Press, 1959.
Joslin P: Joslin's Diabetes Mellitus, 12th ed. Philadelphia, Lea & Febiger, 1985.
King H, Taylor R, and Zimmet P: Non-insulin dependent diabetes in a newly independent Pacific nation: The Republic of Kiribati. Diabetes Care 7(5): 409–415, 1984.
Koplan JP, Caspersen CJ, and Powell KE: Physical activity, physical fitness, and health: Time to act (Editorial). JAMA 262 (17): 2437, 1989.
Lovett RW: Presidential address. Am Phys Educ Rev VI: 300–302, 1901.
Mazess RB and Wheedon, GD: Immobilization and bone: Calcified Tissue International 35(3):265–267, 1983.
Monahan T: Is "activity" as good as exercise? Physician Sports Med 15(10): 181–186, 1987.
Morgan WP and Borg GAV: Perception of effort and the prescription of physical activity. In Graig T (ed): Mental Health and Emotional Aspects of Sports. Chicago, American Medical Association, 1976.
Morris JN, Everitt MG, Pollard R, et al: Vigorous exercise in leisure time: Protection against coronary heart disease. Lancet 2(8206): 1207–1210, 1980.
Nice perk if you can get it. USA Weekend Jan 19–21, 1990.

Nixon JE and Jewett AE: An Introduction to Physical Education. Philadelphia, WB Saunders, 1969.

Nixon PGF: Human functions and the heart. *In* Seedhouse D and Cribb A (eds): Changing Ideas in Health Care. New York, John Wiley, 1989.

Osler W: A Way of Life and Other Selected Writings. New York, Dover, 1958.

Paffenbarger RS and Hale WE: Work activity and coronary heart mortality. N Engl J Med *292*(11): 545–550, 1975.

Paffenbarger RS, Hyde RT, Wing AL, and Chung-Cheng H: Physical activity, all-cause mortality, and longevity of college alumni. N Engl J Med *314* (10):605–613, 1986.

Paffenbarger RS, Hyde RT, Wing AL, and Steinmetz CH: A natural history of athleticism and cardiovascular health. JAMA *252*(4):491–495, 1984.

Paffenbarger RS, Wing AL, Hyde RT, and Jung DL: Physical activity and incidence of hypertension in college alumni. Am J Epidemiol *117*(3):245–256, 1983.

Paganini-Hill A, Ross RK, Gerkins VR, et al: Menopausal estrogen therapy and hip fractures. Ann Intern Med *95*(1): 28–31, 1981.

Pinkston D: Evolution of the practice of physical therapy in the United States. *In* Scully RM and Barnes MR (eds): Physical Therapy. Philadelphia, JB Lippincott, 1989, pp 2–30.

Pollack ML, Jackson AS, and Foster C: The use of the perception scale for exercise prescription. *In* Borg GAV and Ottoson D (eds): The Perception of Exertion in Physical Work. London, Macmillan, 1986, pp 161–176.

Powell KE, Caspersen CJ, Koplan JP, and Ford ES: Physical activity and chronic diseases. Am J Clin Nutr *49*(5): 999–1006, 1989.

Richter EA and Schneider SH: Diabetes and exercise. Am J Med *70*: 201–209, 1981.

Rippe JM, Blair SN, Freedson PS, et al: The health benefits of exercise, Part 1. Physician Sports Med *15* (10): 115–132, 1987.

Salonen JT, Puska P, and Tuomilehto J: Physical activity and risk of myocardial infarction, cerebral stroke and death: A longitudinal study in eastern Finland. Am J Epidemiol *115*(4): 526–537, 1982.

Sheehan G: The three components of sickness: disease, illness, and the predicament. AMAA Q August: 14, 1989.

Sheehan G: The use of exercise in clinical practice. Lecture Notes April, 1987.

Shepard RJ: Can we identify those for whom exercise is hazardous? Sports Med *1*: 75–88, 1984.

Simmons K: The federal government: Keeping tabs on the nation's fitness. Physician Sports Med *15* (1): 190–195, 1987.

Siscovick DS, LaPorte RE, and Newman JM: The disease-specific benefits and risks of physical activity and exercise. Public Health Rep *100*(2):180–188, 1985.

Siscovick DS, Weiss NS, Hallstrom AP, et al: Physical activity and primary cardiac arrest. JAMA *248*(23):3113–3117, 1982.

Stephens T: Physical activity and mental health in the United States and Canada: Evidence from four population surveys. Prev Med *17*(1): 35–47, 1988.

Stephens T, Jacobs DR, and White CC: A descriptive epidemiology of leisure-time physical activity. Public Health Rep *100*(2): 147–158, 1985.

Taylor CB, Sallis JF, and Needle R: The relation of physical activity and exercise to mental health. Public Health Rep *100*(2): 195–202, 1985.

USPSTF: Report of the US preventive services task force. JAMA *263*(3): 436–437, 1990.

Wenger HA and Bell CJ: The interactions of intensity, frequency, and duration of exercise training in altering cardiorespiratory fitness. Sports Med *3* (5):346–356, 1986.

White PD: Walking and cycling save health and money. Hygeia *15*(April): 321, 1937.

Zimmet P, Faaiuso S, Ainuu J, et al: The prevalence of diabetes in the rural and urban Polynesian population of Western Samoa. Diabetes *30*(1):45–51, 1981.

Prevention and Treatment Strategies for Specific Problems

C H A P T E R

4

John M. Barbis

Prevention and Management of Low Back Pain

Sixty to 90% of the United States population will experience low back pain at some time in their lives. About 5% of the population will miss at least 1 day of work within the next year because of back pain. Of this group, 5.4 million workers will go on to be disabled by that injury for 1 year or more. Low back pain treatment and payment for loss of work and disability cost the American public, government, and industry between 6 and 10 billion dollars per year (Frymoyer, 1988; Vanharanta, 1989; Waddell, 1987; Weisel et al, 1985).

ORIGIN OF LOW BACK PAIN

Although over 90% of all low back pain cases are classified as ideopathic—there is no readily identifiable structure producing the pain—there are several structures in the low back that authorities recognize as being causative. The spinal musculature, spinal nerves, ligaments, venous drainage system, disc, facet joints, and sacroiliac joint all have their proponents and detractors as the primary structures of pain production in low back pain. Imaging techniques such as x-ray, computed tomography (CT) scans, myelograms, and magnetic resonance imaging (MRI) or electrodiagnostic testing like electromyograph or nerve conduction velocity testing can provide sufficient evidence to confirm a diagnosis in the less than

10 to 15% of individuals with low back pain. In this small group, the kinds of diagnosis are much more serious and the pathologies producing the pain are most likely to be osseous, neural, or discoid in nature.

In most cases of low back pain, the actual origin of the pain is more of a philosophic statement of the training of the practitioner than hard, scientific fact. Although the most common diagnosis given to clients with ideopathic low back pain is lumbar strain and sprain, there is no reliable method to confirm that diagnosis (Frymoyer, 1988; Waddell, 1987; Waddell and Allan, 1989). The intervertebral disc is now believed to be the most common cause of nontraumatic low back pain (DiMaggio and Mooney, 1987a and 1987b; Frymoyer, 1988; Kraemer, 1981; Vanharanta and Mooney, 1987; Vanharanta, 1989). The most common diagnosis in traumatic low back pain—injury caused by a rapid acceleration or deceleration of either the body or an object as it contacts the body—is lumbar sprain and strain.

Injury to the ligaments, facets, and musculature can be better explained in this kind of event, but again the disc is believed to be an important source of pain in traumatic injuries (Twomey and Taylor, 1989).

The use of the MRI, CT, and discogram has given medicine the ability to recognize many more problems of the disc that were not seen before. The work of Bogduk (1987, 1988) showed that the discs of the cervical and lumbar spines are innervated, and the lumbar disc can be a source of pain not only for the back but down the leg as well. It is no longer believed that the nucleus must first herniate and place pressure on either the posterior longitudinal ligament or the neural structures to produce pain in the leg and back.

Twomey and Taylor's (1989) study of the incidence and location of nondiagnosed spinal injuries after motor vehicle accidents indicates that the facet joints in the lumbar spine may be even more vulnerable to injury during this type of trauma than the disc. According to the authors, small, unrecognized fractures can occur in the articular cartilage on the subchondral bone. Damage can also occur to the joint capsule and the multifidus muscle, which is contiguous with the posterior portion of the joint capsule. Others examined the facet as a potential cause of low back pain in nontraumatic cases, and the view that the facet is an important cause of ideopathic low back pain has waxed and waned over the past two decades (Mooney, 1987).

ANATOMY, PHYSIOLOGY, AND MECHANICS OF THE DISC

Because the disc is such an important potential cause of low back pain, it is important that its anatomy, physiology, and mechanics be discussed. The disc consists of three distinct structures: an outer wall called the annulus, which is made up of thin, concentric layers of fibrocartilage; the nucleus pulposus, which consists of a poorly organized mass of mucopolypeptide and collagen; and the end-plate areas that lie next to the bodies of the vertebrae (Ashman, 1989; Bogduk and Twomey, 1987; Kraemer, 1981). The nucleus does have some structure and is difficult to pull apart, but it does possess fluid-like properties that allow it to change shape and displace its mass with spinal motion and changes in posture (Kraemer, 1981). As the nucleus ages, its consistency changes and becomes more collagenous until the fifth and sixth decades of life when its density differs little from that of the annulus. Most of the loss of water content occurs before early adulthood, and only small changes occur after that. Little change occurs in the hydration of the annulus with age (Kraemer, 1981; Mooney, 1987; Taylor and Twomey, 1987a; Twomey and Taylor, 1987; Vanharanta, 1989).

The outer third of the annulus is innervated by the sinuvertebral nerve (Bogduk, 1987; Bogduk et al, 1981), and its free nerve endings can become irritated either by changes in pressure brought about by deformations in the annular wall or by changes in the chemical environment with injury (Bogduk, 1987; Crock, 1986; Kraemer, 1981; Vanharanta, 1989). The anterior and posterior surfaces of the annulus are supported by the anterior and posterior longitudinal ligaments.

The diurnal pattern of loss and restoration of the hydration of the disc as a result of weight bearing and recumbency plays an important role in maintaining the health of the disc (Adams and Hutton, 1983; Taylor and Twomey, 1987b). The cells within the intervertebral disc receive their nutrition by diffusion through the fluid within the disc. The disc itself does not have a blood supply. Nutrients must diffuse to the annulus and nucleus from the synovium in the end-plate areas of the vertebral bodies. As a result of the relatively long distances between the end-plate areas and the center of the disc, the nutritional environment of the cells in the central parts of the disc and annulus can be poor. Because of the poor nutrition, the cells in the annulus regenerate slowly and are slow to heal. The roles of posture, spinal motion, and fluid movement are critical in disrupting the diffusion gradient that develops as a result of immobilization and in allowing more nutrients to reach the central part of the disc (Adams and Hutton, 1983; Bogduk and Twomey, 1987; Kraemer, 1981; Vanharanta, 1989).

Spinal movement and postures not only move the fluid around within the disc but also move fluid out of the disc. Weight-bearing postures produce pressures within the disc that force water out of the fluid matrix (Adams and Hutton, 1983; Vanharanta, 1989). Upon assuming recumbent postures, these pressures are relieved, and the osmotic pressure within the disc causes the tissue to reabsorb the water. With the new intake of fluid comes additional nutrition. Weight-bearing and spinal movements are necessary for the health of the disc. Prolonged immobilization of the spine and prevention of normal spinal movement can produce significant degeneration of the annulus (Nachemson, 1985).

Another factor in the degeneration of the intervertebral disc is prolonged offset loading resulting from the deforming pressures of sustained postures or repeated movements. Whether these disruptions or fissures in the annular wall are caused by movements of the nucleus, changes in hydration, shear forces upon movement, or a combination of all three is not known (Adams and Hutton, 1981, 1983, and 1985; Hickey and Hukins, 1980; Taylor and Twomey, 1987).

CT-assisted discograms have shown that these disruptions in the annulus exist and do not have to extend through the entire annular wall to produce symptoms (Vanharanta and Mooney, 1987). These defects can occur in anterior, posterior, or lateral directions (Adams and Hutton, 1981 and 1985; Hickey and Hukins, 1980; Kraemer, 1981; Vanharanta and Mooney, 1987; Yasuma, 1990). Although the annular fibers are very effective in resisting compressive forces produced by the vertebrae, they are susceptible to tensile forces that are produced by separating the vertebral surfaces.

The annulus is even more susceptible to damage if the tensile force is accompanied by a rotatory movement (Adams and Hutton, 1981; Bogduk and Twomey, 1987). Aging or osteoarthritic changes seen on x-ray do not, however, appear to be significant contributors to low back pain or disc degeneration. In the fifth and sixth decades of life, the incidence of significant osteoarthritic changes are greatest, but the incidence of low back pain decreases substantially and is much lower than expected (Bogduk and Twomey, 1987; Deyo and Bass, 1989; Kraemer, 1981, Twomey and Taylor, 1987; Vanharanta, 1989).

PRIMARY PREVENTION OF LOW BACK PAIN

Although there are no published studies demonstrating that any singular or combined approach, exercise program, or change in lifestyle can prevent the onset of low back pain (Vanharanta, 1989), most experts believe that the process can be slowed or prevented by the maintenance of good health habits (proper rest, exercise, and the elimination of smoking), frequent movement or unloading of the spine, and proper body mechanics. The prevention of traumatic low back injuries requires attention to safety procedures. Most traumatic low back injuries are the result of either falls or accidents involving moving vehicles. Constant awareness of hazardous situations and activities in the workplace and home and the use of proper safety equipment, the

wearing of seat belts, and vigilance are necessary to avoid these types of injuries (Henker, 1987; States, 1987). Nontraumatic low back injuries are, however, much more common. These injuries usually are not caused by a single incident or movement, but are the result of a series of events that placed the structures of the low back at risk. As a result, an event that by itself would not be injurious to the back now becomes the percipitating factor of the pain. In most nontraumatic back injuries, any of a number of possible interventions leading up to the injurious event most likely would have prevented the occurrence.

To prevent low back pain, therapists must inform clients of those factors that, when combined, are injurious to the back, and they must teach clients how to change or counteract those factors to prevent its onset. The three major areas in which changes can occur to prevent the onset of low back pain are as follows:

1. Adjustment of lifestyle
2. Prevention of prolonged loading or repetitive motions of the low back
3. Maintenance of cardiovascular and musculoskeletal fitness

Adjustment of Lifestyle

Modern industrial societies perceive back pain to be a problem created by heavy labor, lifting, and so on. It is not seen as a problem in societies in which most of the labor force have sedentary jobs involving little lifting and excellent health care. Epidemiological studies of low back pain, however, indicate that its incidence is similar between developed and underdeveloped societies, but the incidence of disability in developed societies may be higher than in underdeveloped societies (Waddell, 1987; Waddell and Allan, 1989).

There must be other factors than heavy work and poor living conditions that influence the incidence of low back pain. Lifestyle factors and attitudes toward low back pain may need to be altered. Those lifestyle areas that presently hold the most promise for producing a reduction in the incidence of low back pain are as follows:

1. A reduction of known risk factors
2. Attention to the early signs of low back trouble
3. Balancing flexion and extension in the lifestyle

Reduction of Risk Factors

Most studies of low back pain identify only four risk factors: truck driving, smoking, extreme height, and extreme obesity (Burton and Tillotson, 1989; Cady et al, 1979; Deyo and Bass, 1989; Deyo and Tsui, 1987; Frymoyer and Cats-Baril, 1987; Kelsey et al, 1984; Vanharanta, 1989).

Truck driving can be made safer by implementing several techniques discussed later, the most important of which is using a seat that has adequate lumbar support (Kelsey et al, 1984). For reasons unknown, smoking contributes to low back pain (Deyo and Bass, 1989; Kelsey et al, 1984). Among the theories that implicate smoking are (a) smoker's cough results in an increase in intra-abdominal pressures and stress on the disc and (b) oxygen delivered to the disc decreases as a result of the influence of the combustion products of tobacco.

The increased incidence of low back pain among tall men and women is probably due to two factors: increased diffusion distances within the disc itself because of its larger size and increased discoid pressures caused by the greater mass (Vanharanta, 1989). Extreme obesity, with its concomitant increased load on the spine and decreased activity level, is a very significant risk factor in the development of low back pain (Deyo and Bass, 1989; Vanharanta, 1989). Being moderately overweight, however, does not significantly increase the probability of experiencing low back pain (Deyo and Bass, 1989).

Another factor that appears commonly in epidemiologic studies but is more difficult to quantify is stress level. Increased stress levels, as measured by job satisfaction, depression, and so on, do appear to significantly increase the probability of low back pain (Berquist-Ullman and Larson, 1977; Bigos et al, 1986a and 1986b; Frymoyer and Cats-Baril, 1987; Nachemson, 1976 and 1983; Spengler et al, 1986; Vanharanta, 1989). Clients with high stress levels also tend to have more frequent and intense bouts of pain. Their discomfort is also more likely to become chronic and lead to disability.

Identification of Early Signs of Back Trouble

A very important aspect of any prevention program is teaching clients to understand the warning signs the low back is providing regarding its health and status. The spine has an intricate sensory and warning mechanism. All too often, we have learned to ignore its early warning signals and begin to pay attention only after a major breakdown has occurred and the pain can no longer be ignored. The signs that indicate potential problems with the back are as follows:

1. Stiffness or tightness
2. The complaint of a "cold in the back"
3. Minor intermittent aches and pains
4. Significant difficulty in rising from sitting or straightening up as a result of stiffness
5. Morning stiffness
6. Low back pain when walking or driving

These are signs that the low back needs more attention and that some change in lifestyle is needed. In addition, it is important to teach clients to associate the pain with the proper cause. All too often exercise is stopped because low back pain develops an hour or so after participating in the activity. In most situations, the exercise is improperly implicated and stopped; it may not be the exercise that is at fault, but rather the positions maintained and the activities performed after the exercise is completed that are the cause. Back pain occurs relatively quickly with and usually during the offending activity.

Balancing Flexion and Extension

The balancing of flexion and extension is an important component of the changes needed in the normal lifestyle to prevent low back pain. Flexion activities dominate most of the normal day. Sitting (unless the lordosis is actively or passively maintained), activities of daily living, most working postures, lifting, cooking, and so on all have strong flexion components, and there are very few activities that contain significant extension components. As a result, unless a conscious effort is maintained to introduce lumbar extension into the daily routine either through exercise or upright sitting, a distinct imbalance develops between flexion and extension. Individuals employed in occupations and those involved in certain sports in which extension activities and postures can dominate (e.g., house painters, wallpaper hangers, volleyball players, gymnasts) need to balance the extension in their activities with flexion. The spine is healthiest when a flexion or extension posture is not maintained for a prolonged period and when it has a balance of movement in both directions. The balancing of flexion and extension maintains the central position of the nucleus and allows the synovial fluid within the disc to maintain the appropriate nutritional status of the cells within the disc.

Prevention of Prolonged Loading or Repetitive Motions in One Direction

In addition to the need for balanced flexion and extension in the lifestyle, prolonged loading of the spine in one position should be prevented. Such prolonged loading—whether sustained or intermittent—can have a deleterious effect on the integrity of the annular wall (Adams and Hutton, 1985; Bogduk and Twomey, 1987; Hickey and Hukins, 1980). Flexion, especially as it is produced by prolonged sitting postures, can produce posterior fissuring, which is probably the most common form of disc disruption (McKenzie, 1987). Prolonged extension positions have also been shown to produce fissures in the anterior anular wall (Kraemer, 1981). Because annular fissuring can occur in the posterior wall with prolonged flexion and in the anterior wall with prolonged extension, it is important to develop programs that encourage people to move frequently and unload the disc by moving in the opposite direction every 20 to 40 minutes. Interrupting long periods of end-range flexion with even a few repetitions to end-range extension can prevent backward bends damage.

Maintenance of Cardiovascular and Musculoskeletal Fitness

A regular exercise program that has as its goals the maintenance of cardiovascular fitness and musculoskeletal flexibility and strength is believed to be effective in preventing low back pain. An often-cited source of evidence is Cady and associates' (1979) work in which direct correlation was found between fitness levels of firefighters and the prevention of low back pain. Further evaluation of the data from that study, however, does produce some skepticism as to the significance of their conclusions (Mooney, 1987). Although no other epidemiological study of low back pain has found a correlation between fitness levels and incidence of low back pain, most authorities still recommend a balanced exercise program that includes aerobic activities, such as walking, jogging, swimming, rowing,

calisthenics, and stretching to help prevent the onset of low back pain (Bigos and Baltic, 1987). Such a program would produce physiologic effects that could both directly and indirectly affect the status of the back, including:

1. Strengthening the musculature that supports the spine
2. Maintaining the length and strength of the ligaments that support the spine
3. Improving the nutritional status of the intervertebral disc through increased spinal movement and cardiovascular status
4. Maintaining the mineral content of the vertebrae and preventing osteoporosis
5. Reducing stress levels and the production of endorphins
6. Increasing the caloric output to help reduce or maintain body weight

Aerobic programs should follow the general standards established by the American College of Sports Medicine (1978) (Table 4–1). This type of program would produce stress on the cardiovascular system sufficient to improve or maintain its efficiency. The stretching or calisthenics program should have two components. First, it should be a gentle, repetitive-movement program involving full flexion and extension to emphasize disc position and health. Such a program

Table 4–1. Quality and Quantity of Exercise for Developing and Maintaining Fitness in Healthy Adults Recommended by the American College of Sports Medicine

1. Frequency of training: 3 to 5 days per week.
2. Intensity of training: 60 to 90% of maximum heart rate reserve or 50 to 85% of maximum oxygen uptake.
3. Duration of training: 15 to 60 minutes of continuous aerobic activity. Duration depends on the intensity of the activity; lower intensity activity should be conducted over a longer period of time. Because of the importance of the total fitness effect, the fact that total fitness is more readily attained in longer duration programs, and the potential hazards and compliance problems associated with high-intensity activity, activity of lower to moderate intensity and longer duration is recommended for the nonathletic adult.
4. Mode of activity: Any activity that uses large-muscle groups, that can be maintained continuously, and that is rhythmic and aerobic in nature (e.g., running, jogging, walking, hiking, swimming, skating, bicycling, rowing, cross-country skiing, rope jumping, and various endurance game activities).

Table 4–2. Musculature Included in a Stretching Program for the Low Back

Lumbar extensors	Hip adductors
Lumbar flexors	Knee flexors
Hip flexors	Knee extensors
Hip extensors	Plantar flexors

should be simple and should be performed several times each day. Second, the program should include sustained stretching of the musculature and the periarticular structures. The musculature should be maintained on a gentle stretch for 20 to 30 seconds. It is not necessary to produce pain during this stretching; in fact, pain may actually be counterproductive. Table 4–2 lists the most important musculature to stretch during this program. It is important to follow the sustained stretching with repetitive spinal movements to prevent excessive loading of the discs. The strengthening program should maintain a balance between the agonists and antagonists of the trunk, hip, and knee.

The strengthening can be accomplished simply through the use of isometrics or home calisthenics, or a more extensive program can be developed at a spa or gym using free-weights or more sophisticated exercise equipment produced by Cybex, Chattanooga, Biodex, and other manufacturers.

SECONDARY PREVENTION OF LOW BACK PAIN

According to Waddell (1987), health-care providers need to develop a new model for back pain, and the disease model that is used to treat other medical conditions is not appropriate for this condition. For most people, low back pain is not a symptom of a disease or degenerative process that could lead to disfigurement or disability. It is a syndrome whose major and sometimes only symptom is pain. The epidemiologic evidence of disability resulting from low back pain in developed and nondeveloped countries indicates that the attitudes of health-care providers and the presence of sophisticated medical technology have a significant impact on the tendency of a functional low back pain client to progress to a disabled low back pain client. The incidence of low back pain in developed and nondeveloped countries is about the same, but the incidence of disability resulting from low back

pain is surprisingly higher in developed countries (Waddell, 1987).

Almost all people will experience low back pain severe enough to affect significantly their level of activity for a few days, and the vast majority will recover without the need for medical intervention. The duration and progression of the condition have been consistent across cultures and through time (Waddell and Allan, 1989). Without treatment, 40% of individuals will recover in 2 weeks; 80% will recover in 6 weeks; and more than 90% will recover in 2 months. However, 35% develop sciatica, but even these clients generally follow these recovery periods (Deyo, 1983; Kraemer, 1981; Nachemson, 1976 and 1985; Vanharanta, 1989; Waddell, 1987; Waddell and Allan, 1989; Weissel et al, 1985). In developed countries where the disease model has been applied to the management of low back pain, the level of disability resulting from low back pain is much higher and has grown with the increasing sophistication of medical care. Low back pain is a condition common to all people, economic groups, and occupations. Disability resulting from low back pain is primarily a condition of a wealthy country with a well-developed health-care delivery system (Waddell, 1987).

The major thrust of any low back pain management program, then, is to prevent the progression from acute pain to chronicity and disability. The typical medical model, which emphasizes rest, modulation, or management of the symptoms and intervention on a biochemical or physical basis, is not relevant to the management of this condition. For most clients whose condition follows the normal progression, the treatment program should emphasize self-care, the judicious use of bed rest, and an early return to activity (Bigos et al, 1986a and b). Passive modalities such as heating pads, ultrasound, massage, and transcutaneous electrical nerve stimulation have not been shown to produce any beneficial effect and are only temporary palliatives (Deyo, 1983; Spitzer, 1987). Their use may even be harmful because they support and reward many of the dependent behaviors that are a part of the chronic pain syndrome (Frymoyer, 1988; Nachemson, 1976 and 1985; Waddell, 1987). Their use can be warranted for the early management of inflammation and pain of traumatic injuries but not for the more common form of idiopathic low back pain.

An early return to light or reduced activity

should also be encouraged as a therapeutic tool (Nachemson, 1983). This has been shown to have a beneficial effect on bone and muscular strength, disc and cartilage nutrition, as well as self-image and stress levels. There is no evidence that an early return to activity is associated with increased pain or a worsening of the condition if clients are properly coached and trained (Berquist-Ullman and Larson, 1977; Nachemson, 1983).

For those who resume employment early, it may be necessary for them to return to a position that does not place as much stress on the back until they regain some strength and endurance and the tissue has healed more thoroughly. A rapid return to tolerated activity levels even in the presence of pain presents many positive benefits and does not pose significant problems if handled carefully (Nachemson, 1983). Clients may also need some lumbar support while sitting, or adaptations in the work area may be necessary to prevent excessive stress on the healing area.

In addition, low back pain clients who have been out of work for more than 6 months have only a 50% probability of returning to their previous level of employment. If the patient has been disabled for more than a year, the probability of returning to the previous level of employment is below 25% (Nachemson, 1983; Waddell, 1987). It is therefore essential that clients try to return to active, functional levels as soon as possible. Such a plan demands a coordinated effort among employers, clients, and all of the health-care providers involved. Research has shown that the willingness of employers to be actively involved in the rehabilitation process can have a positive effect in returning clients to active employment (Bigos et al, 1986a and b).

Therapists must clearly delineate goals and limitations for both clients and employers. They must carefully train clients to use posture, body mechanics, and seating supports to manage the condition. Therapists must also carefully evaluate the environmental factors, such as work postures, work surfaces, furniture, and working conditions (e.g., lifting, exposure to prolonged vibrations), to help clients work at their maximum potential with the least amount of discomfort. In addition, it is important for therapists to begin to develop the confidence of both the employers and the clients.

Self-Care Philosophies

There are essentially two forms of self-care philosophies. One is espoused by most back school programs (Hayne, 1984; Linton and Kamwendo, 1987), and the other is preferred by the evaluation and treatment programs developed by McKenzie (McKenzie, 1987; Oliver et al, 1987). In most back school programs, a standard curriculum is presented to each client, who also receives some individual attention in the instruction of lifting and body-conservation techniques. Each of the major schools (American, Canadian, Swedish, Australian, Californian, and so on) can differ significantly in the information presented and in the techniques emphasized and practiced (Hayne, 1984; Linton and Kamwendo, 1987). Schools can also differ in their emphasis on flexion or extension as preventative philosophies, with their resultant differences in prophylactic exercise, postural instructions, and lifting techniques. Their programs remain essentially the same for all clients, however.

Early studies on the usefulness of back schools were quite encouraging. The work of Berquist-Ullman and Larson (1977) showed a more rapid and successful return to the workplace after clients had attended a back school. Later studies, however, showed that the beneficial effects of back schools on acute low back pain clients may not have been as significant as originally stated (Berwick et al, 1989; Hayne, 1984; Linton and Kamwendo, 1987; Liston, 1987; Spitzer, 1987). Several studies showed no significant effect when the back school was compared with a control group (Berwick et al, 1989; Videman, 1989).

Studies of the system of evaluation and treatment espoused by McKenzie showed that the system may be extremely valuable in managing acute low back pain (DiMaggio and Mooney, 1987a and b; Mooney, 1987; Vanharanta et al, 1986). According to the philosophy espoused by McKenzie, clients should be responsible for following through with an individualized program developed by their physical therapist. As a result, the exercise program and the instruction that clients receive in posture and body mechanics is designed specifically for them and can vary greatly. It does not lend itself easily to the school technique (McKenzie, 1987; Oliver et al, 1987).

Four of the unique characteristics of McKenzie's mechanical approach (McKenzie, 1987; Oliver et al, 1987) are as follows:

1. The reliance on repetitive movements
2. The centralization phenomenon or the proximal regression of symptoms as a joint or disc derangement is reduced

Table 4–3. McKenzie's Classification of Low Back Pain by Location of Symptoms and Response to Repeated Movements

Syndrome	Type of Symptoms	Response to Repeated Movement
Postural	Local and intermittent, no referred pain	No reproduction of symptoms; symptoms reproduced by sustained positioning
Dysfunction	Local and intermittent, no referred pain	Pain reproduced at end range of particular movement; once end-range positions are released, pain decreases or is abolished
Derangement	Local or referred distally, intermittent or constant; possible presence of paresthesia, numbness, diminished reflexes, decreased muscle strength, postural deformities	Symptoms can change their intensity or location with repeated movements; centralization or peripheralization of symptoms is seen; pain is produced during movement, not just at end range

3. The classification of low back problems into three syndromes based on symptoms and response to repeated motions instead of tissue origin (Table 4–3)
4. Four different stages of treatment, with each syndrome emphasizing one or more stages (Table 4–4)

The success of the McKenzie approach in treating low back pain caused by a mechanical problem in the low back is dependent on careful evaluation by therapists to determine the relevant syndrome and careful instruction of clients in correct exercise technique, posture, body mechanics, and symptom-recognition procedures specific for each client.

Bed Rest

Most authorities now propose that low back pain clients receive no more than 2 days of bed rest (Deyo et al, 1986; Frymoyer, 1988; Waddell, 1987). There seems to be no difference in the outcome of clients who received only 2 days and those who received more than 2 days of bed rest. Several days' worth of bed rest have been shown to produce a significant loss in bone mass and a deleterious effect on the cardiovascular system (Deyo et al, 1986; Waddell, 1987).

If clients must be confined to bed, it is important to instruct them carefully in proper sleeping

Table 4–4. Stages of Treatment in the McKenzie System

Stage 1: Reduction of the derangement
Stage 2: Maintenance of the reduction
Stage 3: Recovery of function
Stage 4: Prophylaxis

and lying positions. Sitting up in bed or watching television in bed while propped up can produce sustained flexion postures that have a negative effect on the lumbar spine. Lying with the feet or knees elevated may produce some temporary relief from the symptoms, but its long-term effect may be to delay recovery because it produces a prolonged offset flexion pressure on the disc. Bed rest is most often used during the inflammatory phase after a posterior disc derangement or after a traumatic injury to the low back. In both of these cases, clients should be instructed to use a towel or small pillow to support the low back in as normal a posture as possible. Such normal posture would mean the maintenance of a gentle lordotic curve.

Injury Prevention

After a client has recovered from low back pain, it is essential that a three-part program be developed to prevent reinjury:

1. Recovery of function
2. Education
3. Body awareness

Recovery of Function

Recovery of full function after an episode of low back pain may take anywhere from a few days to stretch some residual tightness after a brief episode to several months for cases in which major damage occurred to the disc and clients need to recover normal motion, strength, and endurance. Recovery of full function is necessary to prevent future injury due to the shrinking of the scar tissue that may limit full recovery of motion and to prevent secondary problems, such as adherences of the nerve root and contractures.

Most of these problems can be successfully managed by clients independently at home with careful guidance and instruction. Aerobic programs, including swimming, walking, jogging, rowing, and bicycling, should be implemented with general and specific stretching and strengthening exercises. Stretching exercises should emphasize the production and maintenance of full lumbar flexion, extension, and rotation. Strengthening should emphasize the abdominal muscles, back, hip, and knee extensors.

Patient Education

Teaching clients to recognize situations that pose a significant risk to the lumbar spine and to correct or modify risk-related activities or positions is a major part of client education. Clients need to know which postures and positions will aggravate symptoms. These instructions will vary depending on the type of problem producing the pain. Clients with histories of posterior disc derangements or significant restrictions in forward flexion as a result of tight tissue need to be aware of the high-risk postures and activities and the resultant corrective actions listed in Table 4–5. High-risk postures and corrective actions for those clients with histories of anterior derangements, stenosis, or extension restrictions as a result of tight tissue are listed in Table 4–6.

Body Awareness

Another component of the education process is to make clients aware of the early signs and symptoms of low back problems. As mentioned earlier, the back has a marvelous system of sensors that provides accurate information about the status of the lumbar structures. It is important for clients to realize that these early warning signals must be heeded and that early intervention can correct the problem in its formative stages. Instituting minor actions such as correcting posture, simple exercises, or correcting faulty body mechanics may be all that is needed at this early stage.

COMMUNITY PREVENTION PROGRAMS

Back pain is not limited to or more common among those people who perform heavy labor. This syndrome affects laborers, managers, and

Table 4–5. Posterior Derangement: High-Risk Postures, Activities, and Corrective Actions

High-Risk Postures or Activities	Corrective Actions
Prolonged sitting, especially in automobiles, soft chairs, and poor desk chairs, and after exercise	Use lumbar roll; stand up and walk once every hour; perform 10 arches of the lumbar spine each hour; increase alertness for poor posture after exercise or when fatigued
Bending or lifting especially after prolonged sitting, after resting for more than 1 hour, or upon the first-time lifting of the day	Maintain gentle lordosis while lifting; lift with legs and not back; make sure that extension is pain-free and unrestricted before and after lifting
Sleeping in a flexed posture (fetal position on a mattress or box spring that lost its firmness)	Sleep on the side with the bottom leg extended; sleep on the back with lumbar support; rotate mattress or box spring every 3 months and purchase new mattress and box spring every 8 to 10 years

nonworkers with about the same frequency (Deyo and Tsui, 1987; Waddell, 1987; Waddell and Allan, 1989). Throughout this chapter, we have emphasized that certain activities and concepts should be implemented to avoid problems

Table 4–6. Anterior Derangement: High-Risk Postures, Activities, and Corrective Actions

High-Risk Postures or Activities	Corrective Actions
Prolonged sitting or standing	Avoid swayback or excessively lordotic positions; use chairs with softer cushioning and less lumbar support
Lifting or bending	Maintain posterior pelvic tilt while lifting and returning from the flexed position
Sleeping on stomach	Use softer mattress or box spring and avoid sleeping on stomach
Walking or running	Maintain posterior pelvic tilt during activities

with the low back, including adjusting the life-style to a healthier pattern by balancing the flexion and extension postures and movements, cessation of smoking, listening to one's body signals, avoidance of positions and repetitive movements that produce a prolonged loading of the spine, and maintaining good aerobic and musculoskeletal fitness. Programs that incorporate these activities and concepts and that are established by industry or by individuals do not demand any significant outlay of funds or time. What most low back pain prevention programs do demand is a commitment to consistency. Caring for the body is a 24-hour responsibility, and the concepts, activities, and exercises must be implemented frequently and consistently.

Good body mechanics, maintenance of good musculoskeletal conditioning, and the development of good health habits are necessary not only to decrease the frequency of low back pain but also to improve job efficiency. A good prophylactic program to prevent all forms of musculoskeletal problems not only prevents pain but is good business. The basic components of a general prophylactic program to prevent low back pain are as follows:

1. An education program to discuss proper care of the back, the prevention or control of high-risk activities, and early intervention techniques if symptoms arise
2. A program to improve the lumbar support of chairs, to improve the efficiency of work surfaces, and to identify proper positioning and support for sitting and work
3. Regular relief periods during the day that not only allow a change in position but that also incorporate gentle stretching and calisthenics. Japanese industry has long used short exercise periods at the beginning of and throughout the workday to prevent injury and increase productivity. Such programs include the activities listed in Table 4–7. Alternative exercises could be incorporated into the program to

---

Table 4–7. Low Back Exercises That Should Be Incorporated Into Work Relief Breaks

Lumbar extensions
Lumbar flexions
Lumbar rotations
Lumbar side flexions
Gentle walking or jogging in place

---

specifically address other musculoskeletal problems.
4. Aerobic exercise three times each week. The characteristics of such a program are listed in Table 4–1.
5. Stress-management program. Although stress does not actually cause back dysfunction, it has been shown to be a factor in its severity and resultant disability.

SUMMARY

Low back pain is a ubiquitous problem. Low back disability is costly not only to society but to individuals and families as well (Snook and Webster, 1987). For the vast majority of clients seen by medical professionals low back pain is self-limiting. The most important role of therapists in the management of low back pain is not in eliminating the pain, but rather in preventing disability. As a result, therapists must become more active in the community, fostering prophylactic programs and focusing treatment not on modulation of symptoms but on function and ability.

References

Adams MA and Hutton WC: The effect of posture on the fluid content of the lumbar intervertebral disc. Spine 8:665–672, 1983.

Adams MA and Hutton WC: Gradual disc prolapse. Spine 10:524–531, 1985.

Adams MA and Hutton WC: The relevance of torsion to the mechanical derangement of the lumbar spine. Spine 5:241–247, 1981.

American College of Sports Medicine: Position paper on the recommended quality and quantity of exercise for developing and maintaining fitness. Med Sci Sports Exerc 10(1):vii–x, 1978.

Ashman R: Disc anatomy and biomechanics. Spine State of the Art Rev 3(1):1–12, 1989.

Berquist-Ullman M and Larson U: Acute low back pain in industry. Acta Orthop Scand (Suppl) 170:1–117, 1977.

Berwick DM, Budman S, and Feldstein M, et al: No clinical effect of back schools in an HMO. Spine 14:338–344, 1989.

Bigos SJ and Battie MC: Acute care to prevent back disability. Clin Orthop 221:121–129, 1987.

Bigos SJ, et al: Back injuries in industry: A retrospective study II. Spine 11:246–251, 1986a.

Bigos SJ, et al: Back injuries in industry: A retrospective study III. Spine 11:252–256, 1986b.

Bogduk N: The innervation of the cervical intervertebral disc. Spine 13:2–8, 1988.

Bogduk N: Innervation, pain patterns, and mechanics of pain production. In Twomey LT and Taylor JR (eds): Physical Therapy of the Low Back. London, Churchill Livingstone, 1987.

Bogduk N and Twomey L: Clinical Anatomy of the Lumbar Spine. London, Churchill Livingstone, 1987.

Bogduk N, Tynan W, and Wilson AS: The nerve supply to the human lumbar intervertebral discs. J Anat 132:39–56, 1981.

Burton AK and Tillotson KM: Prediction of low-back trouble frequency in a working population. Spine 14:939–946, 1989.

Cady L, Bischoff D, and O'Connel E: Strength and fitness and subsequent back injuries in firefighters. J Occup Med 21:269–272, 1979.

Crock HV: Internal disc disruption: A challenge to disc prolapse fifty years later. Spine 11:650–653, 1986.

Deyo RA: Conservative therapy for low back pain. JAMA 250:1057–1062, 1983.

Deyo RA and Bass JE: Lifestyle and low-back pain: The influence of smoking and obesity. Spine 14:501–506, 1989.

Deyo RA, et al: How many days of bed rest for low back pain? N Engl J Med 315:1064–1070, 1986.

Deyo RA and Tsui WU: Descriptive epidemiology of low back pain and its related medical care in the United States. Spine 12:264–272, 1987.

DiMaggio A and Mooney V: Conservative care for low back pain: What works? J Musculoskel Med 4(9):27–34, 1987.

Dwyer AP: Backache and its prevention. Clin Orthop 222:35–43, 1987.

Frymoyer JW: Back pain and sciatica. N Engl J Med 318:291–300, 1988.

Frymoyer JW and Cats-Baril W: Predictors of low back pain disability. Clin Orthop 221:89–98, 1987.

Hayne C: Back schools and total back-care programmes—a review. Physiotherapy 70:14–17, 1984.

Henker FO: Accident proneness and how to prevent it. Clin Orthop 222:30–34, 1987.

Hickey DS and Hukins DWL: Relationship between the structure and function of the annulus fibrosus and the function and failure of the intervertebral disc. Spine 5:106–111, 1980.

Kelsey JL, Githens PB, and O'Connor T: Acute prolapsed lumbar intervertebral disc: An epidemiological study with special reference to driving automobiles and cigarette smoking. Spine 9:608–613, 1984.

Kraemer J: Intervertebral Disc Disease. Chicago, Year Book Publishers, 1981.

Linton S and Kamwendo K: Low back schools. A critical review. Phys Ther 67:1375–1383, 1987.

Linton S, Bradley LA, Jensen I, et al: The secondary prevention of low back pain: A controlled study with follow-up. Pain 36:197–207, 1989.

McKenzie RA: Mechanical diagnosis and theory of low back pain: Toward a better understanding. In Twomey LT and Taylor JR (eds): Physical Therapy of the Low Back. London, Churchill Livingstone, 1987.

Mooney V: Where is the pain coming from? Spine 12:754–759, 1987.

Nachemson A: Advances in low back pain. Clin Orthop 200:266–273, 1985.

Nachemson A: The lumbar spine: An orthopedic challenge. Spine 1:9–21, 1976.

Nachemson A: Work for all, for those with low back pain as well. Clin Orthop 179:77–85, 1983.

Oliver MJ, et al: An interpretation of the McKenzie approach to low back pain. In Twomey LT and Taylor JR (eds): Physical Therapy of the Low Back. London, Churchill Livingstone, 1987.

Snook SH and Webster BS: The cost of disability. Clin Orthop 221:77–84, 1987.

Spengler DM, et al: Back injuries in industry: A retrospective study I. Spine 11:241–245, 1986.

Spitzer W (ed): Scientific approach to the assessment and management of activity related spinal disorders: Report of the Quebec Taskforce on Spinal Disorders. Spine 7(Suppl 7s):1–55, 1987.

States JD: The prevention of injury secondary to motor vehicle accidents. Clin Orthop 222:21–29, 1987.

Taylor JR and Twomey LT: Lumbar posture, movement, and mechanics. In Twomey LT and Taylor JR (eds): Physical Therapy of the Low Back. London, Churchill Livingstone, 1987.

Taylor JR and Twomey LT: The lumbar spine from infancy to old age. In Twomey LT and Taylor JR (eds): Physical Therapy of the Low Back. London, Churchill Livingstone, 1987.

Twomey LT and Taylor JR: Age changes in lumbar vertebrae and intervertebral discs. Clin Orthop 221:97–103, 1987.

Twomey LT and Taylor JR: Unsuspected damage to lumbar zygapophyseal (facet) joints after motor vehicle accidents. Med J Aust 151:210–217, 1989.

Vanharanta H: Etiology, epidemiology, and natural history of lumbar disc disease. Spine State of the Art Rev 3(1):1–12, 1989.

Vanharanta H and Mooney V: The relationship of pain provocation to lumbar disc deterioration as seen by CT/discogram. Spine 12:295–301, 1987.

Vanharanta H, et al: McKenzie exercise, backtrac, and back schools in lumbar syndrome. Abstract of the International Society for the Study of the Lumbar Spine, Dallas, June 1, 1986.

Videman T, et al: Patient handling skills, back injuries, and back pain. An intervention study in nursing. Spine 14:148–158, 1989.

Waddell G: A new model for the treatment of low-back pain. Spine 12:632–644, 1987.

Waddell G, and Allan DB: An historical perspective on low back pain and disability. Acta Orthop Scand 60 (Suppl 234):1–24, 1989.

Weisel S and Rothman R: Industrial Low Back Pain. Charlottesville, VA, Michie, 1985.

Yasuma T, et al: Histological changes in aging lumbar intervertebral discs. J Bone Joint Surg 72A:221–229, 1990.

CHAPTER
5

Wayne W. Rath
Jean Duffy Rath

Prevention of Musculoskeletal Injury

This chapter presents a new and unique system of injury or disorder prevention for the musculoskeletal system. It is a mechanically based approach that attempts to educate the individual and change the postural and movement habits that contribute to cumulative and repeated strain injuries of the musculoskeletal system. We have drawn on our experience with the pioneering work of McKenzie (1972, 1979, 1981, 1983, 1988, 1990) developing our approach to musculoskeletal injury prevention. The postulates of this preventive strategy are listed in Table 5–1.

The McKenzie system of diagnosis, treatment, and prevention of mechanical disorders of the spine should be reviewed by the reader who is interested in understanding the contents of this chapter more thoroughly (McKenzie, 1981, 1990). The McKenzie approach uses clinical strategies to prevent recurrence of a disorder that has required treatment. We take this approach a step further to prevent the development of the disorder in the first place. However, after applying this on a purely preventive level, we quickly determined that many individuals who deny a history of musculoskeletal disorders do not meet our simplest criteria for full mechanical function (the ability to move the joints to end-range repeatedly without pain). Nor have many of the individuals who state that they have recovered from a previous episode met these same stan-

dards, and by our definition these persons have not fully recovered. Thus, they are a problem looking for a place to develop or recur, and they progress toward the disability trap.

We will begin describing our approach to injury prevention by establishing some basic principles and definitions and by reviewing the McKenzie approach. We can then look at the various musculoskeletal regions and discuss the prevention of common mechanical problems. It should be noted that we are addressing only the basic mechanical aspects of musculoskeletal injury prevention. We recognize that the most effective method of injury prevention, especially

---

Table 5–1. Postulates for the Prevention of Musculoskeletal Injury

1. Musculoskeletal disorders are mechanical disorders which require mechanical solutions.
2. Effective treatment strategies can be developed into effective prevention programs.
3. A cause and effect relationship between pain and function is essential in teaching individual responsibility for self-care with mechanical disorders.
4. An analysis of the effect of repeated movements and sustained positions on pain production and pain relief is the most important factor in developing a treatment and prevention strategy.
5. Mechanical disorders can be prevented from developing, recurring, or progressing with understanding and a change of mechanical lifestyle habits.

---

in industry, requires a multidisciplinary approach to address the numerous factors that contribute to these disorders.

BASIC PRINCIPLES

The musculoskeletal system is the mechanical or moving parts system of the body. It is an intricate connection of joints that allows positions to be assumed and movements to occur under a tremendous variation of physical conditions. Problems that arise in this mechanical system present with symptoms, most frequently pain, that are influenced by movements and positions. Thus one issue critical to the concept of musculoskeletal illness prevention is to define normal mechanical function (musculoskeletal wellness). It is from a conceptual framework of normal mechanical function that abnormal occurrences can be prevented or at least recognized in the earlier stages of development and managed more efficiently. *The basis for normal mechanical function in this chapter is the individual's ability to move his or her joint systems through a complete range of motion repeatedly without pain.*

A second issue critical to our concepts in the prevention of musculoskeletal disorders is the recognition that, when disorders develop, most are nonspecific. The pathophysiology of these disorders is not well understood, and despite the diagnostic labeling, the exact structural source of symptoms is invariably unknown. As part of preventive strategy, an understanding of how to classify and manage a nonspecific disorder is essential. This allows a more reliable method of intervening to prevent a recurrence and a progression into a more significant (structurally specific) condition. *The basis for the classification of nonspecific mechanical disorders in this chapter is the mechanism of pain production with repeated end-range movements and sustained end-range positions.* This concept has been pioneered by McKenzie (1981, 1990).

A third issue critical to the prevention of musculoskeletal disorders involves the concept of injury itself. Most musculoskeletal problems are the result of cumulative mechanical stress and strain and not the result of an actual injury (Hadler, 1987). The main clinical findings are pain with an impairment of movement or function (Spitzer et al, 1987). However, there is a strong case in many of these disorders to suggest that there is no tissue damage related to these

findings, no less any actual injury (McKenzie, 1981, 1990). The psychosocial implications of the labels and the wording used to describe these common mechanical disturbances require strong consideration. Musculoskeletal impairment and disability can be influenced strongly by the individual's perceptions, which are nurtured by the diagnostic label and conceptual framework for treatment (Allan and Waddell, 1989; Hadler, 1987; Waddell, 1987). *The preventive strategy in this chapter is based on common sense, is mechanically oriented, and encourages confidence in the patient to regain function and take responsibility for the care of the mechanical parts of his or her body.*

See Table 5–2 for definitions of musculoskeletal injury prevention terms that are used in this chapter.

Mechanical Diagnosis

The title *Mechanical Diagnosis and Therapy* was conceived by McKenzie (1981, 1990) to emphasize the importance of movements and positions in the assessment and management of musculoskeletal disorders. The proposition was that if mechanical forces gave rise to the symptoms and to a loss of function associated with a musculoskeletal disorder, then a meticulous assessment of the effect of mechanical force on the client's symptoms and function would define the disorder and provide the most efficient method of recovery. The understanding of the "mechanics" of the disorder and the procedures that led to recovery would ultimately provide a system that would prevent a recurrence of the same disorder. The clinical success in applying this concept to clients led to the development of a mechanically based system that is logical, measurable, and effective. The classification of the disorder by assessing the mechanics is the diagnostic portion of this system.

McKenzie first applied his concepts to the spinal regions, particularly to the lower back. He recognized that the structure(s) giving rise to the symptoms is not known in most mechanical disorders of the spine. Thus an alternative method of diagnosis (or classification) is required for these nonspecific disorders. The new method that he developed utilized an analysis of the characteristics of the pain response to repeated end-range movements and sustained end-range positions. A pattern of response emerged, which led to the definition of three main mechanical

Table 5–2. Terminology for Musculoskeletal Injury Prevention

Mechanical Pain: the activation of the nociceptive system as a result of sufficient mechanical deformation (distortion) of the pain-sensitive tissues within the musculoskeletal system. Thus, this is pain that develops or is affected by movements, positions, or activities (Cyriax, 1982; McKenzie, 1981, 1990).

Posture: the position in which a joint or series of joints in the musculoskeletal system is held while moving (dynamic posture) or not moving (static posture).

General Mechanical Definitions: The following will aid in our analysis of mechanical function of the body:*

Stress: forces set up between neighboring particles when a tissue is strained (i.e., theory of elasticity is the study of the relationship between stresses and strains).

Strain: the amount of deformation in relationship to the application of stress.

Elasticity: the ability of a body tissue, once strained to return to its original shape. Fluid exhibits elasticity in volume and not shape. Solids exhibit elasticity in shape and size. Is measured as the relaxation time.

Viscoelastic: the strain response is time dependent secondary to the interplay of fluids and solids in relationship to the application of stress. It is measured as the amount of creep deformation of the tissues.

Hysteresis: the phenomenon by which energy is lost when a stress is applied to a body tissue, and as a consequence the strain effect is altered. This plays an important role in understanding fatigue failure of tissues.

Application of Mechanical Forces to a Joint System: The following defines the spectrum of mechanical forces that are applied during the mechanical assessment and treatment of musculoskeletal disorders (Fig. A):

Mid-range: the range of movement or positions in which the soft tissues surrounding and attached to the joint(s) are on slack.

End-range: the range of movement or position in which the soft tissues surrounding or attached to the joint(s) have had the slack removed and are under tension.

End-range with Overpressure: the additional tension applied to the joint(s) once it has reached end-range by pushing it further into that position or direction of motion.

Intermittent Mechanical Stress: the application of mechanical force on a cyclical basis.

Sustained Mechanical Stress: the maintenance of a mechanical force.

Mechanisms of Soft-Tissue Failure: The mechanical system will fail when the soft or connecting tissues are strained beyond the point of elastic deformation. This can happen suddenly or eventually, depending on whether the mechanical forces are cumulative, repeated, or extreme. In either regard, the tissue failure occurs at the end-range with varying amounts of overpressure (Nordin and Frankle, 1989; Panjabi and White, 1990).

Frank Trauma: When the sudden application of a large mechanical force takes the joint tissues to the limit of its extensibility and beyond, sudden tissue injury occurs. The subsequent repair of this injury is guided by the body's stages of healing, and the mechanism of onset is clearly identified. However, most musculoskeletal disorders do not fall into this category, especially in the spine and upper extremities.

Cumulative Trauma: When the application of mechanical forces that are not enough in themselves to cause tissue failure are repeated and sustained in an imbalanced fashion over a sufficient time period, fatigue failure can occur. This is the more common mechanism of onset for musculoskeletal disorders, and the cause is often obscure and its recognition influenced by many nonmechanical factors.

Warning Signs: those transient signs and symptoms that precede the development of a mechanical disorder. Example: aching, discomfort, stiffness, tension, or pain when repeating or performing certain movements or sustaining certain positions.

Musculoskeletal Wellness: refers to the condition in which the mechanical system can move in all intended directions or freedoms of movement to end-range with overpressure repeatedly without pain production. However, wellness also includes the individual's working knowledge of how to strive to maintain this status.

*The stress/strain curve for collagen tissues can be used to explain the effect of mechanical forces acting on the musculoskeletal system (see also Fig. 5–3).

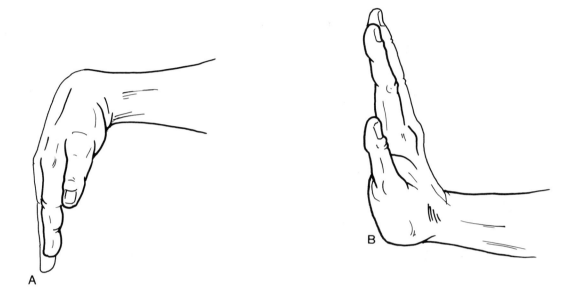

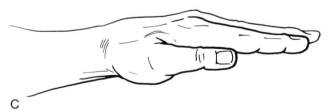

Table 5–2. Wrist joint example. *A,* Wrist joint at end-range flexion. *B,* Wrist joint at end-range extension. *C,* Wrist joint in mid-range flexion-extension. Overpressure at end-range would involve adding force to push the joint further into the motion to test the elasticity of the soft tissues surrounding the joint. This example is used to teach the concepts of normal movement, importance of good posture, and normal joint strain and pain.

syndromes: postural, dysfunction, and derange-ment syndromes. In 1987, an independent group of experts came to the same conclusions regard-ing the classification of activity-related spinal disorders (Spitzer et al, 1987); that is, in most spinal disorders the structure giving rise to the problem is not known (approximately 90%). Thus, the most reliable way of identifying groups of clients in this large category is by the pain (Table 5–3).

In the same year as the Quebec Task Force Report (1987), Hadler published a textbook out-lining the same diagnostic problems in both the spine and the extremities (Hadler, 1987). Also in 1987, Waddell put forth a new clinical model for low back pain, a biopsychosocial model, sug-gesting that much of the recent increase in low back pain disability is actually iatrogenic (Wad-dell, 1987). All three of these publications came to the same conclusion independently by a thor-ough review of the scientific literature. When we can accept the fact that we may not know the exact cause of these common mechanical com-plaints, the alternative classification system of McKenzie becomes extremely valuable. The in-tent is to explore the pain behavior to specific mechanical testing in order to identify the pat-terned response of one or more of the three mechanical syndromes identified by McKenzie (1981, 1990).

Postural Syndrome (McKenzie, 1981, 1990). This syndrome is characterized by a lack of pain production with repeated end-range movements. The joint or joints involved are moved repeatedly to end-range in all the directions they are con-structed to move, and pain cannot be produced with the movement. The only way in which pain can be produced is by placing the joint at end-range and by holding it there for a sustained period of time (perhaps 30 minutes). Then, once the pain is produced, the position is changed and the pain is now abolished. McKenzie uses the ''bent finger example'' to illustrate this mech-anism of pain production (Fig. 5–1). This syn-drome is recognized as a mechanical response in the extremities (sitting with legs crossed) and is managed mechanically (uncross legs). However, when this syndrome occurs in the spine (discom-fort at the base of the neck or lower back when sitting), it is attributed to stress or tension.

Dysfunction Syndrome (McKenzie, 1981, 1990). This syndrome is characterized by a loss of movement with an associated pain at the end-range of movement that neither gets better or worse with repetition. The pain pattern produced at end-range remains fixed in its location and is not present when in mid-range and the joint

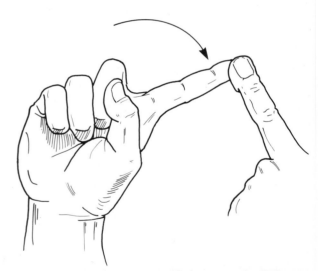

Figure 5–1. McKenzie's bent finger example. Pull your index finger backwards with your other hand until you feel strain. If you were to hold the finger in this position for 30 minutes or repeat the motion too frequently without interruption you would eventually feel pain. Let the finger go and the pain goes away. There is no damage. The pain is a warning that you should interrupt the position or movement more often. If you don't listen to this warning and continue to hold that position for hours a day plus move the finger in that same direction hundreds to thousands of times each day, damage may eventually develop.

Table 5–3. The McKenzie Classification System*

Quebec Task Force Classification	Possible McKenzie Classification
Class I	Derangements 1–4, 7 Flexion, extension dysfunction Postural syndrome
Class II	Derangements 1–4, 7 Adherent nerve root
Class III	Derangements 5–6 Adherent nerve root

*The McKenzie classification system attempts to subdivide the nonspecific (classes I–III) spinal disorders so that a more specific treatment strategy is developed (McKenzie, 1981; Spitzer et al, 1987).

structures are not being stretched. This pattern of response behaves as if the tissues are stiff and have lost their normal elasticity. This condition needs to move the affected joints in the direction that produces the pain to regain a normal end-range response, at a normal point in the range of movement. This syndrome develops as the body repairs itself in response to trauma or to an acute episode of pain, or as a result of disuse. To illustrate the mechanism of pain behavior in this syndrome, the example of a casted elbow can be used. Thus, when one fractures one's arm it is often casted to maintain the alignment of the fractured ends of the bone while these ends heal. After sufficient time for healing has elapsed, the cast is removed and the client notices that the elbow is stiff and hurts when he or she attempts to move to end-range extension or flexion. The pain is no longer due to the fracture, because the fracture has healed. The pain is due to the tightness, or loss of elasticity, in the soft tissues that were injured and have healed as well as the tissues that have not been moved normally during the period of immobilization.

The stiffness that develops as a result of having to wear a cast is easily understood. The need to regain the lost motion after removal of the cast is apparent, and the discomfort with achieving this is expected. However, a cast-like situation exists when an individual's mechanical habits include an exclusion of certain movements in his or her lifestyle. And certainly, after tissue damage (either externally generated or self-imposed) the repaired tissue creates stiffness unless the tissue is stretched appropriately to regain elasticity and strength. However, in many situations the individual is either told, or believes, that if there is pain it should be avoided. But unfortunately in the case of the dysfunction syndrome, this is the wrong conclusion and the stiffness in the tissue is perpetuated and an aberrant learned behavior is reinforced.

Derangement Syndrome (McKenzie, 1981, 1990). This syndrome is characterized by a production of pain during the movement (mid-range as well as at end-range) that can be made both better or worse with repeated testing. The location of the pain often changes, and the individual finds that he or she has an impairment of movement due to pain in a rather sudden time frame (immediately or for hours or several days). This rapid change in function, changing the location of pain and the point in the range of movement in which it is affected, led McKenzie to speculate

that there was an internal derangement of joint tissue.

To illustrate this mechanism of pain production, the trick knee example can be used. When an individual has torn or displaced the cartilage within the knee, the joint complex is now susceptible to bizarre mechanical behavior. Thus, when the person is walking down the street, a sudden twisting motion may lead to immediate pain and locking of the joint. The individual or clinician who has experience with this situation will push, pull, or move the joint in a particular way that will unlock the joint and immediately improve or restore the function and relieve the pain. This mechanical derangement of the joint could be due to an injury or to attrition of the joint over many years of repeated stress. The implications of this problem vary with the severity of the strain on the tissues and the external forces the individual must negotiate in normal (work/home/recreation) function.

The mechanics of the derangement require understanding to resolve the disorder as rapidly as it developed, and the individual must learn how to mechanically prevent its recurrence. The natural history of many of these acute episodic disorders indicates that these problems are temporary and they will resolve spontaneously (Cyriax, 1982; Hadler, 1987; McKenzie 1981, 1990 Waddell, 1987). However, recurrent episodes encourage a progression of the same disorder that may become more chronic and disabling. Thus, it is important that the client should participate in his or her recovery, and that he or she should be instructed with biomechanical education how to individually manage the disorder over the long term. There is evidence that the McKenzie approach provides this mechanism for clients with low back pain disorders (McKenzie, 1979; Roberts, 1989; Stankovich and Johnell, 1990).

Progression from Postural Pain to Dysfunction and Derangement. Unless trauma is the mechanism of onset, these mechanical disorders begin with pain of postural origin. As the bent finger example illustrated, pain of this origin is transient and does not interfere with function. However, when the mechanical system is exposed continuously to these sustained end-range strains, the tissue can become more irritable and can be provoked more easily (less time sustained). This can lead eventually to enough attenuation of the tissue that a normal movement, with sufficient mechanical loading, can cause tissue failure. Thus a derangement syndrome is created as a progression of the postural syndrome. As with trauma, as the tissue repairs itself immobilization and a failure to regain full mechanical function can then lead to development of a dysfunction syndrome.

When poor postural or positional habits encourage movements in one direction and discourage movements in others, stiffness and shortening of the soft tissues develop because of disuse. Thus a dysfunction syndrome is created as a progression of the postural syndrome. If the client continues to function in this mechanically imbalanced fashion, the dysfunction syndrome will then encourage the development of the derangement syndrome.

In either case, pain with movement becomes a part of the mechanical response of adopting certain positions or performing certain movements. In dysfunction, the pain occurs at end range and requires weeks to eliminate. In derangement, the pain occurs throughout the movement, and in the earlier stages it can be very transient or episodic. Clients, and all too often clinicians, do not understand these mechanisms of pain production and consequently create a certain fear of its development. The frequently heard remarks, "if it hurts don't do it," translate into a mechanical behavior pattern that facilitates the vicious mechanical disability cycle (Fig. 5–2).

This is when the importance of the bent finger and the other mechanical analogies are established in helping the client to understand the disorder. This can then be correlated to the client's specific situation and can be used not only to explain the stages of treatment but also to predict the outcome and time frame.

Mechanical Treatment

The strategy of treatment is determined by the mechanical diagnosis (McKenzie, 1981, 1990). The postural syndrome requires postural correction alone; the dysfunction syndrome requires stretching; and the derangement syndrome requires reduction.

The procedures utilized in mechanical therapy are described as a progression of mechanical force (McKenzie, 1981, 1989, 1990). These procedures begin with the client's own positions and movements (*self-generated force*) and progress to include therapist-generated force (*externally generated force*) when required. The general intention is to restore normal movement or mechanical wellness. As mentioned previously, we define this mechanical wellness as the ability to move without pain. As apparent and obvious as that statement may be, it requires much closer inspection to understand.

Restoration of a Normal End-Range Response. As mentioned with the bent finger example, normal joint tissues can give rise to pain. This implies a warning mechanism that the extreme of motion has been reached, and any further movement may cause tissue damage (McKenzie, 1981, 1983, 1988, 1990). This can occur immediately if you bring the finger back very forcefully or it can occur eventually due to viscoelastic response of the tissue to end-range loading.

Mechanical Pain/Disability Cycle

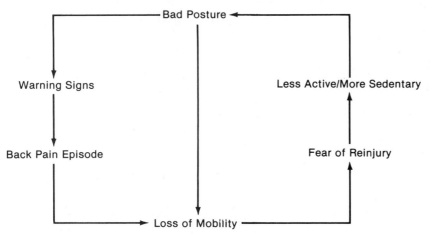

Figure 5–2. The mechanical aspects of pain and disability that require clinical and prophylactic attention.

Figure 5–3. A normal end-range response is found when applying overpressure in the elastic zone, and strain is felt before the perception of pain.

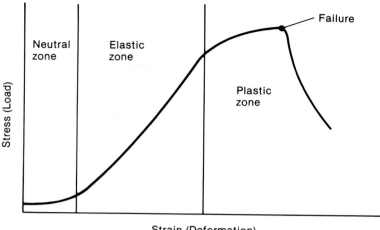

However, if we assess the response more closely, we will see a very distinct pattern of response in normal joint tissue (Fig. 5–3).

In normal tissue there is a healthy amount of motion in this zone of elasticity. Exploration of this mechanical zone has been a major concern of manual clinicians for centuries. Joint manipulation, mobilization, massage, and traction have been historic mechanical procedures to restore this normal end-range response.

In the McKenzie terms, the mechanism of abnormality in this end-range response is more easily understood and managed. In the derangement syndrome, the normal end-range response is obstructed in the mid-ranges, and once the obstruction has been removed, it is immediately restored. However, in the dysfunction syndrome the end-range response is restricted and the zone of elasticity begins prematurely and is abnormally small. The dysfunction syndrome requires remodeling to restore this normal end-range response, and this frequently requires weeks to months of stretching. In the postural syndrome the end-range response is normal, and a strategy to maintain this response is then implemented.

Thus the overall treatment goals are to (1) eliminate pain, (2) restore full "normal" function, and (3) prevent a recurrence and progression of the disorder. However, as is now apparent, the method of achieving this result is quite different in the three syndromes.

Prevention of Recurrence. Prevention is achieved through emphasis on the client's responsibility for his or her recovery and also on a full exploration of self-generated forces before progressing to externally applied forces. Those self-treatment procedures that led to or aided in the recovery of this episode become the main focus of an individualized prophylactic program for the client. Thus the treatment becomes the prophylaxis, and a specific yet simple long-term program is developed. Specific risk and predisposing factors to the disorder are identified. Then, through a correlation of the mechanical cause and effect of pain production and pain relief, the client is provided with a method of controlling the effect of these factors in both the present and the future. There is now evidence that the McKenzie approach can effectively achieve this long-term benefit in the management of mechanical conditions (McKenzie, 1979; Roberts, 1989; Stankovich and Johnell, 1990).

Thus, in summary, the McKenzie approach utilizes the analysis of pain response to movements and positions as a means of classification, treatment, and prevention. An emphasis on client responsibility in the management of the condition is emphasized. The client is taught to understand and control the pain behavior and to use it as a measurement of his or her mechanical wellness.

Musculoskeletal Disorders: Scope of the Problem. Musculoskeletal symptoms and impairment affect approximately 29.7 to 32.6% of the population of the United States, and back pain is the most frequent region to be involved (Cunningham and Kelsey, 1984). Table 5–4 reviews the estimated prevalence of musculoskeletal disorders in the United States as identified by Cunningham and Kelsey.

There is some recent evidence to suggest that the incidence and prevalence of these disorders,

Table 5–4. Estimated Prevalence of Musculoskeletal Disorders in the United States*

	Symptoms	Signs
Back	17.2	15.2
Shoulder	6.7	3.0
Elbow	4.2	1.2
Wrist	3.1	0.9
Fingers	6.8	4.4
Hip	8.2	3.2
Knee	13.3	12.1
Ankle	4.3	0.8
Foot	3.2	0.3

*From Cunningham LS and Kelsey JL: Epidemiology of musculoskeletal impairments and associated disability. Am J Public Health 74(6):574–579, 1984.

Table 5–5. Some Psychosocial Factors Commonly Associated with Increased Risk of Musculoskeletal Impairment and Disability*

Anxiety	Work dissatisfaction
Depression	Stress
Hypochondriasis	Hysteria
Somatization	

*Data from Hadler NM: Clinical Concepts in Regional Musculoskeletal Illness. New York, Grune & Stratton, 1987 and Waddell G: A new clinical model for the treatment of low-back pain. Spine 12(7):632–644, 1987.

especially low back pain, has remained consistent throughout the centuries of recorded medical history (Allan and Waddell, 1989). However, the changing statistic of recent time is the prevalence of musculoskeletal symptoms and impairment leading to disability. This increase in disability appears to be influenced more by psychologic and social factors than particular differences in clinical presentation (Table 5–5). (Allan and Waddell, 1989; Hadler, 1987; Waddell, 1987). Lower back pain is the greatest offender in this regard, with low back pain disability increasing 14 times faster than the population growth between 1971 and 1981 (Frymoyer and Mooney, 1986). Another interesting finding that is relevant to the main concepts of this chapter is the fact that persons reporting involvement of more than one body area are more likely to be disabled than those with only one body area involved (Table 5–6). It is possible that these are simply related regional disorders or referred pain from more proximal structures that can be managed easily if ap-

proached as a regional, nonspecific disorder rather than as an accumulation of specific structural diagnoses.

Regardless of the epidemiologic characteristics of individual musculoskeletal symptoms and impairments, they all have a common bond of symptoms (chiefly pain), a loss of function (aberrant movement), and an actual or perceived inability to participate fully in life's activities (impairment/disability). An understanding of the origins, affectations, and implications of these three factors provide the basis for a proactive strategy of injury prevention. This is regardless of whether the disorder is a result of self-generated forces, as outlined in Table 5–7 (cumulative trauma, repeated strain) or externally generated forces (frank trauma), the interplay of the biologic (mechanical), sociologic, and psychologic factors must be addressed (Waddell, 1987).

PROGRESSION OF A MECHANICAL DISORDER FROM WARNING SIGNS TO STRUCTURAL DIAGNOSIS

The following conceptual model outlines the progression of events from warning signs of im-

Table 5–6. A Prevalence of Impairment and Disability in the United States with Regional Musculoskeletal Disorders

	Moderate/Severe Restrictions of Activity	Change Job	>5 Days Work Loss
Upper extremity, lower extremity, back and neck	37.8	27.4	18.4
Upper and lower extremities	19.1	12.6	8.0
Upper extremity and back/neck	20.0	16.5	7.4
Lower extremity and back/neck	31.0	26.5	17.2
Upper extremity only	7.8	11.6	2.9
Lower extremity only	13.6	12.4	5.5
Back/neck only	17.8	16.3	14.2

Table 5–7. Mechanical Risk Factors for Symptoms in Particular Musculoskeletal Regions*

Low back	Motor vehicle operation
	Vibration
	Prolonged sitting
	Frequent bending/lifting
	Frequent twisting
Neck	Motor vehicle operation
	Vibration
	Prolonged sitting
	Prolonged protruded head position
	Frequent lifting
	Diving
Mid-back	Motor vehicle operation
	Prolonged sitting
	Prolonged protruded head position
	Frequent lifting
Shoulder	Frequent reaching/lifting
	Prolonged sitting/standing
	Frequent throwing movements
	Sustained elevation
Elbow/forearm	Strong/repeated gripping
	Sustained elbow position
	Frequent manipulations with hand
Wrist/hand	Frequent object manipulation
	Sustained wrist/hand positions
Hip	Repeated high-impact loading
	Trauma
Knee	Repeated high-impact loading
	Trauma
Ankle/foot	Repeated high-impact loading
	Trauma

*From Hadler NM: Clinical Concepts in Regional Musculoskeletal Illness. New York, Grune & Stratton, 1987.

pending mechanical problems, to the development of a nonspecific disorder, to an eventual structural diagnosis. The model makes apparent the importance of early intervention within this progression as a logical component of a musculoskeletal wellness program. The role of the identification of McKenzie's three mechanical syndromes (McKenzie, 1981, 1990) becomes apparent in these efforts to prevent both a recurrence and progression (Fig. 5–4).

Initial Warning Signs. The warning signs of a developing mechanical disorder are common, daily occurrences. They are usually described as aching, stiffness, discomfort, tension, or pain. As defined previously, they are transient and do not pose any particular problem with regard to normal mechanical functioning. However, when these signs are ignored or rationalized as the product of emotional stress they can accumulate

into an episode of more acute pain. This acute pain may be associated with muscle guarding or spasm, and movement or function does become painful and sometimes impossible for a short period. This scenario is most classically typified by the sudden back or neck "attack" that develops after a person performs a movement or activity that does not normally cause any difficulties. The individual is usually in a significant amount of pain and has difficulty in moving for a few hours to days, and then the disorder disappears almost as mysteriously as it came. McKenzie's bent finger example is a classic teaching model for this concept of how mechanical warning signs can progress into an acute pain episode (McKenzie, 1981, 1983, 1988, 1990).

Nonspecific Disorders Come Second. This refers to the development of distinct patterns of pain and symptoms, that increase by certain mechanical tests, but the exact structure giving rise to these symptoms cannot be accurately identified. Deduction from the response to the specific tests can put forth a hypothesis regarding the source of the problem. However, this cannot be supported conclusively.

This is unfortunately the most frequent categorization of client seeking treatment for musculoskeletal disorders (Hadler, 1987; Spitzer et al, 1987). However, our proclivity to structural diagnosis compels us to place a label on the disorder, which may or not be right. It is with the utmost discipline that clinicians must refrain from believing they know the actual structure giving rise to the client's symptoms, even if the client gets better during the course of treatment. Nonspecific disorders are mainly self-limiting, and this factor complicates the issue (McKenzie, 1981, 1990; Vanharanta, 1989). The clinician or client, who resolves the pain over a period of time, may ascribe the recovery to the remedies or treatment, when it was merely the passage of time that improved the condition. If we begin to believe that we know the source of the client's problem, we may limit the client's recovery and overlook his or her more specific needs.

Recurrence becomes a major concern with the treatment or management of these nonspecific disorders. It is with the recurrent episodes that the disorder can progress to a more significant problem. Failure to restore musculoskeletal wellness during recovery and failure to control the mechanical factors associated with the mechanism of onset encourage this progression. Worse still, to provide them with a structural label that

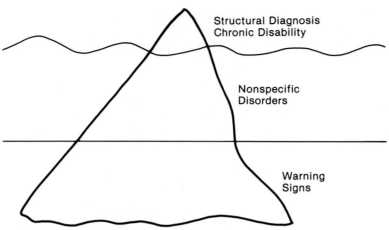

Figure 5–4. Tip of the iceberg: The chronic disabling disorders are few in number and represent the progression over time and the mechanical disorders of poor posture and imbalanced movement.

limits their options may actually facilitate a perception of impairment and disability (Allan and Waddell, 1989; Hadler, 1987; Waddell, 1987).

Structural Diagnosis Follows. The development of a confirmed herniation of the disc or a carpal tunnel syndrome or a rotator cuff tear is often the end result of years of warning signs and more minor nonspecific disturbances. This conceptual model is essential to preventing the incidence and morbidity of mechanical disorders. It is also important for recognition of persons at greater risk for developing a chronic, disabling disorder.

Chronic Disability Comes Last. When a structural label cannot be placed on the client's disorder, or if the subsequent invasive treatment applied to that structure fails, the results are disastrous. This group of clients represents the greatest loss economically, emotionally, and socially. In low back pain alone, only 7 to 10% of all the millions of employees with work-related back incidents represents from 70 to 90% of the cost for this disorder (Snook, 1987). It should be the goal of any preventive strategy not to allow this small group of problems to develop. This is only possible with a proactive strategy that takes more seriously the warning signs and lesser disorders and acts to correct the problem in these earlier stages. In this chapter we have emphasized methods of mechanical identification and correction, but we fully appreciate that there are psychosocial and ergonomic considerations that must also be identified and dealt with.

Trauma Speeds Up the Whole Progression. When an external force causes sudden failure of soft tissues, those lifestyle factors associated with

cumulative trauma disorders can wreak havoc with the injury. McKenzie often illustrates a cut finger analogy to the client to communicate the importance of posture and mechanical stresses in effecting the quality and timing of the repair response to trauma (McKenzie, 1981, 1990). Thus, if you were to cut your finger on the back of the knuckle and then repeatedly bend the finger to end-range thereafter, you would disrupt the repair response and prolong the time for healing. This is what happens to many musculoskeletal injuries when movement and postural habits are not corrected during the initial stages of healing. The most apparent example is the client who sustains a flexion injury and then continues to sit in a slouched fashion and repeatedly moves by flexing the lower back when changing positions and performing activities of daily living. The client interferes with the repair response and delays the recovery not intentionally but by effect of mechanical habits (posture and movements) on the injured tissues.

Management of trauma giving rise to soft tissue injury is guided by the stages of healing and by the severity of the injury: (1) stage 1 is the inflammatory phase (about 1 week) in which signals for repair are initiated; (2) stage 2 is the fibroblastic phase (up to 3 weeks) in which the scar tissues are being laid down; and (3) stage 3 is the remodeling phase, which lasts from 3 weeks on in which the scar tissue is maturing and is being organized to replace the injured tissue (Table 5–8).

The initial stages are concerned with the reduction of swelling and pain. Essential to achieving this is the elimination of mechanical factors

Table 5–8. Stages of Healing with Specific Regard to the Developing Tenacity and Maturity of the Scar Tissue

Inflammatory stage	1–7 days after injury. Rest, reduce pain and swelling.
Fibroblastic stage	7–21 days after injury. Initiate protected reactivation, beginning mid-range and working toward end-range.
Remodeling stage	21 days and thereafter. Progressive recovery of a normal end-range response with overpressure.

that will perpetuate this stage and increase the tissue irritability during this stage and subsequent stages.

The second stage is characterized by a need to initiate careful and appropriate movement. During this stage the new scar tissue is being laid down, and in order to promote a healthy and elastic structure it requires mechanical stress for its development. However, the tissues are not strong, and the mechanical stress should be gentle during this stage so as not to disrupt the process. Most of the movements should be in the mid-range, and by the end of the third week end-range motion should be possible.

Table 5–9. The Progression of a Mechanical Disorder from a Warning Sign to Pain and Loss of Function is Illustrated Utilizing the Three McKenzie Syndromes*

Postural Syndrome	**Warning Signs**
Normal tissue strained for a sustained period of time	↓
↓	
Dysfunction Syndrome	**Stiffness/Loss of Mobility**
	↓
Shortened/inelastic tissue prematurely strained when attempting normal end-range movements	
↓	
Derangement Syndrome	**Pain/Sudden Loss of Function**
Distorted, displaced, or disrupted tissues	

*Data from McKenzie RA: The Lumbar Spine: Mechanical Diagnosis and Therapy. Lower Hutt, New Zealand, Spinal Publications, 1981 and McKenzie RA: The Cervical and Thoracic Spine: Mechanical Diagnosis and Therapy. Waikanae, New Zealand, Spinal Publications, 1990.

The last stage is the remodeling phase and depends completely on mechanical stress and strain. The gradual application of overpressure at end-range from 3 weeks on enables the scar tissue to become fully elastic and organized. This helps to prevent a recurrence of the injury, because an inelastic scar tissue would prematurely give way under greater mechanical stress, as described earlier in defining the McKenzie dysfunction syndrome (McKenzie, 1981, 1990).

Summary of the Mechanical Progression Concept. Regardless of whether the mechanism of onset is cumulative trauma, repeated strain, or frank trauma, there are clear mechanical factors to identify, control, and utilize through their course of events. In some aspects the sudden injury is easier to deal with because it is apparent. However, the cumulative and repeated strain situation provides a greater opportunity to prevent its development and progression. The concept of a mechanical progression of injury is provided in Table 5–9.

REGIONAL STRATEGIES IN PREVENTING MUSCULOSKELETAL DISORDERS

Now that we have developed all the background information, we shall apply these concepts to the prevention of injury. Greater detail is provided regarding the management and prevention of back problems. The same general concepts can then be applied to the extremity disorders.

The musculoskeletal system can be approached as three major regions: (1) the spine or vertebral column, (2) the neck and upper extremity, and (3) the low back and lower extremity. A review of the possible location of symptoms originating in the spine (Cyriax, 1982; McKenzie, 1981, 1990; Spitzer et al, 1987) will emphasize the importance of attacking musculoskeletal disorders from this three-point, regional perspective (Fig. 5–5).

In the treatment of these disorders, it is imperative that a systematic analysis of the mechanical function of all joint systems capable of producing symptoms in the area of complaint be performed in the attempt to localize the origin of the symptoms (Cyriax, 1982; McKenzie, 1981, 1990). Equally as important in the prevention of these disorders is the regular assessment of the mechanical function of all the regional systems. This allows early detection of developing disorders and discourages confusion with regard to

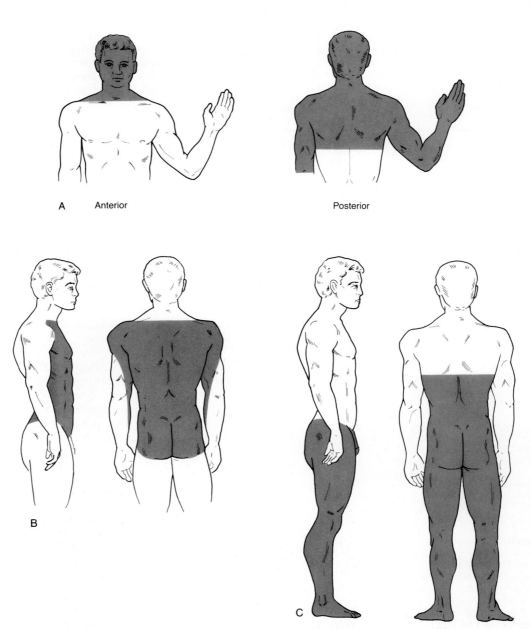

Figure 5–5. Pain pattern possibilities with mechanical disorders of the spine: *A*, cervical; *B*, thoracic; *C,* lumbar.

the origin of the warning signs or symptoms by establishing a repeatable cause and effect in pain behavior with certain movements.

Because the spine or vertebral column provides the foundation from which an assessment of musculoskeletal function begins, it is the first region to be assessed.

Vertebral Column as a Whole

The vertebral column consists of 24 movable vertebrae with three major regions; seven cervical, twelve thoracic, and five lumbar. Each of these regions of the spine is characterized by a curvature, described for its backward concavity (lordosis) in the cervical and lumbar regions and forward concavity (kyphosis) in the thoracic region. When analyzing the mechanical function of these regions, the curved nature of their structure has to be considered. This is especially important in determining end-range and mid-range positions, because they will be influenced by whether the curve is lordotic or kyphotic (Fig. 5–6).

Movements of the Spinal Column. The spinal column moves in all three cardinal planes: sagittal (flexion/extension), coronal (lateral bending), and transverse (axial rotation). The most mobile region is the cervical spine, and the thoracic region is the least mobile (Kapandji, 1976; Panjabi and White, 1990). However, the lumbar region undergoes the greatest amount of mechanical stress and strain due to the greater amount of body weight acting through the lumbopelvic area. Figure 5–7 illustrates the regional mobility of the vertebral column in the three cardinal planes of movement.

The mechanical effect of these movements is most easily understood by looking at the spinal motion segment (Fig. 5–8).

Flexion. This forward-bending motion rounds the spine and is the most frequently performed movement of the spinal column. This motion occurs when a person is slouched sitting, bending, lifting, reaching, bringing the knees towards the chest, protruding the head and neck forwards, or leaning forwards. It has been estimated that this lifting-carrying motion is performed between 3,000 and 5,000 times per day in our modernized society (Wood and Baddeley, 1987).

Extension. This backward-bending motion arches the spine and, in our westernized society, is a relatively infrequent movement. This motion

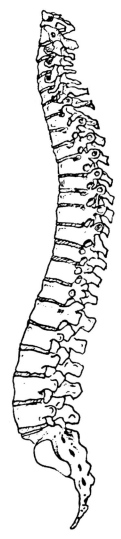

Figure 5–6. Vertebral column: The three main regions are the 7 cervical, 12 thoracic, and 5 lumbar vertebrae. The cervical spine and the lumbar spine have a natural lordosis (posterior concavity), and the thoracic region has a natural kyphosis (anterior concavity). These curves are vital to the strength, flexibility, and resiliency of the spine. They cannot be eliminated but rather are accentuated, reduced, or normalized during posture, movement, and position.

occurs when a person is sitting erect, standing, walking, running, lying on the stomach, propped up on elbows, reaching overhead, or looking upward. This motion of the spine is often stiff in individuals older than 30 years of age secondary to disuse (McKenzie, 1981).

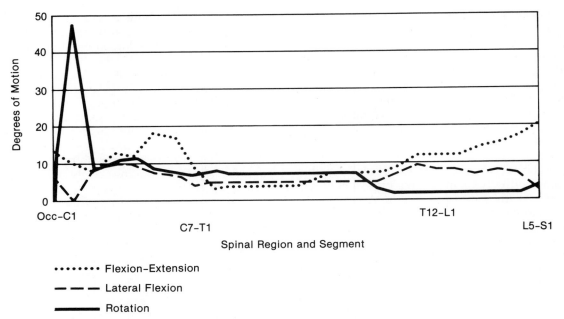

········· Flexion–Extension

— — — Lateral Flexion

———— Rotation

Figure 5–7. General mobility of the spine.

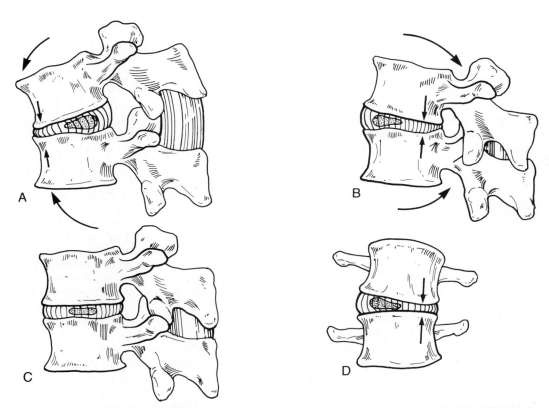

Figure 5–8. Spinal motion segments: *A*, flexion; *B*, extension; *C,* neutral; and *D,* lateral flexion.

Lateral Bending. This sideways motion creates a lateral concavity and convexity of the spine. This is frequently a coupled motion that occurs with rotation and is more prevalent in specific spinal regions (i.e., lower cervical and lumbar). This movement can occur when a person is talking on the telephone or lying on one side and is frequently a mechanical component of asymmetric or twisting movements and positions.

Rotation. This twisting movement is a very important component of general function. Many movements and activities are asymmetric and are influenced especially by hand dominance and by the nature of many tasks. As with lateral bending, rotation is a coupled motion that is more prevalent in certain spinal regions (upper cervical and thoracic spine).

We will first look at the most common and costly musculoskeletal disorder—low back pain.

Low Back Pain

Low back pain is the most common of the musculoskeletal disorders and is estimated to represent an expense of up to $50 billion annually in the United States alone (Frymoyer, 1990). It is the most frequent cause of limited activity in persons under 45 years of age and affects 80 to 90% of the adult population at some point in their lives (Kelsey and Golden, 1987). It is nonspecific in approximately 90% of all cases, and most low back mechanical disorders are believed to involve the bottom two lumbar joints (L4–L5 and L5–S1)(Spitzer et al, 1987).

Mechanical Function of the Lumbar Spine. The lumbar spine undergoes the greatest mechanical stress and strain due to its attachment to the fixed pelvis and to the amount of body weight acting on this lower spinal region (Fig. 5–9).

The position of the pelvis determines the amount of lordosis in the lower lumbar spine and consequently the position of the lumbar joints. Thus a key point of mechanical assessment includes rotating the pelvis forward (increases the lordosis) and backward (decreases the lordosis). A mid-range position of the lumbar spine is with the lumbar lordosis present and thus is dependent on the amount of pelvic rotation (Fig. 5–10).

Lumbar Movements. The primary movements of the lumbar spine are flexion-extension and lateral bending. There is very little rotation in this region of the spine, and that which is present is tested during the lateral-bending movement (Fig. 5–11).

Symptoms. The most common symptom is pain felt in the lower back at about the level of the waist. It is possible for pain to radiate upward toward the mid-back or around the front toward the groin. However, the most common radiation of pain is into the buttocks, posterior or posterolateral thighs, and eventually into the calf, ankle, or foot. These radiating pains are considered nonspecific until they follow a distinct dermatomal pattern with associated neurologic signs (sensory loss, motor loss, or reflex change). It is at this point that the spinal nerve root can be identified as the source of the symptoms and is most frequently associated with entrapment secondary to a disc herniation, extrusion, or sequestration or with stenosis caused by a variety of bony or soft-tissue factors.

Common Mechanical Causes. The most frequent mechanical causes of back pain involve flexion (forward bending) of the lumbar spine, with or without a twisting component to the movements. This is associated with dynamic flexion activities such as lifting, material handling, or twisting or it can be associated with static flexion activities such as sitting, motor vehicle operation, stooping, or standing slightly bent forward.

Although it is certainly possible to create a mechanical back problem extending (bending backward) the spine, the predominance of mechanical activity during one's day at work and home involve bending forward. Thus, balancing the amount of this movement is the lifestyle that is essential to maintaining a healthier low back system.

Progression of the Disorder. In general, low back problems progress from symptoms that are felt locally to the spine, to symptoms that are radiating into the leg but are nonspecific pains, to nerve root pain and symptoms that identify an origin at a specific spinal level. The breakdown into the three categories goes as follows:

Warning Signs. These would be the general aching, discomfort, stiffness, tension, and mild pain felt after being in one position too long, repeating a motion frequently without interruption, or upon straining to lift or move a heavy object. These feelings are not lasting; they are relieved within minutes of ceasing the activity, changing positions, or getting up and moving

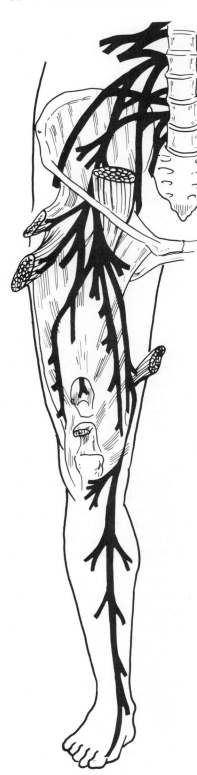

Figure 5–9. The junction of the very mobile lower lumbar joints with the rigid and immobile pelvis creates a convergence of mechanical forces at the lower two lumbar joints (L4–L5, L5–S1) that can lead to mechanical disorders. It is not coincidental that approximately 90% of the lumbar spine disorders occur at these two levels (Cyriax, 1982; McKenzie, 1981).

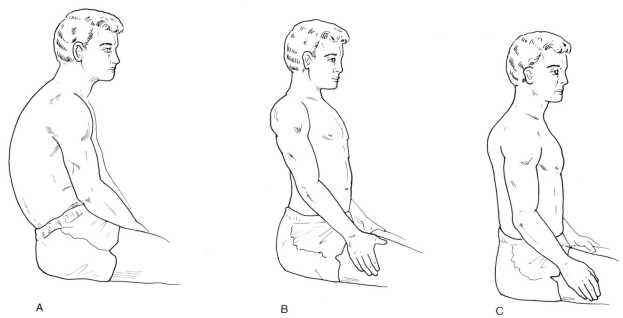

A   B   C

Figure 5–10. McKenzie's slouch-overcorrect-correct exercises demonstrate the effect of the pelvis on the lumbar lordosis (McKenzie, 1988). *A*, Pelvis rotated posteriorly to end-range reduces the lordosis. *B*, Pelvis rotated anteriorly to end-range accentuates the lordosis. *C*, Pelvis rotated in mid-range places the lumbar spine in a mid-lordotic position.

around. When the informed individual checks these warning signs by testing certain movements to end-range, there is no pain produced during the motion. A little stiffness may be felt, but this disappears within several repetitions of the test movement.

Nonspecific Findings. These findings can range in findings from very mild to quite severe. A lot of this depends on when in the development of these symptoms we are assessing them, along with the circumstances of their onset. The pain may be felt locally (central, symmetric, asymmetric, or unilateral) or may radiate into the buttock, thigh, or legs.

The common characteristic separating this level of disorder from warning signs is that movement is now limited secondary to pain, and there is now a pattern of directional preference in which repeated movements either produce and increase or decrease and abolish the symptoms that are now present (Donelson et al, 1991a and b). Muscle guarding or spasm may or may not be present, depending on the severity of the pain and

on the amount of movement loss (more likely when both are greater).

This change of location from local to radiation down the leg represents a worsening of the clinical condition (McKenzie, 1981, 1990; Vanharanta, 1989). Thus, if pain starts locally, all efforts should be made not to allow it to progress toward the leg; or, if present in the leg, all efforts should be made to return the symptoms to the back and reverse the progression. The latter concept is the centralization phenomenon identified by McKenzie (1981, 1983, 1988, 1990). Centralization of pain has been found to be a reliable and highly sensitive indicator that client's with referred pain will respond well to mechanical treatment (Donelson et al, 1990).

Self-treatment booklets and industrial programs teaching the importance of self-management of mechanical disorders can be very successful in treating these disorders (McKenzie, 1983).

Early intervention with mechanical therapy by a well-trained clinician should be initiated if the

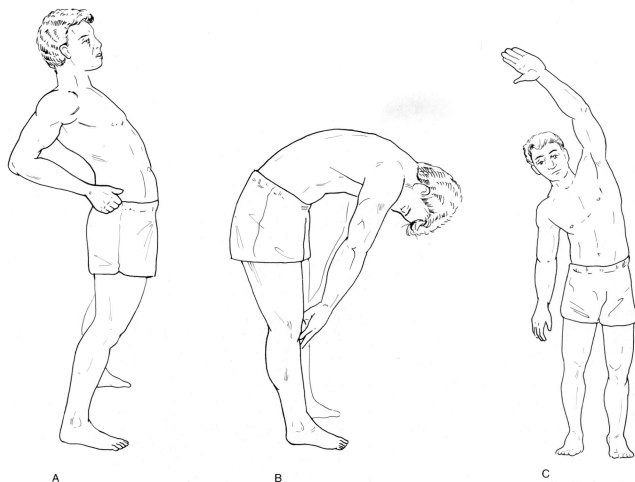

A   B   C

Figure 5–11. The basic movements of the lumbar spine are: *A*, extension, *B*, flexion, and *C*, sidebending. Sidebending can be performed as illustrated or by gliding the hips and shoulders in opposite directions, as described by McKenzie (1981).

individual cannot gain control of the pain within 24 hours. This encourages a more rapid resolution of the problem and less time for the learning of illness behavior.

Structural Findings. Once the low back disorder has progressed to true sciatica (radiating down the leg with an identified nerve root involvement), the lifestyle can be disrupted for a more protracted period of time. Mechanical therapy can often help these disorders despite the presence of severe symptoms and imaging results indicating herniation of the disc (Alexander et al, 1990; Kopp et al, 1986; McKenzie, 1972).

These conservative treatments sometimes work rapidly, but invariably they work eventually. The only clear indications for surgical intervention are progressive neurologic deficit and signs of cauda equina compression (bowel and bladder signs) (Nachemson, 1985; Saal et al, 1990). However, there are suggestions that with specific diagnostic criteria some sciatica will relieve the symptoms and recover function more rapidly with surgery (Weber, 1983). However, the two main drawbacks to this statement is the fact that the same study demonstrates that there is no difference when comparing the surgical group

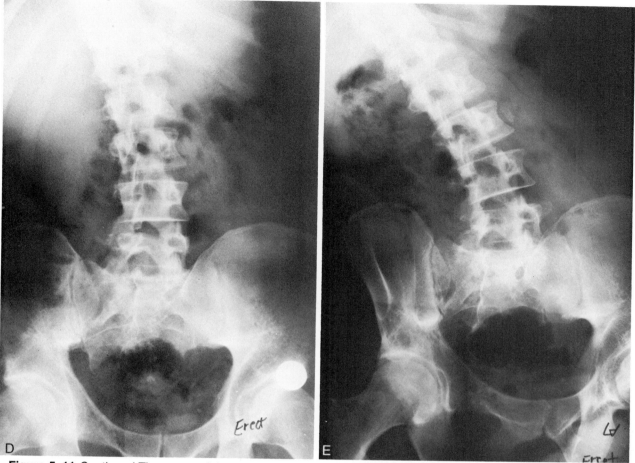

Figure 5–11 *Continued* The x-rays of these two movements demonstrate the similar mechanical effect in *D* and *E*.

with the nonsurgical group on a long-term basis with regard to pain, loss of function, and disability. Furthermore, the possible complications of surgery are greater than the potential complications of conservative treatment (Spitzer et al, 1987).

The questions that arise when a low back disorder progresses to this stage is what could have been done to prevent this from having happened? I suggest the following analysis. One should ask if the sciatica developed suddenly or gradually during this onset of this episode. If it occurred suddenly, the mechanism of onset probably involved a large external load. If so, an ergonomic evaluation of the situation is required. One should ask if the object was too large; was it repeated too often with interruption; were there mechanical factors that set up the problem (prolonged slouched sitting prior to the lift) or a

space/environment problem? Was there a previous history of back problems? Should this individual have been educated more effectively or intensely?

If the sciatica developed gradually and has now become a major functional problem, hindsight can become painfully clear. The client will often report days and weeks (sometimes months and years) of having minor low back or buttock symptoms on a daily basis before the leg pain hits with full force. It is certainly not uncommon for a client to report recurrent episodes of low back pain only, lasting for several days or a few weeks before the sciatica developed. It becomes apparent in both cases that resolving the local pain completely would have reduced the probability for the progression of the disorder. This is why not only eliminating the local pain but also having criteria for achieving wellness (recovery from the episode) is an important part of determining clinical outcomes to treatment and developing an ongoing dynamic assessment tool to prevent onset. **Preventive maintenance requires an ongoing assessment of mechanical function.** Just like caring for a car's moving parts, the body's moving parts require ongoing service and maintenance.

Key Elements for Prevention of Low Back Pain. The most frequent and significant mechanical factors associated with the onset of low back pain involve sustained or repeated flexion in a symmetric or asymmetric fashion. This is a common factor to bending, lifting, sitting, motor vehicle operation, and twisting of the spine. Thus, a return to mid-range from this end-range spinal position involves placing the low back into a more extended posture. Maintenance of the hollow in the back is encouraged, such as the use of lumbar support when sitting, frequent interruption of bending and lifting by backward bending, and a reaction to warning signs that develop in flexion by extending the spine. However, if the warning signs develop with the spinal joints held at the end-range extension, the opposite mechanical procedures should be used.

The essential ingredients for a healthy lower back area are: (1) to maintain a pain-free range of movement in flexion, extension, and side-bending; (2) improved sitting posture by maintaining and supporting the lordosis; (3) improved body mechanics so that poor lifting procedures are more the exception than the rule; (4) frequent interruption of end-range movements by stopping and moving in the opposite direction; (5) improved mechanical environment conducive to improved posture and less mechanical strain to the lower back; and (6) a quick and efficient reaction to warning signs by correcting posture, changing position, or performing opposite movements.

This general conceptual framework is the basis for our preventive strategy for the other musculoskeletal regions.

Neck Pain

The incidence of neck disorders as a source of musculoskeletal impairment or disability is second only to the lower back disorders (Cunningham and Kelsey, 1984). There are similar mechanical factors of imbalanced mechanical stress and strain, and the lower cervical region is the most frequent area of involvement. The cervical spine is particularly interesting in that it can be separated into two functioning mechanical units: the upper cervical unit consisting of the occiput and first two cervical vertebrae, and the lower cervical unit consisting of the remaining five vertebrae (Kapandji, 1976). The cervical spine has a greater range of motion, in more directions, than any other region of the spine (Kapandji, 1976; Panjabi and White, 1990).

Mechanical Function of the Cervical Spine. The mechanical function of the cervical spine is divided into the isolated effect on the upper and lower regions and the interrelated effects that these two regions have upon each other. The upper cervical spine is unique, because it is the most mobile area of the spine and it does not have an intervertebral disc. As a consequence of its unique structure and function, it must be considered as a separate mechanical unit of the head and neck (Fig. 5–12).

The cervical region has a unique ability to protrude forward and to retract backward (Fig. 5–13). This protrusion and retraction has a unique mechanical effect on the upper and lower cervical regions. When the head protrudes forward, the upper region is extended and the lower region is flexed. The opposite occurs when the head and neck are retracted. Thus, in the neck all the cardinal plane movements plus protrusion and retraction have to be checked and maintained (Fig. 5–14).

Symptoms. Symptoms of mechanical origin in the neck can be multiple and varied. The primary symptoms are pain and stiffness that are felt locally in the neck, across the back of the shoulders, into the shoulder blades, and headaches. The pain can radiate into the upper and lower arm or into the wrist, hand, and fingers. As with the lumbar disorders, this will all be considered nonspecific until particular nerve root signs are identified (McKenzie, 1983, 1990; Spitzer et al, 1987).

Common Mechanical Causes. The most common mechanical factors associated with an onset of neck pain are similar to the factors associated with lower back pain. Motor vehicle operation, prolonged sitting, frequent bending and lifting, and frequent VDT operation (Kelsey et al, 1984; McKenzie, 1990). These factors represent an imbalance of flexion strains for the lower cervical unit and extension for the upper cervical unit.

Progression of the Disorder. The cervical disorders progress in the same pattern as the lower

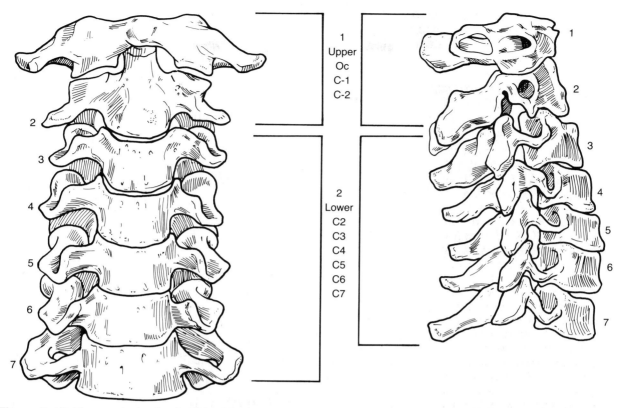

Figure 5–12. The cervical spine is divided into two separate mechanical units: 1, upper, no discs, and 2, lower, the disc segments.

back disorders. The following outlines some of the key indicators of the progressing mechanical disorder in this region.

Warning Signs. These would be the general aching, discomfort, stiffness, tension, and mild pain felt after being in one position too long, repeating a motion frequently without interruption, or upon straining to lift or move a heavy object. These feelings are not lasting. They are relieved within minutes of ceasing that activity, changing positions, or getting up and moving around. When the informed individual checks these warning signs by testing certain movements to end-range, no pain is produced during the motion. A little stiffness may be felt, but this feeling disappears within several repetitions of the test movement.

Nonspecific Findings. These findings can range in findings from very mild to quite severe. A lot depends on when in the development of these symptoms we are assessing them, along with the circumstances of their onset. The pain may be

felt locally (central, symmetric, asymmetric, or unilateral) or may radiate into the scapulae (analogous to buttock radiation in low back problems), across the shoulders, or into the upper and lower arm or hand.

The common characteristic separating this level of disorder from warning signs is that movement is now limited secondary to pain, and there is now a pattern of directional preference in which repeated movements either produce and increase or decrease and abolish the symptoms that are now present. Muscle guarding or spasm may or may not be present, depending on the severity of the pain and on the amount of movement loss (more likely when both are greater). The Quebec Task Force classification system applies to the cervical region just as it did in the lower back. Thus, the first three classes for nonspecific disorders are determined by the location of pain. Class 1 has local pain only; class 2 has proximal arm pain; and class 3 has distal arm pain (Spitzer et al, 1987).

This change of location from an area local to the spine radiating down the arm represents a worsening of the clinical condition. Thus, if pain starts locally, all efforts should be made not to allow it to progress toward the arm. Or, if present in the arm, all efforts should be made to return the symptoms to the neck and to reverse the progression. The latter concept is the centralization phenomenon identified by McKenzie. Centralization of pain has been found to be a reliable and highly sensitive indicator that clients with referred pain will respond well to mechanical treatment (Doneslon et al, 1991; McKenzie, 1990).

Self-treatment booklets and industrial programs teaching the importance of self-management of mechanical disorders can be just as successful in managing neck problems (Mc-

Kenzie, 1983). Again, this is provided the instructions are meaningful to the individual in demonstrating a cause and effect between the mechanical model and relief of pain with the procedures.

Early intervention with mechanical therapy by a well-trained clinician should be initiated if the individual cannot gain control of the pain within 24 hours. This encourages a more rapid resolution and works quickly to prevent the development of disability behavior.

Structural Diagnosis. Once the neck disorder has progressed to brachial neuralgia (radiating symptoms down the arm with an identified nerve root involvement), the lifestyle is disrupted for a more protracted period. As with the low back disorders that have progressed to sciatica, a

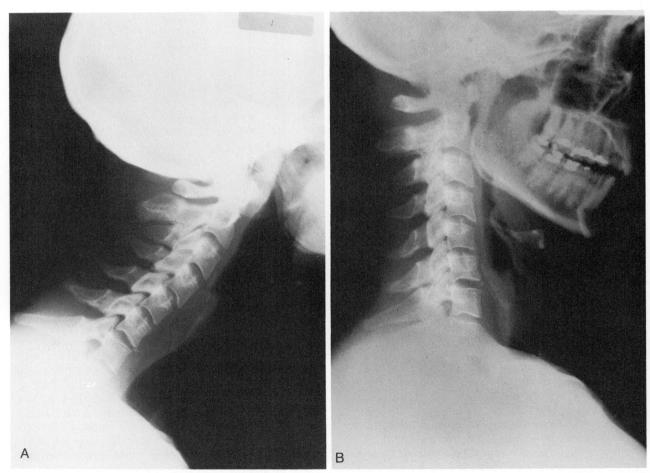

Figure 5–13. The cervical spine has an unusual amount of forward-gliding (*A*, protrusion) and backward-gliding (*B*, retraction) movement. These movements must be considered when one is mechanically assessing the neck.

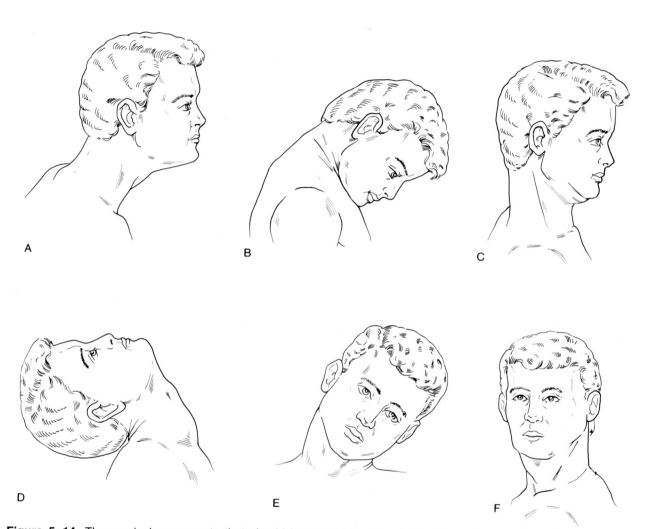

Figure 5–14. The cervical movements that should be serviced and maintained are: *A*, protrusion (flexion lower, extension upper); *B*, flexion; *C*, retraction (flexion upper, extension lower); *D*, extension; *E*, sidebending; and *F*, rotation.

slower clinical recovery is likely regardless of the treatment chosen. The most likely cause of these symptoms is entrapment of the spinal nerve from a severely bulging or extruded disc, with or without bony encroachment on the spinal canal.

The same question arises when a neck disorder progresses to this stage. What could have been done to prevent this disorder from occurring?

Key Elements for Prevention of Neck Injury. The mechanical factors associated with the onset of neck pain are similar to those in the lower back. Sustained and repeated flexion are the major position and movement. The main difference in the method of postural correction and use of opposite movements is the need to retract the neck before extending it. Otherwise, the ingredients for a healthy neck are the same, but there are movements to assess and work on maintaining.

Mid-Back Pain

The frequency of thoracic spine disorders is small compared with the lower back and neck. The incidence rate has been reported at 2 to 4% of reported spine disorders (Kramer, 1981; Rath et al, 1989). However, upper back and scapular pain is a frequent finding with neck problems. This pain and tenderness are referred to the upper back area and do not originate in the thoracic spine.

Mechanical Function of the Thoracic Spine. The thoracic spine is the least mobile region of the spine and has the special consideration of its attachments for the ribs and role in the mechanics of breathing (Fig. 5–15).

The position of the thoracic spine is influenced significantly by the chest and shoulders. This position then strongly influences the position and mechanical function of the head and neck because it provides their foundation for posture and movement. Unlike the cervical and lumbar spine, the thoracic spine has a natural forward curvature or kyphosis (rounded). The movements that require maintenance and evaluation are flexion-extension and rotation (Fig. 5–16).

Symptoms. The primary complaint is pain felt in the mid-back area, which is often increased when the person takes a deep breath. This pain may radiate forward through the chest or around the side of the rib cage toward the front of the chest.

Common Mechanical Causes. Once again there are similar mechanical stress and strains that precipitate mid-back disorders as for the

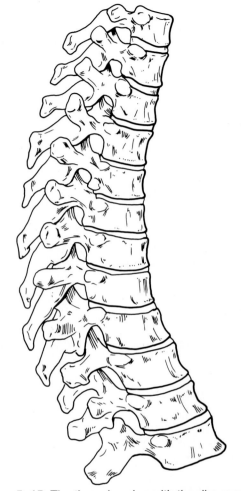

Figure 5–15. The thoracic spine with the ribs removed.

other spinal regions; that is, imbalance flexion activities such as bending, lifting, straining, prolonged sitting, or stooping. Sudden twisting or turning may also be a precipitating factor, which is usually performed from a forward bent or rounded back position.

Progression of the Disorder. Thoracic disorders do not progress with the same pattern as the other spinal regions. However, they can be quite recurrent and interfere with function when present.

Warning Signs. These signs include the same symptoms described for the lumbar and cervical regions, only they are felt in the mid-back area. The mechanisms of onset are also the same as with the other regions.

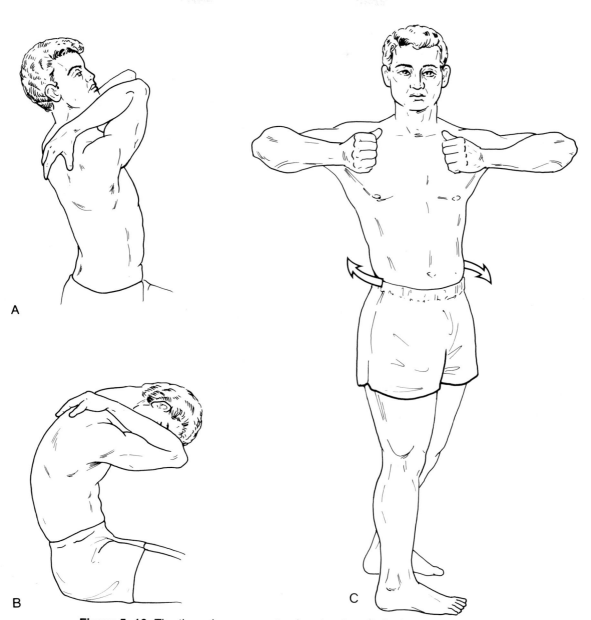

Figure 5–16. The thoracic movements: *A*, extension; *B*, flexion; and *C*, rotation.

Nonspecific Disorder. The nonspecific disorder involves an episode of pain that is usually associated with taking a deep breath or attempting to extend or rotate the thoracic region. The pain may be felt centrally, symmetric, asymmetric, or unilateral in the mid- to lower back region. There may also be radiation around the rib cage toward or to the anterior chest wall, sometimes perceived as directly through the chest to the front. Thus only classes I and II of the Quebec Task Force grouping apply to the thoracic disorders (Spitzer et al, 1987).

Structural Diagnosis. This diagnosis is rare but can include a progression to disc herniation that involves neurologic signs of cord compression.

Key Elements for Prevention. Once again, sustained and repeated flexion is the major mechanical risk factor (McKenzie, 1990). Thus, the same concepts of ingredients for a healthy system apply, but specific emphasis on the position of the chest and upper back is given.

Neck and Upper Extremity Region

The shoulder girdle is the most mobile joint complex of the human body. This enables the hand to function in an extremely large sphere of movement and position. In order to provide this mobility, the shoulder complex sacrifices mechanical stability. Its only joint attachment to the axial skeleton (trunk) is at the sternoclavicular joint, with the remainder of the complex slung from the cervical and upper and mid-thoracic spine by musculature, fascia, and ligaments. Thus movements of the neck and upper back influence the shoulder girdle and vice versa. In conjunction with this, the cervical nerve roots that form the brachial plexus and the major peripheral nerves of the upper extremities undergo length tension change with various neck, shoulder, and arm movements. Thus the mechanical relationship between the neck and upper extremity is inseparable, and this interdependence is an essential consideration in regional musculoskeletal evaluation (Fig. 5–17).

Mechanical Relationship of Neck and Upper Extremity. The soft-tissue structures that mechanically influence the movements of the neck and upper extremity can be separated into the following three main groups.

Neck-Shoulder Structures. These are primarily the muscles that elevate the shoulder or move the head and neck. When the shoulders are

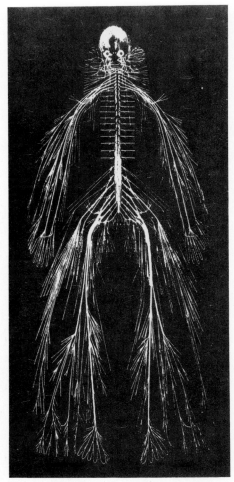

Figure 5–17. The famous dissection of the nervous system by Weaver illustrates the mechanical connection of the peripheral nerves to their attachments at the vertebral column. (Courtesy of Dr. Peter S. Amenta, Hahnemann University, Department of Anatomy, Philadelphia.)

pushed downward (depressed) away from the neck, cervical movements are reduced owing to the passive insufficiency of these muscles.

Neural Structures. The brachial plexus is formed primarily by the fifth cervical to first thoracic spinal nerves. These neural tissues are the connection from the spine to the fingers, providing motor power and sensibility. However, these tissues also provide a mechanical linkage that requires assessment and maintenance in the efforts of the prevention of injury. This neural tissue travels laterally and anteriorly away from the spine and passes anterior to the glenohumeral joint into the arm. As the nerves continue to travel distally to the wrist and fingers, the radial and median nerves pass anterior to the elbow joint and the ulnar posterior. Once in the forearm the radial nerve passes into the wrist posterior to the wrist joints, and the median and ulnar pass anteriorly. Specific testing for adverse mechanical tension on these neural structures has been developed by Elvey (1987), which consists mainly of shoulder girdle depression, glenohumeral abduction and external rotation, elbow extension, forearm supination, and wrist and finger extension. Additional information is then obtained by sidebending the head and neck away from the arm being tested.

Arm and Forearm Structures. Whenever the upper extremity is extended, abducted, and externally rotated the effect on local structures must also be considered. This particularly affects the biceps brachii when considering the arm, because this structure connects the scapula to the radius. The long wrist and finger flexors also need consideration when looking at the mechanical effect on the forearm.

The restoration of full mechanical function to the neck or upper extremity requires an exploration of these special mechanical relationships. This becomes very important when one considers that symptoms felt anywhere in the arm, forearm, wrist, or hand could have a more proximal source or relationship.

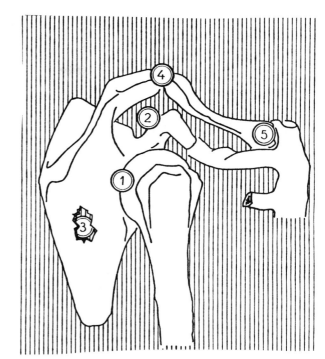

Figure 5–18. The shoulder complex consists of five joint articulations: 1, glenohumeral, 2, subdeltoid, 3, scapulothoracic, 4, acromioclavicular, and 5, sternoclavicular. (From Kapandji IA: Physiology of the Joints. Vol 3: The Trunk and Vertebral Column. New York, Churchill Livingstone, 1976.)

Shoulder Complex

The most frequent mechanism of onset is reaching, lifting, or throwing. Once again we have the mechanical factors of sustained positions, repeated movements, and the efficiency of mechanical function to consider as a mechanism of onset. The shoulder girdle consists of five articulations that require mechanical assessment (Fig. 5–18).

Glenohumeral Joint. This is the main joint of the shoulder complex. It is a ball and socket type of joint formed by the head of the humerus within the glenoid fossa of the scapula. There is a tremendous amount of incongruity of the articular surfaces that allows a great range of movement, but this movement is complex and is achieved with a sacrifice of stability. The shoulder complex has the largest range and freedom of movement of all the extremity articulations. This allows the hand to be placed in a position of function within a large envelope of space. The stability and integrity of this mechanical system depend greatly on posture, position, and muscle function. And, as will be demonstrated, they are influenced strongly by spinal posture and position, which influences the mechanical function of the shoulder complex.

Scapulothoracic Articulation. This articulation is not an actual joint, but rather a functional relationship between the shoulder blade and the rib cage. The position of the scapula is critical to the mechanical function of the shoulder, because it maintains the appropriate orientation of the glenoid fossae and the mechanical relationship of the shoulder girdle musculature. In the process of elevating the upper extremity, there is a 2:1 ratio of glenohumeral movement to scapular movement.

Acromioclavicular Joint. This small joint at the top of the shoulder forms the distal connection with the clavicle and has an important role in elevation and horizontal abduction and adduction.

Sternoclavicular Joint. This joint provides the only direct attachment that the shoulder complex has with the axial skeleton. It provides the proximal attachment with the clavicle and has a limited amount of movement.

Subdeltoid Joint. This is not a true joint, but a functional relationship between the head of the humerus and the coracoacromial arch above it. The mechanical importance of this region concerns the structures that are located in or run through this functional region. The subdeltoid and subacromial bursae and the tendons of the rotator cuff and long head of the biceps are of specific concern regarding mechanical injury. Impingement with subsequent attrition of these particular structures is involved in most shoulder disorders. Thus the maintenance of normal function of the subdeltoid joint is essential to a healthy shoulder complex.

Mechanical Function of the Shoulder Complex. These five articulations can be divided into two main functional units: (1) the shoulder girdle, consisting of the scapulae, clavicles, and the sternoclavicular joint, and (2) the shoulder joint proper, consisting of the glenohumeral joint and the subdeltoid articulation. The movements that should be assessed and maintained are shown in Figure 5–18.

Symptoms. The primary area of symptoms will be felt directly at the shoulder joint for most of the disorders. In this regard, Cyriax (1982) described the shoulder as a very honest joint in which symptoms are perceived by the patient. The pain can refer down the arm, frequently toward the insertion of the middle deltoid, but may include nonspecific radiation (not following a nerve root pattern) to the base of the hand (radial more than ulnar). The acromioclavicular disorders are associated with symptoms at the point of the shoulder at the joint location. The sternoclavicular joint would involve symptoms directly at, or close to, its location. It must be remembered that the cervical spine is capable of referring pain in the same pattern and must be ruled out as a source of the mechanical disturbance.

Common Mechanical Causes. Frequent reaching, lifting, or throwing motions are associated with shoulder disorders. However, so too are the static sitting and standing postures associated with VDT and assembly line operation.

Progression of the Disorder. The shoulder problems follow the same progression as described for the spinal disorders. However, there is now a greater chance of identifying specific muscle/tendon involvement because of the ability to selectively stress these structures in a system of physical examination.

Warning Signs. These signs present as they did with the spinal mechanical system. The symptoms are felt locally and do not interfere with function. They subside quickly once the sustained position or the repeated activity causing them is changed.

Nonspecific Disorder. This presents itself as a pain that is produced on attempting end-range movement. The pain may be felt during the movement, as in a painful arc, or at the very extreme of the motion with overpressure. The structural origin of this pain cannot be determined by isometric contraction of specific muscle groups or by specific structural palpation. The most frequent sign is that of impingement within the subdeltoid region, but the specific structure cannot be determined. Relief of pain and restoration of normal mechanical function are usually rapid when a caudal mobilization of the humeral head within the glenoid fossa is performed.

Structural Diagnosis. This presents itself in one of three basic patterns: (1) tendinitis and tendon rupture, (2) subluxation and dislocation, and (3) bursitis.

Tendinitis and Tendon Rupture. Both of these will be identified by the reproduction of pain with muscle contraction in an isometric fashion with the joint held in a neutral position. However, the distinction between tendinitis and tendon rupture is the ability to exert muscular force. The rupture has weakness and an inability to generate a full contraction and difficulty with active movements if it is severe enough. This weakness in the arm can be distinguished from cervical nerve root signs by the fact that pain is reproduced by shoulder movements and is not influenced by neck movements.

Subluxation and Dislocation. These disorders are characterized by a loss of joint integrity and deformity, almost always associated in onset with a large external force. During the repair process, nonspecific or other specific disorders may be found in association with the injury. However, the injury itself is treatment with rest and immobilization followed by aggressive muscle strengthening to protect the joint. If the injury is too severe or this conservative rehabilitation is inadequate, then surgery is required followed by aggressive rehabilitation. The most common joints to sublux or dislocate are the glenohumeral and the acromioclavicular. Sternoclavicular dislocations are relatively rare and can pose a problem to the mediastinal structures when present.

Bursitis. This inflammation is either in the subacromial bursae or in the subdeltoid bursae. As with the tendinitis disorders, this is frequently a problem of impingement in the subdeltoid joint. A preventive procedure for all these impingement problems is to maintain the caudal gliding of the humeral head to discourage pinching when the arm is elevated (Fig. 5–19).

This is automatically encouraged with good spinal posture, which includes elevation of the chest and retraction of the shoulder girdles.

Elbow Pain

The most frequent mechanical factors associated with elbow and forearm problems involve gripping with the hand, bending of the wrist, twisting of the forearm, with the elbow held in a static position, or moving in a reaching or throwing fashion. This occurs in certain sports, with lifting activities, or the repeated manipulation of objects by the hand. The elbow has three articulations to consider, along with the specific muscle attachments of the forearm, wrist, and hand musculature (Fig. 5–20).

Mechanical Function of the Elbow/Forearm. Movements of the elbow enable the hand to be brought toward or moved away from the body without changing the shoulder position. The rotation motions of the forearm allow the hand to change its relationship in space independent of the elbow position. The movements of the forearm and elbow thus complement the mechanical function of the shoulder and hand (Fig. 5–21).

Symptoms. The symptoms are felt local to the elbow, with or without nonspecific radiation to the forearm, wrist, or hand.

Common Mechanical Causes. The most common causes are associated with repeated throwing movements while sustaining a strong grip or with sustained elbow positions with repetitive movements of the wrist and fingers.

Progression of the Disorder. As with the shoulder, we have the same progression of mechanical disorders for the elbow. There is a greater chance of identifying specific mus-

cle/tendon involvement because of the ability to selectively stress these structures in a system of physical examination.

Warning Signs. Elbow stiffness, aching, and discomfort subsides immediately when an activity is changed. Motions are not affected and do not produce symptoms upon testing.

Nonspecific Disorder. Pain is produced by either moving the elbow or forearm articulation to end-range or upon testing the combined elbow, forearm, wrist, and hand movements to end-range. However, despite the ability to produce symptoms with movements, specific structures are not identified owing to a lack of findings, isometric muscle testing, and special tests.

Structural Diagnosis. As with the shoulder, the most common structural problem is tendinitis. This typically involves the lateral or medial common tendons and occasionally the posterior attachment of the distal portion of the triceps.

Wrist Pain

The most frequent mechanisms of onset are associated with the repeated manipulations of objects (i.e., gripping, pinching, pulling, squeezing). When poor body mechanics are found in association with imbalanced repetitive motions and sustained end-range positions, problems of the wrist can be facilitated. Musculoskeletal disorders of the wrist and hand leading to impairment and disability have received tremendous attention from OSHA, industry, and the health professions. Carpal tunnel syndrome (CTS) alone has become such a problem in some industries that claims for this disorder have forced manufacturing plants to shut down. However, the disorders of the wrist and hand are subject to the same diagnostic problems as the other musculoskeletal regions, and often nonspecific symptoms felt locally at the wrist and hand are labeled CTS without definitive proof. The wrist has four general articulations and two neurovascular tunnels to consider, whereas the hand has the five articular complexes of the digits to mechanically evaluate.

Mechanical Concepts in the Wrist Complex. The wrist complex participates in both movements of the hand and the forearm. The distal articulations ulnar-radial and the ulnomeniscal-triquetral joints are primarily involved in supination and pronation of the forearm. The distal

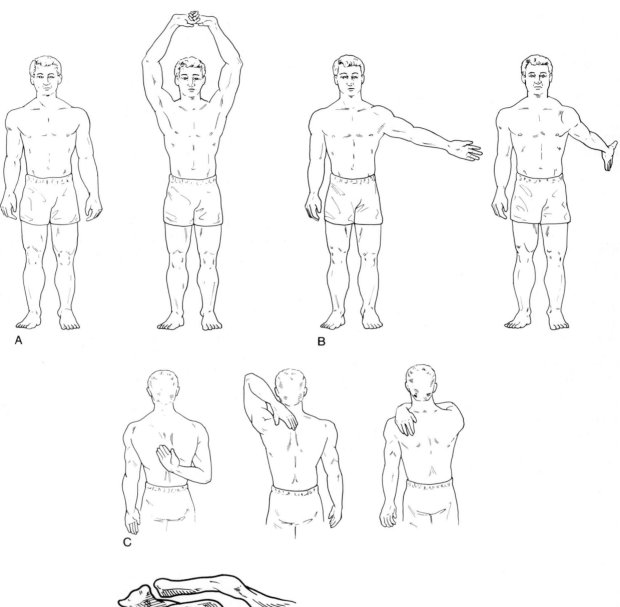

A

B

C

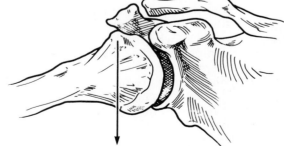

D

Figure 5–19. The shoulder movements are flexion-extension, abduction-adduction, and internal-external rotation. The movement in *A* through *C* cover all of these motions. *D* indicates the importance of caudal gliding of the humeral head in preventing impingement of the rotator cuff tendons and the bursae.

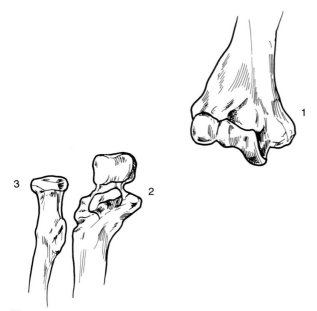

Figure 5–20. The elbow complex is formed by three bones: 1, humerus; 2, ulna; and 3, radius. The three articulations of the elbow are the ulnohumeral, proximal ulnoradial, and the radiohumeral joints.

end of the radius with the proximal row of carpals and the mid-carpal articulation are primarily involved in wrist flexion-extension and ulnar and radial deviations. The two neurovascular tunnels allow passage of the ulnar (Guyon's tunnel) and median (carpal tunnel) nerves, along with blood vessels and tendons that perform flexion of the wrist and fingers (Fig. 5–22).

Symptoms. Symptoms can be felt locally at the wrist but may radiate to include various portions of the hand and fingers. The symptoms may be referred proximally within the forearm but rarely extend above the elbow. When the median nerve is involved, there will be symptoms in the thumb, index, and middle finger on the volar surface. When pressure on the median nerve is sufficient to interfere with conduction to the muscles, wasting (atrophy) and weakness of the intrinsic muscles of the thumb are noted. With regard to entrapment in Guyon's tunnel, there will be symptoms in an ulnar distribution that involve the little and ring fingers.

Common Mechanical Causes. As previously mentioned, occupation, recreational and lifestyle activities involve repetitive manipulation of objects with the hand.

Progression of the Disorder. We have the same progression of mechanical disorders for the wrist as with the other extremity joints. There is a greater chance of identifying specific muscle/tendon involvement because of the ability to selectively stress these structures in a system of physical examination.

Warning Signs. Wrist stiffness, aching, and discomfort that subside immediately when an activity is changed. Motions are not affected and do not produce symptoms when tested.

Nonspecific Disorder. Pain is produced by

Figure 5–21. The movements of the elbow and forearm are: *A*, flexion and extension and *B*, forearm pronation (palm down) and supination (palm up).

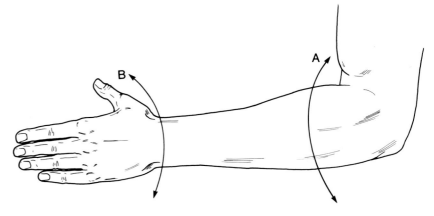

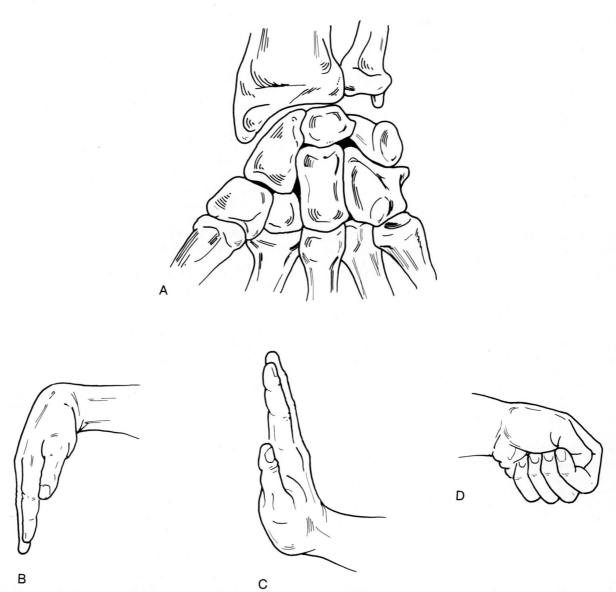

Figure 5–22. The wrist joints and wrist movements are illustrated by: *A,* the multiple articulations of the wrist; *B,* flexion; *C,* extension; and *D,* ulnar deviation (not shown is radial deviation).

either moving the wrist or forearm articulations to end-range or upon testing the combined elbow, forearm, wrist, hand movements to end-range. However, despite the ability to produce symptoms with movements, specific structures are not identified owing to a lack of findings with isometric muscle testing and other special tests.

Structural Diagnosis. The main progression to consider involves the presence of an actual carpal tunnel or Guyon's tunnel syndrome (Fig. 5–23).

Hand and Finger Disorders

The hand and fingers have a tremendous range of mechanical demands placed on them. They are required to have great sensibility and fine control yet must be able to provide strong gripping pressure involved in more strenuous and violent mechanical forces. The volar aspect of the hand is the functional surface, and most movements and activities involve closing the fingers towards the palm of the hand. However, it is the coordinated effort of the extensors of the wrist and the fingers that allows these volar movements to be meaningful and effective. The thumb requires special attention because it has a unique articular design (saddle joint) and provides a much greater freedom of movement than the other fingers.

Mechanical Concepts in the Hand/Finger Complex. The hand consists of five digits, with each of these formed by a metacarpal, proximal, middle, and distal phalangeal bone. There are joint articulations between each of these bones (metacarpophalangeal and interphalangeal joints) within themselves and between the four metacarpal bones of the fingers (excluding the thumb). The former joints allow the movement of the digits themselves, and the latter is more involved with the opening and closing of the hand itself (Fig. 5–24).

The thumb is particularly important because its articulation with the base of the hand and the proximal end of its metacarpal forms a saddle articulation. This allows the thumb to move into opposition, which provides a greater range of function to the hand. The following figure illustrates the movements of the hand and fingers (Fig. 5–25).

Symptoms. These are felt very local to area of involvement as the hand and fingers have a tremendous sensibility with a very large soma-

tosensory representation. Thus disorders are easily localized to the region of the problem with local mechanical assessment. However, problems proximal to the hand can refer or radiate symptoms into the hand and fingers. Thus a disorder of the neck, upper thorax, shoulder, elbow, forearm, or wrist must be considered.

Common Mechanical Causes. As mentioned, imbalanced and repeated use of the hand and fingers is frequently associated with hand and finger disorders.

Progression of the Disorder. We have the same progression of mechanical disorders for the hand and fingers as we do with the other extremity joints. There is a greater chance of identifying specific muscle/tendon involvement because of the ability to selectively stress these structures in a system of physical examination.

Warning Signs. These signs are hand and finger stiffness, aching, and discomfort that subsides immediately when an activity is changed. Motions are not affected and do not produce symptoms upon testing.

Nonspecific Disorder. Pain is produced by specific movements of the fingers with or without the wrist or the forearm and sometimes the elbow in certain positions. However, despite the ability to produce symptoms with movements, specific structures are not identified owing to a lack of findings with isometric muscle testing and other special tests.

Structural Diagnosis. The main progression to consider is the findings associated with trigger finger, DeQuervain's syndrome, and Dupuytren's contracture.

Low Back and Lower Extremity Region

The lumbopelvic region and the lower extremity are subjected to much larger mechanical loadings than the neck and upper extremity. As a result of this mechanical function, movement is sacrificed for stability. There are mechanical interrelationships between the lumbopelvic and lower extremity structures, but they are not as complex as those found in the cervical and upper extremity relationships. However, the mechanical connections are important, and the possibility of lumbar tissues causing symptoms felt in the lower extremity is significant (Fig. 5–26).

Mechanical Relationship of the Low Back and Lower Extremity. The main structures to consider are the sciatic nerve (sacral plexus), femoral

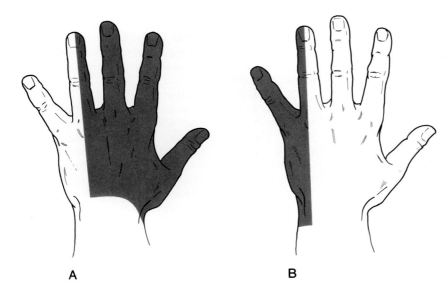

A

B

Figure 5–23. Signs and symptoms of median nerve (carpal tunnel) and ulnar nerve (Guyon's tunnel) entrapment at the wrist are specific. *A*, Median nerve involvement includes sensory changes on the volar surface primarily on the radial side and motor involvement of abductor pollicis brevis, flexor pollicis brevis, opponens pollicis, and 4–5 lumbricales. *B*, Ulnar nerve involvement includes sensory changes on volar and dorsal surfaces of the fifth and fourth digits and motor involvement of palmaris brevis, abductor digiti minimi, flexor digiti minimi.

Figure 5–24. The hand is an intricate connection of joints that allows a tremendous variety of mechanical functions.

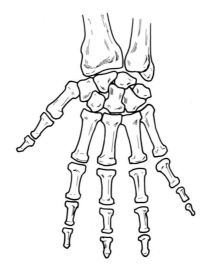
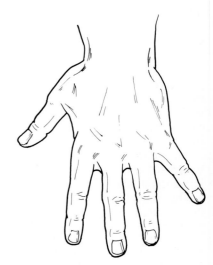

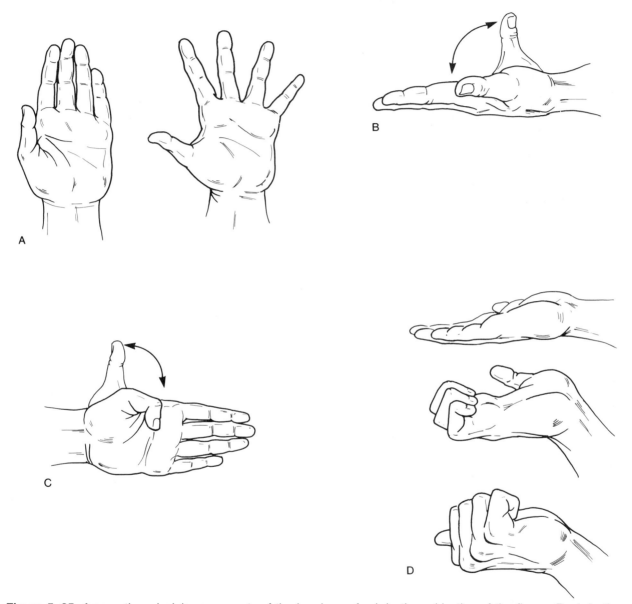

Figure 5–25. Among the principle movements of the hand are: *A,* abduction-adduction of the finger; *B,* abduction-adduction of the thumb; *C,* flexion-extension of the thumb; and *D,* finger flexion-extension.

nerve (lumbar plexus), hamstrings, rectus femoris, and iliopsoas. The sciatic nerve passes behind the hip and knee and as a result influences flexion of the spine and hip when the knee is extended. The femoral nerve passes in front of the hip and knee and as a result can influence extension of the spine and hip with the knee bent. The rectus femorus has the same mechanical effect as the femoral nerve, and the iliopsoas affects the hip and spine extension regardless of knee position.

Mechanical Function of the Lower Extremity. The leg can be separated into three major areas: the hip, the knee, and the ankle/foot. The lower extremity structures are subject to the same mechanical considerations as the upper extremity. However, some of the major differences found in the lower extremity are (1) it has weight-bearing function, (2) it is involved primarily in gross motor function (not prehensile), and (3) it does not have the range of movement of the upper extremity. Thus the movements are similar to the upper extremity, but there is not as much motion to service and maintain (Fig. 5–27).

Table 5–10 summarizes the more common musculoskeletal disorders found in the lower extremity, which can lead to impairment or disability.

MEASUREMENT OF RESPONSE TO PREVENTIVE INTERVENTIONS

Measurement of the effectiveness of the treatment or prevention program is important. There is no one strategy that is effective for all individuals with the same disorder, no less varying disorders. Thus the continuous analysis of the individual's response must be more rapid, and appropriate decisions must be made regarding mechanical strategy. The three main areas of measurement coincide with the three main clinical objectives: (1) pain status, (2) functional status, and (3) prevention of recurrence and progression. Each of these three areas is addressed separately.

PAIN STATUS

The most concerning clinical symptom with which the client with mechanical disorders presents is pain. We have emphasized that in most

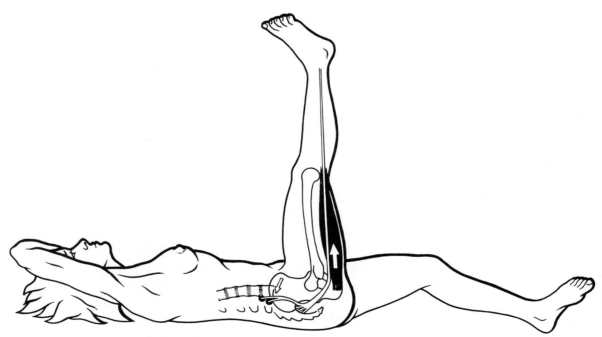

Figure 5–26. Lower limb tension testing by straight leg raising. Additional information can be obtained by adding ankle dorsiflexion and cervical flexion. (Redrawn from Kapandji IA: Physiology of the Joints. Vol 3: The Trunk and Vertebral Column. New York, Churchill Livingstone, 1976.)

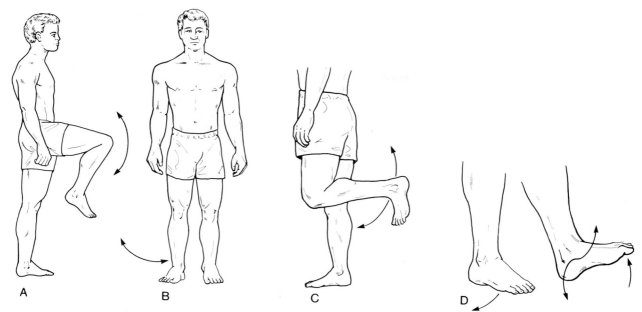

Figure 5–27. Lower limb movements will include: *A* and *B*, hip motions of flexion-extension (*A*), abduction-adduction (*B*), and internal-external rotation (not shown); *C*, knee flexion-extension; and *D*, ankle-foot dorsiflexion-plantarflexion; and inversion-eversion (not shown).

cases it is the only reliable clinical finding with which to classify the client's condition. It is also the most reliable physical examination tool with which to localize the source of the disorder and measure the client's response to treatment (Cyriax, 1982; Deyo, 1988; McKenzie, 1981, 1990). The relief and abolishment of the pain is an important and applicable clinical concern. The

pain status is measured in three ways: (1) its location, (2) its intensity, and (3) its frequency.

Pain Location. The location is recorded with the aid of a drawing. A blank illustration of the body is provided on a sheet of paper, and the individual is instructed to draw in the areas where he or she feels pain. Quantification of the location of pain can be made by applying a grid system to the drawing. The number of grids that encompass the shaded areas identify the extent of the pain (Fig. 5–28). As stressed throughout this chapter, one measure of the progression of a mechanical disorder is the progression of the site or the extent of the pain location.

Pain Intensity. The easiest and most reliable way of measuring an individual's perception of pain severity is a visual analog scale (Huckisson, 1974; Scott and Huckisson, 1979). In this measurement zero means that there is no pain, and 10 means the worst possible pain. The client then rates his or her symptoms in the regional area. It is always more informative to separate body areas (neck, mid-back, low back, arm, leg) to acquire more specific information and look for patterns. McKenzie identified the pattern of centralization in the spine as an extremely valuable predictor of clinical outcome (Doneslon et al, 1990; McKenzie, 1981, 1983, 1988, 1990). Ex-

Table 5–10. Common Musculoskeletal Disorders of the Lower Extremities

Hip:	Bursitis
	Tendinitis and Muscle Strains
	Loose Body
	Osteoarthrosis
Knee:	Bursitis
	Tendinitis and muscle strains
	Ligament sprains
	Internal derangement (menisci)
	Loose bodies
	Patellofemoral syndromes
	Osteoarthrosis
Foot/Ankle:	Tendinitis and muscle strains
	Bursitis
	Fasciitis
	Ligament sprains
	Osteoarthrosis

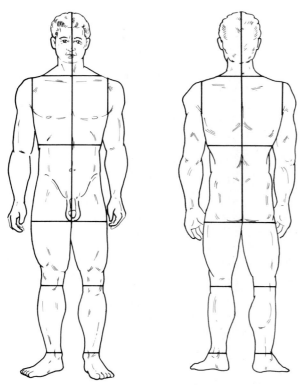

Figure 5–28. Pain drawings can be used to measure the location of the client's pain or discomfort. The illustration incorporates a grid system based on the general classes used by the Quebec Task Force recommendations. (Redrawn from Spitzer WO, LeBlanc FE, Dupuis M, et al: Scientific approach to the assessment and management of activity-related spinal disorders. Spine 12[75]:1–59, 1987.)

plained in analog terms, centralization occurs when the intensity rating is decreasing toward zero in the leg or arm, as it is increasing away from zero in the back or neck.

Pain Frequency. This is the measurement of how often the pain is present during the day; that is, is the pain there continuously or hardly there at all? This is a further qualification of the severity of the condition and is sometimes the only measure that changes to indicate whether a condition has altered for the better or for the worse. An analog scale can be utilized with zero meaning absent all day and 10 meaning continuous all day, regardless of intensity (developed by Rath). As with the intensity rating, it is helpful to separate out the body region for more specific information and identification of patterns.

Functional Status. The client's perceptions of his or her functional ability is an important component to impairment and disability (Deyo, 1988). A technically perfect surgery may have been performed, but if the client's self-reported rating of function (and pain) has not improved, the clinical outcome will be poor. However, we cannot rely on the client's perceptions alone. Thus, the data from the physical tests must be correlated with the client's perceptions of his or her ability. Our system utilizes self-reported questionnaires and repeated motions testing to assess function.

Functional Questionnaires. The questionnaires ask the client to rate his or her perceived functional ability on either a visual analog or on an ordinal scale (Deyo, 1988). It is important that the questions address the mechanical activities that are important to both the body region and to the client's specific function. However, some questions may include more specific information about the client's psychosocial status.

Certainly a most important assessment is whether the individual has had to miss work (how long), change jobs, or avoid certain activities.

Repeated Motions Testing. As the main theme of this chapter, the importance of achieving a normal end-range response with movement is an essential ingredient in musculoskeletal wellness. Thus the most direct and applicable test of this concept is the testing of repeated end-range motions. This has to be applied in all planes of movement that are allowed by the particular region of the body being tested. And 10 repetitions to end-range with appropriate overpressure is a minimum number (McKenzie, 1981, 1990).

Criteria for Clinical Outcome. By utilizing the measurement of pain and functional status, a criteria rating for clinical outcome response to treatment can be formulated. Thus a criteria-based distinction for excellent, good, fair, and poor clinical response can be developed, as suggested by Donleson and associates (1990). This criterion was applied to a consecutive case series investigation of outpatient physical therapy services for spinal patients (Rath et al, 1989). The results of this study suggest that clients with nonspecific spinal disorders respond more favorably than do clients who present with neurologic findings indicative of compression of a spinal nerve root (Table 5–11).

Prevention of Recurrence/Progression. The re-

Table 5–11. Outcome Assessment Study: Mechanical Spinal Disorders*

	Class I–IV (%)	Class I–III (%)
Excellent	54.9	61.4
Good	29.8	29.8
Fair	8.2	6.5
Poor	7.1	2.3

*Consecutive case series—319 patients: acute 9.4%, subacute 26.9%, chronic 63.6%.

Treatment method: McKenzie approach, which includes patient education, self-treatment, and mobilization/manipulation.

currence rate can be assessed through a telephone survey, mail survey, or follow-up examination. The questions should be constructed to provide information about pain and functional status, as well as whether or not the condition returned. The more specific information obtained will indicate whether the condition is recurring in a more or less severe presentation. The longer the follow-up, the more valuable will be the information obtained. However, at least a 3-year period would be recommended.

Prevention of Onset. A wellness program should ultimately target the prevention of onset. This is accomplished through education and methods of early detection. A discomfort survey, analyzed in comparison with known predisposing factors, can identify individuals at greatest risk. Through education, the individual can be taught to assess his or her mechanical function on a daily basis and react appropriately to any identified warning signs.

The prophylactic routines identified in this chapter can be used to check the regional mechanical systems. Known risk situations should be managed with ergonomic and biomechanical principles. Warning signs should be heeded and eliminated immediately with specific mechanical procedures. All of this is the individual's responsibility and requires a daily commitment to wellness that is similar in commitment to brushing one's teeth on a daily basis. The benefit in dental care is better smelling breath and no loss of teeth; in musculoskeletal care, it is no pain or loss of function.

SUMMARY/CONCLUSIONS

This chapter has outlined a mechanical method of assessing pain and function in the moving parts of our body. There has been a conspicuous absence of attention to aerobic fitness and specific strengthening of the muscles. This does not mean that neither of these is important in physical wellness and health. However, we believe that they should have a separate assessment from the more basic evaluation of the moving parts. It doesn't matter how efficient the engine is, or the amount of horsepower, if the wheels don't turn or the tire is flat.

Pain is a measurable, understandable, and predictable response of the soft tissue when it is mechanical in origin. Principles of change in length and tension or mechanical deformation of tissue can render the pain behavior a means of teaching the individual and the clinician when that individual is healthy or otherwise. The McKenzie system allows the individual to use his or her pain constructively and progress toward better health, as opposed to avoidance behavior and further limitation of function (Roberts, 1989).

Prevention of injury is ultimately the responsibility of the individual. The method of musculoskeletal injury prevention described in this chapter emphasizes a conceptual model from which an individual can learn to care for his or her own body. The key to success is the establishment of a cause and effect between pain production and pain relief, a good conceptual model with which to explain the pain response, and early interaction in the progression from warning signs to structural diagnosis. A constructive and caring approach, which is mechanically based, with specific criteria for determining effectiveness and applicability will provide an answer to the treatment and prevention of most musculoskeletal disorders.

References

Alexander AH, Jones AM, Rosenbaum DH, et al: Nonoperative management of herniated nucleus pulposus: Patient selection by the extension sign: Long-term follow-up. Presented at the North American Spine Society Annual Meeting, Monterey, CA, August, 1990.

Allan DB and Waddell G: An historical perspective on low back pain and disability. Acta Orthop Scand 60 (234):1–23, 1989.

Cunningham LS and Kelsey JL: Epidemiology of musculoskeletal impairments and associated disability. Am J Public Health 74(6):574–579, 1984.

Cyriax J: Textbook of Orthopaedic Medicine. Vol I: Diagnosis of Soft Tissue Lesions. London, Bailliere Tindall, 1982.

Deyo R: Measuring the functional status of patients with low back pain. Arch Phys Med Rehab 69:1044–1053, 1988.

Donelson R, Grant W, Medcalf R, et al: Pain response to repeated sagittal spine motion: A prospective, randomized, multi-centered trial. Spine 16: S206–S212, 1991a.

Donelson R, Grant W, Kamps C, et al: Low back and referred pain response to mechanical test movements in the frontal plane: A prospective, multi-centered trial. Presented at the International Society for the Study of the Lumbar Spine, Heidelberg, Germany, May 1991b.

Donelson R, Silva G, and Murphy K: Centralization Phenomenon: Its usefulness in evaluations and treating referred pain. Spine 15(3):211–213, 1990.

Elvey R: The investigation of arm pain. In Grieve G (ed): Modern Manual Therapy of the Vertebral Column. New York, Churchill Livingstone, 1987, pp 530–535.

Farry S, Hawley J, Laslett M, et al: A comparison of the effects of two sitting postures on back and referred pain. Spine (in press).

Frymoyer JW: Magnitude of the problem. In Weinstein JN and Wiesel SW (eds): The Lumbar Spine. Philadelphia, WB Saunders, 1990.

Frymoyer JW and Mooney V: Occupational orthopaedics. J Bone Joint Surg 68-A(3):469–474, 1986.

Hadler NM: Clinical Concepts in Regional Musculoskeletal Illness. New York, Grune & Stratton, 1987.

Huckisson EC: Measurement of pain. Lancet 2:1127–1131, 1974.

Kapandji IA: Physiology of the Joints. Vol 3: The Trunk and Vertebral Column. New York, Churchill Livingstone, 1976.

Kelsey J, Githens P, Walter SD, et al: An epidemiological study of acute prolapsed cervical intervertebral discs. J Bone Joint Surg 66(A):907, 1984.

Kelsey JL and Golden AL: Occupational and workplace factors associated with low back pain. Spine 2(1):7–16, 1987.

Kopp JR, Alexander AH, Turocy RH, et al: The use of lumbar extension in the evaluation and treatment of patients with acute herniated nucleus pulposus. Clin Orthop 202:211–218, 1986.

Kramer J: Intervertebral Disk Diseases. Chicago, Yearbook Medical Publishers, 1981.

McKenzie RA: Manual correction of sciatic scoliosis. N Z Med J 76 (484):194–199, 1972.

McKenzie RA: Prophylaxis in recurrent low back pain. N Z Med J 89 (627):22–23, 1979.

McKenzie RA: The Lumbar Spine: Mechanical Diagnosis and Therapy. Lower Hutt, New Zealand, Spinal Publications, 1981.

McKenzie RA: Treat Your Own Neck. Lower Hutt, New Zealand, Spinal Publications, 1983.

McKenzie RA: Treat Your Own Back, 4th ed. Waikanae, New Zealand, Spinal Publications, 1988.

McKenzie RA: A Perspective on Manipulative Therapy. Position Statement. Wellington, New Zealand, The McKenzie Institute International, 1989.

McKenzie RA: The Cervical and Thoracic Spine: Mechanical Diagnosis and Therapy. Waikanae, New Zealand, Spinal Publications, 1990.

Nachemson A: Advances in low back pain. Clin Orthop 200:266–278, 1985.

Nordin M and Frankle VH: Basic Biomechanics of the Musculoskeletal System, 2nd ed. Philadelphia, Lea & Febiger, 1989.

Panjabi M and White A: Clinical Biomechanics of the Spine, 2nd ed. Philadelphia, JB Lippincott, 1990.

Rath WW, Rath JND, and Duffy CG: A comparison of pain location and duration with treatment outcome and frequency. Presented at the First International McKenzie Conference, Newport Beach, CA, July 1989.

Roberts AP: Nottingham Acute Low Back Pain Study. Preliminary Report. Presented at the First International McKenzie Conference, Newport Beach, CA, July 1989.

Saal JA, Saal JS, and Herzog RJ: The natural history of lumbar intervertebral disc extrusions treated nonoperatively. Spine 15(7):683–686, 1990.

Scott J and Huskisson EC: Accuracy of subjective measurements made with and without previous scores: An important source of error in serial measurement of subjective states. Ann Rheum Dis 38:558–559, 1979.

Snook SH: The costs of back pain in industry. Spine 2(1):1–6, 1987.

Spitzer WO, LeBlanc FE, Dupuis M, et al: Scientific approach to the assessment and management of activity-related spinal disorders. Spine 12 (7S):1–59, 1987.

Stankovich R and Johnell O: Conservative treatment of acute low-back pain: A prospective randomized trial: McKenzie method of treatment versus patient education in "mini back school." Spine 15(2):120–123, 1990.

Vanharanta H: Etiology, epidemiology and natural history of lumbar disc disease. Spine 3(1):1–12, 1989.

Waddell G: A new clinical model for the treatment of low-back pain. Spine 12(7):632–644, 1987.

Weber H: Lumbar disc herniation: A prospective study with ten years of observation. Spine 8(2):131–140, 1983.

Wood PHN and Baddeley EM: Epidemiology of low back pain. In Jayson MIV (ed): Lumbar Spine and Back Pain. London, Churchill Livingstone, 1987, pp 29–57.

CHAPTER

6

Caroline Robinson Brayley
Susan Johnson Lieber

Prevention and Management of Chronic Pain

"Chronic benign pain is one of the most prevalent and resistant of all psychophysiologic disorders and creates severe medical, social, and economic problems for patients, medical personnel, hospitals, insurance companies and industry" (Tollison, 1989, p. 662).

For the past 3 decades, increased attention has focused on the management of individuals who have chronic pain (Bonica, 1988; Little, 1981; Roberts, 1983). When traditional medical management did not meet the needs of these clients, the concept of the multidisciplinary approach was instituted as the best form of medical service to provide comprehensive treatment (Aronoff et al, 1983; Bonica, 1988; Hallett and Pilowski, 1982). The multidisciplinary approach practiced today in many established pain centers throughout the United States is considered the state-of-the-art practice.

MEANING OF PAIN

Pain is subjective. Pain is personal. Pain is a common phenomenon that can occur with trauma such as a broken arm or hitting one's thumb with a hammer, or it can occur with muscle spasms and infections and as a result of surgery or myocardial infarctions. Pain can be due to emotional trauma such as a "broken heart."

Pain is a widespread problem for humans. Estimates of the prevalence of pain indicate that 15 to 20% of the population have some type of pain problems, whereas 25 to 30% have chronic pain dysfunction (Bonica, 1985).

Although pain is a common problem, different people ascribe different meaning to pain. Individuals who have recuperated from a bout with cancer may think that every pain they experience is a recurrence of the disease. Others may think that their pain is something to be expected, and they ignore the symptom until a major problem has developed. These same persons may apply a different meaning to the pain symptom under different circumstances. For example, under one situation an individual may believe that the pain being experienced is "only" indigestion, whereas under different circumstances the same individual may experience the same pain and believe that he or she is having a cardiac arrest.

Pain can be culturally biased. However, one needs to avoid stereotyping individual reactions solely as a function of cultural background. Cultural differences have not been exhaustively studied. However, some studies (Sternbach and Tursky, 1965; Tursky and Sternbach, 1967; Zborowski, 1969; Zola, 1966) have noted ethnocultural differences in pain and illness behavior of Jewish, Italian, Irish, and "Old American" clients. In general, they found that the Irish accepted pain as a matter of fact and often denied its existence. Old Americans tended to be stoic and bear their pain quietly. In contrast, the Jewish and Italian clients expressed their pain openly with emotion, and in some cases tended to exaggerate their pain. Additionally, they found that "people of Mediterranean cultural extraction are more likely to be aware and to communicate symptoms of physical discomfort than Northern European peoples" (Craig and Wyckoff, 1987, p. 102). Detailed descriptions of other ethnocultural groups have been reported by Weisenberg (1982) and Meinhardt and McCaffery (1983).

The effects of individual episodes of pain can far exceed the individual's boundaries. That is, not only can the person's life be totally devastated and dysfunctional, but the immediate family and relatives are also impacted. Employers, fellow employees, and the community are also likely to be affected. Additionally, society as a whole must pay the immense costs for evaluation, medical work-up and treatment, lost work hours, as well as other expenses (Rowlingson and Toomey, 1988).

Pain has been described as "the most complex human experience . . . the most frequent reason patients seek medical counsel" (Bonica, 1985, p. xxxi). It is a complex, personal, subjective, unpleasant experience involving sensations and perceptions that may or may not be related in any way to an injury, illness, or other bodily trauma and is influenced by psychosocial, ethnocultural, biologic, physiologic, and chemical factors (Aronoff, 1983, p. 55). One author defined pain as "an unpleasant sensory and emotional experience associated with actual or potential tissue damage or described in terms of such damage" (Mersky, 1986). Of particular importance in these two definitions is the interrelatedness of both physical and cognitive–affective components regardless if the pain is acute or chronic. This vital aspect must be understood and incorporated in dealing with individuals with pain if one is to provide modern and comprehensive care. More important is the concept that the person with pain must comprehend and accept the combined impact of the body and mind as well (Rowlingson and Toomey, 1988).

There are significant differences between acute and chronic pain. Acute pain is "a biologically necessary physiologic response that, through its function to notify the body of impending or ongoing tissue damage, triggers an escape reaction so that the damage will be diminished or even eliminated" (Rowlingson and Toomey, 1988, p. 47). We all have experienced acute pain in our lifetime and then have been subjected to the stages of injury through relief from acute pain. It is a biologically useful pain warning us of an underlying problem, enabling us to seek treatment and receive relief, frequently through medication. However, when the pain remains after weeks or months of treatment, it is referred to as chronic pain (Bonica, 1985; Mersky, 1986).

Chronic pain is not biologically useful. Some physicians concur that the chronic pain syndrome is a disease entity unto itself, with symptoms of both the original, acute medical problem and a chronic illness (Addison, 1984). It has a negative impact on the individual's lifestyle (physical, psychosocial, vocational, financial, and family) and is generally not effectively treated with medications. Bonica (1982) defined chronic pain as lasting longer than 6 months or beyond the normal course of the disease or injury.

MAGNITUDE OF THE PROBLEM

Chronic benign pain is one of the most serious, challenging, and baffling health problems confronting the health-care establishment and society. Industrial accidents and nonindustrial musculoskeletal injuries result in the chronic disability of thousands of persons each year in the United States. Tons of medications and tranquilizers are prescribed daily, and numerous hospitals provide surgical intervention for the relief of chronic pain. Billions of dollars are spent yearly on lost work time, medications, medical bills, and worker's compensation benefits. The cost for low back pain has been estimated at over 16 billion dollars annually. Yet untold numbers of clients remain unrelieved from their pain and are unable to return to the work force (Brena, 1978; Brena and Chapman, 1983; Crue, 1979; Seres et al, 1981).

Table 6–1 reports the number of selected chronic conditions by race and work age in the United States in 1988. These statistics were gathered by requesting households of the civilian population to respond to an interview survey indicating their chronic conditions.

Snook and Webster (1987) reported that musculoskeletal disorders were the most frequent type of disability (about two thirds of severely disabled and two thirds of partially disabled). They further reported that one of the most com-

Table 6–1. Number of Selected Reported Chronic Conditions by Race and Work Age: United States, 1988*

Type of Chronic Condition	White Population		Black Population	
	Under 45 Years	*45–64 Years*	*Under 45 Years*	*45–64 Years*
Arthritis	5,035	10,337	526	1,154
Intervertebral disc	1,681	1,594	54	114
Bone or cartilage disorders	320	449	24	24
Deformity of orthopedic impairment	13,301	6,048	1,695	700
Back	8,067	3,728	718	285
Upper extremities	1,299	945	160	142
Lower extremities	5,133	2,340	1,024	350
Migraine headache	5,799	1,783	649	193

ªNumber of Chronic Conditions in Thousands
*From National Center for Health Statistics: Current Estimates from the National Interview Survey, 1988 (Department of Health and Human Services publication no. [DPHS] 89–1501). Hyattsville, MD: U.S. Government Printing Office, 1989.

mon musculoskeletal conditions was back pain, estimating that "31 million Americans have back pain and 28 million have some type of back abnormalities" (p. 82).

Figure 6–1 displays the level of disability by the type of disorder. It indicates that musculoskeletal disorders affect a much greater percentage of both severely and partially disabled individuals than any of the other disorders.

Clients with back pain from back injury outweigh by far all other types of chronic pain. The estimates of the number of individuals who will suffer back pain are staggering in terms of cost and work time lost. Waddell (1987) estimated that "at some stage of their lives, 80% of the human race will experience low-back pain" and that "each year 2 to 5% of the at-risk population will seek medical attention or lose time from work because of low-back problems" (p. 632). He further stated that there has been a dramatic increase in low-back disability throughout Western society between the 1950s and 1970s as demonstrated by work-time loss, compensation, certified sick time, and long-term disability. Aronoff (1985) attributed chronic back pain as the most frequent cause of activity dysfunction in young

Figure 6–1. Disability by type of disorder. (Redrawn from Snook SH and Webster BS: The Cost of Disability from Clinical Orthopedics and Related Research. Philadelphia, JB Lippincott, 1987, p 79.)

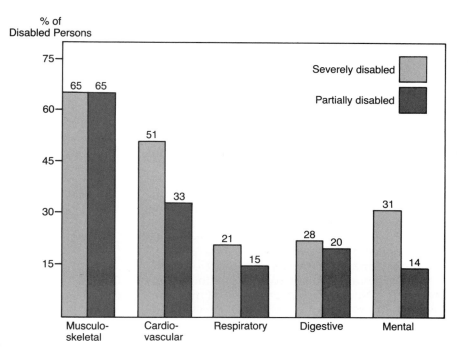

Americans (under age 45). He further stated that it is the third major cause of limitation of activity for older Americans (over age 45).

Beals (1984) estimated that almost 2% of the industrial work force in America suffer a compensable back injury annually. Additionally, a more recent publication by the Institute of Medicine (Osterweis et al, 1987) cited a study that indicated a higher estimation of the problem: Ten to 15% of adults have back pain resulting in some work disability in a given year. Bonica (1982) estimated that there are 8 million partially disabled and 2.4 million totally disabled Americans as a result of low back pain. These statistics for partial and total disability translate into approximately 1.4 lost work days per worker annually or almost one quarter of all disabling work-related injuries in America (Anderson, 1981). When this number of lost work days is compared with the number of work-loss days (5.3) for the entire population with acute and chronic conditions, we can determine that back pain is a significant problem both economically and socially for the clients, health-care service providers, and society.

It also suggests that prevention programs focusing on work-related back injuries and their ramifications would have significant positive effects economically and sociologically.

CHARACTERISTICS OF CLIENTS WITH CHRONIC PAIN

Personality Factors

There is extensive literature about the personality characteristics of clients with chronic pain. Personality testing, specifically the Minnesota Multiphasic Personality Inventory, is widely used in chronic pain centers. Psychosomatic complaints, which are developed in the absence of a physical cause, may be due to various types of psychologic conditions such as conversion symptoms, hallucinations, or tension states. Therefore, it is important to know the extent that personality factors or stress contribute to the expressed symptoms through these mechanisms. However, two very important factors complicate the issue. First, the pain-producing injury itself may be causing the stress and, in turn, the changed personality or emotional state. Second, selection factors such as personality and temperament

contribute to the determination of the persons who will seek treatment (Mersky, 1987).

Physical Factors

Pain is referred to as chronic pain when it has persisted for more than 6 months. Individuals perceive pain differently as a result of a variety of factors; however, regardless of the individual's perception and type of injury, there are common characteristics among the chronic pain clients. West (1988) identified these characteristics as follows:

The person is disabled beyond the scope of the organic disorder. Decreased endurance, strength, and mobility become the result of progressive inactivity.

Time spent resting also is time spent alone. This special isolation can contribute to a person's perception of life as boring and depressing.

Overt pain behavior is customary. This behavior can present in various ways; however, it is most commonly displayed as an antalgic gait, guarded movement, and heavy sighing and groaning. Excessive verbal complaints are the norm in the chronic pain patient populations. In essence, pain becomes the person's central focus and the person's behavior becomes a reflection of this focus.

Preoccupation with pain often paves the way for the person to assume the patient role both at home and in the community. A gradual dependency on others results from this role as other people begin to take on the injured person's responsibilities such as household tasks and parenting. As a result, the person generally is cared for by those around him or her. This type of response from others reinforces the person's inactivity and pain behavior and, consequently, perpetuates the person's chronic pain-dysfunction cycle. Returning to normal responsibilities and activities thus becomes more difficult for the person as the patient role is ingrained (p. 287).

Psychologic Factors

Compensated industrial accident victims may have an exaggerated disability and delayed recovery because of the number of reinforcers that are inherent in the recovery process. "Delayed recovery refers to a group of conditions that prevent injured workers from regaining their productivity or ability to cope at work or in their personal lives'' (Killian, 1988, p. 247). The premorbid behavioral and psychologic factors, in addition to those that developed at the time of and during the process of treatment of the injury, all play a factor in the recovery process. Leedy (1971) indicated that the following seven factors were important indicators to the individual's psychologic set, which could have an impact on injury and recovery: depression, hysterical personality, dependency and immaturity, pseudo–self-sufficient persons, aging workers with a predisposed personality disorder, alcoholics, and sociopathic personalities.

Elton and colleagues (1983) also identified psychologic factors that have impact on the increase of pain. These include anxiety, depression, and low self-esteem, each of which is briefly described next.

Anxiety. Relative to anxiety, numerous studies, both experimental and clinical, have demonstrated that reduction of anxiety levels and increased client control over procedures increased the pain threshold (Hill et al, 1952; Klusman, 1975; Mandler and Watson, 1966; Stam et al, 1984; Wilson-Evered and Stanley, 1986; Wolff and Horland, 1967). These findings indicated that relaxation techniques, biofeedback, and cognitive training can have an important part in the clinical treatment of pain (Elton, 1987).

The literature shows that anxiety plays an important and powerful role in maintaining and augmenting pain. Both experimental and clinical evidence indicate that individuals in pain show considerable anxiety. Psychometric studies point to pre-existing anxiety traits in cases of prolonged and severe pain (Elton, 1987, p. 92).

Elton (1987) of the Department of Psychology, University of Melbourne, further stated that, although both pain and depression may exist in some clients, acute pain clients are predominated by anxiety because of their concern with the pain's implications and worry over potential disability and social problems. Conversely, depression predominates in clients with chronic pain. Sternbach (1978) has theorized that there is a correlation between the biochemical reaction of the body in pain and in depression. ''In both conditions, there was evidence of withdrawal of interests, weakening of relationships, increased somatic preoccupation, appetite disturbance, irritability, sleep disturbance, hopelessness, and despair'' (Elton, 1987, p. 92).

Depression. There are many studies in the literature on the relationship between depression and chronic pain. Although not all studies are conclusive in demonstrating a direct relationship, many studies are. For example, Timmermans and Sternbach (1974) determined that there was a direct relationship between depression and pain and they further argued that when the depression was relieved so was the pain. Although they could not identify the exact mechanism for this correlation, they were convinced that the mechanism of depression may reduce the threshold for pain (Elton, 1987). Other studies (Elton, 1987; Gerschman and Reade, 1987; Joffe and Sandler, 1967; Lesse, 1983) supported these findings. Ward and colleagues (1979) found that many pain symptoms disappear when the clients are administered antidepressant drugs.

Studying the relationship between depression and chronic pain is hampered by the fact that some clients are not aware of their depression. Frequently, clients with chronic pain exhibit anguish, hopelessness, and suffering, the predominant symptoms of depression (Blumer and Heilbronn, 1982). Psychologic testing often shows depression in clients with chronic pain, even though they do not feel depressed, having been masked by somatic complaints. There is significant evidence that masked depression may be heavily related to pain. ''Often when patients attribute their depression to pain, a study of premorbid personality indicates that the depression preceded pain'' (Elton, 1987, p. 94).

Depression is an important factor in the treatment of chronic pain clients because, as Lesse (1983) argued, it is often misdiagnosed and consequently untreated. He described masked depression in terms of sadness, feelings of worthlessness, guilt, dejection, despair, gloominess, excessive criticism of others and self, and negative self-image (Elton, 1987).

Self-Esteem. Elton and associates (1978), Joffe and Sandler (1967), and Lesse (1983) investigated the relationship between chronic pain and self-esteem. They determined that self-esteem may be an important factor in the treatment of clients with chronic pain. Coping with pain is learned in the early years of life. That is, if children learn that they will receive greater attention or rewards by way of increased care and concern by their parents when exhibiting pain, then they will use that symptom to gain what they want (Engel, 1958). Additionally, individuals may find it less difficult to deal with tangible, physical pain than to endure a "state of inner unrest, guilt and low self-esteem. Pain in these patients, may provide a way out of facing difficult situations and decisions" (Elton, 1987, p. 94).

Elton and colleagues' (1978) investigation demonstrated that when treatment was centered on improving self-esteem, the symptom of pain was greatly reduced. Therefore, they deduced that self-esteem was an important factor to consider when treating clients in pain who were not improving with standard medical care.

COSTS

There have been numerous economic studies on disability issues. However, the direct economics of pain as it relates to disability have not been studied. Therefore, we present an overview of the economics of disability so that readers can better comprehend the larger picture of disability programs and the pain problem (Osterweis et al, 1987).

Snook and Webster (1987) defined disability "as a limitation in the amount or the kind of gainful work that can be performed because of a chronic condition or impairment" (p. 77). They went on to classify disability "according to severity or length of time" (p. 77) as in Table 6–2.

The costs for disability include medical care costs, lost wages compensation, and indirect costs such as individual suffering, lost work hours, and production. The first two are usually covered by the three major types of disability insurance in the United States; namely, the federal program, Social Security Disability Insurance (SSDI); the state-regulated program, Workers' Compensation Insurance; and private insurance companies.

Social Security Disability Insurance

The 1935 Social Security Act started providing disability insurance to disabled workers in 1954.

Table 6–2. Classification of Disability

Severity	Length of Time
Severely or totally disabled	Cannot work at all or regularly
Partially disabled	Must do different work or not work full time
Temporary or short-term disabled	Lasts for several months

Since that time the act has changed numerous times so that: (1) it now covers disabled workers of all ages; (2) the eligibility includes those individuals whose disability has or is expected to continue for at least 12 months; (3) the length of work required for eligibility has been reduced to include younger workers; (4) disabled widows (between the ages of 50 and 60 years) of covered workers can receive benefits; and (5) individuals younger than 65 years can receive Medicare benefits if they have been receiving disability payments for at least 24 consecutive months (Grant, 1973).

Because of these increased benefits, the cost of Social Security has risen considerably. By 1985, employees taxes have increased 93 times since 1937. These increased costs have primarily been "due to the disability insurance and hospital insurance programs added to Social Security in later years" (Snook and Webster, 1987, p. 79).

Slightly over 2.5 million disabled workers were granted a monthly check of $469.62 in 1985. Additionally, over 300,000 spouses received an average of $128.97 monthly, and over 900,000 children received an average monthly payment of $138.90. These payments total $16.8 billion annually (Snook and Webster, 1987).

Since 1982 there has been a decrease in the cost of SSDI because of a trend by the federal government to shift the cost from the public to the private sector. SSDI typically reviews its disability cases every 3 years, and in 1982 it terminated over 45% of its cases (Snook and Webster, 1987).

Workers' Compensation Insurance

All 50 states have enacted Workers' Compensation Insurance laws requiring employers to pay for job disability insurance regardless of fault. This included 77.8 million or 87.5% of all wage and salaried workers in the United States in 1982. Exempted workers often include state and local government employees, farm workers, casual laborers, domestics, and those employed in small companies.

Workers' Compensation Insurance benefits include (1) impairment and disability cash benefits; (2) unlimited dollar and time medical benefits; and (3) medical and vocational rehabilitation benefits for severe disabilities. Most employers subscribe to this type of insurance from private insurance companies; in some states, however, employers may insure with a public fund. Still other employers, if financially capable, may chose to self-insure their employees. The cost to the employers in the United States in 1982 was just over $22.5 billion (Snook and Webster, 1987).

The total cost of workers' compensation benefits in the United States in 1982 was $16.1 billion. Of this, $4.8 billion was spent on medical costs and $11.3 billion was compensation for lost wages (Chamber of Commerce of the United States, 1985). Individuals classified as temporary total disability received more than 70% of the cash payments; however, workers with permanent partial disabilities received the largest amount of money (Price, 1984).

Private Health Insurance

Private health insurance comes in various forms, for both individuals and groups. There are insurance plans for hospital expenses (the most common form) and surgical, physician, and dental expenses. "Major medical expense insurance covers a wide range of medical expenses with few internal limits and a high overall maximum benefit. Major medical insurance is often subject to some form of deductible and co-insurance payments by the insured" (Snook and Webster, 1987, p. 81).

There is also disability income protection insurance, which provides a vehicle for the worker to replace lost income in cases of accident, illness, or pregnancy. Short-term protection enables the worker to collect benefits for up to 2 years. Long-term protection provides benefits for a minimum of 5 years and even for life. Disability income protection is offered only by insurance companies (Health Insurance Association of America, 1982–1983).

In the United States, there are over 1,000 insurance companies providing private health-insurance coverage. Blue Cross offers hospital coverage plans; Blue Shield covers surgical and medical care by the physician. Health-maintenance organizations (HMOs) provide health-care coverage with plans directed by employers, unions, communities, fraternal societies, and both consumer and rural health cooperatives (Snook and Webster, 1987).

In 1981, Americans spent $84.9 billion for private health-insurance plans. During the same year, private insuring organizations paid a total of $75.9 billion in health-insurance benefits, rep-

resenting a 13.1% increase from 1980 and 4 times the amount paid in 1970. Higher medical costs, increased benefits, and increased user rates are attributed to this increase (Health Insurance Association of America, 1982 to 1983).

As already stated, musculoskeletal disorders are the leading cause of disability among the working-age population (aged 18 to 64 years). Back pain is the most common musculoskeletal disorder and economically results in almost $16 billion in expenditures annually (Grazier et al, 1984). Workers' compensation spends nearly $5 billion for back pain in the United States (Snook and Jensen, 1984). "The average cost of compensable back pain is approximately $6,000 per case (median cost, $750). The large discrepancy between the mean and median indicates that back pain costs are not normally distributed. A few high-cost cases account for most of the cost" (Snook and Webster, 1987, p. 82).

PAIN CENTERS: A HISTORICAL PERSPECTIVE

The early writings of Mandel (1938) and Leriche (1939) apprised the medical community that anesthesiologists were able to provide treatment of pain by administering a local anesthetic to block the nerve pathways. After World War II, a small number of pain clinics emerged that used the nerve blocks as the primary form of intervention. Simultaneously yet separately, the unique strategy of multidisciplinary treatment was being developed by Bonica in Washington, Alexander in Texas, and Livingston in Oregon. Despite Alexander's (1954) and Livingston's (1943) endorsement of the multidisciplinary model, Bonica has been heralded as the forefather of the multidisciplinary chronic pain treatment center.

Bonica recognized the value of multidisciplinary intervention when his clients were being treated more effectively as a result of gathering his consultants to collaborate on treatment plans. In 1953, he published *The Management of Pain*, which elaborated on the multidisciplinary model; the differences between acute and chronic pain; the anatomic, physiologic, and psychologic bases of pain; classification of pain syndromes; nerve block techniques; and therapeutic modalities.

Similarly, the fields of physical medicine and rehabilitation experienced growth and development after World War II because of the recognition that allied health professionals were qualified to address the needs of the rehabilitation population (DeLisa et al, 1988). As a result, multidisciplinary treatment became the standard for rehabilitation. The parallels in growth patterns between physical medicine and the field of chronic pain can be attributed to the growth of the allied health professions and the physicians' recognition that the complex needs of their clients were optimally addressed by a variety of specialists dedicated to coordinating their energies to obtain maximal functional outcomes.

As previously stated, Bonica and White established a multidisciplinary pain clinic at the University of Washington in 1961. Since then, there has been a tremendous growth in the number of pain clinics, many of these modeled after Bonica and White's. In 1976, 17 pain clinics were listed in *Medical World News*; currently, the American Academy of Pain Medicine and the American Pain Society estimate that there are over 1,000 pain clinics in the United States.

In recent years, the concept of interdisciplinary treatment has been introduced as a similar yet uniquely different type of intervention than the multidisciplinary model. Newman and Seres (1986) suggested the differentiating feature of the interdisciplinary team is that the members operate as a democratic unit with integration of therapeutic modalities and without deference to some arbitrary hierarchy. Aronoff and Wagner (1987) and Segraves (1989) also suggested that for a team to address the needs of the chronic pain population they must act as a cohesive unit. Despite the authors' consistent emphasis on the highly interactive team, they have not reached a consensus on whether the type of team should be called inter- or multidisciplinary or labeled another term to describe the treatment model.

The development of a cohesive interdisciplinary team has been challenged or delayed by a variety of interrelated factors. First, if the physician or allied health professional is accustomed to acute care intervention, the transition to rehabilitation can be a difficult adjustment because of the involvement of additional personnel and because progress is generally made at a slower pace. Second, the interdisciplinary or the multidisciplinary approach is not consistent with the traditional medical model because the physician is called on to manage the team rather than direct their actions. Some physicians may experience difficulty in altering their approach to the other professionals. Most have had little or no training in team-management skills (Currie and Marber-

ger, 1988). Third, a loss of autonomy is experienced by all team members to assimilate the multiplicity of theories into a single common approach to client care (Newman and Seres, 1986; Segraves, 1989). The willingness to accept the identity of a team is facilitated by the actions and attitudes of each team member. The effectiveness of the team is promoted by team members who can abandon their notion of territorial rights, recognize the benefits of melding their professional knowledge and experiences, and demonstrate allegiance to the team. The development of an effective team is obstructed when team members fail to recognize the benefits of a harmonious team and when membership values the identity of their sole profession over the identity of the team.

Because interdisciplinary treatment is considered state of the art, it is imperative that the individual health-care providers join together to define the goals and objectives of the clinic and develop a plan to meet the goals. In addition, a method for evaluating programmatic outcomes is crucial to determine the effectiveness of treatment and the need for programmatic revisions.

TREATMENT MODALITIES

The regulation of pain and suffering has been a preoccupation since the beginning of time. There are references to strategies to ameliorate pain in the Egyptian papyri, the Koran, and the Bible. Philosophers, religious leaders, health care providers, and layman alike have speculated as to the nature and cause of pain while seeking effective means of relief. The therapeutic armamentarium has consisted of a dizzying array of modalities. Consider the following melange: surgery, dorsal column stimulation, hot packs, cold packs, traction, massage, cupping, trephining, palliative radiotherapy, nerve blocks, steroid injections, manipulations of the spine, transcutaneous nerve stimulation, muscle relaxants, antiinflammatory medication. This list includes just some of the treatment modalities administered by the many different kinds of health care professionals who work with patients with chronic pain . . . Many other approaches have been employed outside the purview of medical practitioners; for example, copper bracelets, faith healing, distraction, "rational repudiation" through logical means, and the use of "patent" medicine, to name only a few (Turk and Holzman, 1986, p. 257).

According to Turk and Holzman (1986), there are two important factors about this statement. First, some clients seem to have received relief from their pain with each of these treatment modalities, whereas others have not been relieved of their pain no matter what treatment was attempted. Perhaps, it might be speculated, those who were relieved from pain had a "psychologic pain," an unreal pain. Even with all the increased knowledge, the medical field does not thoroughly understand pain and its control, nor does it have adequate treatment protocols.

Out of frustration with existing inadequate treatment of pain, pain centers came into existence to deal with the complexity of problems of clients with pain, particularly chronic pain. Many types of pain centers exist: modality-oriented unidisciplinary clinics, where the primary treatment is predominantly transcutaneous electrical neuromuscular stimulation (TENS) and nerve blocks; syndrome-oriented unidisciplinary or multidisciplinary clinics, which primarily treat low back pain or headaches; and multidisciplinary pain clinics, which treat chronic pain syndrome (Aronoff and Wagner, 1987).

APPROACHES TO CHRONIC PAIN MANAGEMENT

Two different philosophies are discussed here: operant behavioral and cognitive behavioral.

Operant Behavioral Approach

The interest in the operant behavioral approach (also known as operant conditioning; Gil et al, 1988) to the management of clients with chronic pain started when Fordyce published his description in 1968 (Fordyce, Fowler, and DeLateur, 1968; Fordyce, Fowler, Lehmann, et al, 1968; Roberts, 1986). The operant approach focuses on the behavior exhibited by the clients and family members and not on the reduction of pain. It does not presume necessarily an underlying psychiatric or medical determinant for the disability. Therefore, the goal of the treatment is to enable clients to improve their function and to reduce their disability by changing their behavior.

The underlying premise of this approach is the belief that the behaviors of some chronic pain clients are reinforced by social factors. That is, "patients may learn that pain behavior results in positive reinforcement such as the solicitous attention from a spouse, or provides a legitimate excuse for avoiding unwanted responsibilities" (Gil et al, 1988, p. 378). These clients do not exhibit pain connected to specific tissue damage or any specific neurologic diagnoses. Consequently, their pain is viewed as excessive. As previously stated, the goal of the treatment is not to reduce pain, even though many clients report decreased pain after receiving operant conditioning treatment, but to reduce "excess disability" (Roberts, 1986). It should be noted, however, that the degree of excessive disability is not easy to discern.

The protocol of the operant behavioral approach is assessment, treatment, and discharge.

Assessment. First, medical participation is warranted for both the start and continuation of the operant program. Second, a functional behavior interview is conducted with the clients and their family members to identify the environmental and social reinforcers impacting on the degree of pain disability. The assessment is designed to discern the limitations of the clients' daily activities as a result of pain, the frequency and duration of pain, and the clients' mood and attitude as related to pain. Some clients are requested to keep a pain diary for several days. Clients are observed by the health-care personnel using a standardized pain behavior observation form to corroborate the clients' pain behavior.

Information from family members is assessed. This is frequently very useful for determining the clients' operant behavior pain patterns. The family members often provide clues to the clients' behavior patterns in the home. They can report on the clients' activities and interests, which are often lacking or have greatly decreased. Frequently, they report that the clients' life is primarily focused on their pain and visits to the doctor. Usually psychologic tests (Minnesota Multiphasic Personality Inventory) are administered to clients and their spouses to screen for depression, anxiety, psychopathology, ego strength, dependency, and so on (Roberts, 1986).

The results of the assessment determine whether clients should be treated and what parts of the program should be engaged. The assessment should provide answers to the following questions: "How disabled is the client? How much time, effort, and expense is the client and his or her family willing to put into a treatment program? Which components of a management program are necessary to increase function and which ones can be dispensed with? How long should a treatment program continue? How much follow up is needed?" (Roberts, 1986 p. 20).

Roberts (1986) purported that the assessment will also include the answers to these questions:

> Will the patient need special treatment of attention for depression? In addition to the withdrawal of medications and focus on increasing activity and function, what special problems, such as alcohol, weight, or marital problems, need to be addressed? If the patient has a weight problem that is medically significant, will diet need to be a component of the program or can it be managed by exercise alone? What are the marital and family relationships contributing to the disability? Can intervention change these sufficiently to assure reasonably that the patient will not only increase his/her activity but also maintain these changes? If marital stress is involved, are interventions possible or appropriate to reduce these stresses? (p. 20)

Treatment. After the assessment, the client is told about the prescribed operant conditioning treatment program, which is described in general terms, and rationale for this type of treatment is provided. The treatment protocol is designed to obtain sanction and support from a medical physician, discontinue unnecessary medications, increase levels of physical activity, teach the client to functionally adopt methods of dealing with the pain, and engage the family in facilitating physical activity and withholding reinforcements of disability (Roberts, 1986). Physical therapy is used to recondition the client and to teach him or her to rest between bouts of activity. This principle of activity and rest cycles is inherent in the philosophy of the operant behavioral approach.

The issue of reinforcers is prevalent throughout this choice of treatment. Individual positive reinforcers are selected for each client and incorporated into the treatment plan by all health-care workers providing care. "The most common reinforcer is praise and attention from members of the health care team and family members" (Roberts, 1986, p. 23). Other reinforcers may include appropriate refreshments, activities that the client likes to do as provided by the occupational therapist, rest, and so on.

The important factor here is that negative reinforcers be decreased and withdrawn. No attention is paid when the client presents or expresses pain symptoms. Roberts (1986) reported that initially, when pain symptoms are ignored by the health-care team members, they increase, only to decrease later on. Also "failure is never reinforcing" (Roberts, 1986); therefore, goals are never set too high or increased too soon to result in failure.

Shaping and molding are other aspects of the treatment procedure. In the aspect, shaping the desired behaviors are broken into graded steps, which are sequentially taught. Each step is then rewarded and the client moves on. Eventually, he or she will learn a new pattern of behavior, approximating normal activity. Molding involves therapists and family members participating in exercise programs and activities with the client. The family is then encouraged to participate in the client's home program.

Clients are provided with their own personal copy of graphs depicting improvement in their activities to carry with them while in the treatment areas. The purpose of these graphs is as a self-reinforcer as well as an indicator for team reinforcement.

Discharge. The client is discharged when he or she has developed "alternate and more functionally adaptive ways to manage pain" (Gil et al, 1988, p. 382). A more detailed description of the operant approach can be found in *Pain Management* by Holzman and Turk (1986) or *Chronic Pain* by France and Krishman (1988).

Cognitive-Behavioral Approach

This approach was developed when the effects of the operant approach were difficult to generalize beyond the treatment clinic and found to be more theoretically based on Melzack and Wall's (1965) theory of pain (Turk and Kerns, 1983). The aspects of the program include screening, assessment, treatment, and discharge.

Screening. Almost all clients referred to cognitive-behavioral treatment programs are accepted for treatment except those who meet the following criteria for exclusion: (1) plans for other medical or surgical procedures; (2) reported pain for less than 4 months; (3) acute psychiatric care needed; and (4) pain from terminal illness (Holzman et al, 1986).

Clients are interviewed to discern their complaints relative to their pain and its duration, a brief medical history, and mental status evaluation. Then if clients are deemed to be acceptable candidates, the program is explained in detail. Emphasis is on informing the clients that they will be taught coping mechanisms to deal with and control their pain. It is important that clients' attitudes and motivation for changing their behavior be addressed directly.

During the screening process, any misconceptions clients have about the treatment are addressed. Clients are informed that they must be active participants in the treatment process and that no guarantees are given for success; however, they are given a positive outlook for success.

Assessment. The assessment includes data gathering through interviews with the clients and their significant others; questionnaires, psychophysiology, and behavioral observation. The purpose of such data collection is to (1) determine if clients are appropriate for the treatment program; (2) develop a baseline from which to determine progress; (3) develop an individualized treatment plan; (4) acquire knowledge of the problems and situations that can later be used in treatment; and (5) develop a basis for goal setting and assignments for homework (Holzman et al, 1986).

Multiple cognitive-behavioral assessments are used to determine factors about the clients' pain, including its effect on their lifestyle and also their coping mechanisms. Other factors such as the specific impact the pain has on the clients' attitude and psyche are determined during the assessment.

During the assessment phase, and central to this approach, is the notion that the clients are seen as collaborators in the intervention process and that the therapists are facilitators of the process. This concept is initiated during the goal-development stage, usually the end of the assessment phase of the program. Goals were individually determined for clients and negotiated with them. The goals must be measurable, obtainable, observable, and agreed upon by clients and staff. The goals are "developed in consideration of the individual's current status, of his or her particular limitations or disabilities, and of the more general goals for treatment" (Holzman et al, 1986, p. 17).

Treatment. The underlying philosophy of the cognitive-behavioral treatment program is that clients must reconceptualize their beliefs and thoughts about pain. The desired change is that clients forgo the belief that they suffer from an uncontrollable medical all-encompassing pain to

one over which they have control. Thus, the intervention is designed to teach clients how to control their pain through coping mechanisms. Clients must be able to give up old habit patterns and ineffective responses by learning new methods of compensation such as problem solving, control of affect, and changing behavior (Kanfer and Karoly, 1982). Individuals must be actively involved in their own treatment and learn to "recognize and alter the association between thoughts, feelings, behaviors, environmental stimuli, and pain" (Holzman et al, 1986, p. 38).

According to Holzman, Turk, and Kerns (1986), the treatment process consists of four elements: education, acquisition of skills, cognitive and behavioral rehearsal, and generalization and maintenance. These are usually presented to clients simultaneously, offering the opportunity of elements interacting with each other.

The first aspect—education—has already been presented under assessment. That is, clients collaborate in the development of individualized goals in relation to their competencies, limitations and strengths, and situation.

The second aspect—skills acquisition—deals with a variety of strategies and techniques used to meet the goals. Such procedures include relaxation training, cognitive distraction or attention diversion, and cognitive restructuring. The object of skills acquisition is to teach clients to reconceptualize their pain problems by learning new coping strategies.

During the third phase of the intervention program—cognitive and behavioral rehearsal—clients practice the skills they have learned and apply them to everyday situations. Clients accomplish this rehearsing through mental imagery, role-playing, and homework activities. Each of these are designed to provide opportunities to experience managing and controlling pain. They assist clients in meeting the stated goals and achieving success.

The final aspect—generalization and maintenance—helps to prevent a relapse of previous symptoms and behaviors. During this phase, the therapists help clients identify future situations or factors that may cause them to revert to old patterns and thoughts. Successful coping mechanisms are then reinforced, and problem solving is promoted.

Discharge. The final meeting before discharge is spent reviewing all prior training. Time is spent reinforcing clients' abilities and recognizing their efforts to achieve the goals. Clients are encouraged about their progress and informed that the therapists believe that this progress will be maintained (Holzman et al, 1986).

PAIN EVALUATION AND TREATMENT INSTITUTE

The Pain Evaluation and Treatment Institute is located in an outpatient facility sponsored by the University of Pittsburgh Medical Health Care Division and Presbyterian-University Hospital in Pittsburgh. The institute is a major comprehensive pain center committed to the evaluation and treatment of a variety of pain and rehabilitation problems. The philosophical foundation of the treatment offered at the institute is the cognitive-behavioral approach discussed earlier. The primary emphasis of the treatment provided by the staff is on aiding individuals in developing their maximum functional level through various types of physical and psychologic interventions.

Referrals to the institute may be initiated by clients' primary physician, insurance adjusters, rehabilitation specialists, or on occasion by the clients. Before scheduling treatment, referrals are screened to determine the most appropriate type of evaluation and to obtain authorization of reimbursement from either workers' compensation, private insurance, automobile liability insurance, medical assistance, Medicare, or the clients themselves.

Clients with chronic pain generally undergo a 5-hour comprehensive evaluation conducted by the physician, psychologist, and physical therapist. As part of the evaluation process, clients are asked to complete a series of psychometric tests that are used to examine the impact of pain on each client's life, the response of others to their communication of pain, and their general activity level. In addition, the clients' significant others or family members are interviewed by the psychologist to ascertain the impact that the pain has had on family functioning.

For clients with acute pain, the evaluating team consists of the physician, physical therapist, occupational therapist, and the nurse. If there appear to be psychosocial issues at the time of the evaluation, the psychology staff will be consulted. The differences between the chronic and acute teams' membership results in examining the unique needs of each group and designing a program to best serve each population.

After each type of assessment, the evaluating team convenes to discuss their findings and outline treatment recommendations. Immediately thereafter, the evaluation findings and recommendations are reviewed with clients and their significant others, if present, to ascertain their willingness to participate in treatment. Correspondence with the auxiliary team members occurs within 48 hours to report the evaluation findings and treatment recommendations and to obtain authorization from the third-party payer.

Treatment is rendered by an interdisciplinary team of health-care professionals dedicated to assisting clients in identifying the thoughts, emotions, and behaviors that contribute to their experience of pain and to teaching them alternate coping strategies. Implementation of the management strategies enables clients to cope with their routine levels of pain as well as any flare-up or exacerbation of the pain when it occurs. The treatment goal is to prevent the long-term effects of inactivity often associated with an increase in pain and to prevent future flare-ups. Prevention is facilitated by establishing a regular exercise program, pacing daily activities, using body mechanics for the performance of activities of daily living, and incorporating relaxation techniques into the daily routine. It also includes monitoring and adjusting the clients' thoughts about their chronic pain and using medications appropriately.

The Institute's treatment team consists of representatives from various specialties including anesthesiology, physical medicine, physical therapy, occupational therapy, nursing, and psychology. In addition, clients, their significant others, insurance adjusters, rehabilitation nurses, and vocational counselors are considered to be auxiliary members of the team. Consistent communication among the team members is critical for successful and effective implementation of interdisciplinary treatment.

At the institute, the communication process is reinforced by regularly scheduled team meetings to discuss each client's progress, identify factors impeding progress, and develop strategies to produce successful outcomes. Contact with the auxiliary team members may occur during formal meetings or through written or verbal correspondence with clients.

There are two types of client meetings. The first one occurs before the initiation of treatment when the team members meet with clients to collaborate on the establishment of treatment goals. The second type of meeting is scheduled to discuss the clients' progress and to outline the emphasis for future treatment sessions.

The interdisciplinary treatment approach is further augmented by informal daily interactions among the team members and at general staff meetings. Each setting provides the team members with an opportunity to discuss treatment philosophies and to refine their perpetually developing approach to this unique population. This process is necessary in order for all the staff, regardless of their professional identity, to be able to present a consistent message to the clients regarding the holistic management of their chronic pain.

Recommendations may include individual appointments with a specific team member or treatment through one of the Institute's programs discussed next.

Intensive Pain Rehabilitation Program

This group-oriented program requires the clients' presence daily for 3½ weeks, 8 hours a day. The schedule of the program is predetermined to include daily rounds, exercise periods twice daily, and a variety of educational and discussion-oriented sessions provided by each of the team members. For example, anatomy is covered by the physical therapy staff, body mechanics by the occupational therapy staff, healthful living by the nursing staff, stress management by the psychology staff, and medication usage by the physicians. Management of flare-ups or exacerbations is addressed by all team members. There is an intentional overlap of the information presented to clients for the purpose of reinforcing the message that pain can appropriately and effectively be managed by implementing the recommended strategies into daily living.

Back Injury Clinic

This program is designed to address the needs of the acute or subacute spinal injury client. The treatment offered usually is a combination of physical therapy and occupational therapy but may also involve nursing and psychology. If clients do not progress as anticipated and their pain has persisted beyond 6 months since onset, they are referred to the psychologist for an evaluation. During a team meeting, the results of the

evaluation and response to treatment are discussed to determine if a modification in treatment is indicated. The members may recommend a transfer into the aforementioned program to assist the clients in developing effective strategies for managing their chronic pain.

Work Performance Assessment and Rehabilitation (WPAR) Program

This is often the final form of treatment rendered to injured workers before being released to return to work. When maximum medical improvement has been attained, clients are referred for an evaluation of their current physical tolerances and a determination of their ability to perform work-related tasks. If the tolerances demonstrated are not compatible with the job demands, a 4- to 6-week work-hardening program may be indicated. If a job is not available through the individual's former employer, obtaining alternate employment is either facilitated by the rehabilitation specialist or the individual is referred for vocational rehabilitation services.

Participation in the pain-oriented treatment programs previously described is desirable before being referred to the WPAR program for work hardening when pain is the primary factor limiting the individual from returning to gainful employment. The programs provide individuals with the opportunity to understand the anatomic and psychologic factors contributing to their pain and to learn effective management techniques. Thus, the focus of the WPAR program is on reinforcing the implementation of the strategies while developing the necessary job-related tolerance to return to work. The staff are able to provide the reinforcement because most are responsible for providing services to more than one program.

CASE STUDY

H.P., a 42-year-old male steel worker with multiple work-related back injuries, was referred to the Institute for a comprehensive evaluation. Medical history was remarkable for an injury that occurred 6 years ago while lifting and resulted in a spinal fusion to stabilize the spondylolisthesis at L5 to S1. He returned to work for 1 year when he was involved in a second accident in which he fell backward, striking his back on some poles that were protruding from the floor, and he had been unable to work since then. Data obtained during the evaluation resulted in issuing the following diagnoses: depression, mechanical back pain with resultant posture and gait disturbances, and deconditioning.

H.P. agreed to participate in a treatment program comprised of individual sessions with the psychologist, physical therapist, and occupational therapist. The psychologist worked with the client on identifying the thoughts and beliefs that were hindering his ability to manage his pain (e.g., "As long as I am in pain, I'll never be the person I was before I got hurt"). The psychologist also assisted him in reconceptualizing his thinking to measure improvement in terms of functional gains rather than on pain intensity and duration. The physical therapist's treatment focused on educating the client about the musculoskeletal factors affecting his condition, developing an appropriate exercise routine that emphasized flexibility, and instructing the client in the use of heat and ice for the management of routine pain and exacerbations. The occupational therapist's treatment was devoted to assisting H.P. in learning proper body mechanics, problem-solving skills for integrating the concepts, and recognizing that the pacing of daily activities was an integral part of maintaining or decreasing his daily pain as well as preventing future flare-ups.

As a result of the treatment, H.P. reported a decrease in pain severity, a decrease in the amount the pain interfered with his daily life, an increase in activity level, an increase in sense of control over his life, a decrease in worry and depression as well as an overall increase in mobility, endurance, and strength. On the basis of H.P.'s desire to return to work without restrictions, the occupational therapist contacted the employer to obtain data regarding the critical physical demands of the job before scheduling a work-capacity evaluation. A comparison of these data revealed deficiencies in H.P.'s use of body mechanics, lifting strength, pushing and pulling strength as well as endurance to work an 8-hour shift. Therefore, he was enrolled in a daily work-hardening program that increased the demands on him not only in the number of hours worked, but also the amount of work performed over the course of 4 weeks. Midway through treatment, H.P. began to express maladaptive beliefs about the chronicity of his pain. This setback warranted additional sessions with the psychologist to aid the client in reconceptualizing his beliefs about his progress and ability to return to work. At the completion of treatment, the team recommended that he be released to return to work without restrictions and that H.P. monitor his thoughts to increase the probability that he will continue to implement the strategies taught over the previous months.

FUTURE DIRECTIONS IN CHRONIC PAIN MANAGEMENT

Research

Of the various types of pain management programs that exist, it appears that comprehensive multidisciplinary rehabilitation helps to reduce the disability and dysfunction associated with chronic pain. However, major research efforts are needed to determine the efficacy of this type of management. The focus of such an effort should be on both the clinical aspects and the country's economic and social policy. The clinical research should concentrate on both the process and outcome of various rehabilitation treatments (Osterweis et al, 1987).

Research should also continue on the criteria for client selection for chronic pain centers. It should determine which clients would best respond to which treatment, although the criteria should not be so stringent that individuals who might receive partial benefit would be eliminated from treatment (Dickerson, 1989).

Research should also continue on increasing the knowledge of the physiologic and behavioral management of pain. Understanding the role of brain mechanisms and endorphins in relation to the behavior and physiologic aspects of pain has been cited by Dickerson (1989) as important research areas. Additionally, she stated "an immediate need for a more accurate means of measuring physical capacities" (p. 676).

A research of the existing policies should be expanded to determine the feasibility of early identification of pain in clients and the effects of early rehabilitation "hold promise for preventing long-term disability" would add significantly to our current knowledge of the prediction of long-term disability, the optimal timing and content of rehabilitation and the relative costs and benefits of early versus late intervention (Osterweis et al, 1987, p. 275). Earlier recognition and prevention are important to employees, employers, and society. Methods of preventing chronicity must be found.

Communication

Increased education of the public, health-care providers, and third-party payers is the key to improved overall pain management. Increased communication with these three populations will enable referral of clients to appropriate care sooner, thus avoiding unnecessary analgesics and inappropriate or excessive medical treatments while being shuffled from one health-care provider to another.

Workers should be educated about the workers' compensation law to know what benefits they are entitled to. If the worker were fully informed, his or her anxiety about dealing with the legal system would be greatly alleviated, and the negative effects of compensation factors on treatment would be decreased.

In summary, "chronic pain represents a disease in itself, with characteristics and associated treatments very different from any other set of problems within the field of medicine, including psychiatry. Because the human wastage represented by this disease is massive, it is the challenge of the health professional from every medical and paramedical specialty to recognize it, understand its unique concepts, and help prevent it and treat those who suffer from it so that they can be restored to healthy and productive lives" (Brena and Chapman, 1983, pp. 234–235). Chronic pain has an enormous impact on society today. Its costs in financial terms, societal ramifications, and personal losses are staggering. To reduce this inflating problem, work-related injuries must continue to decrease and their chronic long-term effects prevented.

References

Addison RG: Chronic pain syndrome. Am J Med 77:54–58, 1984.

Alexander FAD: Anesthesiology. In Hale D (ed): Control of Pain. Philadelphia, Davis, 1954.

Anderson GBJ: Epidemiologic aspects of low back pain in industry. Spine 6:53–60, 1981.

Aronoff GM: The role of the pain center in the treatment for intractable suffering and disability resulting from chronic pain. Semin Neurol 3(3):377, 1983.

Aronoff GM: Psychological aspects of non-malignant chronic pain: A new nosology. In Aronoff GM (ed): Evaluation and Treatment of Chronic Pain. Baltimore, Urban and Schwartzenberg, 1985.

Aronoff GM, Evans WO, and Enders PL: A review of follow-up studies of multidisciplinary pain units. Pain 16:1–11, 1983.

Aronoff GM and Wagner JM: The pain center: Development

and dynamics. In Burrows GD, Elton D, and Stanley C (eds): Handbook of Chronic Pain Management. Amsterdam, Elsevier Science Pub, 1987.

Beals RK: Compensation and recovery from injury. West J Med 140:233–237, 1984.

Blumer D and Heilbronn M: Chronic pain as a variant of depressive illness. Br J Psychiatr 138:37–39, 1982.

Bonica JJ: Introduction. In Aronoff GM (ed): Evaluation and Treatment of Chronic Pain. Baltimore, Urban and Schwarzenberg, 1985.

Bonica JJ: Introduction to narcotic analgesics in the treatment of cancer and postoperative pain. Acta Anaesthesiol Scand 26(Suppl 74):5–10, 1982.

Bonica JJ: Evolution of multidisciplinary interdisciplinary pain programs. In Aronoff GM (ed): Pain Centers: A Revolution in Health Care. New York, Raven Press, 1988.

Bonica JJ: The Management of Pain. Philadelphia, Lea & Febiger, 1953.

Brena SF: Chronic Pain: America's Hidden Epidemic. New York, Atheneum/SMI, 1978.

Brena SF and Chapman SL: Management of Patients with Chronic pain. New York, Spectrum Publications, 1983.

Chamber of Commerce of the United States: Analysis of Workers' Compensation Laws (publication no. 6803). Washington, DC, U.S. Chamber of Commerce, 1985.

Craig KD and Wyckoff MG: Cultural factors in chronic pain management. In Burrows GD, Elton D, Stanley C (eds): Handbook of Chronic Pain Management. Amsterdam, Elsevier Science Pub, 1987.

Crue B: Chronic Pain. New York, Spectrum Publications, 1979.

Currie D and Marburger R: Writing therapy referrals and treatment plans and the interdisciplinary team. In DeLisa J (ed): Rehabilitation Medicine, Principles and Practice. Philadelphia, JB Lippincott, 1988.

DeLisa J, Martin G, and Currie D: Rehabilitation medicine: Past, present and future. In DeLisa J (ed): Rehabilitation Medicine, Principles and Practice. Philadelphia, Lippincott, 1988.

Dickerson CC: Pain centers: A survey and analysis of past, present, and future functioning. In Tollison CD (ed): Handbook of Chronic Pain Management. Baltimore, Williams & Wilkins, 1989.

Elton D: Emotional variables and chronic pain. In Burrows GD, Elton D, and Stanley GV (eds): Handbook of Chronic Pain Management. Amsterdam, Elsevier Science, 1987.

Elton D, Stanley GV, and Burrows GD: Psychological Control of Pain. Sydney, Grune & Stratton, 1983.

Elton D, Stanley GV, and Burrows GD: Self-esteem and chronic pain. J Psychosom Res 22:25–30, 1978.

Engel GL: Psychogenic pain. Med Clin North Am 26:1481–1496, 1958.

Fordyce WE, Fowler RS, and DeLateur B: An application of behavior modification technique to a problem of chronic pain. Behav Res Ther 6:105–107, 1968.

Fordyce WE, Fowler RS, Lehmann JF, et al: Some implications of learning in problems in chronic pain. J Chron Dis 21:179–190, 1968.

France RD and Krishman KRR (eds): Chronic Pain. Washington, DC, American Psychiatric Press, 1988.

Gerschman JA and Reade PC: Management of chronic orofacial pain syndromes. In Burrows GD, Elton D, and Stanley GV (eds): Handbook of Chronic Pain Management. Amsterdam, Elsevier Science, 1987.

Gil KM, Ross SL, and Keefe FJ: Behavioral treatment of chronic pain: Four pain management protocols. In France

RD and Krishman KRR (eds): Chronic Pain. Washington, DC, American Psychiatric Press, 1988.

Grant HE: Disability insurance under social security. IMJ 144:76, 1973.

Grazier KL, Holbrook TL, Kelsey JL, et al: The frequency of occurrence, impact and cost of musculoskeletal conditions in the United States. Parkridge, IL, American Academy of Orthopaedic Surgeons, 1984.

Hallett EC and Pilowski I: The response to treatment in a multidisciplinary pain clinic. Pain 12:365–374, 1982.

Health Insurance Association of America: Source Book of Health Insurance Data (24th ed. Washington, DC, Health Insurance Association of America, 1982–1983.

Hill HE, Kornetsky CH, Flanary HG, et al: Studies of anxiety associated with anticipation of pain. I: Effects of morphine. Arch Neurol Psychiatr 67:612–619, 1952.

Holzman AD and Turk DC: Pain Management: A Handbook of Psychological Treatment Approaches. Elmsford, NY, Pergamon Press, 1986.

Holzman AD, Turk DC, and Kerns RD: The cognitive-behavioral approach to the management of chronic pain. In Holzman AD, and Turk DC (eds): Pain Management: A Handbook of Psychological Treatment Approaches. Elmsford, NY, Pergamon Press, 1986.

Joffe WG and Sandler G: On concepts of pain, with special reference to depression and psychogenic pain. J Psychosom Res 11:69–75, 1967.

Kanfer FH and Karoly P: The psychology of self-management: Abiding issues and tentative directions. In Karoly P and Kanfer FH (eds): Self-Management and Behavior Change. Elmsford, NY, Pergamon Press, 1982.

Killian LE: Psychological barriers to recovery. In Isernhagen SJ (ed): Work Injury: Management and Prevention. Rockville, MD, Aspen, 1988.

Klusman LE: Reduction of pain in child birth by alleviation of anxiety during pregnancy. J Consult Clin Psychol 43(213):162–165, 1975.

Leedy JJ: Compensation in Psychiatric Disability and Rehabilitation. Springfield, IL, Charles C Thomas, 1971.

Leriche R: Surgery of Pain. Baltimore, Williams & Wilkins, 1939.

Lesse S: The masked depression syndrome—results of a seventeen-year study. Am J Psychother 37:457–475, 1983.

Little TF: Chronic pain: Modern concepts in management. Aust Fam Physician 10:265–270, 1981.

Livingston WK: Pain Mechanisms: Physiologic Interpretation of Causalgia and Its Related States. New York, Macmillan, 1943.

Melzack R and Wall PD: Pain mechanisms: A new theory. Science 150(3699):971–979, 1965.

Mandel F: Di Paravertebrale Blockage. Vienna, Springer, 1938.

Mandler G and Watson DL: Anxiety and the interruption of behavior. In Spielberger CD (ed): Anxiety and Behavior. New York, Academic Press, 1966.

Meinhardt NT and McCaffery M: Pain, a nursing approach to assessment and analysis. East Norwalk, CT, Appleton-Century-Crofts, 1983.

Mersky H: Classification of chronic pain: Description of chronic pain syndromes and definition of pain terms. Pain 26(Suppl 3):1–225, 1986.

Mersky H: Pain, personality and psychosomatic complaints. In Burrows GD, Elton D, and Stanley GV (eds): Handbook of Chronic Pain Management. Amsterdam, Elsevier Science, 1987.

National Center for Health Statistics: Current Estimates from the National Interview Survey, 1988 (DHHS publication no. [PHS] 89–1501). Hyattsville, MD, U.S. Government Printing Office, 1989.

Newman R and Seres J: The interdisciplinary pain center: An approach to the management of chronic pain. In Holzman A and Turk D (eds): Pain Management, A Handbook of Psychological Treatment Approaches. Elmsford, New York, Pergamon Press, 1986.

Osterweis M, Kleinman A, and Mechanic D: Institute of Medicine's Committee on Pain and Disability: Clinical, Behavioral and Public Policy Perspectives. Washington, DC, National Academy Press, 1987.

Price DN: Workers' compensation: 1976–80 benchmark revisions. Social Security Bulletin 47(7):3.

Roberts AH: The operant approach to the management of pain and excess disability. In Holzman AD and Turk DC (eds): Pain Management: A Handbook of Psychological Treatment Approaches. New York, Pergamon Press, 1986.

Roberts MTS: Pain relief clinics. Patient Management 8:25–32, 1983.

Rowlingson JC and Toomey TC: Multidisciplinary approaches to the management of chronic pain. In Ghia JN (ed): The Multidisciplinary Pain Center Organization and Personnel Functions for Pain Management. Boston, Kluwer Academic Pub, 1988.

Segraves K: Bringing it all together: Developing the clinical team. In Camic P and Brown F (eds): Assessing Chronic Pain: A Multidisciplinary Clinic Handbook. New York, Springer-Verlag, 1989.

Seres JL, Painter JR, and Newman RI: Multidisciplinary treatment of chronic pain at the Northwest Pain Center. In Ng IKY (ed.): New Approaches to Treatment of Chronic Pain: A Review of Multidisciplinary Pain Clinics and Pain Centers (NIDA research monograph 36). Rockville, MD, National Institute on Drug Abuse, 1981.

Snook SH and Jensen RC: Cost of occupational low back pain. In Pope MH, Frymoyer JW, and Anderson G (eds): Occupational Low Back Pain. New York, Praeger, 1984.

Snook SH and Webster BS: The cost of disability. Clin Orthop 221:77–84, 1987.

Stam HJ, McGrath PA, and Brooke RI: The treatment of temporomandibular joint syndrome through the control of anxiety. J Behav Ther Exp Psychiatry 15:41–45, 1984.

Sternbach RA: The Psychology of Pain. New York, Raven Press, 1978.

Sternbach RA and Tursky B: Ethnic differences among housewives in psychophysical and skin potential responses to electric shock. Psychophysiology 4:67–74, 1965.

Timmermans G and Sternbach RA: Factors in human chronic pain: An analysis of personality and pain reaction variables. Science 184:806–807, 1974.

Tollison CD: Assessment and treatment at pain therapy centers programs. In Tollison CD (ed): Handbook of Chronic Pain Management. Baltimore, Williams & Wilkins, 1989.

Turk DC and Holzman AD: Commonalities among psychological approaches in the treatment of chronic pain: Specifying the meta-constructs. In Holzman AD and Turk DC (eds): Pain Management: A Handbook of Pyschological Treatment Approaches. New York, Pergamon Press, 1986.

Turk DC and Kerns RD: Conceptual issues in the assessment of clinical pain. Int J Psychiatry Med 13:15–26, 1903.

Tursky B and Sternbach RA: Further physiological correlates of ethnic differences in responses to shock. Psychophysiology 4:67–74, 1967.

Waddell G: A new clinical model for the treatment of low-back pain. Spine *12*(7):632–644, 1987.

Ward NG, Bloom VL, and Friedel R: The effectiveness of tricyclic antidepressants in the treatment of coexisting pain and depression. Pain *7*:331–341, 1979.

Weisenberg M: Cultural and ethnic factors in reaction to pain. *In* Al-Issa II (ed): Culture and Psychopathology. Baltimore, University Park, 1982.

West JL: Chronic pain management. *In* Isernhagen SJ (ed): Work Injury: Management and Prevention. Rockville, MD, Aspen, 1988.

Wilson-Evered E and Stanley GV: Stress and arousal during pregnancy and childbirth. Br J Med Psychol *59*:57–60, 1986.

Wolff BB and Horland AA: Effects of suggestion upon experimental pain: A validatonal study. J Abnorm Psychol *72*:402–407, 1967.

Zborowski M: Cultural components in response to pain. J Soci Issues *8*:16–30, 1969.

Zola I: Culture and symptoms: An analysis of patients presenting complaints. Am Soc Rev *31*:615–636, 1966.

CHAPTER
7

Julie Moyer Knowles
Theresa Cappelli Calibey

Prevention, Treatment, and Rehabilitation of Sports Injuries

Sports medicine involves the prevention, evaluation, immediate treatment, and rehabilitation of injuries incurred to athletes. Applying traditional medical techniques to athletes does not constitute sports medicine; sports medicine often involves modifications to traditional treatment approaches. Many times the athlete works closely with the sports medicine specialist before the injury insult; therefore, prevention of disorders is maximized. Then if any injury does occur, the individual's medical history is already known, the mechanism of injury is frequently seen by the practitioner, and treatment may be initated immediately on the field. Soon thereafter, the athlete receives further treatment and rehabilitation in a training room or sports medicine clinic.

The health-care provider who most frequently provides on-the-field care is the athletic trainer. Certified athletic trainers complete 4 years of college in an approved athletic training curriculum, complete practical internship hours, and pass a national examination. When a qualified health-care provider is not immediately available to treat the athletic or nonathletic client, therapy is frequently not initiated for at least 24 hours post-insult. This hesitation in treatment initiation can increase total rehabilitation time and delay return to normal activities.

In recent years, as sports medicine gained in popularity, more health-care providers have become actively and holistically involved in athletic care. In additional to physicians and athletic trainers, such practitioners include physical therapists, occupational therapists, dentists, nurses, physiologists, biomechanists, nutritionists, and sports psychologists. The American Physical Therapy Association now has national specilization requirements for therapists interested in working in sports physical therapy. Alternatively, occupational therapy in sports medicine is still very new, and no requirements for sports specialization have been established. However, there are many physical therapists and some occupational therapists who are also certified in athletic training, making them very qualified in the treatment of athletic injuries.

Another very obvious difference in sports medicine versus traditional medicine is insurance reimbursement. In increasing numbers, high schools, colleges, and professional sports teams are hiring health-care practitioners, primarily athletic trainers, to treat their injured athletes and to help with the prevention of such injuries. In these cases, health insurance is not a consideration (i.e., no insurance company is billed for services), and the athlete often receives two to

Figure 7–1. The preparticipation physical determines if the athlete may safely participate in a sport without medical complications.

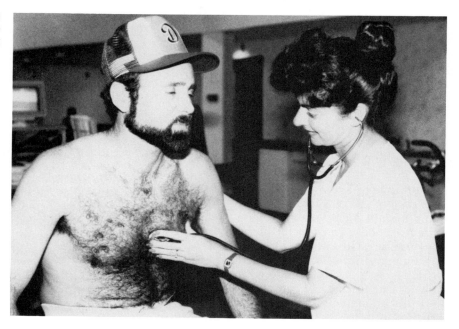

five sports therapy treatments a day at no cost every day of the week. The salary for the athletic trainer is usually fit into the school's athletic budget similar to a coach's salary, or in some cases the salary is partially supported by the school's booster club. Because many athletic trainers are also certified in teaching, the schools frequently combine some teaching responsibilities with athletic training services.

GOALS

The primary goal in sports medicine is the prevention of injuries to athletes. This can be achieved by (1) a comprehensive preparticipation physical and screening, (2) year-round conditioning, (3) a well-balanced diet, (4) education of the athletes, coaches, and parents, (5) psychological management of the athlete, and (6) understanding environmental risk factors, proper equipment fitting, and rules of sport.

The second goal of sports medicine is the return of injured athletes to their previous competitive level as quickly yet as safely as possible. This is best achieved by a proper initial evaluation, immediate treatment, and a comprehensive rehabilitation program using a multidisciplinary team approach including the athlete, physician, athletic trainer, sports therapist, and coach.

PREVENTION

Screening and the Preparticipation Physical

The best way to treat an athletic injury is to prevent it from occurring. This form of prevention can be assisted through the use of a comprehensive preparticipation physical (Fig. 7–1).

It is important to obtain medical clearance from the physician before participation in sports so that the athlete may safely participate without medical complications. This examination must be performed by a physician familiar with the physical demands placed on the body by the sport. It should be performed 4 to 6 weeks before the beginning of the season so that, if necessary, adequate time is given to initiate a rehabilitation program and establish playing restrictions.

To reduce the chance of injury by identifying predisposing factors, the preparticipation physical should ideally include the following components: (1) past and current medical information concerning the athlete; (2) a general medical examination including height, weight, heart and lung status, eye and dental screening, dermatologic review, palpation of internal structures, and laboratory tests as needed; (3) a musculoskeletal examination including range of motion, strength, body type, percentage of body fat, girth measurements, posture, level of maturation, and ligament laxity; (4) cardiovascular endurance; (5) an evaluation focusing on injuries specific to the athlete's particular sport and position; and (6) review of medical information by a physician to determine if sports participation should be allowed, disallowed, or modified (Kibler et al, 1989; Moyer, 1990a).

Conditioning

Conditioning is an excellent means of injury prevention. A comprehensive conditioning program should include seven major areas: (a) the warm-up phase to prepare the body for upcoming stresses, (b) range of motion promotion through stretching, (c) strengthening and power activities, (d) endurance exercises for both involved and uninvolved areas, (e) sport specific and functional activities, (f) a warm-down, and (g) relaxation techniques to speed fatigue recovery time (Moyer, 1990b).

The primary purpose of the warm-up is to provide an initial stretch and flexibility of tissues and, most important, to initiate an increased blood supply to the heart to prepare the cardiovascular system for increased work output. Warm-ups vary depending on the athlete's physical status, sport, and psychology. Although some research suggests that the internal rise in body temperature and increased metabolism from warm-ups enhance human performance, others have found detrimental effects of preactivity heat on strength and power (Carlisle, 1956; Hall et al, 1947; Nukuda, 1955, cited in Grose, 1958; Robins, 1942; Sargeant and Jones, 1978; Sedwick and Whalen, 1964).

Stretching is the second phase of a comprehensive exercise program. A common method of performing stretching exercises is progressively to stretch a muscle as much as possible and then sustain that position for 30 to 60 seconds, repeating it 3 to 5 times. Stretching may be performed in other ways through techniques such as proprioceptive neuromuscular facilitation. Regardless of the technique used, stretching should first be performed in a gross manner throughout the body, followed by the lengthening of sport-specific muscles. Stretching increases joint range of motion and reduces the potential for injury.

The strengthening phase actually encompasses both strengthening and power exercises. In past years, the words *strength* and *power* have been frequently used interchangeably. Lumex Incor-

porated has used the measurements of 60 degrees per second and less on the Cybex (an isokinetic strength testing device) to describe strength and measurements greater than 60 degrees per second to denote power. In turn, these definitions of strength and power have been carried over into research (Gleim et al, 1978; Lesmes et al, 1978; Londeree, 1981). The more accurate definition for strength is the force of a single maximal contraction measured in units of the pound, newton, and kilogram (Heusner, 1978; Hislop and Perrine, 1967; Moffroid and Kusiak, 1975; Scudder, 1980). Power is the product of force times velocity or the strength of a muscle times the velocity of the limb through the range of motion. Power can also be considered to be the amount of work performed per unit time.

There are several factors to consider while conditioning in the strengthening phase: intensity, frequency, duration, types, and age and sex differences. Intensity involves a progressive systemic increase in total work. Increased muscular strength and hypertrophy will occur when a muscle is resisted with a force significantly above normal muscular demands. Total work increases can also be accomplished by decreasing the total time required to perform the strengthening phase. Repetition of the exercises with progressively heavier weight allows for increased strength production and increased involuntary actions; this is especially necessary with exercises that are sport-specific. For maximum effectiveness and minimization of fatigue, a muscle group should be exercised at a frequency of alternate days.

There are three main types of strength and power exercises: isometrics, isotonics, and isokinetics. All three should be incorporated into an off-season program to achieve maximal conditioning effectiveness. Exercises should be performed both eccentrically and concentrically.

Multiple definitions are also found when describing isometrics, isotonics, and isokinetics. Many researchers defined an isometric contraction or static strength as a muscular contraction in which there is an increase in muscular tone without a change in muscular length. An isotonic contraction or dynamic strength/power has been defined as a muscular contraction during which time joint motion occurs (Coplin, 1971; Gleim et al, 1978; Heusner, 1978; Pipes, 1977; Werner, 1980). Isokinetics is thought to be a form of dynamic power where maximal resistance is applied throughout the entire range of motion by accommodating resistance against a lever moving at a fixed speed (Fig. 7–2) (Coplin, 1971; Gleim et al, 1978; Heusner, 1978).

There are sex and age differences in strength that must be considered as well. Women possess about one half the strength of men with comparable size and weight (Klafs and Arnheim, 1977). Most of this strength difference is in the woman's upper body, with only minimal strength differences in the legs (Kulund, 1982). Maximal strength is achieved around 25 years of age and decreases thereafter at a rate of approximately 1% per year (Kulund, 1982).

The endurance phase of the conditioning program should involve both aerobic and anaerobic activities. Fatigue increases the risk of injury acquisition by decreasing the body's ability to generate repetitive short bursts of high-level muscular activity (anaerobic) or maintain movements over an extended time frame (aerobic). Thus, the body's ability to avoid injurious situations is impaired.

Anaerobic fitness depends mainly on energy derived from the muscle's phosphate reservoir. The reservoir, based on adenosine triphosphate creatine phosphokinase (ATP-CP), is the primary source of energy for high-power, short-duration exercises. A second form of anaerobic energy known as anaerobic glycolysis is used for activities of longer duration (½ to 2 minutes) but lower intensity work loads. Interval training involving repeated maximum bursts of work for 5 to 10 seconds followed by a 30- to 60-second rest between bouts is an excellent way to enhance the ATP-CP energy capacity of the specific muscles (Kulund, 1982; Margaria, 1972).

Aerobic energy is primarily based on the oxidation of fat or carbohydrate, producing ATP with extremely long-lasting duration but relatively lower power. The power is significantly lower because of its dependence on the rate at which oxygen can be delivered to the muscles by the cardiovascular system. Therefore, the two primary goals of aerobic training should be to enhance the capacity of the central circulatory system and to improve the aerobic capacity of the sport-specific muscles (Kulund, 1982; Margaria, 1972).

As with the strengthening phase, the development of an aerobic conditioning program is based on three variables: intensity, duration, and frequency. Generally, the aerobic phase should last a minimum of 20 minutes, at an intensity of 70 to 80% of the maximum heart rate, and at a minimum frequency of 3 to 4 days a week.

The fifth phase of the conditioning program is sport-specific/functional activities. This phase allows athletes to meet the special demands and skills of their sport. The effects of the program

Figure 7–2. Isokinetic training allows for maximum strength output by applying accommodating resistance against a lever moving at a fixed speed.

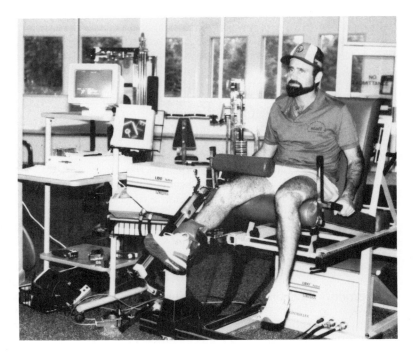

are very specific to the muscles exercised, the physiologic system that is overloaded, and the types of muscle fibers used to perform the exercises. Other sport-specific exercises include activities in proprioception, balance, timing, coordination, agility, biomechanical motions, and anatomic alignment.

Diet and Nutrition

A good, well-balanced, natural diet should be practiced by both the athletic and nonathletic population. A proper diet includes high-fiber, low-fat, well-balanced foods from the milk, meat, breads and cereal, and fruits and vegetable food groups. Fifteen per cent of all ingested food should be in the form of protein, 25% in fats, and 60% in carbohydrates (Moyer, 1990a). During sports participation, caloric requirements may double (from approximately 1,500 calories/day for sedentary persons to 3,000 calories/day for active athletes); therefore, caloric intake during the sport season must increase.

Psychology of Sport

Sport psychology is an important component of both injury prevention and rehabilitation. Injuries can be devastating because they can take away from the physical capabilities that form the athletes' identity. In general, athletes are very motivated and will do whatever they can do to return to or excel in their activity (Faris, 1985; Samples, 1987). This can be beneficial, but the aggressive attitude can also hinder a healthy season. For example, athletes may overexert themselves, thus causing or exacerbating an injury. It is therefore important for the health-care provider to identify these overmotivators and closely monitor their conditioning and rehabilitation programs. It is also important for the medical provider to dispel myths associated with sports such as "no pain, no gain." Some discomfort associated with training and rehabilitation should be expected; however, pain is a signal of bodily distress. A more appropriate saying is "strain but no pain."

Equipment, Environment, and Rules

Three responsibilities of the sports medicine practitioner are to (1) study environmental risk factors, (2) ensure safe playing facilities and equipment, and (3) understand sport rules and how they relate to injury treatment.

Weather conditions, especially heat and lightning, can be life threatening for athletes. Body signs must be constantly observed to avoid heat cramps, heat exhaustion, and heat stroke. When playing in rain, health-care providers must voice their opinion if the conditions are not appropriate for reasonably safe play. If one can count 15 seconds or less between the time lightning is seen and thunder is heard, the competition should be postponed (Moyer, 1988).

Fields of competition should be free from trash and other injurious substances. All athletes should wear properly fitting equipment and clothing, and rules regarding protective padding, on-the-field treatment, and injury re-entry must be enforced.

Education

Educated athletes are healthy athletes. Educated athletes will maintain good off-season conditioning (including exercise and nutrition), study proper mechanics and sport techniques, ensure proper equipment fitting, and be familiar with injury prevention and treatment procedures. Educated athletes understand rules as they affect sport, including rules associated with abuse of nontherapeutic drugs. This knowledge not only helps prevent injury to the athletes, but, through the sharing of knowledge, it also makes for a healthier team and athletic program.

EVALUATION, TREATMENT, AND REHABILITATION

One of the major focuses in sports medicine is the implementation of a proper and adequate rehabilitation program (Harvey, 1985). The rehabilitation of athletes must involve the evaluation of specific demands to facilitate their return to a high level of function. The process of returning athletes to their previous activity level can be separated into three phases: (1) evaluation, first aid, and initial treatment, (2) rehabilitation of the injury to a "competitively functional state" including the use of modalities and exercise, and (3) continuation of the exercise program to maintain safe athletic participation.

Specific Adaptations to Imposed Demands

The application of the specific adaptations to imposed demands (SAID) principle is imperative to the rehabilitation of athletes (O'Donoghue, 1976). The SAID principle states that the rehabilitation program must be adapted to the specific demands placed on athletes during athletic participation (Fig. 7–3). Therefore, the rehabilitation program must be specific to the athletes' sport, position, age, and sex.

In terms of adaptations needed according to sport and position, different lower extremity strengthening exercises would be used for a punter versus a quarterback, and treatment of a baseball pitcher's throwing arm would differ from that of a shoulder injury to a soccer player (the arms are not used by soccer players, except the goalie). Each specific physical characteristic needed for the sport and position within the sport must be considered.

Many differences exist between male and female athletes. Some differences in injury distribution can be attributed to biologic differences between the sexes; however, many injury differences in the female athlete can be attributed to sociologic training.

According to Clarke and Buckley (1980) and the National Collegiate Athletic Association (NCAA) Injury Surveillance System (NCAA, 1989a, 1989b, 1989c, and 1990), the following statistical observations were noted between male and female athletes: (1) more injuries occurred in practice versus games in both sexes because of the increased time spent in practice; (2) similar sports had similar common areas of injuries despite the sex; (3) strains and sprains were the most prevalent injuries; (4) sports such as gymnastics that involve different equipment and rules for each sex had different types of injuries (e.g., female gymnasts had more knee injuries, whereas male gymnasts had more shoulder and arm injuries); (5) because of a wider pelvis, increased quadriceps "Q" angle of pull, and increased ligament laxity, women were more prone to knee disorders; and (6) men had more contusions, whereas women had more fractures and knee injuries.

Treatment modifications must also be made according to the athletes' age. As more and more older athletes participate in physical activities, therapists will become increasingly more involved with their rehabilitation. Matheson and colleagues (1989) found that athletic injuries among the older athlete (51 to 63 years old) were most commonly associated with racquet sports, walking, and low-intensity activities; whereas young adult athletes (22 to 49 years old) com-

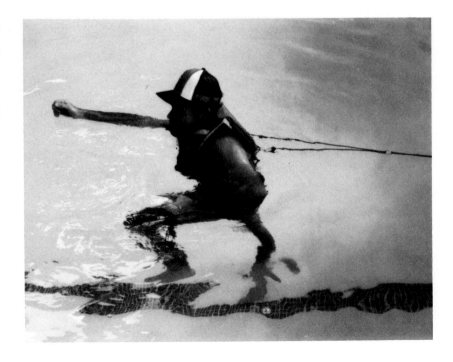

Figure 7–3. The SAID principle states that the athlete's rehabilitation program should be adapted to the specific demands placed on the patient during athletic participation. An example of such adaptations includes exercising a runner in the water in order to minimize stresses to the lower extremities.

Table 7–1. College Athletic Injuries*

Variable	Football 1988	Football 1989	Soccer (Spring) Men's 1989	Men's 1988	Men's 1989	Women's 1988	Women's 1989	Field Hockey 1988	Field Hockey 1989	Volleyball Women's 1988	Volleyball Women's 1989	Wrestling 1989
Total no. injuries per 1000 exposures	6.7	6.9	10.6	7.2	7.7	8.3	7.5	5.8	3.8	4.5	4.6	9.5
Injuries during games†	41	43	7	60	49	52	58	46	44	38	35	33
Injuries during practice†	58	57	93	40	51	48	42	54	56	60	65	67
Common injuries												
Hip/thigh	—	10	—	21	17	17	15	13	8	-	—	—
Ankle/foot	14	14	16	21	20	27	21	14	—	27	27	—
Forearm/wrist/hand	—	—	—	—	—	—	—	—	18	—	—	—
Knee	20	19	24	17	14	16	21	14	—	18	11	26
Torso	—	—	—	—	—	—	-	—	17	8	—	—
Shoulder/arm	11	—	10	—	—	—	—	—	—	—	11	15
Head/neck/spine	—	—	—	—	—	—	—	—	—	—	—	—
Face/scalp	—	—	—	—	—	—	—	—	—	—	—	9
Type of injury												
General trauma	—	—	—	—	—	—	—	—	—	—	—	—
Sprains	31	27	34	31	27	36	31	20	27	42	34	32
Strains	19	21	17	21	24	15	23	24	21	20	29	18
Fracture	—	—	—	—	—	—	—	—	—	—	—	—
Neurotrauma	—	—	—	—	—	—	—	—	—	—	—	—
General illness	—	—	—	—	—	—	—	—	—	—	—	—
Musculoskeletal	17	17	13	27	22	15	15	18	16	5	8	—
Thermotrauma	—	—	—	—	—	—	—	—	—	—	—	—

monly experienced injuries in running, fitness class, and field sports. Older athletes sustained a higher rate of metatarsalgia, plantar fasciitis, and meniscal injury compared with the younger adult group, who had patellofemoral pain syndromes, stress fractures, and periostitis. Tendinitis was common to both age groups. Overuse injuries constituted 85% of the injuries. The most common body parts involved were the foot and the knee for the older and younger adult athletes, respectfully (Matheson et al, 1989).

The older athletes should be encouraged to continue participation in physical activities with the least amount of risk for injury. Physical activity has been shown to increase functional independence by decreasing age-related problems. In addition, the sport injury in the older athletes is usually compounded by several factors including cardiovascular disease and longer healing time. Therefore, rehabilitation of the older athlete is very important (Matheson et al, 1989).

Young children are susceptible to sports injuries and need special attention secondary to the physical and psychologic immaturity, overall poor conditioning, inadequate or improper coaching, decreased tolerance to environmental changes, improper equipment and officiating, mismatching of the opponents, and decreased physiologic tolerance to extreme hot and cold (Moyer, 1990b).

In terms of treatment and rehabilitation to the prepubescent athletes, care should be taken

when applying temperature-altering modalities. Excessive temperatures affect children to a greater extent than adults; therefore, treatment duration and intensity may need to be lowered. Diathermies and electrical stimulation can adversely affect the epiphyses of young athletes, thus causing a limb-length discrepancy; therefore, their use over the epiphyseal plates of young children is not encouraged (Moyer, 1990b).

Exercise adaptations should also be instituted for young athletes. Exercises should be performed equally and bilaterally. Range of motion and mobilization techniques should be performed cautiously because of possible ligamentous damage from excessive stress. Exercises should encourage normal postural alignment. Isotonics should be performed concentrically, submaximally, and throughout the full available range of motion (Moyer, 1990b).

General Statistics Relating to Sports Injuries

The National High School Injury Registry conducted by the National Athletic Trainer's Association (NATA) has estimated that 1 million injuries occur to high school athletes (NATA, 1987a). The surveys were performed at schools that have athletic trainers; therefore, the statistics were obtained under favorable conditions (less

Table 7–1. College Athletic Injuries* *Continued*

Variable	Ice Hockey 1989	Basketball		Lacrosse		Gymnastics		Baseball 1989	Softball 1989
		Men's 1989	Women's 1989	Men's 1989	Women's 1989	Men's 1989	Women's 1989		
Total no. injuries per 1000 exposures	5.5	4.9	5.6	60	3	5.5	7.9	3.3	3.8
Injuries during games†	68	35	37	40	30	19	23	58	48
Injuries during practice†	31	64	63	60	70	81	77	41	51
Common injuries									
Hip/thigh	10	7	—	—	17	—	—	10	—
Ankle/foot	—	31	26	15	19	13	19	14	9
Forearm/wrist/hand	—	—	—	—	—	9	—	—	—
Knee	16	14	20	15	15	—	19	—	12
Torso	—	—	6	—	—	—	—	—	—
Shoulder/arm	17	—	—	13	—	14	—	19	16
Head/neck/spine	—	—	—	—	—	—	—	—	—
Face/scalp	—	—	—	—	—	—	—	—	—
Type of injury									
General trauma	—	—	—	—	—	—	—	—	—
Sprains	23	39	36	24	23	35	26	21	23
Strains	16	19	15	22	30	26	27	26	27
Fracture	—	—	—	—	11	—	8	—	—
Neurotrauma	—	—	—	—	—	—	—	—	—
General illness	—	—	—	—	—	—	—	—	—
Musculoskeletal	—	10	8	19	—	13	—	14	16
Thermotrauma	22	—	—	—	—	—	—	—	—

*Information obtained from National College Athletic Association (1989a, 1989b, 1989c, 1990). All statistics are percentiles unless otherwise noted.

†May be due to increased time spent in practice.

than 15% to 18% of high schools have athletic trainers). Boy's football and girl's basketball teams experienced the highest incidence of injury (37% and 23%, respectfully). Over half of high school football injuries and girl's basketball injuries occurred during practice compared with actual competition. The position that the athlete played influenced the incidence of injury and the total time lost from the injury. Experience did not appear to significantly affect the frequency of injury for the high school football player (Tables 7–1 and 7–2) (NATA 1987a, 1987b, 1988b, 1989a, 1989b, and 1989c).

In a study by Derscheid and Feiring (1987) involving 1,707 clients attending a sports medicine clinic, injuries were hierarchically arranged based on most common diagnoses and length of hospitalization. Anterior cruciate ligament reconstructions were the lengthiest, averaging 39 visits over 15½ weeks. This was followed by lateral release (21 visits), patellar debridement (20 visits), lateral meniscectomies (17 visits), medial meniscectomies (15 visits), anterior cruciate ligament sprains (15 visits), plical removal (14 visits), rotator cuff impingements (14 visits), chondromalacia (14 visits), and biceps tendonitis (13 visits). The remaining eight diagnoses—patellar tendinitis, medial collateral ligament sprains, cervical sprains and strains, lateral ankle sprains, plantar fasciitis, lateral epicondylitis, sacroiliac joint dysfunctions, and lumbar strains—required fewer than 12 therapy treatments. In general, one sixth of the 18 diagnoses occurred to the neck and trunk, one sixth occurred to the upper extremities, and two thirds occurred to the lower extremities (Derscheid and Feiring, 1987).

Sports Therapy Versus Traditional Therapy

As discussed previously, prevention of athletic injuries is the ultimate goal of sports medicine; however, when athletic injuries do occur, the main objective is to return the athletes to their previous level of function as quickly and as safely as possible. This is best achieved through the cooperative effort of the entire sports medicine team.

The rehabilitation of athletes must be specifically geared to the type of injury, severity of the injury, psychologic status of the athlete, and the sport and position to which the athlete is returning (Fig. 7–4). The timing of the rehabilitation process is also very important. The results obtained from an early evaluation are less likely to be contaminated or obscured by inflammation, edema, and diffuse pain. The entire rehabilitation process can be shortened by early evaluation and

Table 7-2. High School Athletic Injuries*

Variable	Football 1986	Football 1987	Football 1988	Basketball Boy's 1988	Basketball Boy's 1989	Basketball Girl's 1987	Basketball Girl's 1988	Basketball Girl's 1989	Wrestling 1988	Wrestling 1989
Number of participants (projections)	1,048,100	1,021,685	1,041,721	379,864	—	441,441	318,043	—	273,334	—
Players sustaining injuries	37.2	36.7	35.2	23	—	23	23	—	30	—
Injuries during games†	62	60	—	60	—	63	55	—	68	—
Injuries during practice†	38	40	—	40	—	37	45	—	32	—
Injuries during the second half of game	—	—	—	65	—	60	67	—	—	—
Common injuries										
Hip/thigh	17.9	17.0	17.3	11.3	11	12.4	12	13	6	7
Ankle/foot	16.6	15.7	15.5	43	42	29.7	34.2	31	8.6	8
Forearm/wrist/hand	14.6	15.2	15.3	11.1	11	14.8	17.3	12	17.2	14
Knee	14.6	14.2	14.8	9	12	15	9	19	14.2	16
Torso	10.0	10.2	9.5	7	7	8.6	6	6	17	15
Shoulder/arm	9.7	11.0	10.1	2	2	1.9	3	4	16.5	16
Head/neck/spine	9.0	9.9	10.5	2	2	2.5	3	3	8	10
Face/scalp	2.8	2.3	2.5	10	9	5.4	10	6	8	11
Percent of minor injuries	74.9	72.3	69.9	74	—	73.5	71	—	68	—
Percent of moderate injuries	16.5	16.6	17.1	14	—	16.5	17	—	17	—
Percent of major injuries	8.6	11.1	13.0	12	—	10	12	—	15	—
Type of injury										
General trauma	28.8	27.5	28.3	22	21	17.6	18	18	28	28
Sprains	28.8	27.3	28.7	43	43	41.4	44	39	30	30
Strains	21.3	21.7	20.7	14	14	15.1	19	12	23	22
Fracture	6.6	7.7	7.8	9	8	6.5	6	8	8	7
Neurotrauma	5.7	7.2	6.4	2	1	2.4	3	3	2	2
General illness	5.1	4.6	3.2	6	7	9.7	4	9	6	5
Musculoskeletal	2.9	3.1	3.4	4	5	6.5	5	11	3	6
Thermotrauma	1.4	0.9	1.5	1	1	.6	1	1	1	1
Catastrophic injuries‡	0	0	0	0	—	0	0	—	0	—
Mechanism of injury										
Direct impact	43.9	—	—	35	—	—	39	—	34	—
Stretched muscles	12.7	—	—	11	—	—	12	—	20	—
Torsion	11.2	—	—	25	—	—	30	—	20	—
Indirect force	9.1	—	—	—	—	—	—	—	—	—
Overuse	3.9	—	—	—	—	—	—	—	—	—

*Information obtained from Powell (1987) and National Athletic Trainers Association (1987a, 1987b, 1988a, 1988b, 1988c, 1989a, 1989b, and 1989c). All statistics are percentiles unless otherwise noted.
†May be due to increased time spent in practice.
‡Catastrophic injuries in the group surveyed, but an average of 24 catastrophic injuries in football and 36 catastrophic injuries in all high school sports.

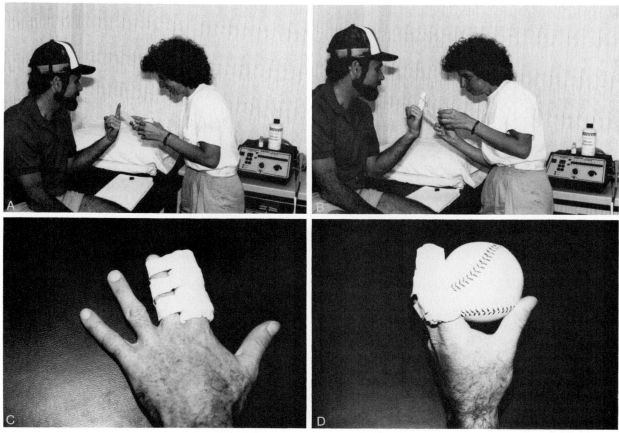

Figure 7–4. *A–D,* Rehabilitation and protective equipment must be geared toward the type of injury, sport, and rules governing the sport. For example, a fractured phalanx may be splinted through the use of silicone cement, combined with gauze and taped in order to provide protection without endangering other players (From Dewey TJ and Gallapsy JB: The use of percutaneous pinning and a silicone splint for a fractured proximal phalanx. Athletic Training 25(1):55–56, 1990).

treatment (O'Donoghue, 1976). Hocutt and associates (1982) found that individuals who sprain their ankle to the severity that they could not initially bear weight reached full activity with early use of cryotherapy (within 36 hours postinsult) almost 2½ times faster than those starting cryotherapy after 36 hours or those receiving heat-therapy treatments.

Consequently, athletes who have athletic trainers at their school have many advantages. Athletic trainers play an important role in the immediate evaluation and treatment of the athlete because they are frequently available during practice and competition. In addition, athletic trainers in the school setting are usually available to provide services more than once a day 7 days a week if necessary. In this setting, insurance does not dictate the type and quantity of therapy the athletes receive.

Evaluation of Injuries

Many sports-related injuries have the advantage of immediate, on-the-field evaluation as opposed to the traditional 36-hour delay or more in therapy initiation. The evaluation should be a systemic process performed as soon as possible to obtain the most reliable results. This includes history of injury, inspection, palpation, and tests. Although emergencies will not be addressed here, it is important to note that an emergency is not a time for a turf battle between health-care providers. Even though emergencies receive initial care and stabilization from the team physician or athletic trainer, most ambulance attendants are very well trained in transportation of the injured and therefore should be allowed to perform this service.

History should include information such as previous injuries, mechanism of injury, pre-existing conditions, type of pain, unusual sensations, presence of an immediate disability, and the production of sounds and feelings such as popping or cracking (Faley, 1986; O'Donoghue, 1976).

Inspection should include discoloration, body movements, posture, gait, apprehension, deformity, swelling, general appearance of the athlete, damage to the skin or signs of a direct blow, and signs of shock (Faley, 1986; O'Donoghue, 1976). Comparison of the injured area to the opposite, noninjured side will provide a baseline value.

Palpation should be performed systemically to correlate point tenderness with anatomy. Palpation should include soft tissues, tendons, ligaments, muscles, joints, and boney structures. Signs of inflammation and crepitation must be noted.

Several tests may be indicated including active and passive range of motion, strength, joint stability (ligament and capsular stress tests), agility, neurologic tests, girth measurements, injury-specific tests, and possibly x-rays. All athletes must undergo functional tests before returning to competition.

Immediate testing such as stress examinations can often recognize bodily damage that may be masked later by swelling and spasm (Staples, 1965 and 1972). This immediacy of testing allows for a more accurate evaluation, quicker initiation of treatment, and less total rehabilitation time.

Immediate Treatment

Treatment optimally begins on the field in the form of first aid and continues that day in the training room or clinic. Control of inflammation is a major issue in the treatment of acute injuries, such as strains, sprains, and contusions. The mnemonic commonly used to recall effective treatment phases for acute athlete injuries is PRICE: *p*rotection, *r*estricted activity, *i*ce, compression, and *e*levation. Protection from further injury can be assisted through techniques such as protective strapping or bracing. Varying degrees of restricted activity may be indicated as

well for the injured area. The type of restriction may vary from total immobilization and crutches to light activity and a modified position (e.g., a shortstop who sprains an ankle may play at first base instead).

Ice or cold is universally accepted for acute injuries to decrease edema, bleeding, hematoma formation, tissue metabolism, inflammation, and pain (Spain, 1985). Cold also decreases muscle spasms, tissue temperature, muscle and nerve excitability, blood flow, and capillary permeability (Hillman and Delforge, 1985). Cold therapy can be applied through ice massage, chemical cold packs, ice packs, cold whirlpools, iced wet towels, intermittent cryotherapy compression units, and cold sprays (Spain, 1985; Torg et al, 1987).

Compression applies external pressure to decrease the accumulation of edema or decrease existing edema. Methods of applying compression include elastic wraps, adhesive tape, air splints, and intermittent compression devices. Elevation by raising the involved body part above the heart level uses gravity to assist in decreasing edema.

Rehabilitation

The rehabilitation of athletes is basically comprised of therapeutic exercise (including manual therapy) and physical modalities. The purpose of therapeutic exercise is the restoration of injured tissue to its previous functional level (Allman, 1989). Therapeutic exercise is the fundamental part of the rehabilitation of athletes. As previously stated, there are seven major areas in the exercise/conditioning program; however, depending on the type and severity of the injury, all seven areas may not be initially included in the rehabilitation program.

Modalities are beneficial in the early stages of rehabilitation to enhance the therapeutic exercise program (Davis, 1986; Hillman and Delforge, 1985; Torg et al, 1987). The modalities used during the rehabilitation process vary depending on the specific goal, experience of the health-care provider, contraindications, availability of the equipment, and type and severity of injury. The major difference in the types of modalities and treatment plan used by physical and occupational therapists in sports medicine is that sports medicine concentrates on the therapeutic exercise program, with modalities used more as a supplement to that exercise program (Torg et al, 1987). Modalities are used to increase the athletes' ability to participate in the therapeutic exercise program. For example, by interrupting the vicious cycle of swelling, pain, and muscle spasm, athletes will progress quicker through the exercise rehabilitation program and lessen total recovery time.

CONCLUSIONS

As noted by the editors of this volume, the two main causes of bodily insult are accidental injuries and voluntary lifestyle choices. In terms of sports and athletics, unintentional injuries frequently occur but may sometimes be avoided through proper implementation of sport technique, abidance of rules, proper equipment fitting, education, and recognition of environmental risk factors. Two of the more common causes of sports-related injuries—overstress syndromes and the "overnight athlete"—are considered voluntary lifestyle choices and are easy to prevent through good conditioning, education, screening/preparticipation physical, and a well-balanced, natural diet. If an injury does occur, initial treatment in the form of PRICE should begin immediately after a good initial evaluation.

Applying traditional physical and occupational therapy practices does not constitute sports medicine. In sports medicine, a bicyclist with a fractured arm may have his or her handlebars casted to the forearm so that training can continue; a football player with a sprained ankle may receive three treatments a day, which is often cost-prohibitive to the general public; or a wrestler with weak cervical musculature may be evaluated in a preparticipation physical examination and placed on a strengthening program to minimize the risk of future injury.

The primary goals in sports medicine are the prevention of injuries and, if an injury does occur, the safe return of the athletes to their previous level of competition as quickly as possible. When treatment is performed, the SAID principle must be strictly enforced by the sports medicine practitioner. The rehabilitation program must not only be specific to the athlete's age and sex, but it must be specific to the athlete's sport and playing position as well.

References

Allman FL: Rehabilitation of sports injuries: A practical approach. *In* Ryan AJ and Allman FL (eds): Sports Medicine. San Diego, CA, Academic Press, 1989.

Carlisle F: Effects of preliminary passive warming on swimming performance. Res Q 27:143–152, 1956.

Clarke KS and Buckley WE: Women's injuries in collegiate sports. Am J Sports Med 8(3):187–191, 1980.

Coplin TH: Isokinetic exercise: Clinical usage. Athletic Training 6(3):110–114, 1971.

Davis JM: Rehabilitation of sports injuries: A practical approach. *In* Bernhardt DB (ed): Sports Physical Therapy. New York, Churchhill Livingstone, 1986.

Derscheid GL and Feiring DC: A statistical analysis to characterize treatment adherence of the 18 most common diagnoses seen at a sports medicine clinic. J Orthop Sports Phys Ther 9(1):40–46, 1987.

Dewey TJ and Gallaspy JB: The use of percutaneous pinning and a silicone splint for a fractured proximal phalanx. Athletic Training 25(1):55–56, 1990.

Faley TD: Athletic Training Principles and Practice. Palo Alto, CA, Mayfield Publishing, 1986.

Faris GJ: Psychologic aspects of athletic rehabilitation. Clin Sports Med 4(3):545–551, 1985.

Gleim GW, Nicholas JA, and Webb JN: Isokinetic evaluation following leg injuries. Phys Sports Med 6:75–82, 1978.

Grose JE: Depression of muscular fatigue curves by heat and cold. Res Q 29:20, 1958.

Hall VE, Muniz E, and Fitch B: Re-education of the strength of muscular contraction by application of moist heat to the overlying skin. Arch Phys Med Rehabil 28:493–499, 1947.

Harvey JS: Foreword. Clin Sports Med 4(3):403–404, 1985.

Heusner W: The Theory of Strength Development. New Orleans, Isokinetics, Inc, ASCA Clinic, 1978.

Hillman SK and Delforge G: The use of physical agents in the rehabilitation of athletic injuries. Clin Sports Med 4(3):431–438, 1985.

Hislop HJ and Perrine JJ: The isokinetic concept of exercise. Phys Ther 47(2):114–117, 1967.

Hocutt JE, Jaffe R, Rylander CR, et al: Cryotherapy in ankle sprains. Am J Sports Med 10(5):316–319, 1982.

Kibler WB, Chandler TJ, Uhl T, et al: A musculoskeletal approach to the preparticipation physical examination. Am J Sports Med 17(4):525–531, 1989.

Klafs CE and Arnheim DD: Modern Principles of Athletic Training. St. Louis, C. V. Mosby, 1977.

Kulund DN: The Injured Athlete. Philadelphia, JB Lippincott, 1982.

Lesmes GR, Costill CL, Coyle EF, et al: Muscle strength and power changes during maximal isokinetic training. Med Sci Sports 10(4):266–269, 1978.

Londeree BR: Strength testing. J.P.E.R. 52:44–46, 1981.

Margaria R: The sources of muscular energy. Sci Am 26:84–91, 1972.

Matheson GO, Macintyre JG, Taunton JE, et al: Musculoskeletal injuries associated with physical activity in older adults. Med Sci Sport Exerc 21(4):379–385, 1989.

Moffroid MT and Kusiak ET: The power struggle. Phys Ther 55:1098–1104, 1975.

Moyer JA: Playing in lightning is risky business. Softball News 6(7):2, 1988.

Moyer JA: Rehabilitation goals in sports medicine. *In* Prentice WE (ed): Rehabilitation Techniques in Sports Medicine. St. Louis, C. V. Mosby/Yearbook, 1990a.

Moyer JA: Unique factors in rehabilitating the young athlete. *In* Grana WA, Lombardo JA, Skarkey BJ, and Stone JA (eds): Advances in Sports Medicine and Fitness. Chicago, Yearbook 1990b.

National Athletic Trainers Association: Cold facts on basketball, wrestling injuries. Athletic Training 23(4):383–388, 1988a.

National Athletic Trainers Association: Final report shows prep injuries most likely in practice, during late stages of game. Athletic Training 24(4):368–370, 1989a.

National Athletic Trainers Association: Injury toll among prep athletes at one million. Athletic Training 2(3):273–277, 1987a.

National Athletic Trainers Association: Injury toll in prep sports estimated at 1.3 million. Athletic Training 24(4):360–367, 1989b.

National Athletic Trainers Association: Picture brightens, but injuries to prep football players still at 37%. Athletic Training 23(2):185–187, 1988b.

National Athletic Trainers Association: Study shows 35 football injuries per school under "good" conditions. Athletic Training 23(2):1988c.

National Athletic Trainers Association: Study shows 23% of girls who play prep basketball injured this year. Athletic Training 22(3):267–271, 1987b.

National Athletic Trainers Association: Three-year study finds "major injuries" up 20% in high school football. Athletic Training 24(1):60–61, 1989c.

National Collegiate Athletic Association: Injury rate for football reaches a seven-year high. NCAA News January 24, 1990.

National Collegiate Athletic Association: Report released on injury trends in spring sports. NCAA News July 5, 1989a.

National Collegiate Athletic Association: Report shows injury trends in association's winter sports. NCAA News May 3, 1989b.

National Collegiate Athletic Association: Study shows injury trends in fall sports for '88 season. NCAA News February 1, 1989c.

O'Donoghue DH: Treatment of Injuries to Athletes, 3rd ed. Philadelphia, WB Saunders, 1976.

Pipes TV: The acquisition of muscular strength through constant and variable resistance strength training. Athletic Training 12(3):148–151, 1977.

Powell J: 636,000 injuries annually in high school football. Athletic Training 22(1):19–22, 1987.

Robins AC: The effect of hot and cold shower baths upon adolescents participating in physical education classes. Res Q 13:373–380, 1942.

Roy S and Irvin R: Sports medicine prevention, evaluation, management, and rehabilitation. Englewood Cliffs, NJ, Prentice-Hall, 1983.

Samples P: Mind over muscle: Returning the injured athlete to play. Physician Sports Med 15(10):172–180, 1987.

Sargeant AJ and Jones NL: Effect on power output of human muscle during short term dynamic exercise. Med Sci Sport 11:39, 1978.

Scudder GN: Torque curves produced at the knee during isometric and isokinetic exercise. Arch Phys Med Rehabil 61:68–73, 1980.

Sedwick AW and Whalen HR: The effect of passive warm-up on muscular strength and endurance. Res Q 35:49–59, 1964.

Spain J: Prehabilitation. Clin Sports Med 4(3):575–585, 1985.

Staples OS: Ligamentous injuries of the ankle joint. Clin Orthop 42:21–35, 1965.

Staples OS: Result of study of ruptures of lateral ligaments of the ankle. Clin Orthop 85:50–58, 1972.

Torg JS, Vegso JJ, and Torg E: Rehabilitation of athletic injuries—an atlas of therapeutic exercise. Chicago, Yearbook 1987.

Werner JK: Neuroscience: A Clinical Perspective. Philadelphia, WB Saunders, 1980.

Williams M and Stutzman L: Strength variation through the range of joint motion. Phys Ther 39:145–152, 1959.

GLOSSARY

Athletic trainer: Generally is a graduate of a bachelor's or master's program that emphasizes the prevention, evaluation, treatment, and rehabilitation of athletic injuries.

Isokinetic muscular contraction: Maximal contraction is applied throughout the entire range of motion by accommodating resistance against a lever moving at a fixed speed.

Isometric contraction: A contraction where there is an increase in muscular tone without a change in muscular length.

Isotonic contraction: A muscular contraction during which time joint motion occurs.

NATA: National Athletic Trainers Association, which is the certification and governing body for certified athletic trainers.

NCAA: National Collegiate Athletic Association.

PRICE: Protection, restricted activity, ice, compression, and evaluation is commonly used for the treatment of acute athletic injuries.

Power: Product of force times velocity; amount of work performed per unit time; strength of a muscle times the velocity of the limb through the range of motion.

SAID: Specific adaptations to imposed demands principle; conditioning or rehabilitation program must prepare the athlete for the specific demands of the sport. The athletes' sport, position, age, and sex must be considered when a conditioning or rehabilitation program is designed.

Strength: The force of a single muscle contraction measured in units of the pound, newton, and kilogram.

CHAPTER

8

Julie Belkin
Susan M. Blackmore

Injury Prevention Through Splinting

Splinting the hand or upper extremity to prevent acute injury or to relieve chronic impairment is suggested for the treatment of cumulative trauma disorders (CTDs) and sports-related injuries. This chapter presents splinting strategies and patient-education principles for three stages of intervention. Primary prevention deals with the asymptomatic clients; secondary intervention, clients with intermittent or acute symptoms; and tertiary intervention, clients returning to work or sports participation.

Webster's Third New International Dictionary defines splint as "a rigid or flexible material used to protect, immobilize or restrict motion in a part." The literature is replete with examples of splints designed to maintain or improve the position of the hand affected by disease or injury. One can go as far back as the 1600s for a description of splints designed to mobilize and immobilize parts of the hand and upper extremity. In 1944, Sterling Bunnell gave us a series of custom-designed splints that are still used today for postoperative immobilization and rehabilitation.

Ten years ago, splints began to change so that they support and limit motion rather than fully immobilize a part (Henshaw et al, 1989). Limiting the extremes of motion became very important in industries in which workers are required to perform job duties repetitively and with their hands in positions that may compromise nerve and tendon function. Fitting the work task to the person to facilitate maximum productivity without excessive risk of injury is the study of ergonomics.

The development of the field of ergonomics has brought with it a recognition of the mechanical forces humans experience during activity. This field has emphasized workplace design to facilitate prevention of industrial injury (Armstrong, 1986; Blair and Allard, 1983; Tichauer, 1966). Splinting the hand or arm as a measure of prevention against occupationally induced injury has more recently been described by Rossi (1988) and Henshaw and associates (1989).

As just defined, a splint may be used to immobilize, to restrict, or to protect. The philosophy of preventive medicine dictates that, as therapists, we seek out methods to stop injury or disease from occurring. Extending that philosophy to the practice of splinting, one must take into consideration the concept of a splint as a support. When a support is defined as an assist to motion or as a prop to hold a part in place, splints take on another purpose. For example, an elastic elbow band may serve as a reminder to limit the extremes of elbow motion (Fig. 8–1).

The concept of splinting as supporting motion requires us to examine the materials used in fabrication. Metal, wood, and leather are the ancestors of the materials we use today. The introduction of copolymer plastics in the fields of orthotics and in therapy greatly influenced

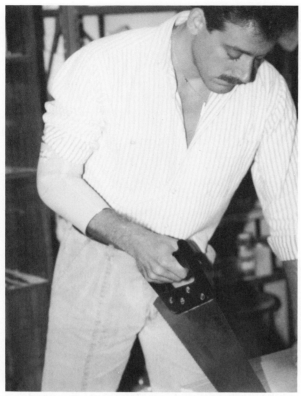

Figure 8–1. A Neoprene elbow band limits the extremes of range of motion at the elbow.

fabrication techniques in the 1960s and 1970s. A new revolution has begun in the 1990s with the marketing of semiflexible materials that allow motion while retaining conformity and support around a body part.

PROGRAM DESCRIPTION

A program of splinting for injury prevention includes consideration of the neurologic, muscular, and skeletal components of the upper extremity. Programs designed to address prevention of CTD and sports injuries include the following objectives:

1. Identification of target populations
2. Design and fabrication of splints for use during and after activity
3. Evaluation of splint selection to ensure that its use does not compromise performance of an activity and to ensure client compliance and acceptance of the splint

4. Client education of injury-prevention measures and possible risk factors

Primary Prevention Program

Primary prevention uses splints for the asymptomatic client. Client selection is based on epidemiologic studies that link high-risk individuals and activities with certain injury categories. Clients will continue to participate in the activity but will wear a splint during the activity or during rest after completion of the activity. An education program accompanies the fitting of a splint to increase the client's awareness of potential symptoms and knowledge of recommended musculoskeletal conditioning techniques.

Goals of splinting for primary prevention include the following:

1. Prevention of upper extremity trauma in at-risk populations during high-risk activities
2. Education of clients to identify risk factors and implement appropriate risk-reducing strategies

Secondary Intervention Program

Secondary intervention involves splinting as a corrective measure directed toward relieving acute or intermittent symptoms. Splinting in this stage may aid in alleviating an acute injury and in allowing continued participation in an activity. As with primary prevention, splints may also be used for rest after activity.

Goals of splinting for secondary intervention include the following:

1. Correction or relief of symptomatic injuries to allow continuing participation in activities
2. Facilitation of participation in activity while preventing further injury or an increase in symptoms
3. Education of clients on potential for reinjury and of techniques to reduce symptoms if they are exacerbated

Tertiary Intervention Program

A tertiary splinting program focuses on prevention of recurrent injury or on splinting that allows activity participation in an adapted manner. In this stage clients may present with an irreversible limitation, and splinting must be designed to maximize capabilities to allow for participation in the desired activity. Splints may provide stability to an injured area, protect a hypersensitive part, or assist movement to augment strength and range of motion. At this stage, clients may use one splint designed for use during activity and one for rest after activity. For example, a client with a radial nerve injury uses a dynamic finger-extension splint during functional tasks and a resting-hand splint at night.

Goals for a tertiary splinting program include the following:

1. Facilitate participation in activity through use of a splint designed to support, protect, or assist motion as indicated by anatomic limitations
2. Provide client education designed to enhance understanding and performance of adapted techniques for successful participation in activities.

POPULATION IDENTIFICATION

It seems that we live in a medical community beset with diseases, known only by their call letters. Our clients and family ask what we know about CTS, TOS, CTD and UCL tears. Carpal tunnel syndrome (CTS), thoracic outlet syndrome, CTD, and ulnar collateral ligament tears are compression neuropathies and ligamentous injuries that appear to be on the rise.

In truth, CTDs, although not named as such, were described in the literature over 200 years ago (Ramazinni, 1940). Ligamentous injuries were likely seen, if not recorded, when humans first lifted and threw rocks.

In the past 2 to 3 decades, both CTDs and sports-related injuries have been brought to the forefront of medicine. Various media focus the public's attention on the ball player whose shoulder has been repaired through surgery and therapy, allowing resumption of a million-dollar career. CTS may be known on almost every assembly line in America.

Target populations for at-risk groups have been identified in the literature on industrial and sports medicine. Tendinitis, tenosynovitis, ligamentous injury, and chronic nerve entrapment are described for both work-related and sports-related activities in which the hand and upper extremity are used in a repetitive manner. What varies for the activity is not symptomatology, but the causative factor and the suspected high-risk population.

Female workers in the fourth and fifth decades of life whose jobs require repetitive wrist and finger motion are most often cited as high-risk candidates of CTD, particularly CTS (Armstrong and Chaffin, 1979; Phalen, 1972; Tanaka et al, 1988). Occupational neuritis of the ulnar nerve is found in both men and women whose jobs require sustained gripping with compression over the hypothenar eminence of the hand (Hunt, 1911) and in professional bicyclists. An increased incidence of ligamentous sprains and tendinitis in both men and women in the second and third decades of life is attributed to expanding interest and opportunities for participation in organized sports. Where the at-risk population for sports-related injuries was once solely men between the ages of 15 and 30 years, we now treat 50-year-old women tennis players and 70-year-old golfers for such injuries. This expansion of participation in both work- and sports-related activities does broaden the areas in which prevention programs using splints can be effective. Specific at-risk populations, their identification of relationship to injury prevention programs, and treatment are described later.

REFERRAL

Therapists play an ever-expanding role in industrial medicine and sports medicine. Many large industries have on-site clinics that provide medical intervention for on-the-job injuries. These clinics also seek to prevent injury through the implementation of exercise programs, ergonomic redesign of equipment, and job modification. Sports clinics are often multidisciplinary settings using the expertise of doctors, trainers, coaches, and therapists.

Referrals for splints may be generated from direct involvement in such clinics. The media have helped to expand the public's awareness of symptoms and treatment of CTDs. Both hospital-based and private-practice–based therapists can use media attention to their advantage because it may generate referrals. Part of the education program must be aimed at community medical personnel and sports and industrial clinics to increase awareness of the potential for splints to be part of a treatment program.

OVERVIEW OF TREATMENT

It is beyond the scope of this chapter to present any but the basic concepts of anatomy, biology, and mechanics as they relate to the fabrication of preventative splints. There are many basic texts, and all therapists working with the hand should have a thorough understanding of the splinting and treatment principles as presented by Brand (1985), Fess (1987), and Bunnell (1956) among others. Therapists whose practice includes injury-prevention programs must have a thorough understanding of the normal hand and how its mechanics may be affected by external supports. Therapists who understand the mechanics of the normal hand are in the position to best determine when and how a splint should be used. In addition to splinting, ergonomic intervention may redesign the manner in which work is performed (Armstrong, 1986; Armstrong et al, 1987; Tichauer, 1966). Splinting and ergonomic redesign may reduce occupational risk factors that contribute to CTDs and ligamentous injuries.

The hand is a mobile instrument that conforms to many shapes and tasks. It is exquisitely sensitive to texture and yet can tolerate and transmit tremendous force. Splints fabricated to support the hand must interfere with hand function as little as possible. The volar surface of the digits must be free from straps and material whenever possible.

Gloves that cover the entire finger will reduce the function of the hands by limiting sensory feedback. The hand's bony arches allow it infinite changes in shape. The hand can move from a flattened position to a slightly curved shape to a complete ball fist. Maintenance of these transverse arches of the hand at the metacarpal heads and the distal carpal row is a basic splinting principle that must be observed. These arches transmit strength to the grasping hand and allow the fingers to converge into flexion.

The joints of the thumb, as we see later in this chapter, are often the site of stress injuries. The carpometacarpal (CMC) joint of the thumb allows for rotation and circumduction as seen with palmar abduction and adduction of the thumb. Limiting motion at the CMC joint is often called for in splinting. With proper positioning of the thumb in opposition to the digits, function will not be limited while providing rest and support to the CMC joint (Fig. 8–2). The wrist joint complex is also capable of circumduction through a combination of motions. Wrist motions involve an intricate interplay among the carpal bones, the radius, and the ulna. All forearm-based splints will cross and affect these joints. In so doing, splints also alter in some way the mechanics of the hand.

A splint that restricts motion at one joint will affect the mechanics at the joints proximal and distal to the splinted joint. A splint that is comfortable, rests the affected joint, and allows functional motion of the unaffected joints will be worn and thus will be effective. The splint that does not meet these criteria will be discarded.

SPLINTS: PREFABRICATED VERSUS CUSTOM FABRICATED

Prefabricated splints for the hand and upper extremity are available in a vast array of styles, materials, and sizes. Therapists may choose from dozens of companies manufacturing a variety of splints designed for one purpose. One must

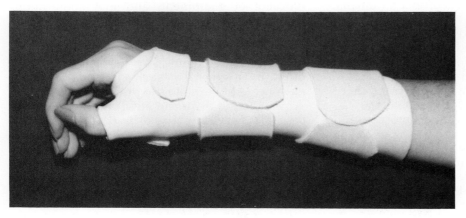

Figure 8–2. A thumb spica splint limits the motion at the thumb carpometacarpal joint. It is used to limit thumb motion for the patient with de Quervain's disease and to limit thumb and wrist motion for the patient with scapholunate dissociation.

assume that, when there are dozens of splints available for one purpose, no particular splint is superior to all others and no one splint can be used in all cases. Therapists must closely evaluate the advantages and disadvantages of prefabricated splints.

One size that fits all generally fits no one well. Hands do not come in small, medium, and large sizes. These splints can be adjusted for proper fit, but therapists must be prepared to adjust splints individually to meet specific needs. A prefabricated splint must fulfill the requirements of proper fit as described by Fess (1987) and Malick (1976). If a proper fit can be obtained, a prefabricated splint may prove expedient and cost-effective, especially if time is of major importance.

Therapists must learn to make custom splints from low-temperature thermoplastic materials or from materials such as neoprene. Therapists, with their knowledge of anatomy and kinesiology and their understanding of injury and disease, are uniquely qualified to design and fabricate preventive splints. The ability to perform task analysis and determine an individual's specific physical requirements is essential in splint design. In short, a custom-designed and fabricated splint is a superior way to meet an individual's need.

In the case of secondary prevention, directed toward preventing impairment once symptoms of injury or disease are evident, a splint may be custom made to alleviate those specific symptoms while not interfering with task performance. Custom-fabricated splints are perhaps most necessary when tertiary prevention is considered. When medical management of injury or disease is complete, individuals may have anatomic or mechanical limitations that obviate the fitting of a splint. Custom-designed splints, along with re-education or retraining, may provide support and increased function so that clients will resume job-related tasks or develop independent daily living skills.

Choosing to fit a prefabricated splint versus a custom-fabricated splint depends largely on the experience of the treating therapist. In today's atmosphere of cost accountability, the financial implications, including reimbursement, also need consideration. The general public can obtain off-the-shelf splints from their local pharmacy or medical supplier. Therapists' service in providing prefabricated splints must include expertise in fitting the splint, adapting the splint, and educating clients to the splint's proper use. Also therapists must recognize when a prefabricated splint will not suffice. At the very least, we suggest that therapists fitting prefabricated splints have the equipment (heat gun and sewing machine in particular) available to customize the fit of these splints.

TREATMENT

The topic of splinting the hand and upper extremity is vast when one considers the variety of diagnoses that occur as a result of trauma or overuse and the array of splints designed to treat these diagnoses. This section presents suggestions for primary, secondary, and tertiary treatments as they relate to three major diagnostic categories:

1. Nerve compression
2. Tendinitis
3. Ligamentous injuries

From each of these categories we have chosen one or two diagnoses frequently seen in industrial settings and in sports-related activities.

Nerve Compression Syndromes

Compression of nerves in the upper extremity is often linked to CTDs. CTDs may be defined as "disorder of soft tissue due to repeated exertions and movements of the body" (Armstrong, 1986, p. 553). All soft tissue can be affected; however, compression of the median nerve at the wrist is often cited as a cause of impaired hand function. This compression is known as CTS. Early symptoms include impaired sensibility such as tingling over the median nerve distribution and night pain with numbness. Late symptoms of CTS include atrophy of thenar musculature and impairment in autonomic nerve function resulting in loss of sweat patterns.

The cause of CTS has been linked in the literature to many factors, including developmental anomalies, fractures, hormonal influence, and local tumors. Occupational factors such as repetitive use, force, mechanical stresses, vibration, and posture are implicated in the development of CTS (Armstrong, 1986). Of these, one cannot isolate the factors of posture and vibration from those of repetitiveness, force, and stress.

Job analysis and restructuring can be used to reduce repetitiveness, force, and stress. Force and mechanical stress may be best addressed through the use of ergonomically designed tools and workstations to reduce or eliminate harmful effects. Splinting can assist in reducing the effects of vibration and posture.

Primary Prevention in CTS. Primary prevention for CTS focuses on the at-risk population and seeks to prevent the occurrence of even mild symptoms. A controversy exists, however, as to how we choose the at-risk population. Many authors believe that given occupations cause or exacerbate CTS (Birkbeck and Beer, 1975; Smith et al, 1977). Armstrong (1983) called CTS "one of a family of occupational illnesses" (p. 1).

Other authors maintain that CTS may not be job related. Phalen (1972), in a retrospective study of 598 clients maintained that occupationally caused CTS was rare. Nathan and colleagues (1988) were unable to establish in their study of 471 employees "any consistent association between the occurrence of impaired sensory conduction of the median nerve and occupational class or the level of hand activity" (p. 169). McCormack and associates (1990) found no significant correlation between five job categories and CTS.

Therapists who want to prevent CTS can rely on evidence that supports the hypothesis that occupation and epidemiologic factors (sex, age factors) can be used to determine at-risk populations.

The common design of a wrist support used for CTS is prefabricated canvas or woven elastic with a metal or plastic bar constructed to hold the wrist at 20 degrees to 30 degrees of extension (Fig. 8–3). Studies have shown that pressure within the carpal tunnel is reduced with the wrist positioned in 0 degrees to 45 degrees of extension compared with 30 degrees to 60 degrees of flexion (Smith et al, 1977; Tanzer, 1959). These studies support the practice of splinting the wrist in slight extension to minimize pressure within the carpal tunnel. Often a custom-fabricated volar or dorsal thermoplastic wrist splint may provide a more comfortable and effective fit. Splints that support or limit wrist motion must be designed and fabricated to interfere with adjacent joints as little as possible. The metacarpophalangeal (MP) joints of the digits must not be limited in flexion or extension. Thumb circumduction at the CMC joint should be free as possible.

A semiflexible splint may be advisable because the digits will experience an increased load with immobilization of the wrist. The splint will limit extremes of motion while still permitting mid-range motion.

Using a support fabricated from elastic materials provides compression, warmth, and a tactile reminder to avoid positions of extreme wrist flexion or extension. Splinting as a primary prevention strategy combined with a conditioning program to maximize clients' flexibility and strength of muscles may reduce the development of CTS in populations at risk. There are, however, no retrospective data to support this supposition.

Secondary and Tertiary Intervention for Carpal Tunnel Syndrome. The basic tenets of splinting the wrist do not change significantly in the presence of acute symptoms (secondary interven-

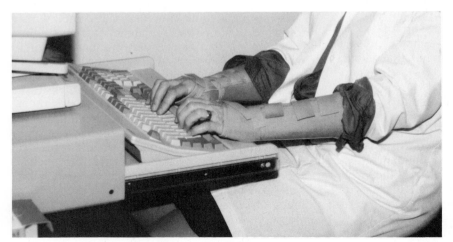

Figure 8–3. A prefabricated wrist splint can be used in primary prevention of carpal tunnel syndrome if a good fit can be obtained.

tion) or after surgical decompression of the median nerve (tertiary intervention). Custom-fabricated splints are used more often than prefabricated splints during these phases of treatment. Splints are worn full time (day and night) until symptoms subside. The splint is removed for skin care as needed. As symptoms are relieved, the splint is removed during daytime activity. Night splinting may be continued as needed to prevent clients from sleeping with a fully flexed or extended wrist, because these positions compress the median nerve at the wrist. Education is aimed at increasing awareness of activities that may exacerbate symptoms and teaching problem solving to elicit adaptive behaviors. Frequent rest periods are recommended during activity. Nerve-gliding exercises performed on a regular basis are suggested as a tertiary intervention strategy to prevent adhesions of surgically released nerves and tendons (Baxter-Petralia, 1990).

Ulnar Nerve Compression at the Wrist

Entrapment neuropathies of the ulnar nerve at the wrist occur most frequently in or near Guyon's canal. Symptoms of compression vary depending on whether the ulnar nerve or one of its branches is involved. Three types of compression were described by Shea and McClain in 1969. Classification of type is dependent on the site of compression and the nerve branch involved. Type 1 is defined as pressure on the nerve just proximal to Guyon's canal. Type 2 is pressure on the nerve where it exits from Guyon's canal; and in type 3 a compressive lesion is noted in or at the end of the Guyon's canal.

Guyon's canal is bordered proximally and medially by the pisiform, laterally and distally by the hook of the hamate, and distally by the volar carpal ligament and the medial attachment of the transverse carpal ligament. There are no tendons that pass through the canal. Within the canal the ulnar nerve bifurcates into a superficial and deep branch. The superficial branch supplies sensation to the hypothenar eminence and to the ring and little fingers. The deep motor branch innervates the hypothenar muscles and travels across the deep palmar arch to innervate the interossei, the flexor pollicis brevis, and the first dorsal interosseus.

Two commonly reported causes for compression of the ulnar nerve in the wrist and hand are ganglions and occupational trauma. Of these two causes, occupational trauma (and avocational trauma) is most amenable to conservative treatment, including splinting. Numerous occupations require static pressure over the hypothenar eminence and sustained gripping of the ring and small fingers. The occupations cited as causative were jeweler, machinist, and brass polisher. Hunt, in 1908, described this occupational neuritis as that of the deep palmar branch of the ulnar nerve. In 1911, Hunt described similar symptoms in people who opened oysters routinely. These professions exist today and are performed in the same manner as they were years ago. In addition, avocational sports as a causative factor includes long-distance bicycling.

What has changed today is the development of shock-absorbing materials, which can be used to reduce the stress imposed over the hypothenar eminence when pushing a press machine, when holding an oyster-shucking knife, or while riding a bicycle. Occupations causing repetitive trauma over the ulnar border of the hand along with professions requiring sustained gripping with the ulnar two fingers are easily identified. For example, the jackhammer operator and a person operating a paper-cutting machine have incidences of ulnar nerve compression at the wrist.

Primary Prevention. Fingerless gloves or molded hand-based splints incorporating shock-absorbing materials such as Sorbothane, PPT, and silicone gels are available commercially. A primary intervention strategy of requiring gloves for workers involved in targeted occupations and long-distance cyclers has excellent potential to prevent the symptoms of ulnar neuropathy (Fig. 8–4).

Secondary and Tertiary Intervention. As a strategy for both secondary and tertiary interventions, the proper fitting of gloves or splints that incorporate shock-absorbing materials may allow a person to continue working or make return to work possible. Client-education programs, as presented later in this chapter, are helpful to determine necessary job and equipment modifications to allow safe return to activity. Although splints or gloves may alleviate obvious symptoms, they are only one segment in a comprehensive prevention program.

We mentioned early in this chapter that the 1990s have brought a new focus on materials used in splinting the upper extremity. Flexible shock-absorbing foams and thermoplastics have been used for decades by prosthetists and ortho-

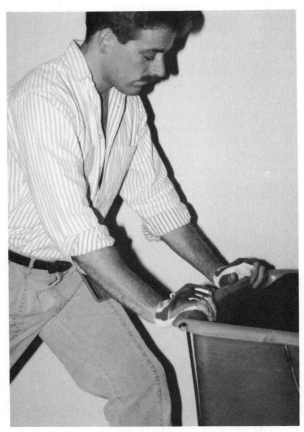

Figure 8–4. Gloves that have silicone gel as a shock-absorbing material are available through medical suppliers or sporting goods stores. The gloves can assist to disperse pressure, which is applied to the ulnar nerve at the wrist.

tists. Some of these materials are moldable only at high temperatures (300° F and higher) and must be draped or vacuum-formed over a positive mold. The materials described in this chapter can be formed directly on the body part, thereby reducing fabrication time and cost.

Materials are described in Tables 8–1 and 8–2 according to their properties, suggested application, fabrication process, and available styles.

Tenosynovitis

The development of stenosing tenosynovitis in the first dorsal compartment of the wrist is often associated with activities requiring sustained pinching in combination with ulnar or radial deviation of the wrist. The condition was first described in 1895 by Fritz de Quervain, and the disease entity bears his name. The onset of de Quervain's disease is usually gradual. Symptoms include pain about the radial styloid, which may or may not radiate down the thumb and up the forearm (Finkelstein, 1930). Movement of the thumb into extension or abduction and ulnar deviation of the wrist usually exacerbates the pain. Supination of the forearm is often found to elicit pain. A positive result on Finkelstein's test—pain elicited by placing the thumb in palmar flexion and the wrist in simultaneous ulnar deviation—is a strong indicator of de Quervain's tenosynovitis.

Readers are referred to several excellent texts that describe in detail the anatomy and pathophysiology of the tendons in the first dorsal compartment: Boyes (1970), Froimson (1988), and Hamilton (1976). This chapter concerns itself with identification of at-risk populations for primary prevention and with splinting as part of the treatment regime to relieve de Quervain's disease in primary, secondary, and tertiary prevention.

Primary Prevention. Symptoms of tenosynovitis at the wrist are common among workers performing intense, repetitive maneuvers with their hands. As noted, deviation of the wrist and sustained pinching are implicated in the development of de Quervain's disease. Armstrong and colleagues, in 1987, cited repetition and forcefulness as the most important factors in the development of tendinitis in the wrist and hand. Women were found be at 4.6 times greater risk than men of developing hand and wrist tendinitis (Armstrong et al, 1987), and a ten-fold risk factor has also been reported (Kirkpatrick, 1990). Some specific risk tasks include tool use in the electronics industry, assembly line packagers, and food processors.

Prevention through the use of ergonomically designed tools and redesign of workstations is rapidly becoming accepted in industry (Armstrong, 1986; Tichauer, 1966). Although many researchers discuss the use of splints to ensure rest after the onset of acute symptoms, rarely are splints prescribed as a preventive technique. This technique could prevent the onset of symptoms (Finkelstein, 1930; Froimson, 1988; Lipscome, 1951).

The preventative splint supports the thumb in a functional position (CMC joint at 45 to 50 degrees of abduction, MP joint at 5 to 10 degrees of flexion, interphalangeal joint free) in opposition to the index and long fingers to allow per-

Table 8–1. Soft, Moldable Plastics

Material	Properties	Applications	Process	Styles
AliPlast	Soft closed-cell foam, lightweight, easily cleaned, antishear, low durability	Used predominantly as a lining material; can be a soft, lightweight splint for nonindustrial use	Heat in convection oven at 285° F; mold over stockinette-covered body part	3/16"–1/2"; white and buff; self-adhesive available
Plastizote	Closed-cell polyethylene, autoadhesive in dry heat; easily cut and sanded; shock absorbing but compresses with weight bearing; moderate durability	Interface material custom-molded splints for nonindustrial use	Heat in convection oven less than 1 minute, mold over stockinette	3/16"–1"; pink, white, black; perforated; self-adhesive available
AliSoft	Flexible, cloth-lined AliPlast; durable nylon cover; straps can be sewn on material	Semiflexible custom-molded wrist and thumb supports	Heat at 275° F convection oven; can be formed against skin	3/16" sheets; beige nylon
Neoprene	Flexible, elastic material; lycra covered, washable, waterproof	Flexible, custom-designed or prefabricated supports; used for wrist, thumb, and elbow supports	Fabricated from custom-designed patterns; seams can be sewn or glued	1/8"; multiple colors

formance of prehension activities. It is possible when splinting for prevention in the absence of symptoms to use a hand-based splint (short opponens) as an alternative to immobilization of the wrist (Figs. 8–5 and 8–6). The rationale is that the thumb is protected from palmar flexion, and a free wrist limits the possibility of transferring stress to the unencumbered joints. If the wrist is to be included, we suggest a semiflexible support (Henshaw et al, 1989) or one of the prefabricated neoprene splints that are available (Sports Support) (Fig. 8–7).

Use of the splint is recommended during activity only. It is important, as in all phases of primary prevention, to allow nerves and tendons to glide when the hand is out of the splint. A program of gentle range of motion, both passive and active, is recommended to maintain motion in all planes of thumb and wrist movement.

Secondary Intervention. A conservative approach of rest and gentle exercise is recommended, with an emphasis on reduction of pain and inflammation. A splint designed to support the thumb in the position described previously

Table 8–2. Interface Materials

Material	Properties	Applications	Process	Styles
PPT	Frothed cellular urethane; does not bottom out; washable, highly durable; excellent shock absorption	Shock-absorbing lining; can be used to pad bony prominences	Self-adherent sheets or glued with orthotic cement	1/16"–1/2", blue color, nylon or felt, covered or uncovered perforated and nonperforated
Sorbothane	Viscoelastic polymer; does not bottom out; excellent shock absorption; durable, washable	Shock-absorbing lining; used as padding over bony prominences	Adheres with orthotic cement	1/8"–1/4" sheets
AliCover	AliPlast 4E laminated to nylon fabric; durable, washable	Cushions rigid splints	Adheres with glue or self-adherent sheets; can be vacuumed or heat formed	1/32" blue nylon

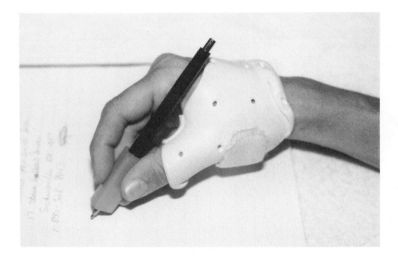

Figure 8–5. A short opponens splint immobilizes the thumb MP joint. It can be used in some cases for primary prevention of de Quervain's disease and for treatment of thumb MP ulnar collateral ligament injuries.

should be used, and should include the wrist in a position of 15 to 20 degrees of extension. A long opponens splint, fabricated as a radial- or volar-based splint, must avoid pressure over the superficial branch of the radial nerve and the ulnar digital nerve of the thumb (Rayan and O'Donoghue, 1983) (see Fig. 8–2).

Exercises included in a secondary intervention program are performed to prevent the formation of adhesions between the tendons and synovial sheaths (Totten, 1990). A conservative range of motion program is designed to prevent forceful motions that may exacerbate symptoms. A program of gentle progressive exercise and activity is suggested to restore strength and endurance to facilitate return to work (Herbin, 1987; Totten, 1990). Continuing use of a supportive splint is an important adjunct to a successful and pain-free return to activity.

Tertiary Intervention. Surgery is recom-mended in cases where a program of secondary intervention does not relieve symptoms after 4 to 6 weeks. Splinting will continue after surgical release of adhesions and decompression of tendons. The long opponens splint described for secondary prevention is worn full time between exercise periods performed 3 times a day. Additions to the splinting program may include elastomer molds to assist with scar-tissue remodeling and desensitization. A gentle progressive range of motion and strengthening program proceeds according to client tolerance (Totten, 1990).

Ligamentous Injuries

Ligamentous injuries are among the most common injuries to occur during sporting activity (McCue, 1974; Ruby, 1983). Injuries occur at all levels of athletic competition including the week-

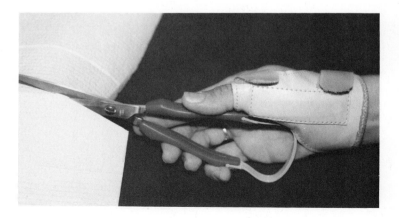

Figure 8–6. A prefabricated short opponens splint can limit thumb palmar flexion for select patients who have early symptoms of de Quervain's disease.

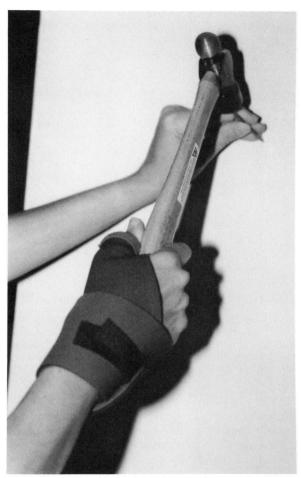

Figure 8–7. A semiflexible Neoprene support is used to limit the extremes of wrist and thumb motion for the patient with de Quervain's disease.

end athlete as well as the professional competitor. Clients with clinically stable injuries can return to athletic competition days after injury if a protective splint is worn. Those clients who required surgery may also return to sports participation after the required immobilization time if splinted.

Ligamentous injuries to the wrist occur from falling on an outstretched hand or flexed wrist. Frequently, the scapholunate (SL) ligament is injured (Ruby, 1983). Individuals who play contact sports such as football, basketball, or volleyball are injured most often.

Finger MP and proximal interphalangeal (PIP) joint injuries may involve the volar plate and collateral ligaments. If the MP joint sustains a dorsal dislocation, the characteristic posture that ensues is MP ulnar deviation and hyperextension. Even more frequently injured is the PIP joint, which results in pseudoboutonnière or a swan-neck deformity. Injuries to the fingers occur most often in ball sports. The fingers sustain an axial compression or a hyperextension force. If a palmar dislocation occurs at the PIP joint, there is a high risk for disruption of the central slip of the extensor tendon along with ligamentous injury. If this is left untreated, the PIP joint will assume a boutonnière deformity.

Injuries to the thumb MP joint most often involve tearing of the ulnar collateral ligament, which may occur when skiing or from a fall on the outstretched hand (Ruby, 1983). In a skiing accident, a radial deviation force is applied from the ski pole, resulting in an injury. After the injury, the client experiences pain and weakness with pinching activities and laxity of the thumb MP joint.

Primary Prevention. The use of external supports, such as taping and gloves, are well accepted in the sports literature to prevent injuries. Soft prefabricated splints are considered less effective as a primary prevention because they may unnecessarily restrict motion and may cause chafing of the skin. In college and professional sports, there are regulations that apply to the types of splints and wraps used. Thus, splinting for primary prevention may be limited to coaches and athletic trainers.

Secondary Intervention. Splinting after an acute partial ligament tear is the treatment of choice to facilitate an early return to activity. Therapeutic management often accompanies a splinting program. We suggest splints for several types of injuries.

Scapholunate Ligament Dissociation. Many styles of semiflexible wrist supports are available for S-L dissociation. The Duke (Dobson et al, 1971) splint, the soft playing splints as described by Bergfield and colleagues (1982), and a variety of neoprene supports are commonly used. In cases of severe injury, the client may wear a thumb spica splint at all times except during competition (see Fig. 8–2). In almost all cases, clients with S-L dissociation require surgery.

MP and PIP Collateral Ligament and Volar Plate Injury. Extension block splinting is used both during and between competition for volar plate injuries. The final 10 to 20 degrees of full digit extension is blocked with these splints (Fig. 8–8A). For PIP volar plate and collateral ligament injuries, a figure-of-8 splint is suggested (Fig. 8–

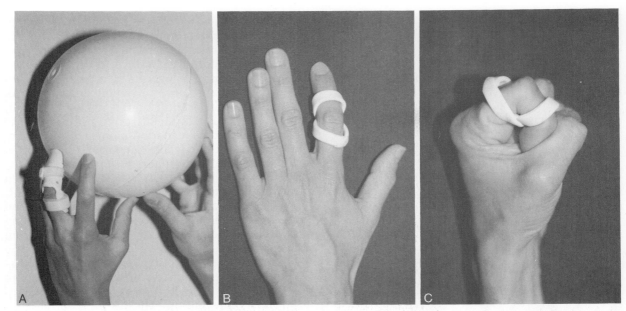

Figure 8–8. *A*, The dorsal extension block splint is designed to limit PIP joint extension to 10 degrees and to allow full PIP joint flexion for treatment of a volar plate injury. The patient can return to activities with the splint in place approximately 3 weeks after the injury. *B* and *C*, A figure 8 splint can limit PIP joint extension and allow full flexion. This splint can also limit lateral stresses applied to the PIP joint for treatment of volar plate and collateral ligament injuries.

8*B* and 8–8*C*). If stress to the joint can be avoided during activity, buddy-taping adjacent fingers and restricting heavy activities will provide the necessary limits to motion (Fig. 8–9). Night splinting with the joint in full extension may be required to prevent the development of PIP joint flexion contractures, which is the most common sequela after these injuries.

Ulnar Collateral Ligament Injuries to the Thumb. An effective secondary intervention strategy for ulnar collateral ligament tears, grades 1 and 2, is the use of a short opponens splint. These splints are available in a variety of prefabricated styles or can be quickly fabricated from low-temperature thermoplastics (see Fig. 8–5). A short opponens splint, which immobilizes the thumb MP joint only, does not significantly limit hand function, and clients can often return to activity. Clients often wear a short opponens splint or a splint fabricated circumferentially around the MP joint under a ski glove. A grade 3 ulnar collateral ligament tear will require surgery.

Tertiary Intervention. Splinting to minimize disability after a ligamentous injury that may or may not have required surgery involves the principle of long-duration, low-intensity stretch.

Splinting may use serial static splints, including cylindric casting, or dynamic splints (Colditz, 1990). Splints that immobilize a joint or limit motion, such as those suggested for primary prevention, can prevent further damage to lax ligaments. Strengthening within a pain-free range is also an essential intervention to promote hand function.

Splint selection in this phase must also consider any adjacent structures that may limit motion. Secondary tightness of the muscle tendon units or joint capsular tightness must be considered. Readers are referred to other sources that address the wide spectrum of splints suggested to resolve resultant deformities (Colditz, 1990; Fess and Philips, 1987).

EDUCATION

Splinting is but one strategy to be used in prevention programs for clients with nerve compression, tenosynovitis, or ligamentous injury. Clients must be educated to the causes of injury and to their involvement in prevention. It is well known among therapists that motivated, cooperative, and knowledgeable clients have a better

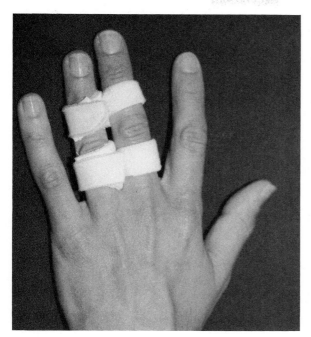

Figure 8–9. Velcro buddy tapes prevent lateral stresses to the PIP joints and allow for full range of motion. This simple splint can be used for select patients with a volar plate or collateral ligament injury.

chance at successful rehabilitation than those who are passive and expect the therapist alone to "cure" them. The education principles presented for the three phases of prevention are suggested for clients ranging from the assembly line worker to the semiprofessional athlete.

Primary Prevention

The principle behind education in the primary prevention phase involves increasing clients' awareness of potential problems. The program may involve education for early symptom awareness, instruction in warm-up and stretching techniques, and instruction in the proper use of work or sports equipment. Education to alert clients to the motions or postures that place the hand or upper extremity at risk for injury is important as well.

Clients who understand the rationale behind the fitting and wearing of a splint are more likely to be compliant with a splint-wearing schedule. Similarly, they will recognize and appreciate the advantages of a prevention program that may

include a physical fitness program, ergonomic design of equipment, and preventive splinting.

Secondary Intervention

Education for secondary intervention requires client understanding of the mechanism of injury, the sequence of treatment, and the expected outcome. Preventive education programs build upon themselves. Results improve if knowledgeable clients seek treatment soon after injury or symptom appearance.

As in the primary prevention phase, injured clients who understand the cause of their injury or symptoms are in a position to participate in rather than just receive treatment. Clients who are aware of the activities and postures that bring on symptoms may be the best persons to suggest intervention strategies, including splints, that reduce symptoms or job modifications. Sports-injured clients may have the "no-pain, no-gain" philosophy and unknowingly undermine conservative management by placing stress on healing structures. Players, however, who are educated by therapists to the basic anatomic and physiologic aspects of their injury are more likely to see the value in warm-up exercises and in the use of splints for protection from further injury.

Tertiary Intervention

The educational program in the tertiary prevention program involves clients' understanding of their abilities and limitations. Clients must be educated about activities that are likely to cause recurrence or exacerbation of symptoms or injuries. Instruction in sensory precautions may be required if sensibility is diminished as a result of nerve compression. The rationale behind the use of protective splints on a more permanent basis to protect insensate skin or to support reconstructed ligaments must be understood to ensure compliance. Adaptive equipment and techniques are presented as needed to allow safe participation in activities.

Finally, clients with similar limitations may benefit from group support to learn problem-solving techniques. As with all phases of prevention, a therapist's visit to the job site or playing field may provide insight to the employer or coach as to how to return a worker or player to activity safely.

FINANCIAL IMPLICATIONS

In an age of cost accountability, one must consider the cost of providing a service or a commodity. Inherent in the price of a splint is the therapist's time involved in evaluation, education, and fabrication and fitting of the splint. Many third-party payers have fee schedules based on what they consider to be reasonable and customary charges for splints. These schedules will not take into account the experience level of the provider or the cost of overhead, but they can help to establish a baseline for charges.

Splinting is likely to be but one strategy in a thoroughly marketed prevention program. Unlike client education, evaluation, or consultation, a splint is a commodity. As such, a splint is a tangible product the consumer (the client) leaves your office with or wears at work. A commodity is often paid for with less questioning by the client or a third-party payer than is a service (e.g., a 30-minute therapy session). To debate the logic in this is futile, but it can be used to a program's advantage.

Third-party payers may reimburse for a splint when they will not reimburse for a therapy treatment. The therapist must be aware of what is and is not reimbursable whether they bill the third party directly or the client does the billing. The fact that the majority of third-party payers do reimburse for splints can be a boost for a prevention program. A client or an employee may be more willing to accept a program with the assurance that a portion of the program's costs are reimbursable. Additionally, we project that a preventive splinting program will decrease medical costs by preventing injury.

The major drawback to preventive splinting is the difficulty of defining the at-risk population and the lack of prospective data on the value of preventive splinting programs. Cost justification is difficult. Therapists must be prepared to participate in research to facilitate justification for service effectiveness.

PROGRAM EVALUATION

As discussed previously, the therapist's follow-up after splint fabrication and client education may be limited. This may be due in part to the financial implications just presented.

If follow-up can be obtained, pre- and postintervention measurements can be used to determine the effectiveness of the splinting program:

1. Edema: volumetric measurements
2. Strength: grip, pinch, dynamic strength testing with equipment such as the BTE work simulator or the Cybex
3. Pain: subjective pain analog scale
4. Range of motion
5. Ligamentous laxity
6. Splinting compliance
7. Work productivity
8. Symptom intensity and onset
9. Electromyograph and nerve conduction studies
10. Physical capacity evaluation

Acknowledgments

The authors thank Drs. Lloyd A. Hoffman and Richard R. McCormack for their contributions to this chapter and to Marge Lloyd for her time and patience.

References

Armstrong ER: Some aspects of stress on forearm and hand in industry. J Occup Med 8(2):63–71, 1966.

Armstrong ER and Chaffin BD: Carpal tunnel syndrome and selected personal attributes. J Occup Med 21(7):482–486, 1979.

Armstrong TJ: An Ergonomics Guide to Carpal Tunnel Syndrome. Akron, Ohio, American Industrial Hygiene Association, 1983.

Armstrong TJ: Ergonomics and cumulative trauma disorders. Hand Clin 2(3):553–565, 1986.

Armstrong TJ, Fine LJ, Goldstein SA, et al: Ergonomic considerations in hand and wrist tendinitis. J Hand Surg 12A(5, Pt. 2):830–836, 1987.

Baxter-Petralia P: Therapists management of carpal tunnel syndrome. In Hunter JM, Schneider LH, Mackin EJ, and Callahan AD (eds): Rehabilitation of the Hand, 3rd ed. St. Louis, CV Mosby, 1990.

Bergfield J, et al: Soft playing splint for protection of significant hand and wrist injuries in sports. Am J Sports Med 10(5):293–296, 1982.

Birkbeck MQ and Beer TC: Occupation in relation to the carpal tunnel syndrome. Rheumatol Rehabil 14:218–221, 1975.

Blair SJ and Allard KM: Prevention of trauma: A cooperative effort. J Hand Surg 8(5, Pt. 2):649–653, 1983.

Boyes JH (ed): Bunnell's Surgery of the Hand. Philadelphia, JB Lippincott, 1970.

Brand PW: Clinical Mechanics of the Hand. St Louis, CV Mosby, 1985.

Bunnell S: Surgery of the Hand, 3rd ed. Philadelphia, JB Lippincott, 1956.

Colditz JC: Anatomic considerations for splinting the thumb. In Hunter JM, Schneider LH, Mackin EJ, and Callahan AD (eds): Rehabilitation of the Hand, 3rd ed. St Louis, CV Mosby, 1990.

de Quervain F: Uber Eine Form Von Chronicler Tendovaginitis. Correspondenz, Blatt F. Schweizer Aerzte 25:389–394, 1895.

Dobson JL, et al: Exhibit presented at the meeting of the American Academy of Orthopaedic Surgeons and American Medical Association, San Francisco, 1971.

Fess EE and Philips C: Hand Splinting: Principles and Methods. St Louis, CV Mosby, 1987.

Finkelstein H: Stenosing tendovaginitis at the radial styloid process. J Bone Joint Surg 12(3):508–540, 1930.

Froimson AI: Tenosynovitis and tennis elbow. *In* Green DP (ed): Operative Hand Surgery, Vol 3. New York, Churchill Livingstone, 1988.

Hamilton WJ: Textbook of Human Anatomy. St Louis, CV Mosby, 1976.

Henshaw JL, Fatren JW, and Wrightsman JA: The semiflexible support: An alternative for the hand-injured worker. J Hand Ther 2(1):35–40, 1989.

Herbin ML: Work capacity evaluation for occupational hand injuries. J Hand Surg 12A(5, Pt. 2):958–960, 1987.

Hunt JR: Occupational neuritis of the deep palmar branch of the ulnar nerve. J Nerv Ment Dis 35(11):673, 1908.

Hunt JR: The thenar and hypothenar types of neural atrophy of the hand. Am J Med Sci 141(2):224–241, 1911.

Kirkpatrick WH: de Quervain's disease. *In*: Hunter JM, Schneider LH, Mackin EJ, and Callahan AD (eds): Rehabilitation of the Hand, 3rd ed. St Louis, CV Mosby, 1990.

Lipscomb PR: Stenosing tenosynovitis at the radial styloid process. Ann Surg 134(1):110–115, 1951.

Malick M: Manual Static Hand Splinting, Vol 1, 3rd ed. Pittsburgh, Hamerville Rehabilitation Center, Inc, 1976.

McCormack RR, Inman RD, Wells A, et al: Prevalence of tendinitis and related disorders of the upper extremity in a manufacturing workforce. J Rheum 17(7):958–964, 1990.

McCue FC, et al: Ulnar collateral ligament injuries of the thumb in athletes. Sports Med 2(2):770–780, 1975.

Nathan PA, Meadows KD, and Doyle LS: Occupation as a risk factor for impaired sensory conduction of the median nerve at the carpal tunnel. J Hand Surg 13B(2):167–170, 1988.

Phalen GS: The carpal tunnel syndrome. Clin Orthop 83:29–40, 1972.

Ramazinni B: The diseases of workers (Wright W., Trans). Chicago, University of Chicago Press, 1940 (originally published 1717).

Rayan GM and O'Donoghue DH: Ulnar digital compression neuropathy of the thumb caused by splinting. Clinical Orthop 175:170, 1983.

Rossi J: Concepts and current trends in hand splinting. *In* Cromwell FS and Bear-Lehman J (eds): Occupational Therapy in Health Care, Vol 4. New York, Haworth Press, 1987, pp 53–67.

Ruby LE: Common hand injuries in the athlete. Clin Sports Med 2(3):609–619, 1983.

Shea JD and McClain EJ: Ulnar nerve compression syndromes at and below the wrist. J Bone Joint Surg 51A(6):1095–1102, 1969.

Smith EM, Sonstegard DA, and Anderson WH: Carpal tunnel syndrome: Contribution of flexor tendons. Arch Phys Med Rehabil 58:379–385, 1977.

Tanaka S, et al: Use of workers compensation claims dates for surveillance of cumulative trauma disorders. J Occup Med 30(6):488–492, 1988.

Tanzer RC: The carpal tunnel syndrome: A clinical and anatomical study. J Bone Joint Surg 41A(4):626–634, 1959.

Tichauer ER: Some aspects of stress on forearm and hand in industry. J Occup Med 8(2):63–71, 1966.

Totten PA: Therapist's management of de Quervain's disease. *In* Hunter JM, Schneider LH, Mackin EJ, and Callahan AD (eds): Rehabilitation of the Hand, 3rd ed. St Louis, CV Mosby, 1990.

Margaret E. Rinehart
Debra S. Zelnick

Prevention of Spinal Cord Injury

The desired outcome of rehabilitation for clients with traumatic spinal cord injuries (SCI) has been functional independence and prevention of complications after discharge. Physical and occupational therapists have provided therapy in the rehabilitation setting but have not been as active with other issues involving this population. In the model systems approach to treatment of SCIs, physical and occupational therapists play a major role in the prevention of secondary and tertiary complications. It is one of the few programs available that provides a means to incorporate prevention along with treatment. This chapter reviews the roles therapists can play in the prevention of SCIs, treatment of clients with traumatic SCIs, and prevention of lifetime complications.

INCIDENCE

The annual incidence of traumatic SCI is estimated to be 30 to 32.1 cases per million persons in the United States or 10,000 new SCIs each year (National Spinal Cord Injury Statistics Center [NSCISC], 1988). Currently, there are over 200,000 individuals with SCI living in this country (Buchanan, 1987).

The Spinal Cord Injury National Data Base recognizes 38 different causes of injury, which have been classified into five major categories: motor vehicle accidents, falls, acts of violence, recreational/sporting activities, and other causes (Fig. 9–1).

Motor vehicle accidents, the majority of which are automobile accidents, make up 45.2% or almost half of all SCIs. Falls account for 21.5% of all traumatic SCIs. This includes any type of fall such as down stairs or in the bathtub. Interestingly, being struck by a falling object is included in this category. A little over 15% of SCIs are caused by acts of violence. Gunshot wounds and stabbings are the most common, and these tend to occur more frequently in large urban areas. Sports/recreational injuries account for 13.4% of SCIs. Most (two thirds) of these injuries are caused by diving, followed by football, snow skiing, and surfing (NSCISC, 1988).

COSTS

The present costs to society for SCIs are estimated at $6.2 billion per year. This includes direct costs of $2.5 billion and indirect costs of $3.7 billion (DeVivo, 1989).

Direct costs include lifetime expenses for all rehabilitation services, emergency medical services, hospitalizations, and supplies. Costs during the first year after injury are much higher than those incurred in subsequent years because of the initial acute care hospitalization, the equip-

Figure 9–1. Causes of spinal cord injury. (From the National Spinal Cord Injury Statistical Center: Spinal Cord Injury: Fact Sheet. Birmingham, AL, University of Birmingham, 1988.)

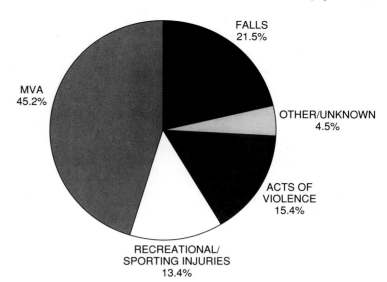

ment, and environmental adaptations required for the home. Indirect costs—the value of expected earnings lost since the injury occurred—are also high.

Direct costs for clients treated in model SCI centers (see section on Model Systems) after January 1, 1988 ranged from $71,980 for those with incomplete paraplegia to $153,312 for those with complete quadriplegia. (This reflects costs adjusted to the 1989 dollar.) The length of stay is longer and hospital costs are higher for clients whose admission to a model SCI center or facility accredited by the Commission for Accreditation of Rehabilitation Facilities (CARF) for SCI is delayed. Available data also indicate that earlier admission to a system of care is associated with a higher rate of discharge to home or noninstitutional settings (Gibson, 1989). Institutional and attendant care contribute significantly to the long-term costs, especially for persons with complete quadriplegia. Based on data reported by Young and colleagues in 1982, the average costs of care postdischarge are $4,962 for persons with incomplete paraplegia and $12,756 for those with complete quadriplegia. (Costs reflect adjustment to 1989 dollar.) Lifetime direct costs for persons with SCI can be estimated by multiplying the annual cost of care by life expectancy.

Because most injuries occur among young men, the indirect costs resulting from lost wages and productivity frequently exceed direct costs. Data from the NSCISC revealed that only 33% of people with incomplete paraplegia and 14% of those with complete quadriplegia are working in the competitive labor market 5 years after injury (DeVivo, 1989). More emphasis must be placed on having people with SCIs return to the work force so that they can remain productive members of society.

PREVENTION

The prevention of SCIs is an area of concern for everyone, from the community and local hospital to the state and federal government. Efforts are being made to educate the public about ways to prevent SCIs and about the need for proper emergency care and medical care throughout one's lifetime to prevent further complications.

In 1988 the federal government charged the Centers for Disease Control (CDC) with the task of initiating a program to prevent primary and secondary disabilities in the United States. The objectives of the program included the development of local and state disability prevention programs, the establishment of a public health surveillance system for the high-priority disabilities (SCI, head injury), and the use of epidemiologic studies to determine priorities and target effective interventions (Houk and Thacker, 1989). Examples of existing programs are listed in Table 9–1.

MODEL SYSTEMS

As part of efforts to prevent SCIs and to provide the best medical care to those who are injured,

Table 9–1. Prevention and Educational Programs

Educational Programs for High-Risk Groups

Researchers in Oregon studied the use of shoulder belts by high school drivers before and after an educational program was offered. They found no change in behavior (use of shoulder belts) or attitudes of students; however, there was evidence of increased knowledge on the post-test. The task now is to determine an effective way to change attitudes and behaviors (Neuwelt et al, 1989).

Professionals at the Southeastern Michigan Spinal Cord Injury (SCI) System Rehabilitation Institute evaluated the violent behaviors of teenagers in response to altercations. These altercations frequently led to the use of handguns. A graphic video was the end product of the evaluation and study. The video shows the injuries that result from the use of handguns and how teenagers can avoid becoming victims of violent behavior (Graham and Weingarden, 1988).

Sports and recreational activities are also the cause of many SCIs. Recreational vehicles such as all-terrain vehicles (Maynard and Krasnick, 1988) and ultralight aircraft (Zwimpfer and Gertzbein, 1987) are used primarily by teenagers and young adults. Better safety guidelines were adopted in New Jersey, and educational programs are recommended. Sales are banned to individuals younger than 16 years.

Diving is another recreational activity that warrants special attention. There are continuing efforts to educate the public about diving into shallow water. Swimmers are urged to check water depth and to jump feet first in unfamiliar waters. Most of the regional spinal cord injury centers have "Feet First" educational programs.

Trauma centers/SCI centers are providing educational programs for elementary and high school children about the prevention of catastrophic accidents. Individuals who have had an SCI or head injury participate in these programs to share their experiences about living with a disability.

This provides more credibility for the presentations.

Examples of improvement in care for the person with an SCI are:

1. Determination of the cause, prevalence, and location of SCIs. States are establishing registries as well as surveillance systems to monitor the incidence and prevalence of SCI (U.S. Department of Health and Human Services, Public Health Services, 1988). This information is required to determine the actual incidence and cause of SCIs. When better information is available, states will know where to focus their energy and money for prevention, treatment, and lifelong care.
2. On-going educational programs presented to emergency medical technicians and community-based ambulance services. Educational programs for the public are used to reinforce the need for proper handling of victims at the accident site.
3. The prevention of lifetime complications is very important, and individuals with an SCI are taught to follow the prescribed guidelines for continued medical follow-up because this can help prevent readmission to the hospital (see Discharge and Follow-Up sections).

a coordinated approach to treatment provides the best results. In 1970 the Department of Health, Education and Welfare (DHEW) designated the first model system center for the treatment of individuals with SCIs. Since then, as many as 17 other centers have been funded by the federal government for treatment and research. A national SCI data base was developed to gather information from the designated centers. Since its initiation, the data base has been modified and is now monitored by the federally designated centers. To be funded, the model system center provides the injured person with an organized system of care from the accident site to the emergency room to the acute care setting, with a smooth transition through the rehabilitation hospital and into the community. An integral part of the model system approach to treatment is the availability of an organized system for lifetime follow-up. Data from the model centers show there has been a decrease in the length of stay in the acute hospital and

rehabilitation center if individuals with an SCI are admitted to an SCI center within 24 to 72 hours of injury (Buchanan et al, 1990). This has resulted in a significant reduction in the cost of care for these individuals.

Although it would be ideal to have all individuals with an SCI treated in a model center, that is unrealistic because there are only 13 models centers in existence today. CARF is now providing accreditation for rehabilitation centers that have units for SCI clients. CARF accreditation standards have been based on the model system center standards, and those are the standards that should be used to determine if the hospital/rehabilitation center can provide quality care for SCI clients.

The components of the model center system are listed in Table 9–2. The model system of care has been developed to provide a holistic approach to care of the clients. There is an effort to address every area of the clients' life that has been affected by the SCI. The overall goal is to

Table 9–2. Components of the Model Center System

Emergency services, which include evacuation from the vehicle and transportation from the accident site and care in the emergency room of the hospital

Acute care in the hospital where the multidisciplinary approach to treatment is used

Rehabilitation services that encompass not only the physical needs of the client but also psychosocial, vocational/educational, and preparation for community reintegration

Comprehensive lifetime follow-up, which includes medical, physical and occupational therapy, social, psychologic, and vocational follow-up on a regular basis

Research to improve the care, function, or potential of the individuals with spinal cord injuries

---

have clients live a normal lifespan and be a productive member of society.

EMERGENCY SERVICES

Good emergency care for accident victims is imperative to prevent further injury and complications. Paramedics have been trained to monitor the stability of the spine as well as other life-support functions, and emergency services at hospitals are becoming better equipped to cope with trauma victims. Public education has stressed the importance of not moving the victim until medical help has arrived.

ACUTE CARE

When the individual is admitted to the hospital, the multidisciplinary team of health professionals is notified, and a coordinated plan of care is instituted. The team members include physicians (neurosurgeons, orthopedic surgeons, physiatrists), nurses, physical and occupational therapists, psychologists, social workers, nutritionists, and other professionals as required. The coordinated team approach, if based on the rehabilitation team model (Rinehart, 1990), can help to prevent complications and help clients achieve their goals.

The goals of acute care are to maintain medical stability and prevent complications; increase the function of the client, using muscle strengthening and range of motion (ROM) exercises; maximize respiratory status; and begin the process for discharge planning. Family and client education is also a goal at this time. There are many

aspects of care, coping, and rehabilitation that may require attention, and it is important to have support teams readily available.

The physical and occupational therapists work closely with the nurses in the acute setting to prevent complications and to improve function. The therapists evaluate clients to establish a baseline and then develop a treatment program. Because nurses provide care 24 hours a day, it is important for all team members to communicate with the nurses on a daily basis.

The evaluation should include measurements of passive and active ROM, muscle strength, endurance, sensation, respiratory status, ability to perform activities of daily living (ADL), skin condition, and emotional response to the injury. It is helpful to understand what impact family dynamics may have on the total rehabilitation of the clients.

The bedside treatment program includes:

1. ROM to maintain joint mobility. This can include active as well as passive ROM.
2. Education about proper positioning in bed and in the wheelchair to prevent joint contractures and skin breakdown. Schedules for turning and weight shifts should be adhered to closely.
3. Strengthening exercises using manual resistance, when appropriate, to maintain and increase strength.
4. Respiratory exercises to help prevent pulmonary complications. The exercises can include incentive spirometry, blowing bubbles, sip 'n puff shuffleboard using straws and cotton balls, and diaphragm and accessory muscle strengthening; review of coughing techniques and chest physical therapy are also part of the respiratory program.
5. Education about the SCI for the clients and their families. Clients' responsibility for directing their self-care is emphasized.
6. Elevation of the head of the bed when clients are medically and orthopedically stable. The head of the bed is elevated to help clients adapt to the upright position, which helps prepare them for transfer out of bed to a wheelchair.
7. Adaptive equipment to assist clients with functional activities.

The nurses help to promote these activities on a daily basis as well as inform the therapists and other team members of the individual's medical condition and coping strategies.

TRANSITION TO REHABILITATION

Transfer to a rehabilitation center usually occurs when there are no medical complications and the individual is able to tolerate sitting in a wheelchair for 1 hour. The goals at the rehabilitation center are to maximize individual independence, to understand their injury and possible complications to adapt to community living, and to resume premorbid life roles.

When clients are transferred to the rehabilitation center, there should be communication with the team members from the acute hospital. This helps to ensure continuity of care and also helps the rehabilitation team members to understand better the medical course and complications each client has had. An additional benefit is that the transition to the rehabilitation center will be less traumatic for clients if they feel that the team already knows something about them. Any acute care hospital that transfers SCI clients to a rehabilitation center should send discharge summaries from the therapists in the disciplines who treated them.

REHABILITATION

Adherence to the rehabilitation team model (Rinehart, 1990) is crucial to ensure that clients are functioning at the highest level possible based on their physical capabilities.

When clients are admitted to a rehabilitation hospital, a complete evaluation must be done before treatment can begin. The areas evaluated in acute care should be re-evaluated and improvements or changes noted. Additional areas to be evaluated include sitting balance and mobility skills. Therapists should also note clients' medical and social history. Home environment, job or school situation, occupational roles and leisure interests become more important during rehabilitation because clients will be discharged, ready for life in the community. When possible, it is helpful if the physical and occupational therapists perform the evaluation together.

The acute care goals are reinforced during rehabilitation, with more emphasis placed on functional activities that lead to increased independence and clients' ability to direct their own care. Prevention of medical complications is a lifetime goal. The clients should be active participants in the goal-setting process. They should have a clear understanding of the significance of the goals and the rationale for treatment, which will help them to return to their premorbid lifestyle.

CLIENT AND FAMILY EDUCATION

Client and family education is a collaborative process between clients, families and rehabilitation teams. Clients and their family members share their concerns about the impact the injury has had on their life and their ability to lead a normal lifestyle. Each member of the rehabilitation team educates clients about their area of expertise. This allows clients to develop skills and use the resources available to return to community living. This information should be supplemented by written materials. Having the information in a written format is helpful, because clients and family members often have trouble remembering everything they learn while in the hospital. Clients and family members should be encouraged to use the written material as a reference throughout the hospitalization and when questions arise after discharge.

RANGE OF MOTION, STRENGTH, AND ENDURANCE

Maximizing ROM, strength, and endurance is the basic building block for improving functional activities. A formal passive ROM program is not necessary if ROM can be maintained through clients' participation in functional activities. If clients lack full ROM, they should be taught to perform self-ROM. If self-ROM is not possible, someone else will need to perform it; however, clients should be able to instruct others correctly about the proper procedure.

Increasing strength and endurance can be accomplished using standard exercise programs as well as functional activities. Standard exercise programs can include progressive resistive exercises, free weights, or the use of other strengthening equipment. Examples of functional activities include wheelchair mobility, self-feeding, grooming, and mat and bed mobility.

WHEELCHAIR POSITIONING AND SKIN CARE

Good positioning in the wheelchair is important to maintain proper alignment of the body and help to provide even weight distribution. Adaptations to the wheelchair, including a solid seat or back, lateral trunk supports, headrests, armrests, and lapboards, can help promote good positioning. It may take time for clients to adjust to the positioning adaptations that help to compensate for impaired or absent trunk and lower extremity muscle strength.

When clients are in a wheelchair, weight shifting is crucial. Clients and families are taught that the best treatment for pressure sores is prevention. The principles of positioning and skin care should be adhered to not only when clients are in a wheelchair but also when they are in bed or sitting in a car or shower chair.

WHEELCHAIR MOBILITY

Initially, all clients use a manual wheelchair. The clients' upper extremity strength and endurance will determine what type of adaptive devices will be required for propelling the wheelchair. Initially some clients may require lugs or quad pegs to make propulsion easier; however, as rehabilitation progresses, clients may not need them to propel the chair. Clients with high-level quadriplegia will be trained in the use of a power wheelchair. Clients and therapists will decide on the most appropriate type of control mechanism for the wheelchair. Two popular methods are a sip 'n puff control, which is operated by blowing into a straw-like device, and a chin-control device that is operated by moving a joystick with the chin. All clients will be taught how to maneuver safely when in the wheelchair and about wheelchair maintenance. Wheelchair propulsion is also used as a way to build endurance and help with aerobic conditioning.

ACTIVITIES OF DAILY LIVING

Independence in ADL is emphasized during the rehabilitation phase, because clients are expected to do more for themselves as their strength and endurance increase. Clients are taught to assist with grooming, bathing, and dressing. Various pieces of adaptive equipment may be recommended to assist clients in performing functional activities. Adaptive equipment that can be used includes universal cuffs, wash mitts, long-handled sponges, dressing sticks, reachers, and transfer boards. This equipment should be re-evaluated as strength and endurance increase.

For example, a person with C5 quadriplegia may initially require the use of an overhead sling and a dorsal wrist splint for self-feeding. As shoulder strength and endurance increase, the sling may be discontinued. If the person develops sufficient wrist strength, a universal cuff can be substituted for the dorsal wrist splint. It is important to start ADL training early so that clients will be less likely to become dependent on others.

SEXUALITY

Sexual activity is an ADL, and therapeutic intervention may be required for clients to become as independent as possible. Therapists may adapt equipment to make birth-control devices easier to use or offer suggestions about ways to attain comfortable positions for sexual activity.

Sexuality concerns are addressed throughout the entire rehabilitation process. However, clients may have more specific questions and concerns that should be answered before discharge. They may have specific questions about performance, fertility, or sexuality in general. Frequently, clients feel comfortable discussing their questions and concerns with their occupational or physical therapist.

Therapists can use the PLISSIT model (Annon, 1976) to assist them when counseling about sexual issues. The model helps the therapists to understand their own limitations when working with these clients. The model is based on four levels—permission, limited information, specific suggestions, and intensive therapy—and each level requires the health-care professional to have increasing degrees of knowledge, training, and skill. If therapists do not feel comfortable or knowledgeable enough to answer more specific questions, they should refer their clients to an appropriate member of the rehabilitation team.

HOME MANAGEMENT

The home-management activities addressed vary depending on the level of the injury and clients' premorbid roles and responsibilities. Some areas that may be addressed include meal preparation, house cleaning, and financial management. Although all clients do not have primary responsibility for home management, they should at least be able to maneuver in the kitchen and retrieve items from the refrigerator. This is especially important if there are times when they are home alone.

HOME-VISIT EVALUATION

Early in the rehabilitation process, clients, their family, and the rehabilitation team visit the clients' homes to evaluate accessibility. Ideally, it is done early so there will be time to make the necessary modifications to the home. It also gives the treatment team the opportunity to address concerns identified during the home visit. If a client is discharged before the home modifications are complete, temporary living arrangements have to be made. This could involve using a living room for a bedroom, constructing a temporary ramp to get into the house, or staying at the home of a friend or family member until renovations are complete.

Available funding must be considered when recommending changes because, in some situations, modifications may not be possible or the cost of the recommended modifications is prohibitive. In this case, the ideal situation is for the client and family to move into a more accessible home. However, if it is not possible for the client to move, the therapists must use their ingenuity and creativity to adapt the environment for the client. Another option for clients without financial resources or family support is to move to a residential facility for the physically handicapped.

THERAPEUTIC PASSES

Clients should be encouraged to use therapeutic passes when they are medically stable. A therapeutic pass allows clients the opportunity to explore the environment by leaving the rehabilitation center for a few hours. This may involve exploring the area around the hospital or going home. This is an excellent opportunity for clients to identify potential problem areas before discharge. The potential problems can then be addressed by the appropriate member of the rehabilitation team.

DRIVING

If clients are planning to resume driving, they should be evaluated before being discharged from the hospital because reimbursement may be easier to obtain while the client is still in the rehabilitation center. This is handled most efficiently through a referral to a well-established driving program where a predriving assessment can be completed. If the results of the assessment indicate that certain clients will not be able to drive, they will need to be instructed in how to maximize their independence and safety as passengers. If the assessment indicates that clients are able to drive, the process continues with driver's training. The clients must have a current driver's license or learner's permit before training is initiated. Training should continue until a certified driving instructor determines that the individual is a safe driver. The client must then pass the state driving test.

The final step is to select a van or automobile that meets the client's needs. The financial resources and personal needs will determine the type of vehicle to be purchased.

RECREATION AND LEISURE

Participation in recreational and leisure activities is beneficial for everyone. In recent years, there has been an emphasis on health promotion and wellness evidenced by an increasing number of health clubs and wellness programs that are in operation. These areas should be addressed during the rehabilitation process, and it can be introduced during the acute rehabilitation process.

A recreational therapist can help clients realize that they will be able to participate in recreational and leisure activities that were meaningful to them before this injury. The recreational therapist should work closely with the occupational therapist to adapt tools and equipment so that clients can engage in activities or hobbies such as painting, woodworking, or ceramics. Later in the rehabilitation process, the recreational therapist may schedule clients to go on outings to movies, restaurants, or sporting events. This provides an opportunity for clients to explore new ways to complete these activities or to become more assertive, which will enable them to have their needs met. For example, clients may have to ask a waiter for assistance when cutting food, or they may have to ask an usher for assistance when maneuvering in a theater.

Participating in wheelchair sports is another example of how people confined to wheelchairs enjoy recreational and competitive activities. This also enables them to maximize their physical strength and endurance and promote good health. One way of introducing sporting activities is through "Sports Night," during which members of wheelchair sports teams are invited to speak about their participation in sport activities, such as track and field, weight lifting, and basketball. Adaptations of sports equipment for people with disabilities are displayed. The program has been successful in increasing awareness about the sporting activities possible for people in wheelchairs. Many communities, rehabilitation centers, and universities have wheelchair sports teams, and people should be encouraged to explore these resources in their community. Other activities that clients may have engaged in before their injury can also be adapted, such as swimming, rowing, tennis, and hunting.

National and international travel has become more accessible to people using wheelchairs, and there are organizations and agencies specifically geared to address these issues. Frequently, it is the occupational and physical therapists who make clients aware of these opportunities. All kinds of adaptations are possible, and people should not let their disability get in the way of participating in meaningful activities.

VOCATIONAL REHABILITATION

Vocational rehabilitation is the process of helping to prepare a person with a disability to become a productive member of society. This may involve:

Preparing clients to return to the job they held before the injury after modifications to the work environment and job description have been completed
Finding a new job that will better meet the person's functional abilities
Returning to primary homemaker responsibilities
Returning to school to complete education or receive technical training.

There are many components of vocational rehabilitation that include:

Job site or school evaluation
Analysis of how a job is performed
Vocational counseling
Training and educational assistance
Identifying funding resources

The vocational rehabilitation counselor evaluates clients to identify an appropriate vocational plan. This information is communicated to the rehabilitation team so that they can assist clients to achieve the vocational goals. It has been documented that employment, regardless of financial remuneration, may have a positive influence on life satisfaction (Decker and Schultz, 1985).

DISCHARGE

Discharge planning actually begins upon admission to the acute care hospital, but the final step of inpatient rehabilitation is the completion of the discharge plan. Clients may feel anxious about leaving the rehabilitation hospital where there are many people with physical disabilities and the environment is designed to accommodate wheelchairs. In addition, the staff are knowledgeable about and comfortable interacting with disabled people.

The patient and family education that began in the acute setting and continued throughout rehabilitation is completed. Families participate in therapy and assist with nursing care to finalize the care plans and review questions. Families should be knowledgeable about and comfortable with all aspects of care. If clients will have an attendant, the attendant should also attend the teaching session before discharge. The clients must be knowledgeable about all aspects of care, especially those in which they require assistance.

Equipment orders are finalized, and durable medical equipment, such as beds and bathroom equipment, are delivered directly to the client's home. Wheelchairs should be delivered to the hospital to ensure that the prescription was filled accurately. If a customized wheelchair was ordered, clients may be sent home with a rental chair until the permanent chair is ready.

Smaller adaptive equipment issued during hospitalization should be re-evaluated and upgraded if necessary. Clients should not be sent home with equipment that they no longer need.

FOLLOW-UP

The main goal of a follow-up program is to provide services and guidelines to help the individual maintain good health and maximize independence and to assist with reintegration into the community. Follow-up for a person with an SCI should be a lifelong process because there are many issues and concerns that will continue to arise throughout the person's lifetime.

One model center uses a follow-up system that has been successful in maintaining a continuum of care. Clients are seen by their physician and follow-up nurse in a clinic in the rehabilitation hospital four times during the first year after discharge and then yearly thereafter. Clients may also see the other rehabilitation team members for consultation during the follow-up visit. For example, they may request to see the physical therapist for a new wheelchair or the occupational therapist for a new splint.

During the follow-up appointment, medical tests are performed to ensure that clients are in good health. If serious problems are identified, clients can be admitted to the acute care hospital affiliated with the model system or to a local hospital. Staff at community hospitals are now more aware of how to treat individuals with SCIs because the model systems have provided educational opportunities for them and act as resources for the community hospitals.

The model systems have established satellite programs so clients who live far away from the center can still access the follow-up system. Key members of the rehabilitation team participate in the follow-up clinic held at a local hospital.

The follow-up programs have been extremely successful in identifying potential problems and evaluating and upgrading equipment. This helps to ensure that the clients maintain good health and function at the highest possible level of independence.

MEDICAL CARE AFTER DISCHARGE

If the person with an SCI has had rehabilitation at a model center or CARF-accredited rehabilitation center, there is a system in place for at least a yearly follow-up evaluation. However, for day-to-day medical care, the person with an SCI must identify their own family physician. This is especially important because clients do not always live in close proximity to the center where they initially received treatment. If the family physicians are knowledgeable about medical issues pertinent to this population, the number of visits to the emergency room for primary care will

decrease as will the number of hospital readmissions.

Along with basic medical care, other professional services should be available in community settings. Physical and occupational therapists who work in community hospitals or who provide home care need to develop a knowledge base about issues particular to this population. Areas such as skin care, respiratory problems, overuse syndromes, and equipment issues are just some of the areas that will be of concern throughout the clients' life. Not everyone can be an expert when treating individuals with SCIs; however, therapists should tap the knowledge of their colleagues who have expertise in this area or use the resources of the model centers for more specific information (see Appendix I for a list of model centers). It is the responsibility of the health-care professionals who work with this population to maintain current knowledge of new treatment techniques and research. They can do this by attending continuing education courses and reading current literature.

It is the responsibility of persons with an SCI to follow the medical guidelines given to them upon discharge from the rehabilitation center. The medications prescribed and home-exercise program should be continued. The daily home programs to maintain skin integrity and a healthy respiratory and urinary tract system should be followed because these systems are the source of potential medical problems.

Most problems with skin breakdown can be prevented by following a consistent pressure-relief program and close monitoring of the skin. Improperly fitting clothing or orthotics, weight gain or loss, or changes in muscle tone that affect sitting posture can contribute to skin breakdown. Adaptations to clothing or to the wheelchair may be required to prevent complications.

The urinary tract system can be a constant source of infection and may require the use of antibiotics or rehospitalization. Clients should take the medications prescribed for them and follow the bladder/bowel program given to them when discharged from the hospital. Diet and fluid requirements should be adhered to.

Respiratory problems can arise when clients are discharged. It is helpful if clients continue to use the incentive spirometer they received in the hospital, because it can help monitor respiratory status and encourages the use of the diaphragm for deep breathing. If clients have a change in their ability to use the spirometer, the physician should be notified, because this is often an early sign of infection or respiratory distress.

It is important to acknowledge the early warning signs of any potential medical complication. The goal is to prevent illness and complications that require admission to the hospital as well as time lost from work, school, or home management.

PSYCHOLOGIC SUPPORT

While SCI clients are in the hospital or rehabilitation center, they receive on-going psychologic support. The support is not only from the psychologist but also from the team members who work with them on a daily basis. When clients are discharged from the hospital, psychologic support is not always available or easily accessible. Qualified professionals with an understanding of the needs of the SCI population may also be limited. Not all clients will require the intervention of a psychologist for individual treatment on a regular basis. Others may benefit more from a less formal intervention such as stress-reduction classes or a karate course. Before clients are discharged from the rehabilitation center, they should be made aware of the psychosocial resources available to them as well as to their family or support system.

CLIENT AND FAMILY SUPPORT

Counseling may be required for the family unit, and a family therapist can be recommended. The impact of an SCI on the family unit is addressed during the rehabilitation stay, but it is possible that many issues will not be identified until clients start living a "normal" life at home. The roles of each family member may change, temporarily or permanently.

Family therapists can play an important role with the SCI population. There are so many adjustments to be made with an injury of this magnitude, and the family unit should not be overlooked.

CASE STUDY

A 37-year-old man became a C7 quadriplegic after a diving accident. Before the injury, both he and his wife had full-time jobs. They had two children, aged 4 and 7 years. The couple was fortunate to have an insurance policy that would pay for an aide to help with morning care. The client's wife helped with his evening care and also had to prepare the children for bed. At times the wife saw herself in the situation of having three children. The client used home-care services, which included an aide for morning care, an occupational therapist, and a physical therapist. Home therapy helped the client to identify other areas in the home that required modifications that would allow him to be independent. The therapists also provided a support system for the client to help him learn how to problem solve when he was confronted with a new or difficult situation. For a short time, the client continued seeing the psychologist from the rehabilitation hospital; however, he was unable to keep the appointments when he returned to work. Eventually the client learned how to drive, purchased a van, and was able to return to work. Although he gained more independence over time, his wife still had the same responsibilities. The children also had difficulty in dealing with the changes in the family, and the older child had difficulty in school. This is a situation in which family therapy may be able to help the family cope with these changes.

RESEARCH

There is much research being done on the topic of SCI. Physical and occupational therapists should be familiar with current research because clients will undoubtedly have questions about advances in the field. These research outcomes can help to prevent costly complications and help therapists to use all resources available to them when treating individuals with SCIs. Therapists will also be part of the research team when evaluating the changes in muscle strength and then strengthening the muscles and improving function as soon as possible. A few of the more recent studies that address improvements in neurologic recovery and the use of functional electrical stimulation (FES) are discussed next.

Methylprednisolone

Bracken and colleagues (1990) published a controlled, randomized study using methylprednisolone, naloxone, or placebo in the treatment of acute clients with SCI. They found that acute clients with SCI who were treated with methylprednisolone within 8 hours of injury had significant improvement in neurologic recovery. Treatment with naloxone, following their protocol, did not improve neurologic recovery.

Localized Spinal Cord Cooling

Jansssen and Hansbout (1989) reviewed the pathogenesis of SCI and the newer treatments available. They reviewed the chemical, anatomic, and functional changes associated with an SCI. They also reviewed current treatments being used to improve neurologic recovery. Along with the two drugs mentioned previously, they presented a summary of the information available about localized spinal cord cooling. If begun within 8 hours of acute SCI, cooling is beneficial. The blood flow to the spinal cord is decreased, which delays the effects of ischemia and, therefore, helps to decrease neurologic impairment.

Functional Electrical Stimulation

FES is being used to enhance fitness and training of SCI clients who have upper motor neuron lesions. Initial research (Pollack et al, 1989; Ragnarsson, 1988; Ragnarsson et al, 1988) shows that FES can increase muscle strength, endurance, and bulk of the stimulated muscles. This is very costly, and much research is needed to determine the long-term benefits of FES.

Axonal Regeneration

Researchers are studying the possibility of neurologic recovery below the level of injury through axonal regeneration (Cohen et al, 1988; Mackler and Selzer, 1987; Villegas-Perez et al, 1988). The studies provide promising results that axonal regeneration may be possible in humans; therefore, the person with an SCI may gain improved functional ability.

Conclusion

There are many other areas related to SCI that warrant research. Therapists can play an integral part on the research team because they are most familiar with the clients' functional abilities. As clients with SCI age, there are many changes in their functional abilities. It is not clear why some

of these changes occur: Is it from overuse syndromes, decreased endurance, psychosocial issues, or other related issues? Therapists can assist with the evaluation of these changes over time and help develop innovative treatment programs and research studies that address these issues.

References

Annon JS: The PLISSIT model: A proposed conceptual scheme for the behavioral treatment of sexual problems. J Sex Educ Ther 2:1–15, 1976.

Bracken MB, Shepard MJ, Collins WF, et al: A randomized, controlled trial of methylprednisolone or naloxone in the treatment of acute spinal-cord injury. N Engl J Med 322:1405–1411, 1990.

Buchanan LE: An overview. In Buchanan LE and Nawoczenski DA (eds): Spinal Cord Injury: Concepts and Management Approaches. Baltimore, Williams & Wilkins, 1987.

Buchanan LE, Ditunno JF, Osterholm JL, et al: Spinal cord injury: A ten-year report. P Med 93:36–39, 1990.

Burry HC and Calcinai CJ: The need to make rugby safer. Br Med J 296:149–150, 1988.

Cohen AH, Mackler SA, and Selzer ME: Functional regeneration in the lamprey spinal cord. Trends in Neurosci 11:277–231, 1988.

Decker SD and Schultz R: Correlates of life satisfaction and depression in middle-aged and elderly spinal cord-injured persons. Am J Occup Ther 39:740–745, 1985.

DeVivo MJ: What is known about the costs of spinal cord injury? In Proceedings from the National Consensus Conference on Catastrophic Illness and Injury. Washington, DC, 1989.

Gibson DJ: Criteria for evaluating performance of the system. In Proceedings from the National Consensus Conference on Catastrophic Illness and Injury. Washington, DC, 1989.

Graham PM and Weingarden SI: Targeting teenagers in a SCI violence prevention program. Am Spinal Injury Assoc Abstracts 1988, p. 91.

Houk VN and Thacker SB: The Centers for Disease Control program to prevent primary and secondary disabilities in the United States. Public Health Rep 104:226–231, 1989.

Janssen L and Hansbout RR: Pathogenesis of spinal cord injury and newer treatments—a review. Spine 14:23–32, 1988.

Kennedy EJ (ed): Spinal Cord Injury: The Facts and Figures. Birmingham: University of Alabama at Birmingham, 1986.

Mackler SA and Selzer ME: Specificity of synaptic regeneration in the spinal cord of the larbal sea lamprey. J Physiol 388:183–198, 1987.

Maynard FM and Krasnick R: Analysis of recreational off-road vehicle accidents resulting in spinal cord injury. Ann Emerg Med 17:30–33, 1988.

National Spinal Cord Injury Statistics Center: Spinal Cord Injury: Fact Sheet. Birmingham, University of Alabama at Birmingham, 1988.

Neuwelt EA, Wilkinson AM and Avolio AE: Oregon head and spinal cord injury prevention program and evaluation. Neurosurgery 24:453–458, 1989.

Pollack SF, Axen K, Spielholtz N, et al: Aerobic training effects of electrically induced lower extremity exercises in spinal cord injured people. Arch Phys Med Rehabil 70:214–219, 1989.

Ragnarssen KT: Physiologic effects of functional electrical stimulation-induced exercises in spinal cord injured individuals. Clin Orthop 233:53–63, 1988.

Ragnarsson KT, Pollack S, O'Daniel W, et al: Clinical evaluation of computerized functional electrical stimulation after spinal cord injury: A multi-center pilot study. Arch Phys Med Rehabil 69:672–677, 1988.

Rinehart ME: Early mobilization in acute spinal cord injury, a collaborative approach. Crit Care Nurs Clin North Am 2:1–7, 1990.

U.S. Department of Health and Human Services, Public Health Services: Diving-associated spinal cord injuries during drought conditions—Wisconsin, 1988. MMWR 37:453–454, 1988.

Villegas-Perez MP, Vidal-Sanz M and Bray GM: Influences of peripheral nerve grafts on the survival and regrowth of axotomized retinal ganglion cells in adult rats. J Neurosc 8:265–280, 1988.

Young JS, Burns PE, Bowen AM, et al: Spinal Cord Injury Statistics: Experience of Regional Model Spinal Cord Injury Systems. Phoenix, AZ, Good Samaritan Medical Center, 1982.

Zwimpfer TJ and Gertzbein SG: Ultralight aircraft crashes: Their increasing incidence and associated fractures of the thoracolumbar spine. J Trauma 27:431–436, 1987.

Bibliography

Access Tours, 720 N Bedford Rd, Bedford Hills, NY 10567.

Durgin RW and Lindsey N: Physically Disabled Traveler's Guide. Toledo, OH, Resource Directories, 1986.

Ford JR and Duchworth B: Physical Management for the Quadriplegic Patient. Philadelphia, FA Davis, 1987.

Johnson DL, Giovannoni RM, and Driscoll SA: Ventilator-Assisted Patient Care—Planning for Hospital Discharge and Home Care. Rockville, MD, Aspen Publications, 1986.

National Wheelchair Athlete Association, 3595 East Fountain Boulevard, Suite L 10, Colorado Springs, CO 80910, (719) 574–1150.

Trieschmann RB: Aging with a Disability. New York, Demos Publications, 1987.

Trieschmann RB: Spinal Cord Injuries: The Psychological, Social, and Vocational Adjustment. New York, Demos Publications, 1987.

Whiteneck G, Adler C, Carter RE, et al: The Management of High Quadriplegia. New York, Demos Publications, 1989.

APPENDIX I: MODEL SPINAL CORD INJURY SYSTEMS 1991

Samuel L. Stover, MD
University of Alabama
Birmingham, SCI Care System
520 SRC
Birmingham, AL 45294
(205) 934-3450

Robert L. Waters, MD
7601 E. Imperial Highway
Building 121
Downey, CA 90242
(213) 940-7161

David F. Apple, Jr., MD
Georgia Regional SCI System
Shepherd Spinal Center
2020 Peachtree Rd., NW
Atlanta, GA 30309
(404) 352-2020, ext. 2575

Paul R. Meyer, Jr., MD
Northwestern University Medical Center
Northwestern Memorial Hospital
250 E. Chicago Ave., Suite 619
Chicago, IL 60611
(312) 908-3425

Frederick M. Maynard, MD
University of Michigan Model SCI System
University of Michigan Hospitals
300 N. Ingalls Building
Ann Arbor, MI 48109-0491
(313) 763-0971

Bruce Gans, MD
Southeast Michigan SCI System
261 Mack Blvd.
Detroit, MI 48201
(313) 745-9731

Joel A. Delisa, MD
Kessler Institute for Rehabilitation
Pleasant Valley Way
West Orange, NJ 07052
(201) 731-3600

Kristijan T. Ragnarsson, MD
Mt. Sinai Medical Center
One Bustave Lane, Leby Place
New York, NY 10029
(212) 241-9657

John F. Ditunno, Jr, MD
Regional SCI System Harriman Delaware Valley
Thomas Jefferson University
111 S. 11th St.
Room 9243, New Hospital
Philadelphia, PA 19107
(215) 955-6573

R. Edward Carter, MD
Texas Regional SCI System
The Institute for Rehabilitation and Research
Texas Medical Center
1333 Moursund Ave.
Houston, TX 77030
(713) 797–5910

Diana D. Cardenas, MD
BB 919 Health Science Building
Rehabilitation Medicine
University of Washington
1959 NE Pacific St.
Seattle, WA 98195
(206) 543–8171

Conal B. Wilmot, MD
Northern California SCI System
Santa Clara Valley Medical Ctr
751 South Bascom Ave.
San Jose, CA 95128
(408) 299–5643

Robert R. Menter, MD
Craig Hospital
3425 South Clarkson St.
Englewood, CO 81110
(303) 789–8220

CHAPTER
10

Mary Winegardner Voth

Prevention and Management of Temporomandibular Joint Dysfunction

Prevention and management of temporomandibular joint (TMJ) dysfunction can be accomplished only through careful biomechanical assessment of its causes. Essential to assessment is consideration of surrounding areas, including the spine, shoulder girdle, and cranium, and their contribution to the symptoms. All of these areas may produce symptoms in the TMJ and teeth, a fact that has earned TMJ its nickname of the "great imposter" (Morgan et al, 1977).

Modern TMJ dysfunction prevention and management are in a state of flux (Farrar, 1982). Confusion and chaos exist in standards of evaluation, practice, and management among practitioners, researchers, and insurance carriers. Therefore, communication and cooperation are difficult and often frustrating.

Controversy abounds in this field for the following reasons:

1. The anatomy is complex, as is the interrelation of the function of the cranium and cervical spine; the anterior, posterior, and lateral cervical spine and shoulder; and the maxillary mandibular complex.
2. The signs and symptoms noted are interpreted by the philosophy of each researcher or combination resulting in a multiplicity of

terms. This includes the philosophy of causative agents being from occlusion versus muscular imbalances or musculoskeletal conditions.
3. Pain is a dilemma. It is uniquely individual, subjective, and difficult to measure. Studies based on subjective pain complaints or on pain elicitations by palpation have limited validity and value. Pain is known to have a constant threshold, but responses vary according to perceptions (Wilson and Schneider, 1987).

Eighty-five per cent of hospitalizations in the world today are the result of stress-related diseases (Carr, 1988). TMJ dysfunction is lumped in this group along with hypertension, myocardial infarctions, cerebrovascular accidents, gastrointestinal disorders, cancer, and asthma. The cost of these to U.S. companies alone is over $100 billion per year. Chronic pain accounts for $70 billion of this amount (Fricton et al, 1987). Therefore, it is imperative not only to assess properly the problem of TMJ dysfunction but also to teach prevention and management of the biomechanical and psychologic stress factors.

Joint mechanical analysis of the TMJ is discussed in this chapter, along with pathology, evaluation, treatment, and prevention. A gestalt approach is used; that is, the whole is seen as greater than the sum of its parts.

ANATOMY AND BIOMECHANICS

Musculoskeletal disorders may affect the cervical and craniomandibular areas together. Headache and TMJ pain can be caused by referred pain from cervical muscle imbalances, segmental facilitation (Korr, 1973), and occupational and postural habits. Widespread involvement of the muscles of the upper quarter is often noted with TMJ problems.

Thorough anatomic understanding of the TMJ and the masticatory system, and their intimate relation with the upper quarter (cranium, cervical, upper thoracic spine, and shoulder girdle), is necessary for biomechanical and physiologic evaluative analysis. The masticatory system—responsible for chewing, swallowing, and speaking—is part of the stomatognathic system. The stomatognathic system consists of the masticatory system and related organs and tissues such as the salivary glands and the muscles of expression. The components of this system are the cranial bones, mandible, hyoid, clavicle, sternum, masticatory muscles and ligaments, dental alveoli (teeth joints), and the craniomandibular joint as well as the vascular and lymphatic systems, teeth, and a very complex neurologic controlling system.

Like a class III lever system, with the joint as the fulcrum, the TMJ consists of the bony articulation between the mandible and cranium. The disc between these two bony structures is fibrocartilagenous in nature. It functions as a shock absorber in weight bearing; the thickest portion is located at the eminence and is used for chewing. In contrast, the non–weight-bearing section at the roof of the glenoid fossa is the thinner portion.

The joint has synovial membrane with hyaluronic acid lubricating the structures in the form of synovial fluid. This makes it unique among synovial joints because its cartilage is fibrocartilage, not hyaline (Dubrul, 1980; Mansour and Mow, 1972; Rees, 1954; Sicker, 1949).

The joint receptors are predominantly type II, which are active in movement through the midrange. They regulate motor unit activity of phasic or prime movers of the craniomandibular joint and are fast adapting. Type I receptors are also present in the posterior joint capsule of the TMJ, and these types are also predominantly in the cervical and shoulder joint areas. They are tonic reflexogenic, static, and dynamic at the beginning and end of movement and give information about coordination of muscle activity and awareness of joint (mandibular) position. They give reciprocally coordinated facilitative and inhibitory reflex effects on motor unit activity of the mandibular muscles (Clark and Wyke, 1974).

To a lesser extent, type III receptors are located in superficial layers in the joint capsule and are activated by a strong stretch to the capsule and ligaments. These are activated by excessive tension in the lateral TMJ ligament. This results in pterygoid and mylohyoid muscle spasms with inhibition of the temporalis and masseter muscles (Clark and Wyke, 1974).

Type IV nociceptors are present as well. These are nonadapting, pain-provoking receptors. They are located in the joint capsule, blood vessels, and connective tissues such as the retrodiscal pad and TMJ ligament. (They are also located in the articular fat pads, the anterior dura mater, the anterior and posterior longitudinal ligaments, and the iliolumbar ligament. They are not found in the blood vessels in the brain.) They are simulated by a firm stretch, inflammation, or high temperature equal to or greater than 44.8° C (Wyke, 1972). Respiratory and cardiovascular effects result from their stimulation as well as from pain provocation.

Five ligamentous structures support the TMJ: capsular ligaments, TMJ ligament, stylomandibular ligament, sphenomandibular ligament, and malleomandibular ligament. The capsular ligament controls the medial, lateral, and inferior forces and separates the articular surfaces. Its blood supply is the superior temporal artery and anterior tympanic artery, which also supplies the retrodiscal area. The TMJ ligament is the suspensory mechanism of the mandible, limiting downward movement in posterior displacement. Its outer division limits normal rotational components in mandibular opening, whereas the inner division limits the posterior movement of the disc and condyle. The TMJ ligament acts to limit excessive posterior glide of the condyle, thus protecting the retrodiscal tissue from condyle impingement. As a specialized division of the deep cervical fascia, the stylomandibular ligament runs to the pterygoid muscles. It is taut with mandibular protrusion and relaxed with opening and acts as a stop for the mandible and lessens the anterior drift of the mandible during outer opening. The sphenomandibular ligament from the spine of the sphenoid and tympanosquamous fissure runs downward and lateral to the medial surface of the mandibular ramus called the *lingula*. This is part of the remnant of the Meckel's cartilage. It checks the mandibular angle from sliding as far forward as the condyles do during translation (Friedman and Weisberg, 1985). Its nerve supply is the auricular temporal and masseteric branch of the mandibular nerve, which is the third and only motor branch of the trigeminal nerve. The final supporting ligament is the malleomandibular ligament, or Pinto's ligament, which runs from the malleus of the inner ear to the posterior TMJ capsule and disc and blends with the sphenomandibular ligament. According to Erm Shar, the malleomandibular ligament is the cause of associated ear symptoms with TMJ dysfunction (Pinto, 1962).

MUSCLES ASSOCIATED WITH THE TEMPOROMANDIBULAR JOINT

. As with skeletal muscles, two muscle types are associated with TMJ: tonic muscle types (type I) and phasic movers (type II). The type I muscle fibers contract slowly and resist fatigue, whereas the type II fibers are able to contract faster. Type II fibers have two subcategories: Type IIA are fatigue resistant, and type IIB fibers fatigue quickly.

The masticatory muscles contain type I and type IIA and IIB fibers. Consisting of 50 to 60% of type IIB fibers, the masseter muscle can contract rapidly but fatigues easily (Manns et al, 1979). The lateral pterygoid muscle, alternatively, consists of approximately 70% of the type I slow-twitch fibers, indicating that it is very resistant to fatigue (Taylor et al, 1973).

A brief description of each muscle intimately and indirectly associated with the TMJ is given in Figure 10–1. This is not meant to be a complete description of the muscular functions but will aid in TMJ dysfunction evaluation.

The *temporalis muscle* originates in the temporal fossa and fascia and, via a tendon, inserts into the medial surface in the apex and anterior border of the coronoid process and the anterior border of the ramus of the mandible (see Fig. 10–1*A*). Its anterior fibers are vertical, although the middle fibers become increasingly oblique and the posterior fibers horizontal. The nerve supply is the anterior and posterior deep temporal nerve branches from the anterior division of the mandibular branch of the trigeminal nerve. Blood supplies are the middle and deep temporal arteries. The temporalis muscle is responsible for mandibular elevation and closure. The posterior fibers are responsible for retrusion and lateral deviation to the ipsilateral side, whereas the anterior fibers are responsible for closure to edge-to-edge position.

Superficial and deep divisions are noted in the *masseter muscle*. Its origin is from the zygomatic process of the maxilla and zygomatic arch to the external surface of the angle of the mandible and to the inferior half of the ramus; the deep fibers go to the superior half of the ramus. Its nerve supply is the masseteric nerve in the anterior branch of the mandibular division of the trigeminal nerve. Blood supplies are from the masseteric artery branch of the maxillary artery. Its action is elevation of the mandible and clenching. The superficial fibers, which are at a 90-degree angle to the occlusal plane of the molars, are responsible for grinding forces, whereas the deep fibers are responsible for retrusion.

The *medial pterygoid* functions as a sling, along with the masseter muscle, to support the mandibular angle. It originates from the medial lip of the lateral pterygoid plate of the sphenoid and pterygoid fossa as well as parametal process of the palatine bone; these fibers are inferior, lateral, and posterior, and they insert into a strong tendinous lamina in the ramus and angle of the mandible. The nerve supply is the medial pterygoid from the mandibular division of the trigeminal nerve, and the blood supply is from the maxillary artery branch. Kinesiologically, the medial pterygoid assists the temporalis and masseter muscles with elevation of the mandible and shows increased activity with protrusion during elevation. Unilaterally, it acts to deviate the mandible laterally to the opposite side and assist the lateral pterygoid with protrusion (Carlsoo, 1952).

The *lateral pterygoid* has two heads: inferior and superior. The larger, inferior head originates from the lateral lip of the pterygoid plate, and a smaller, superior head originates from the infratemporal surface of the greater wing in the sphenoid. The superior head attaches into deep articular capsule and the anterior border of the articular disc. The remaining superior and inferior fibers insert into a roughened anterior surface in the neck of the mandibular condyle. Its nerve supply is the lateral pterygoid from the

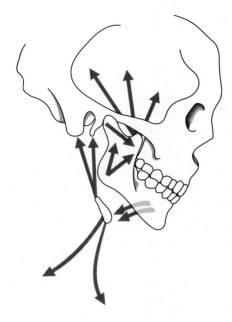

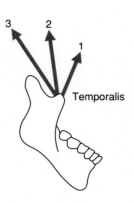

Temporalis muscle
1. Vertical pull by the anterior fibers
2. Temporalis oblique pull by the middle fibers
3. Horizontal pull via the posterior fibers

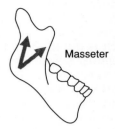

Masseter muscle
Grinding is accomplished by:
1. Superficial fibers of masseter
2. The deep fibers of masseter cause retrusion

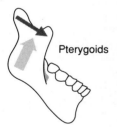

Pterygoid muscles
1. The lateral pterygoid has a superior and interior head functioning as reciprocating muscles. The interior head elicits mandibular opening, protrusion, and lateral deviation to the opposite side. The superior head is active during closing, rotating the disc on the condyle.
2. The medial pterygoid assists with mandibular elevation and protrusion during elevation. Unilaterally, it laterally deviates the mandible to the opposite side and assists the lateral pterygoid with protrusion.

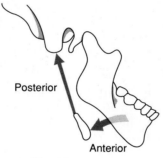

Digastrics

Digastric muscles
As a suprahyoid muscle, the digastric assists with mandibular depression with the hyoid fixed. With the mandible fixed, it elevates the hyoid. Acting bilaterally, it assists with mandibular retrusion.

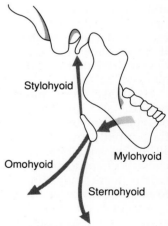

Suprahyoid muscles
Stylohyoid and mylohyoid (inferior to mylohyoid and not pictured geniohyoid)

Infrahyoid muscles
Omohyoid and sternohyoid with the sternothyroid and thyrohyoid muscles running deep to the sternohyoid

Figure 10–1 *See legend on opposite page*

anterior division of the mandibular branch of the trigeminal nerve, and blood supply is from the branches of the maxillary artery. The lateral pterygoid functions as two separate and reciprocating muscles. The inferior lateral pterygoid is responsible for forward, inward, and downward pulls on the mandible, which causes mandibular opening, protrusion, and deviation of the mandible to the opposite side. This is considered as one muscle functioning unilaterally. The superior belly is inactive during opening (McNamara, 1973), but as it inserts into the condyle and disc it causes rotation of the disc on the condyle during closing. It rotates the disc anteriorly and only as far as the width of the articular disc permits (Mahan et al, 1983).

Thus far, muscles discussed have been mandibular movers. If these muscles or joints with which they are associated become injured, each will be affected. Resisted movements or stretching the muscle in the opposite direction will give information about the degree of soft-tissue involvement. Joint involvement is noted with passive movement and reproduction of pain. Chewing and speech would be affected.

As a group, the suprahyoid muscles are at- tached from the mandible to the hyoid. The infrahyoid muscles are attached from the hyoid to the scapular areas and sternum. Together, these two groups of muscles coordinate mandibular function.

The geniohyoid muscle originates from the mental spine and inserts into the hyoid. Its nerve supply is via the ventral rami at the lesser occipital nerve of C_1. It pulls downward and backward on the mandible along with the digastric muscle.

The *digastric muscle* has an anterior and a posterior belly. The posterior belly attaches into the mastoid notch as the deepest attachment; the longissimus capitis, splenius capitis, and sternocleidomastoid muscles are the superior attachments on the mastoid process. The anterior belly attaches to the inferior border of the mandible close to its midline symphysis. The posterior belly is innervated by the facial nerve, whereas the anterior belly is innervated by the mylohyoid nerve, which is a division of the posterior division of mandibular nerve and third division of the trigeminal nerve. It assists with mandibular depression when the hyoid is fixed. With the mandible fixed, the digastric muscle elevates the hyoid. Bilaterally, it assists with mandibular re-

Figure 10–1. Component force couples of mandibular posture. These muscles control mandibular motion while the suprahyoid and infrahyoid muscles stabilize and move the tongue and hyoid bone, facilitating proper swallowing, deglutination, and speech.

Temporalis Muscle
1. Vertical pull by the anterior fibers.
2. Temporalis oblique pull by the middle fibers.
3. Horizontal pull via the posterior fibers.

Masseter Muscle
Grinding is accomplished by 1. Superficial fibers of masseter, 2. Deep fibers of masseter cause retrusion.

Pterygoid Muscles
1. The lateral pterygoid has a superior and interior head functioning as reciprocating muscles. The interior head elicits mandibular opening, protrusion and lateral deviation to the opposite side. The superior head is active during closing, rotating the disc on the condyle.
2. The medial pterygoid assists with mandibular elevation and protrusion during elevation. Unilaterally, it laterally deviates the mandible to the opposite side and assists the lateral pterygoid with protrusion.

Digastric Muscles
As a suprahyoid muscle, the digastric assists with mandibular depression with the hyoid fixed. With the mandibular fixed, it elevates the hyoid. Acting bilaterally, it assists with mandibular retrusion.

Suprahyoid muscles
Stylohyoid and mylohyoid (inferior to mylohyoid and not pictured geniohyoid).

Infrahyoid muscles
Omohyoid and sternohyoid with the sternothyroid and hydrohyoid muscles running deep to the sterbigtiud.

trusion. The digastric muscle is essential for maximum depression such as with coughing or swallowing.

The *mylohyoid muscle* originates from the mylohyoid line of the mandible and symphysis menti to the last molar tooth, and the posterior fibers run medially and inferiorly to insert into the body of the hyoid bone. It is innervated by the inferior alveolar branch of the mandible division of the trigeminal nerve along with a small artery. It functions as a stabilizer and an elevator of the tongue during swallowing.

Stylohyoid muscle arises from the posterolateral surface of the styloid process and inserts into the body of the hyoid bone just superior to the omohyoid muscle. It is innervated by the facial nerve. Its function is drawing the hyoid bone backward and upward during swallowing. Interestingly, the anteroposterior position of the hyoid is determined by muscle functioning of the stylohyoid, geniohyoid, and infrahyoid muscles.

The infrahyoid muscle group consists of a sternohyoid, omohyoid, sternothyroid, and thyrohyoid. They are often referred to as strap muscles because they cover the front and much of the sides of the larynx, trachea, and thyroid gland. Along with the geniohyoid muscle, they form a continuation of the cervical region of the muscle mass and fascial investments that connect the mandible to the symphysis pubis.

As their names suggest, the *sternohyoid* and *omohyoid* muscles attach into the hyoid region. The sternohyoid muscle ascends from the posterior surface of the manubrium sterni and sternal end of the clavicle to the hyoid. The omohyoid muscle runs from the hyoid to the superior border of the scapula just medial to the notch.

The *sternothyroid* and *thyrohyoid* muscles are deep to the sternohyoid muscle. The sternothyroid muscle originates from the posterior aspect of the manubrium and attaches obliquely into the thyroid cartilage. The thyrohyoid muscle arises from the thyroid cartilage and attaches into the hyoid.

The suprahyoid and infrahyoid muscles function to stabilize and move the tongue and hyoid bone, facilitating proper swallowing and deglutition as well as speech. Hypotension or hypertension of these muscles would affect those functions and, in time, TMJ health.

The strap muscles are innervated by the upper cervical nerves; the nerves to the lower muscles are given off from the ansa cervicalis, the cervical loop. These are containing fibers from the second and third cervical nerves. As this loop descends, it joins with a superior root, which seems to originate from the hypoglossal nerve or the 12th cranial nerve.

The hyoid muscles are responsible for depression of the larynx and hyoid and for function such as singing low notes followed by elevation of larynx and hyoid. Along with the suprahyoid muscles, they fix the hyoid as a stationary base for tongue and mandibular movements.

A final division of muscles vital for functioning of the mandible are the cervical muscles. Muscles such as the sternocleidomastoid and anterior and posterior cervical muscles play a vital role in stabilizing the skull for controlled mandibular movements. The anterior division of muscles includes the infrahyoid muscles and deep prevertebral muscles, the longus capitis, and longus cervicis muscles. The lateral group includes the scalenes and sternocleidomastoid muscles and levator scapulae. The posterior division consists of four separate layers; the deepest layer is the rectus major and minor and superior and inferior obliques. The next division includes small, deep muscles along the spine of the multifidus, rotatores, intertransversarii, and the interspinales.

The second deepest layer is comprised of the semispinalis cervicis and semispinalis capitis. Increased tension of the semispinalis capitis can entrap the greater occipital nerve from the posterior ramus of C_2. The splenius muscles form the third layer, and the last, most superficial layers are formed by the ligamentum nuchae and the cervical part of the trapezius muscle.

These muscles are responsible for movement of cervical spine flexion, extension, rotation, and lateral sidebending. Because these muscles structurally are so close to the TMJ, there seems to be a functional correlation among cervical spine, TMJ, and occlusion. Therefore, changing head posture from these muscles influences mandibular position. For example, with hypertonicity of the levator scapulae, a cervical sidebending may result that would involve mandibular compensation. This compensation takes the form of lateral deviation to the opposite side for postural equilibrium. The client would, therefore, appear to have a crossbite, which in fact originated from hypertonicity of the levator scapulae on the opposite side.

GROWTH AND DEVELOPMENT

Growth and development involve an interrelation with other anatomic area systems. The cranium, nasomaxillary, and mandibular complex constantly interact and are affected by the cervical spine and shoulder relation as well as head posturing and the amount of cervical lordosis present, physiologic or nonphysiologic. Postural equilibrium is a delicate balance between these areas. Other immediate concerns in growth and development of the TMJ are the cranial bones, the midfacial bones, and the mandibular complex. Each of these is dependent on the others for growth, development, and function, as are the muscles of the scalp, mastication, and facial expression. Correlations of upper airway obstruction to head posturing and craniofacial growth are imperative. Early recognition of abnormalities or deficiencies in growth and development is imperative in preventing TMJ problems.

Craniofacial growth is dependent on these complex relations (Enlow, 1982), and the maxilla and mandible are constantly affecting each other throughout life, adapting throughout the aging process. There may also be psychologic implications as well as learning abilities and dysfunctions not yet scientifically correlated with physical growth and development.

The TMJ, flat at birth, develops with age (Grimsby, 1987). The maxilla is formed as a result of bone deposition on the lingual surface and that bone taking away a reserve from the nasal surface. This is responsible for the vertical facial growth that occurs in all humans. Horizontal growth begins in the fetus through direct deposition to the surfaces of the maxilla in both the anterior and posterior directions. This growth continues for the first 2 years of life such that the dental arch is sufficient to accommodate dentition. From 6 months to 2½ years, this mandibular fossa increases its depth from 2 mm to 4 to 5 mm as the dentition develops (Wright and Moffett, 1974). Functional requirements for the TMJ are changing throughout this time as well.

According to Wolff's law, (Enlow, 1968), bone will change its internal architecture according to the forces placed on it. Therefore, bone remodeling occurs in response to changes in soft tissue, mechanical stress, and subsequent remodeling of the bone. An example is an infant who is bottle-fed or who does not get optimal sucking time. Therefore, maxillary and mandibular growth is affected.

To satisfy the physiologic need for sucking 120 to 130 min/day, the child may begin sucking the thumb or other fingers. This directly affects mandibular growth. As the tongue presses against the rugae, it is flattened, thus allowing the tongue to move forward pushing against the upper gumline and causing the gumline or teeth to protrude. Because the tongue continues to push against the palate, it moves up, narrowing the lateral margins and causing further protrusion of the anterior teeth. The upper lip responds by curling up. Normally, the buccinator and the internal and external orbicularis oris muscle forces are counterbalanced by the tongue position and pressure under the palate.

As the infant grows, lip incompetence or a lips-apart posture is observed. This generally means the mandible will be opened and the teeth will be apart. To keep this position, the lateral pterygoid muscles as well as the anterior cervical muscles must increase their activity. Thus, the mandible will not have a clockwise rotation resulting from the rotational forces placed on it by the masseter, temporalis, and medial pterygoid, balanced by the lateral pterygoid holding the condyle against the articular eminence. The child will have a counterclockwise, rotational, and downward force. Over time, the alveolar bone will compensate posteriorly, resulting in an open-bite occlusion.

During this process of compensation, the tongue also responds by falling to the floor of the mouth, pressuring the lower gum and teeth. These begin protruding, and the lower lip curls down as well (Grimsby, 1987).

Occurring simultaneously is the respiratory pattern of mouth breathing. The results decreased the anteroposterior development of the nasal pharynx and are accompanied by a forward-head posturing with flexion in the midcervical area and a high hyoid bone position (see Fig. 10–24). Other findings, according to Rickets' respiratory obstructive syndrome, are as follows: (1) a primary unilateral or bilateral crossbite; (2) functional unilateral crossbite with mandibular deflection; (3) history of enlarged adenoids or tonsils; (4) open bite; (5) a lower tongue position; (6) tongue thrust; (7) a narrow upper arch; (8) chronic mouth breathing; (9) secondary problems with TMJ and maxilla; (10) pseudo +1 condition in bilateral crossbite with anterior mandibular deflection; (11) head backward on cervical column; (12) narrow nasal cavity; and (13) opening of the mandibular angle (Rickets, 1968).

Rickets' findings are consistent with those of other clinicians. The best controlled and notable work in controlled animal experimentation was that of Harvold and colleagues (Harvold, 1975 and 1975b; Harvold, Chierici, and Vargervik,

1972; Harvold, Vargervik, and Chierici, 1972). These studies involving rhesus monkeys demonstrated reproducibility of direct cause-and-effect relationships.

Mouth breathing entails forward mandibular translation to decrease resistance of the increased air volume. Therefore, open-mouth and forward translation of the mandible results. The lateral pterygoid compensates for this. This may be damaging in children because the condyle eminence could be stunted in growth. The smaller eminence affects posterior movement during lateral deviation, and condylar damage may inhibit vertical mandibular growth. This would lead to a decreased posterior facial height and a deficient skeletal relationship.

The condyles are also subject to trauma as a result of any fall or blow on the chin and mandible, driving the mandible into the condyle or articular fossa. Intraoral trauma also affects the health of the condyles as a result of loss of both occlusion and tooth support. This is most common with children learning to walk and play and falling off or into objects. Affectations of the chondrogenic areas of the condyle may lead to degenerative joint disease and may directly affect the growth of the condyles, resulting in growth deformation or condylar resorption. Growth deformity results in a flat eminence or small condyle and a large fossa. The ramus of the mandible therefore shortens through remodeling.

An example of this is a 3-year-old child who is kicked by a horse, resulting in a fracture of the symphysis and dislocation of the condylar head. This resulted in decreased condylar growth and decreased mandibular range of motion by 5 years of age. A neuromaxillary arch and possible development of posterior crossbite were also noted. The body compensated with the upper molars flaring buccally, causing interference lingually with those cusps tilted down. Lateral deviation was also decreased. To affect the growth of the mandibular head biomechanically, soft-tissue stretching was initiated as well as re-establishing normal physiologic joint axis position and normal TMJ range of motion. Correct tongue positioning for swallowing and proper rest position of the mandible were also taught. The child required orthodontic evaluations at proper intervals.

Occlusal problems may be reversed with early intervention. The total respiratory system, craniomandibular system, and occlusion must be addressed for proper growth and development.

Nasal respiratory distress is also of immediate concern with growth and development. This primarily concerns allergies. Marks, a prominent pediatric allergist (Marks, 1965), attributed many allergies of infants and children to cow's milk. Children's immune systems are unable to cope with the large amount of proteins contained in cow's milk, thus causing allergies.

Smith (Smith and Ware, 1972) attributed most cases of otitis media to cow's milk allergies as well. He also studied hyperkinetic children and reported that diet and allergies are contributing factors affecting behavior.

Children with chronic nasal congestion are noted to develop a nasal crease from rubbing the nose upward to relieve itching. This may also contribute to nasal septum deviations. Mouth breathers are noted to have a narrow external nares as a result of atrophy. With congenital premaxillary, dental, or palatal malformations, a narrow nose is often noted because embryologically the upper incisor teeth and portions of the palate and nasal septum arrive from the premaxillary area (Smith and Ware, 1972).

Children with chronic allergies often are found to have "shiners" or darkened areas under their eyes. Their eyes tend to tear frequently, and their faces tend to take on a dull, sad expression.

The nasal septum is labeled as deviated if it is not in the midline. The normal position of the nasal septum is equal by section of the nares. The turbinates should be glistening pink. With chronic allergic rhinitis, they are pale, bluish, and often edematous.

Bushey described nasal patency tests (Bushey, 1979). Nasal patency is easy to test by sealing the lips for 1 to 2 minutes to determine if the person is able to breathe through the nose. It is also easy to test which passage may be blocked by alternately collapsing each nostril to evaluate nasopharyngeal viability. Humming also makes it more apparent. Breathing into a pocket mirror with one nostril blocked will also prove functional abilities. Facial balance and symmetry should be examined for normal function.

Most notably, in evaluating growth and development sequences, social factors of less active children must be taken into consideration. They commonly sit in school, sit while doing homework, and sit watching television. This stresses the head, neck, and shoulders. There is tremendous pressure to perform and excel in our industrialized society, which creates stressful psychologic conditions for these children and results in hypertonia of the facial and neck areas and may lead to skeletal or dental malformation.

In evaluating and treating children, the main

goal is to promote balance of the craniomandibular and craniocervical structures. This includes optimal development and function during the growing years and stable function via balance through the adaptive years of aging.

OCCLUSION

The purpose of this chapter is not occlusal evaluation, but the identification of certain aspects of occlusion to understand prevention and treatment.

There are three general classes of occlusion. Normal occlusion, class I, is the symmetrically shaped upper and lower dental arches, with the teeth in maximal interdigitation. The buccal aspects are outside of the lower teeth throughout the dental arch (Fig. 10–2).

Class II occlusion (Fig. 10–3) is equivalent to an overbite. The posturing that accompanies the class II occlusion is usually a retrognathic lower face with mandibular deficiency. The face is vertically long. TMJ arthritis, forward-head posturing, and myofascial conditions result in class II occlusion. They may or may not have disc dysfunction or distal condylar displacement.

Class III occlusion is a protrusive mandible (Fig. 10–4). With the amount of soft-tissue compression and TMJ distraction, this may also lead

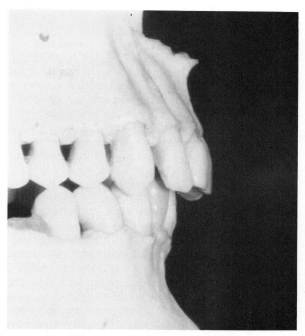

Figure 10–3. Class II occlusion.

to TMJ arthritis as well as forward-head positioning and myofascial dysfunction. Other conditions that may apply to the classes of occlusion include open bite. In this condition, the teeth do not overlap vertically when the mandible is closed. It can occur both in the anterior and posterior regions or both. Crossbite occurs when the buccal aspects of the teeth are not outside the lower teeth.

Centric position is the initial tooth contact on a closure of the mandible, and it is a postural position. In centric occlusion, the cusp of the mandibular and maxillary teeth interdigitate maximally. Centric occlusion and centric position are subject to change with change in postural equilibrium.

The freeway space or the interocclusal distance is necessary physiologically but cannot be scientifically determined. The norm is a 1:3 ratio between the vertical dimension of occlusion and the vertical dimension of rest. The 1-mm distance is measured between the tips of the cusp of the posterior molars, whereas the 3-mm measurement is the distance between the tips of the incisors.

The vertical dimension of occlusion designates the distance from the base of the nose to the base of the chin and is dependent on the occlusal

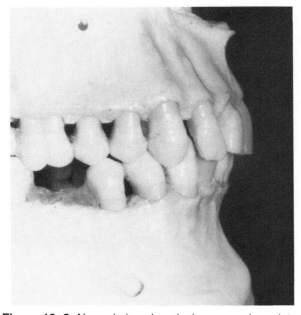

Figure 10–2. Normal class I occlusion, normal overjet.

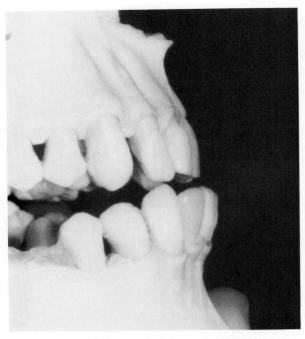

Figure 10–4. Class III occlusion: open bite anteriorly.

stop. With the teeth in centric occlusion, there should be approximately a 1½-mm overbite in relation to the lower incisors.

The vertical dimension of rest is the rest position of the mandible. It is genetically and physiologically determined. It can be considered the most important functional position of the mandible because:

1. All movements of the mandible begin and end from this position
2. The stomatognathic system is in homeostasis and postural equilibrium results
3. The vertical dimension of rest position is the basis for the vertical dimension of occlusion

Maintaining the vertical dimension of rest depends on posture and should be the final goal of treatment (Kraus, 1989).

MOBILITY

The mandibular rest position and trajectory of jaw closure are influenced by the cervical spine. Both are influenced by intraoral orthotic relation. TMJ range of motion can be described in three

ways. First, it is limited, in which an individual is moving in an unphysiologic zone and impeded. The movement is about a nonphysiologic axis. According to Cyriax (1981) mobility would be classified as grade 0 (fused), grade I (moderate to marked limitation), and grade II (mild limitation). Second, range of motion that is functional, symmetric, and pain- and friction-free, and is classified as grade III mobility. It can enable an individual to perform all daily stomatognathic functions. Third, range of motion can be excessive, classified as a grade IV or slight increase in motion, a grade V, which is a moderate to marked increased motion, or a grade VI, which is unstable. These movements also occur in unphysiologic zones in which the individual is confronted with varying degrees of loose jointedness and loss of neuromuscular control.

Joint mobility is not age dependent, but it does vary with facial types: short and horizontal brachyfacial, long and narrow dolichofacial, and combinations of the two (Grummons, 1989).

	Opening	Lateral deviation
Brachyfacial	50–55 mm	12–15 mm
Mesofacial	45–52 mm	9–12 mm
Dolichofacial	42–50 mm	8–10 mm

Youths may have approximately a 2-mm difference or may be the same as their adult counterparts.

TMJ motion is instantaneous, with about a three-dimensional center and the lever arm changing during movement. The first 15 to 20 mm are nearly pure rotation; from 15 to 50 mm the motions are combinations of rotation and translation (Nordin, 1989).

The articular disc rotates posteriorly as the condyle moves anteriorly during translation. If superior joint adhesions increase, condylar translation results in the lower joint, and increased friction is also produced in the lower joint. This leads to decreased elasticity of collateral ligaments. In treatment, the joint is positioned as close as possible to the resting position. This is the loose-pack position where the ligaments, muscles, and capsule are as relaxed as possible and there is maximum joint space. The mandibular resting position is maintained by the position of the tongue against the palate of the mouth. The anterosuperior tip of the tongue is placed in the palate posterior to the back side of the upper incisors. The first half of the tongue is also in the palate. The posterior portion of the tongue forms the anterior wall of the pharynx. It should stay there unless the person is talking, chewing, yawning, coughing, or licking the lips.

The back teeth should be apart to lessen muscle activity. Breathing should be nasal diaphragmatic with the lips together. A negative pressure is created in the oral cavity, reducing muscle activity in this position. Swallowing normally should be occur with the tip of the tongue in the roof of the mouth.

In the closed-pack position, the joint space is decreased and the soft tissues and capsule are tight. If the joint was hypermobile, the treatment would initiate as near as possible to the resting position with stabilization techniques of splinting and exercises. Neuromuscular stabilization would be the goal in this position. There is no treatment in the case of a class VI hypermobile joint. In addition, there is no treatment for a grade 0 mobility joint because life would be difficult in this condition. However, the ultimate goal for classes I and II hypermobile joints would be to return to a normal physiologic axis of movement and to the resting position of the mandible.

Mandibular movements guided by activities of the TMJ and muscles occur in interrelated series of three: dimensional, rotational, and translational. These movements depend on four factors: the initiating position, movement types, movement directions, and degree of movements (Neff, 1980).

The initiation of movement is determined by a maximum intercuspated position or tooth-to-tooth position. From this position—the proprioceptive awareness—two types of movements are possible: rotation and translation. Rotation involves movement of the mandible around the glenoid fossa, and translation or gliding movement occurs among the inferior surface of the articular fossa, the eminence of the temporal bones, and the superior surface of the articulating disc. The third factor—direction of movement—is related to all planes of movement. Three planes of movement are associated with the TMJ: the frontal plane, the sagittal plane, and the horizontal plane. The final factor of the degree of movement concerns mandibular function such as chewing and talking, which occur at lesser degrees of opening. Therefore, opening and closing movements of the jaw are combinations of rotary and translatory movements of the mandible and disc. For normal movements to occur, it is vital that the rest position of the mandible be established as well as normal disc condyle translation without displacement.

RESPIRATION PATTERNS

Optimal breathing patterns involve maximum diaphragmatic excursion, physiologic head-on-neck positioning and spinal posturing, as well as full-rib mobility. Less than optimal breathing patterns have intimate effects on the nasomaxillary function and development and will in time affect other areas of the musculoskeletal system.

The diaphragm is the major muscle of inspiration, working in synergy with the pelvic diaphragm. When it contracts, the intrathoracic pressure decreases, the intra-abdominal pressure increases, and the lower ribs elevate, thus increasing the transverse diameter of the thorax. As the central tendon pulls down, the vertical dimension increases and the anteroposterior dimension decreases with the help of the sternum.

The abdominals function to bring the diaphragm down with the abdominal viscera providing resistance to the action of the diaphragm. Diaphragmatic tone increases while abdominal tone decreases. Both sets of muscles are also in active contraction. Inspiration is associated with extension postures. Accessory muscles of inspiration are the sternocleidomastoid, scalenus, pectoralis major and minor, latissimus dorsi, and other deep spinal muscles.

Expiration is normally passive as a result of recoil effects of the elastic components. The abdominals are strong, forced expirators and reduce the three dimensions of the thorax. Decreased diaphragmatic tone is noted while abdominal tone increases. Expiration is associated with a flexion posture. Because mouth breathing has been the subject of much discussion, it is interesting to discuss once again the consequences of this respiratory pattern. Possibly, additional studies may be needed to examine fully its physiologic consequences. Mouth breathing seems to create a socially unacceptable appearance. The mouth is open, and many postural changes are associated with an insufficient respiratory pattern. The general musculoskeletal appearance is that of forward-head posturing, flattened facial features, as well as a decreased capacity for exercise and sports ability (Grimsby, 1987). The person generally seems to present with less self-esteem and often has behavior problems (Keleman, 1975 and 1985; Lowen, 1975). It is important to teach clients proper diaphragmatic excursion and breathing patterns along with postural tone.

PATHOLOGY

Volumes could be written on any one subject of this chapter, not to mention pathology. These afflictions are internal or external consequences. They require recognition in diagnosis and differential management. Because prevention is not always possible, awareness is necessary. A brief outline is offered, along with evaluation and treatment guidelines.

Some pathologies concerning the TMJ are associated with growth disorders. These can occur any time from the 14th week of development. The TMJ derives from two cell layers: one for the mandibular condyle and the other for the temporal bone. A third cell group forms the disc. Most commonly, the time period for development is during weeks 8 through 12 (Keith, 1982; Moffett, 1966; Symons, 1952).

Condylar hypoplasia is rare. It is not painful, but it may cause problems if the mandible ipsilaterally is small or if the ramus has lessened vertical height. Treatment may be orthodontic. At times, condylar hypoplasia occurs in conjunction with various syndromes. The most recent syndrome noted in clinical experience is Nager syndrome, in which the mandible may be in various stages of development or may not be developed at all. For example, a 3-year-old boy who had no mandible, closed ears, and radial limb hypoplasia presented for clinical evaluation. He breathed through a tracheal tube and was fed through a stomach tube. The child is in the process of surgical correction, including creation of a mandible from rib grafts. Because the tongue and the teeth were in the posterior throat before its creation, one can imagine the implications for the developmental sequencing yet to follow such as tongue patterns and positionings necessary for sucking, swallowing, speech, chewing, and many other functions and muscle responses for the same and mandibular movement. Determining a normal physiologic axis for condylar movement of the TMJ in this child involves many changes. Treatment of children such as this involves a multidisciplinary approach that includes musculoskeletal evaluation; proprioceptive training; physical, occupational, and speech therapies; and surgical or orthodontic intervention.

Condylar hypoplasia usually occurs in adolescence, causing facial asymmetry with the mandible growing downward and laterally. Occlusal changes are eminent. Treatment is surgical or orthodontic in nature. It may involve physical therapy for musculoskeletal affectation and intervention and for improvement of function.

Neoplasms cause signs and symptoms similar to other TMJ dysfunctions. They are not common. Neoplasms should be suspected when pain either does not change or increases with treatment. Benign tumors are more common than malignant ones. These, of course, involve surgical intervention and diagnosis.

Arthritic disorders are numerous. They include infectious arthritis, traumatic arthritis, metabolic joint disease (gout), degenerative joint disease, rheumatoid arthritis, psoriatic arthritis, and osteochondritis. Treatment includes dental surgery, rheumatologic or medical management, as well as physical therapy.

Degenerative joint disease demands the most attention from the general population. The primary symptom is pain with condylar translation during movement at any point. Maximum opening is usually decreased, and the mandible deviates to the affected side. Joint noises are palpable and can be auscultated. They are often confused with popping.

Typically, affectations are to one joint and symptoms last 9 to 12 months, gradually fading. A small percentage of cases may continue with pain and dysfunction despite conservative management, however.

Treatment of degenerative joint disease involves education, reassurance, medications, physical therapy for muscle imbalances of the mandible and cervical spine, and possibly splint therapy by the dental specialist. The joint-rest position is important. Physical therapy should include modalities and exercise to unload the TMJ.

Total or partial joint replacement surgery is indicated in 2 to 12% of clients with degenerative joint disease (Benson, 1988). Type of replacement surgery should be carefully selected for the desired favorable responses. Postsurgically, occlusal and muscle hyperactivity problems should be addressed with splint therapy via dental care or physical therapy.

Other *immune disorders*, including lupus erythematosus, psoriasis, and Reiter's syndrome, may be implicated in TMJ pathology. Still others may also give rise to symptoms but are less common.

Neurologic disorders affecting neuromuscular control of the TMJ must be recognized as causes of TMJ disorders. The most common of these may be multiple sclerosis, which attacks the myelination of the nerve sheath. These clients generally have considerable pain and should be taught proper rest positions and avoidance of fatigue.

Trauma disorders for TMJ can be both acute and chronic in nature. They include fractures, TMJ dysfunction, disc condyle derangements, disc displacements, anteriorly displaced with or without reduction, capsular tightness, condylar subluxation, and condylar dislocation.

TMJ dysfunction is further defined as a problematic functioning of that area not related to growth disorders, disease, or trauma. This category includes myalgia, myofascial dysfunction syndrome, fibromyalgia, the disc, and condyle.

EVALUATION

History and clinical examination of TMJ disorders are the basis for differential diagnosis and objective treatment. The differential diagnosis may include work-ups from neurologic, otolaryngologic, psychologic, cervical, and dental perspectives to determine the client's status and to make appropriate referrals. This ensures a positive response to treatment and the client's confidence and commitment. (As Moffett, 1964, stated, "If all else fails, try making a diagnosis.") TMJ is a place, not a diagnosis. It is important to know the gross anatomy, neuroanatomy, and neurophysiology to correlate signs and symptoms to their sources. It is impossible just to memorize these findings. Correlation and assessment skills are of major importance.

The subjective portion of the evaluation includes the client's chief complaint. It gives details of progression of the symptoms including the onset, the acute or subtle phase, and the chronic phase, if involved. It defines what the client believes is most problematic and should be the central theme of discussion at the end of the evaluation. It is important to acknowledge the client's complaint in this way to assure him or her that the clinician has listened. If the chief complaint is not in the professional's area of competence, the client should be referred to the appropriate health specialist.

A medical history should be taken that includes identification of system disorders related to the chief complaint. This will alert the health professional to cardiac disorders, which may require prophylactic or antibiotic treatment, and it identifies the client who is medically compromised by, for example, cardiac pain with angina; myocardial infarctions; and cardiac pain from the substernal, jaw, throat, back, shoulder, or arm areas. It may also identify systemic autoimmune disorders or endocrine disorders, such as diabetes.

During the subjective interview, clinicians should find out the origin of pain; its onset, nature, and intensity; and what exacerbates and what relieves the pain. A separate history should be taken for the initial onset and each subsequent onset up to the present incident and reason for which the client seeks help.

There are many excellent questionnaires such as the Visual Analog Scale, the McGill Pain Questionnaire (Terezhalmy et al, 1982), the Ransford Quantified Pain Drawing, and the Modified Somatic Perception Questionnaire that may be completed before the interview or history taking. These should be used as screening tools only, reviewed in the presence of the client, and used in the final correlation as it applies to the client. The questionnaires are not a diagnosis, but they help to quantify objective measures of perceived pain and decreases of the same. Pain thresholds remain constant while perception varies. It is not the cause of the problem: it is part of the symptoms.

The anatomy, function, and pathology of the TMJ must be related to a total examination and treatment of (1) posture, (2) congenital deformities, (3) developmental anomalies, (4) respiration, (5) speech, (6) function of the lips, (7) function of the tongue, (8) chewing and swallowing patterns, (9) position of the teeth, and (10) behavior patterns (Grimsby, 1987).

Postural considerations concern the position of the head and neck in relation to the mid-dorsal spine, giving information about the loss of physiologic lordosis or increased cervical lordosis. It also provides information about backward bending over, sidebending, and rotation of head, as well as thoracic kyphosis. Because of the intimate relation of the musculoskeletal elements in the cervical nerve root, elevation of the first rib is of extreme importance as a result of its association with the head and neck. Finally, functional limitations of movement of the cervical spine and the upper thoracic region are also important.

The muscular system should be evaluated for muscle spasm of the facial muscles or masticatory muscles as well as the muscles of the paralateral, prelateral, or lateral neck muscle. Dysfunction of the tongue, lips, and cheeks should be assessed. Muscle hypertrophies, mainly of the masseter, temporalis, and sternocleidomastoid, must also be evaluated (Fig. 10–5 to 10–23).

Respiratory dysfunction as related to the optimal breathing pattern should be assessed to identify upper thoracic respiration or short insufficient breathing patterns influencing hyperactivity of the accessory muscles of respiration or mouth-breathing patterns. Lip flexibility and ability to close are important for resting mandibular posture, speech, chewing, and swallowing. Vital to the success of these functions are tongue posturing and usage. Occupational therapists have excellent opportunities to evaluate these conditions early during feeding sessions.

Ear, nose, and throat conditions and performance should be checked as they relate to the TMJ. These areas may include: (1) hyperacusia, (2) sounds such as clicking, grindings, and pops, (3) sinus syndromes, (4) changes in the voice, (5) tight throat, and (6) difficulty swallowing. The mandibular pattern and its range of motion should be assessed including the position of the mandible as it is altered in space in all planes as a result of occlusion, muscle activity, and head and neck posturing (Fig. 10–24). Dynamic dysfunctions caused by muscle, capsula, and ligament muscle should also be assessed in the objective findings.

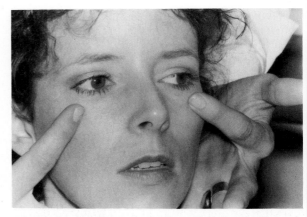

Figure 10–6. Palpating the infraorbital rim, testing pain response. This should not be painful.

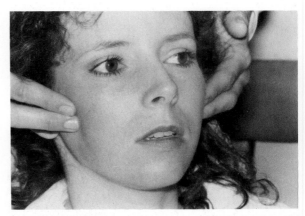

Figure 10–7. Palpation of the superficial masseter.

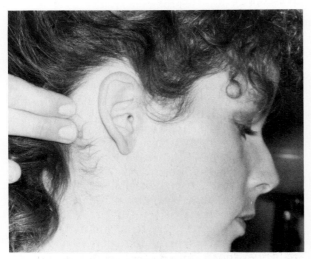

Figure 10–5. Palpating the posterior mastoid process avoiding the sternocleidomastoid and cervical muscles, testing pain response. This should not be painful.

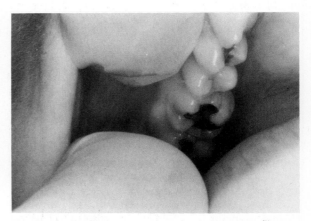

Figure 10–8. Palpation of the deep masseter fibers.

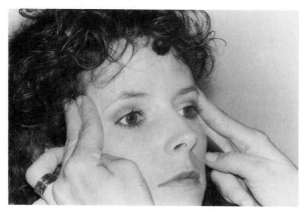

Figure 10–9. Palpation of the anterior temporalis fibers *(vertical)*.

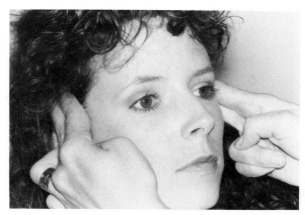

Figure 10–10. Palpation of the middle temporalis fibers.

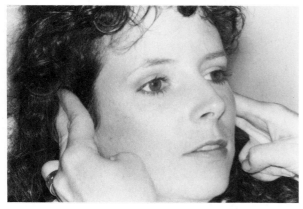

Figure 10–11. Palpation of the posterior temporalis fibers *(horizontal)*.

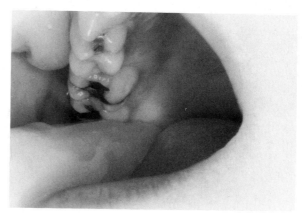

Figure 10–12. Palpation of the coronoid process.

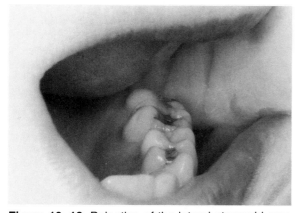

Figure 10–13. Palpation of the lateral pterygoid area.

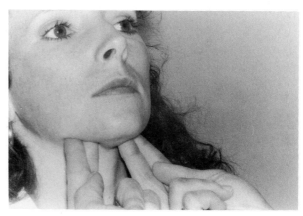

Figure 10–14. Palpation of anterior belly of the digastric muscle.

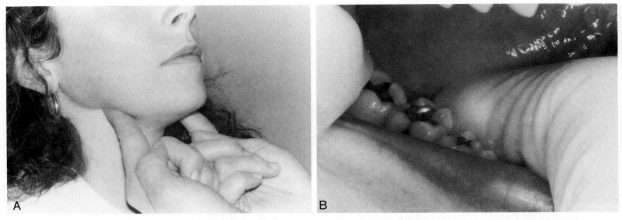

Figure 10–15. *A,* Palpation of the medial pterygoid insertion. *B,* Palpation of the medial pterygoid insertion.

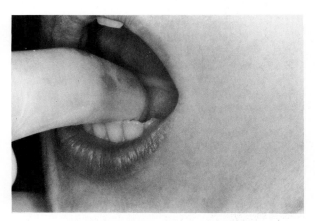

Figure 10–16. Palpation of the mylohyoid muscle.

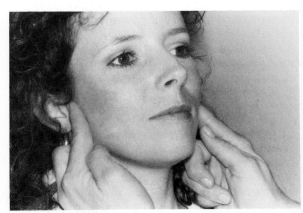

Figure 10–17. Bilateral palpation over the lateral pole of condyle.

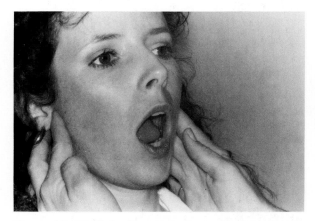

Figure 10–18. Palpation posterior to the lateral pole, with the mouth opened.

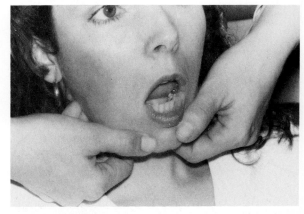

Figure 10–19. Superior loading of the TMJ should also be done with a stethoscope.

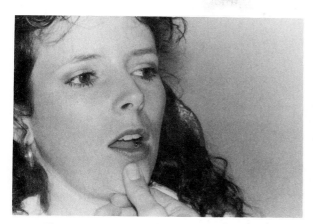

Figure 10–20. Posterior loading of the TMJ.

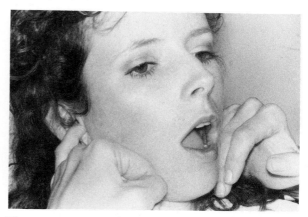

Figure 10–21. Palpation through external auditory meatus.

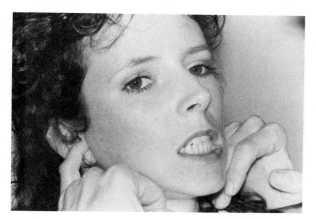

Figure 10–22. Palpation through the external auditory meatus, with the teeth together.

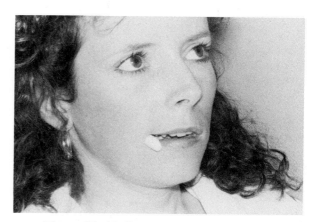

Figure 10–23. Dynamic loading the left TMJ.

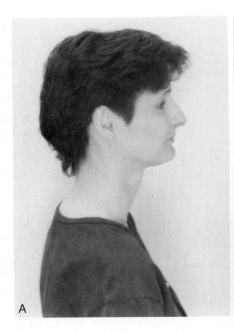
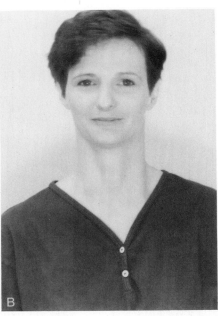

Figure 10–24. *A* and *B,* Forward head posturing with increased sternocleidomastoid tension bilaterally; levator scapula tension to the left; crossbite posterior to the right; hyoid tension; and decreased facial symmetry in the lower third of the face.

Dental occlusion should be briefly checked, although it is a complicated area for nondental professions. One should also check for malocclusion, loss of vertical dimension (Fig. 10–25), and bruxism. In addition, psychologic patterns of behavior should be noted, including anxiety, depression, and frustration. Although physical therapists and occupational therapists are not the professionals to perform psychologic evaluations, recognition of potential problems may be of vital importance for successful treatment of clients with TMJ.

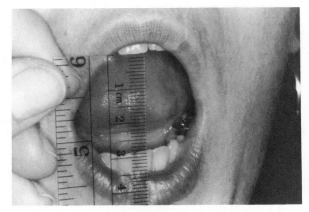

Figure 10–25. Measuring the vertical mandibular opening between the maxillary and mandibular incisal edges.

Another consideration in the evaluation of any musculoskeletal problem and particularly TMJ is that habitual overloading of the system will cause it to respond and adapt. Muscular atrophy resulting from disuse, immobilization, and starvation (i.e., lateral pterygoid) causing decreased contractile and sarcoplasm proteins must be considered. Atrophy occurs more quickly in the slow-twitch muscles than in the fast-twitch muscles. With unequal tone, shortening of the muscular tissues results in lengthening of other antagonistic groups. The joint then positions itself in a new angle where tensions are equal (Brooks, 1983). This adapted change in the tonic stretch reflexes affects reciprocal inhibition reflexes required to hold a joint in a physiologic position. Finally, gamma bias affecting muscle-spindle sensitivity results in poor sensory motor integration. Sensory perceptions are based on edited versions of the sensory input and are, therefore, the key to motor control.

CORRELATIONS OF FINDINGS

The questions to be answered in the correlation are: (1) What are the causative sources of irritation and (2) What is the optimal stimulus necessary for the desired tissue response? Treatment direction can therefore be defined.

Bony problems respond to compression or decompression because either one activates protein synthesis of the osteoclast and osteoblast. If the joint is not receiving optimal biomechanical energy in the line of stress, atrophy results (i.e., osteoporosis as evidenced in Skylab 4 Research). Bony problems may be the consequence of abnormal muscle compression, trauma from fracture, capsular tightness, or decreased range of motion. Wolff's law deals with the interaction between muscle function and bone development (Enlow, 1968).

Trauma from fracture and its possible consequences of degenerative joint disease have been previously discussed in the case of the 3-year-old. The earlier trauma is recognized and treated, the greater the chance of preventing dysfunction.

If capsular tightness is at fault, then decreased blood flow is noted in the capsule with less oxygen supply and nutrients. This in turn causes a decreased amount of synovial fluid and waste product accumulation, leading to cartilage cell atrophy (Cotta and Puhl, 1978; Larrson and Thilander, 1964). This may initiate degenerative joint disease (Salter and Field, 1975). Clients often describe capsular tightness as feeling as though "their bite is off." Mechanoreceptor activity from the anterior joint capsule is affected, causing lack of proprioceptive feedback and increased supramandibular muscle activity and thus influencing initial tooth contact (Clark, 1976; Kraus, 1988).

Improper loading of the articular cartilage also affects its health. The optimal stimuli for regeneration of cartilage are intermittent compression and decompression with glide. Muscular function and balancing are optimal for influencing cartilage specifically to unload the cartilage but then at times also to apply the proper amount of compression and decompression (Mansour and Mow, 1972) along with gliding movements such as occur with lateral deviation and optimal amounts of mandibular opening.

Disc material is both cartilage and collagen (Hansson et al, 1977). Regeneration of this tissue is stimulated with modified tension in the line of stress with compression and decompression. Gliding techniques are not used because they create shearing. Obviously, disc material is not easy to regenerate, but these are the optimal conditions for it. Therefore, proper posturing of the head and neck as well as optimal occlusion and muscle function are vital for disc health.

Muscle, tendon, ligament, and collagen tissue respond to modified tension in the line of stress. Inflammation results if the tension is too great, such as with hypertonicity of muscles or accumulation of habitual overload over time (Cummings and Tillmon, 1989), or if the force of tension is too sudden, as with whiplash.

Biochemical and biomechanical changes occur in the capsule when joint motion is lessened either completely or partially. Biomechanically, decreased water and glycosaminoglycan (GAG) results in less capsular lubrication via collagen fibers. Without the free gliding of the collagen fibers biomechanically, the capsule becomes tight. Classically, this is the response to immobilization (Akeson, 1961; Akeson et al, 1968 and 1980; Donarelli and Owens-Burkhart, 1981; Rocabado, 1981).

Massive concentrations of macrophage cells are present with trauma. These act as catalysts for fibroblastic activity, facilitating fibroblastic overproduction. Prostaglandin E is produced with macrophage cells in response to pain. This contributes to excessive fibroblastic activities. Adhesions begin forming within 2 to 3 days.

At approximately 4 to 14 weeks after injury, myofibroblasts become active, shortening or contracting the cross-links between the fibroblast (Cummings and Tillmon, 1989). Modified tension without pain in a line of stress is necessary along with modified tonic stretch reflex response so as to avoid inflammation. This may include gentle distraction of the atlanto-occipital joint to improve posterior cranial circulation and decrease phasic mandibular closure tension that results with forward-head posturing. Another consideration may be gravity-assisted lateral deviation of the mandible with gentle finger guidance on the mandible open to approximately 11 mm (the rest position). Finally, it may include shoulder elevation exercises to improve circulation and decrease levator scapulae tension.

The manual therapist can make a vital contribution toward primary healing. Knowing that modified tension in the line of stress stimulates GAG, production and original tissue regeneration can result. The half-life of GAG is 1.7 to 7 days, whereas the half-life of collagen fibers is 300 to 500 days. Therefore, early mobilization is most desirable.

If chronic inflammation persists for 7 to 8 months, irreversible covalent bondings occur. This tissue is avascular. Treatment options at this time are limited and without totally desirable affects. If progressive, prolonged stretch occurs, plastic elongation results along with hypermobility of the joint. Because GAG production decreases, hypermobility and lack of physiologic axis movement results, leading to degeneration. This scenario is not advisable.

Heating of the tissues to 40° C to melt cross-links of hydroxyglycine is not advisable either. Range of motion is gained, but it is hard on the tissues because protein coagulates at 44.4° C.

Therefore, the preferable method is early intervention with manual therapy procedures to increase elasticity and plasticity of tissues and scar, thus affecting increased protein synthesis and regeneration of tissues. This may be preceded by pain-control procedures including modalities such as ice, heat, ultrasound, electrical stimulation, transcutaneous electrical nerve stimulation application, spray and stretch, electromyographic relaxation techniques, and laser application. All of these modalities must be seen in terms of tissue response solicited by application. Certainly, compromises in plasticity of tissues and elasticity of fibers must be considered, especially if ultrasound is used. Excessive heating of the tissues, which may result from either ice or heat application, should also be considered for optimal tissue response.

Other considerations to be noted in the correlations are the possibility of different related tissue system involvement. These may include involvements in the levator scapulae. This muscle causes the cervical spine to sidebend, which creates a compensatory crossbite and scoliosis. Thoracolumbar compensation and TMJ symptoms are noted. However, the TMJ is not the cause of the symptoms. Another example is decreased atlanto-occipital space, which results in increased masseter and medial pterygoid tone as well as temporalis tension. TMJ symptoms are noted, but again the TMJ is not the cause. Omohyoid contraction and hypertonicity results in the scapula being protracted and elevated. The pectoralis minor brings the shoulder in a protracted position as well. Because of the omohyoids and the blendings with the deep cervical fascia and subclavius muscle, and because the sternocleidomastoid is a synergist, symptoms may be elicited from the TMJ, but again it is not the causative agent.

Also keep in mind that if the bite is opened 8 mm beyond the clinical rest position with splint therapy, the cervical spine will go into extension. This may cause both cervical and TMJ symptoms, but here again the TMJ is not the cause of these problems. With acquired tongue thrust, suboccipital muscle contraction accompanies swallow-

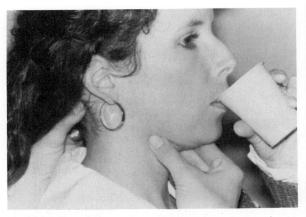

Figure 10–26. Evaluating for anterior tongue thrust. These are signs of altered swallowing sequence, possibly from forward head posturing, slow hyoid bone movement, contraction of the suboccipital muscles, head extension on the neck, excessive lip activity, or perception of the tongue pressing against the front teeth. A combination of these signs confirms altered swallowing.

ing (Fig. 10–26). If this is a severe tongue thrust, forward movements of the entire head and neck occur (Kraus, 1988). Again this results in TMJ symptoms, but TMJ is not the cause. Excessive lip activity is noted with tongue thrust as well. The treatment sequence should include correction of head on neck position and teaching normal sequence of swallowing.

TREATMENT, EXERCISES, AND ACTIVITIES OF DAILY LIVING INSTRUCTION

Treatment should be based on causative elements determined by a thorough examination of the upper quarter. This most likely will be accomplished via a team approach including medical, dental, psychologic, physical, occupational, and speech therapies.

The belief that malocclusion, loss of teeth, and occlusal interferences cause TMJ dysfunction is not consistently supported (Dworkin et al, 1990). Muscular imbalances have many different causes. In attributing occlusion to these imbalances of the upper quarter and TMJ dysfunction, one has failed to recognize much literature with contrary documentation.

Each person on the "team," including the professionals and the clients, should set goals before treatment initiation and should make these goals known to all. This ensures better communication and helps set a time line of expectations. Goals and time lines can be revised as necessary. This also makes a great difference in reimbursement, because progress can be quantified. Client commitment should be higher with set goals and expectations known among all.

The treatment is based on correlations of findings. It may include (1) proper tongue positioning to enhance swallowing, speech, and therefore physiologic joint position and alignment; (2) physiologic breathing instructions to enhance respiratory diaphragm function; (3) manual therapy to restore normal physiologic joint axes along with neuromuscular stabilization and functional synergies, taking into consideration the visual, perceptual, emotional, and physical aspects of the client's dysfunctions; (4) body mechanics instructions or the ''do's and don'ts.''

The list of ''do's'' should include the following: (1) Chew on both sides of the mouth when eating, not the same side constantly, (2) drink from a straw rather than a glass, (3) cut food, including sandwiches and apples, into small pieces and even slicing corn off the cob to control the bite, avoiding a forward position of the jaw; and (4) postural instructions in activities of daily living specific for each individual. For instance, most clients with TMJ protrude their chins, causing compensations in the neck and mandible; this should be avoided. Second, clients should avoid crossing their legs and position their feet flat on the floor to keep from slouching. Third, clients should stand with both feet even and with weight evenly distributed. Fourth, clients should sleep with a good supportive mattress for support of physiologic spinal curves, and they should use a pillow, preferably sleeping on the back and not the side because of pressure on the jaw. Fifth, if using a computer, observation of good posture must be observed and a good, ergonomic workstation should be created. Sixth, posture should be frequently checked in front of a mirror. Seventh, clients should check their breathing rhythm especially in stressful situations and while eating.

Included on the ''don't'' list are the following: (1) Do not hold the breath; (2) do not chew ice, (3) do not chew gum; (4) in acute and subacute stages, do not chew steaks, tough meats, potato chips, crispy tortillas, raw vegetables, hard bread, peanuts, lettuce, or any other chewy foods (avoiding tough, crunchy, or chewy foods will

decrease strains on the TMJ capsule) (Clark and Wyke, 1975); (5) do not rest the chin in the hand while sitting; (6) do not yawn widely, but control the yawn by positioning the fingertips below the chin; (7) do not hold the telephone on the shoulder; (8) do not carry heavy items on one side of the body; (9) do not fall asleep without proper neck support, especially in an airplane or automobile; (10) never open the jaw in a manner that will cause a pop, a click, or pain.

Beginning exercises and instruction in proper exercise for specific problems may include:

1. Stretching exercises in opening and in lateral deviation
2. Isometrics for opening and lateral deviation as well as protrusion and retrusion
3. Rhythmic stabilization or contract-relax techniques
4. Postural exercises and regular fitness training
5. Proprioceptive training exercises
6. Gentle long-axis distraction
7. Self-distraction (Rocabado, 1989).

The exercise program is designed for optimal tissue stimulation and optimal tissue response (Figs. 10–27 through 10–35).

Myofascial releases or craniosacral treatment enhances soft-tissue function and circulation. In the case of craniosacral rhythm facilitation and treatment, cerebrospinal fluid and circulation

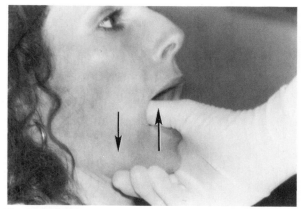

Figure 10–27. Distraction used for an evaluation or for treating distraction joint play; recapturing an anterior disc dislocation not reducing; unloading the joint to differentiate capsulitis or retrodiscitis. The force direction is the thumb pressure downward on the molars as the rest of the hand lifts up minimally on the anterior mandible.

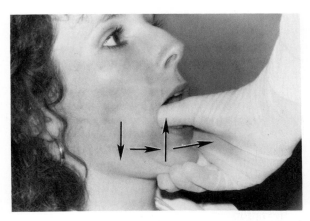

Figure 10–28. Translation with distraction used to evaluate and treat translation and distraction as joint play movements; recapturing an anterior disc dislocation not reducing, emphasizing translation; relocating a dislocated condyle. Translation is in the posterior direction; distraction is as previously described. The hand also pulls the mandible forward and minimally across the midline.

may be enhanced. Both of these treatment techniques prepare clients for more normalized musculoskeletal function by facilitating or inhibiting soft-tissue tone. These treatment techniques can be quite influential, and the desired outcome must be calculated before their use (Upledger and Vredgewood, 1983).

Pain modulation and control involve appropri-

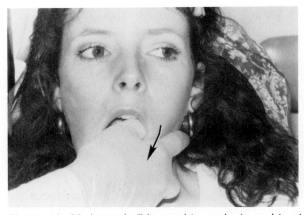

Figure 10–29. Lateral glide used to evaluate and treat lateral glide joint play movement. The force direction is with the thumb on the lingual side of the molars pressing buccally and slightly down and forward. The hand continues to pull the mandibular tip across the midline, in the opposite direction of the mobilized joint.

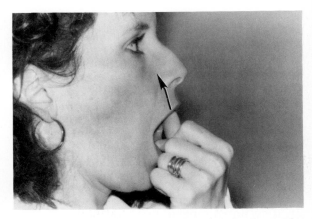

Figure 10–30. Active/passive exercise for increasing mandibular opening. Opening is active, then after relaxing, the thumb and index fingers apply a depression force to the mandible.

ate use of pain-control modalities previously discussed. Diaphragmatic breathing instruction and practice are vitally important for pain and stress control as well. Practitioners must keep in mind that the therapy will frequently involve dealing with the perception of pain. This was recognized long ago in the *Canterbury Tales* in the story of the faith healer.

There was a faith healer from Deal
Who said, although my pain is not real,
When I sit on a pin and it punctures my skin,
I dislike what I fancy I feel.

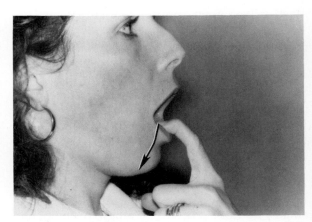

Figure 10–31. Active/passive exercise for increasing mandibular opening. After actively closing against the resistance of the index finger and relaxing, the index finger applies a depression force to the mandible.

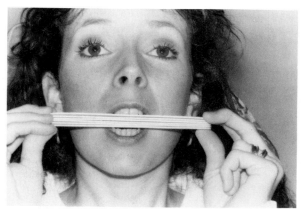

Figure 10–32. Active exercise to increase mandibular protrusion, supported with 11 mm of opening by tongue blades. Protrusion is done to increase translation. Unilateral translation may be worked on by protruding the mandible forward and opposite the side of the involved joint.

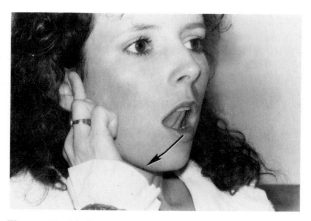

Figure 10–34. Proprioceptive retraining exercise to control excessive translation with use of the index finger on the lateral pole of the TMJ (progression from Figure 10–33).

Preventive exercises for avoiding TMJ dysfunction include proper tongue positioning in the upper soft palate, influencing the resting position of the joint and muscle tension; diaphragmatic breathing; and cervical posturing fostering physiologic lordosis and the avoidance of forward-head posturing, thus affecting resting-muscle tension. Exercises enhancing tongue position in the roof of the mouth include drinking through a straw, placing foods such as peanut butter on the roof of the mouth and swallowing, and holding small candies to the roof of the mouth. All of these techniques require tongue elevation while swallowing. Tongue-stretching exercises may be indicated at the time it is limited in its ability to protract or retract. This can be done using a wet washcloth. Contract-relax exercises can also be incorporated into these stretching techniques. Another exercise that may be valuable for enhancing correct swallowing and chewing patterns is lip stretching if the upper lip is short. Clients should stretch the upper lip down over the upper maxillary teeth and hold this position for at least a count of 10. Lip-strengthening exercises may involve the use of buttons

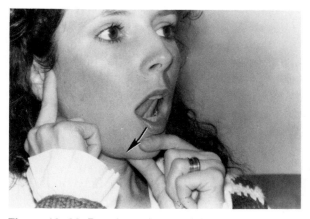

Figure 10–33. Proprioceptive retraining exercise to control excessive translation. The tongue is placed up against the palate; the index finger is placed lightly on the chin; and the other finger is placed on the lateral pole of the TMJ.

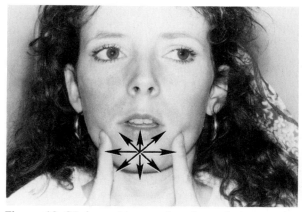

Figure 10–35. Isometric exercises to control excessive translation with the tip of the tongue up against the palate. The index fingers offer light resistance only in all directions.

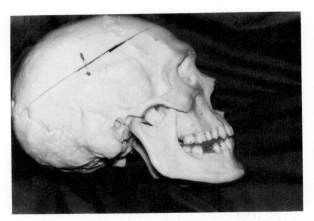

Figure 10–36. Example of a repositioning splint used to pull the mandible forward, opening the joint space, and for relocating the disc.

held between the lips and teeth, with elastic bands providing resistance from outside the mouth. This type of elastic strength may be used (Gelb, 1977). In addition, proper postural instructions should be given including postural awareness and clients' avoidance of overusing the accessory muscles of respiration and especially the sternocleidomastoids for controlling head-on-neck movements.

Therapists must understand dentists' splint therapy goals, which are to free up occlusion and unload muscles and the joint or affect disc position. There are multiple types of splints (Fig. 10–36). They can be positioned in a tripod, dipod, or unipod (Grummons, 1988) position or as modified pivotal appliances. It is most important that dentists convey their goals of treatment to clients and therapists as well as the expectations and length of time that clients should be involved in the splint therapy.

Diet and nutritional concerns are another area that is often forgotten in discussions of return to health and TMJ. A professional visit with a qualified nutritional counselor or dietitian is recommended.

Generally, foods with high complex carbohydrates derived from fruits or vegetables (ideally eaten fresh), moderate proteins, and low saturated fats are recommended (Nestle, 1987). Cooked foods should be prepared by broiling, baking, or pressure cooking or by crockpot preparation.

Foods and habits to avoid include:

Fried foods
Carbonated and alcoholic beverages
Fatty meats
Dairy products other than skim milk, buttermilk, and cottage cheese
Cakes, candy, pies, and other sweets
High-fat nuts, not including seed-type nuts
All caffeinated foods and drinks
Smoking
All hydrogenated fats (oleo, margarine, and hard cooking fats)
Cooked cabbage, brussels sprouts, and cauliflower because they produce gas

Foods to eat include:

Fresh juices
Cooked vegetables
Lean meats
Natural cereals
Bread, not including white bread
Brown rice
Fresh fruits
Fresh vegetable salads
Fresh vegetable oils (not hydrogenated)
Fresh fish and seafoods
Pastas

Another important area is stress management, which is largely avoided by many Americans. It reaches into near and remote corners of clients' lives and includes adjustment to changes. Clients' ability to adjust to change depends on their reactions, perception of the change, and the attitude toward the change.

Therapists need to be aware of clients' coping abilities. Wellness is nebulous in the face of perceived overwhelming stress. It is important to calm anxieties and fears and provide proper coping tools. Psychologic intervention and counseling by a licensed counselor or along with biofeedback may be of significant importance for wellness and recovery.

PREVENTION

Insurance groups pay for treatment in varying amounts of reimbursement. Many insurance companies are disallowing TMJ dysfunction claims altogether. How often a therapist treats an actual TMJ problem is debatable in view of the fact that there are so many opinions regarding the cause of the problem. Prevention or wellness is generally not in the realm of the game of the insurance provider. However, more and more corporations realize the necessity of providing wellness programs ("wellness equals prevention"). Therapists can be involved in community service wellness programs as paid professional consultants and as living examples.

Wellness and prevention challenge clients to be responsible and take control of their lives and health. Understanding and coping with stress-management tools as well as fitness conditioning and observing proper activities of daily living are excellent action plans.

It is ideal to promote prevention among parents with young school-age children, pediatricians, pediatric dentists, and adolescents. Young people's self-esteem, stress management, education, and physical fitness level contribute extraordinarily to their success in maturation as a contributing member of society. Perception of motor dysfunction has long been researched as a problem along with learning disabilities. More endeavors and correlations in these areas are necessary.

Education at an early age and clients' ability to control internal or external factors will help set lifetime aspirations of health. This may be the greatest gift that the health-care provider can provide to young persons.

Prevention in the workplace, home, office, or health club is important as well. Job analysis for the worker as well as education of proper body mechanics and posturing is vital to health management, both in function and dysfunction. (Preventive tips can be found under the Treatment, Exercises, and Activities of Daily Living Instruction section of this chapter.)

The biggest question looming in prevention of TMJ is "What tips the scale to TMJ dysfunction if structure is nonphysiologic or less than ideal?" Many individuals of all ages, sizes, and shapes are functioning without pain because their bodies have had time to adapt and compensate for their structural shortcomings. They will, most likely, functionally stay in homeostasis with their environments, internal and external, unless a significant life stressor assaults and upsets their system.

CONCLUSIONS

It is imperative for clients to receive the proper diagnosis for early treatment and intervention. This early treatment should be correct and based on a full subjective and objective evaluation, along with correlation of the findings for optimal treatment planning for desired effects and results. It is equally important to set goals and expectations on a time line for clients and to communicate these goals to the team of health-care providers. This ensures greater client commitment and responsibility toward healthiness and continued wellness. It is also equally important to re-evaluate and assess goal completions and expectations to ensure that clients have not plateaued and that proper treatment is being derived for the money spent.

Therapists have vital roles in prevention and treatment of TMJ dysfunction, especially in this aspect of such a large function. The TMJ is used over 1,500 times a day for swallowing, not to mention speech and eating functions.

Wellness programs include more client or potential client involvement and responsibility. They have heavy implications for society and sociologic, psychologic, family, and ergonomic health. Young people need to develop self-esteem and responsibility along with musculoskeletal health, good posturing, stress management, and fitness programs. Adults largely need the same. Although this is rather simply stated, regardless of age, every person needs the same relative survival tools psychologically and physically. Individuals merely adapt as best as their system allows with aging. The challenge of the health professional is to enhance well-being and health for those persons seeking help.

Acknowledgments

I offer special thanks to Gayle V. Voth and Ola Grimsby for their technical advice and to Richard R. Riggs for photography.

References

Akeson WH: An experimental study of joint stiffness. J Bone Joint Surg (Am) 43:1022, 1961.

Akeson WH, Amiel D, LaViolette D, et al: The connective tissue response to immobility: An accelerated aging response. Exp Gerontol 3:289, 1968.

Akeson WH, Amiel D, and Woo S: Immobility effects of synovial joints: The pathomechanics of joint contracture. Bromheology 17:95, 1980.

Benson F: TMJ Disorders Management of the Craniomandibular Complex. New York, Churchill Livingstone, 1988.

Brooks VB: How posture and movements are governed. Phys Ther 63(5):664–673, 1983.

Bushey R: Adenoid obstruction of nasopharynx. In McNamara JA (ed): Naso-Respiratory Function and Craniofacial Growth, Craniofacial Growth Series, monograph no. 9. Ann Arbor, University of Michigan, Center for Human Growth and Development, 1979.

Carlsoo S: Nervous coordination and mechanical function of the mandibular elevators: An electromyographic study of the activity and an anatomic analysis of mechanics of the muscles. Acta Odontol Scand 11:1, 1952.

Carr S: TMJ Symptoms and Solutions. Dallas, Texas, Myodata, 1990.

Clark R: Neurology of the temporomandibular joints: An experimental study. Ann R Coll Surg Engl 58:43, 1976.

Clark RKF and Wyke BD: Contributions of temporomandibular articular mechanoreceptors to the control of mandibular posture: An experimental study. J Dent 2:121, 1974.

Clark RKF and Wyke BD: Temporomandibular arthrokinetic reflex control of the mandibular musculature. Br J Oral Surg 13:196, 1975.

Cotta H and Puhl W: The pathophysiology of damage to articular cartilage. Prog Orthop Surg 3:20, 1978.

Cummings G and Tillmon L: Inflammation in the Development of Postimmobilization Contractures. Atlanta, Dogwood Conference, 1989.

Cyriax J: Diagnosis of Soft Tissue Lesions. Textbook of Orthopedic Medicine. London, Balliere Tindal, 1981.

Donarelli R and Owens-Burkhart H: Effects of immobilization on the extensibility of periarticular connective tissue. J Orthop Sports Phys Ther 3:67, 1981.

DuBrul EL: Sicher's Oral Anatomy, 7th ed. St. Louis, CV Mosby, 1980.

Dworkin SF, LaResche L, and Truelove E: Epidemiology of signs and symptoms in temporomandibular disorders: Clinical signs in cases and controls. J Am Dent Assoc 120(3):288, 1990.

Enlow DH: Handbook of Facial Growth. Philadelphia, WB Saunders, 1982.

Enlow DH: Wolff's law and the factor of architectonic circumstance. Am J Orthod 54:803, 1968.

Farrar WB: Craniomandibular practice: The state of the art definition and diagnosis. J Craniomandib Prac 1:1, 1982.

Fricton JR, Bromaghim C, and Hathaway KM: Interdisciplinary management of patients with TMJ and craniofacial pain: Characteristics and outcome. J Craniomandib Dis: Facial Oral Pain 1(2):115, 1987.

Friedman MH and Weisberg J: TMJ Disorders. Chicago, Quintessence, 1985.

Gelb H: Clinical Management of Head, Neck and TMJ Pain and Dysfunction: A Multidisciplinary Approach to Diagnosis and Treatment. Philadelphia, WB Saunders, 1977.

Grimsby O: Advanced cervical, thoracic and temporomandibular manual therapy (Course notes). Dallas, Sorlandets Fysikalske Institut, 1987.

Grimsby O: Temporomandibular Dysfunction. J Manuell Terapi issued by Noreisk Spesialgruptte for Manuell Terapi, 1987.

Grummons D: Orthodontic dysfunction finishing procedures. Lecture at the Second World Conference of International College for Craniofacial and Vertebral Therapeutics, Atlanta, 1989.

Grummons D: Stabilizing the occlusion: Finishing procedures TMJ disorders—Management of the Craniomandibular Complex. New York, Churchill Livingstone, 1988.

Hansson T, Carlson GE, Oberg T, et al: Thickness of the soft tissue layers and the articular disc in the temporomandibular joint. Acta Odontol Scand 35:77, 1977.

Harvold EP: Experiments on mandibular morphogenesis. In McNamara JA (ed): Determinants of Mandibular Form and Growth, Craniofacial Growth Series, monograph no. 4. Ann Arbor, University of Michigan, Center for Human Development and Growth, 1975a.

Harvold EP: Normal and morphological adaptations in experimentally induced oral respiration. In McNamara JA (ed): Naso-Respiratory Function and Craniofacial Growth, Craniofacial Growth Series, monograph no. 9. Ann Arbor, University of Michigan, Center for Growth and Development, 1975b.

Harvold EP, Chierici G, and Vargervik K: Experiments on the development of malocclusion. Am J Orthod 61:38, 1972.

Harvold EP, Vargevik K, and Chierici G: Primate experiments on oral sensation and dental malocclusion. Am J Orthod 61:38, 1972.

Keith DA: Development of the human temporomandibular joint. Br J Oral Surg 20:217, 1982.

Keleman S: Emotional Anatomy. Berkeley, CA, Center Press, 1985.

Keleman S: Your Body Speaks Its Mind. Berkeley, CA, Center Press, 1975.

Korr IM: The Facilitated Segment: A Factor in Injury to the Body Framework. The Collected Papers of Irvin M. Korr. Newark, Ohio, American Academy of Osteopathy, 1979.

Kraus S: Physical Therapy Management of TMJ Dysfunction, TMJ Disorders—Management of the Craniomandibular Complex. New York, Churchill Livingstone, 1988.

Kraus SL: Cervical Spine and Craniomandibular Relationships. Lecture at the Second World Conference of International College for Craniofacial and Vertebral Therapeutics, Atlanta, 1989.

Larrson L and Thilander B: Mandibular positioning: The effect of pressure on joint capsule. Acta Neurol Scand 40:131, 1964.

Lowen A: Bioenergetics. New York, Penguin Books, 1975.

Mahan PE, Gibbs CH, Wilkinson TM, et al: Superior and inferior bellies of lateral pterygoid muscle: EMG activity at basic jaw positions. J Prosthet Dent 50:589, 1983.

Manns A, Miraldes R, and Palazzi C: EMG bite force and elongation of the masseter muscle under isometric normal voluntary contractions and variations of vertical dimensions. J Prosthet Dent 42:159, 1979.

Mansour JM and Mow VC: The permeability of articular cartilage under compressive strain and at high pressure. J Bone Joint Surg 53:59, 1972.

Marks MB: Allergy in relation to orofacial dental deformities in children: A review. J Allergy 36:293, 1965.

McNamara JA Jr: The independent function of the two heads of the lateral pterygoid muscle. Am J Anat 138:242, 1973.

Moffett BC: The morphogenesis of the temporomandibular joint. Am J Orthod 52:401, 1966.

Moffett BC Jr, Askew HC, Johnson LC, et al: Articular remodeling in the adult human temporomandibular joint. Am J Anat 115(1):116, 1964.

Morgan DH, Hall WP, and Vamvas VJ: Diseases of the Temporomandibular Apparatus. St Louis, CV Mosby, 1977.

Neff PA: Occlusion and Function: A Teaching Aid, 4th ed. Washington, DC, Georgetown University, 1980.

Nestle M: What should Americans eat? From public policy to patient care. J Craniomandib Dis: Facial Oral Pain 1(2):123–126, 1987.

Nordin M: Biomechanics in Theory and Practice. Lecture at the Second World Conference of International College for Craniofacial and Vertebral Therapeutics, Atlanta, 1989.

Pinto OF: A new structure related to the TMJ and middle ear. J Prosthet Dent 12:95, 1962.

Rees LA: The structure and function of the mandibular joint. Br Dent J 96:125, 1954.

Rickets R: Respiratory obstructive syndrome. Am J Orthod 54:495, 1968.

Rocabado M: Biomechanical Effect of Periarticular Connective Tissue (Course notes). Santiago, Chile, Rocabado Institute, 1981.

Rocabado M: Physical Therapy for the Postsurgical Maxillofacial Patient. Lecture at the Second World Conference of the International College for Craniofacial and Vertebral Therapeutics, Atlanta, 1989.

Salter RB and Field P: The effects of continuous compression on living articular cartilage: An experimental investigation. J Bone Joint Surg *57A*:570, 1975.

Sicker H: Oral Anatomy, 7th ed. St Louis, CV Mosby, 1949.

Smith L and Ware L: Embryology applied anatomy and physiology. *In* Bluestone C (ed): Pediatric Otolaryngology, Vol 2. Philadelphia, WB Saunders, 1972.

Symons NBB: The development of the human mandibular joint. J Anat *86*:326, 1952.

Taylor A, Bosley MA, and Cody FW: Histochemical and mechanical properties of the jaw muscles of a cat. Exp Neurol *38*:281, 1973.

Terezhalmy GT, Pellen GB Jr, and Ross GR: The language of pain associated with temporomandibular joint—myofascial pain dysfunction syndrome. Ear Nose Throat J *61*:620–625, 1982.

Upledger JE and Vredgewood JD: Craniosacral Therapy. Seattle, Eastland Press, 1983.

Wilson ES and Schneider CJ: The Origin of Pain and Its Perpetuating Factors. Human Adaptivity—A Primer of Psychobiology. Unpublished manuscript, 1987.

Wright DM and Moffett BC: The post-natal development of the human temporomandibular joint. Am J Anat *141*:235, 1974.

Wyke BD: Articular neurology—a review. Physiotherapy *58*:94, 1972.

C H A P T E R

11

Rodney S. Taylor

Prevention for Cardiac Patients

Coronary heart disease (CHD) has had the dubious reputation as one of the most prevalent causes of mortality of our times. In recent years, a leveling off or fall in the rate of CHD mortality has begun in many countries. For instance, since 1968, both the United States and United Kingdom have reduced their CHD death rates by 53% and 12%, respectively, among individuals aged 35 to 74 years (World Health Organization, 1982). Although the precise explanation for this decrease has not been fully established, advances in surgical and medical treatment have certainly contributed to some extent. Moreover, the results of primary prevention studies suggest that lifestyle modifications, such as reduced smoking behavior and better dietary habits and physical activity patterns, lead to a reduction in cardiac risk factors, thereby contributing to a lower CHD mortality rate (Multiple Risk Factor Intervention Trial Research Group, 1982).

Despite these encouraging declines in CHD mortality, the cost of the long-term effects of CHD remains high. Survivors of myocardial infarction (MI) often have problems such as emotional distress and difficulty in returning to work and to a normal pattern of social life, and they experience excessive caution in physical activities (Mayou, 1979). Angina pectoris sufferers' lifestyle is limited considerably by the recurring onset of chest pain at times of physical and mental strain. The economic costs of the long-term effects of CHD are equally dismal. It has been estimated that illness through CHD in the United Kingdom is responsible for 12% of all lost working days, which in 1987 accounted for some 40 million days at an enormous cost in lost earnings (Coronary Prevention Group, 1990). The annual cost of cardiovascular disease in United States, including medical treatment and labor output losses, has been calculated at approximately $85 billion (American Heart Association, 1987). This drain on economic resources and reduction in quality of life emphasizes the importance of a structured program of long-term care program for cardiac clients.

The last 10 to 20 years have seen the inception and development of a number of cardiac rehabilitation programs throughout the world. The aims of these programs have been both secondary and tertiary prevention; in other words, to reduce the incidence of mortality and morbidity in clients with CHD as well as to restore cardiac clients to optimal levels of physiologic, psychosocial, educational, and vocational function (Wenger, 1986). A 3-year phase approach has been adopted by many cardiac prevention centers. An inpatient (phase I) program is begun in the hospital, usually in the coronary care unit. An outpatient (phase II) program is initiated within a few weeks after discharge from the hospital. Clients completing the outpatient program are encouraged to begin a home or unsupervised community-based program (phase III). Some centers may provide only one or two of these phases.

Studies have used differing measures of outcome to evaluate the effectiveness of cardiac prevention programs. Nine controlled trials have measured changes in cardiac mortality. In only one of these studies was there a statistically significant reduction in mortality. Pooling the results of these studies has shown that prevention program clients have a significantly lower (32%) mortality compared with controls who receive conventional cardiac treatment (May et al, 1982). Although these results indicate that the efficacy of cardiac prevention in terms of secondary prevention is still rather equivocal, in terms of tertiary prevention, they have been extremely encouraging. A number of studies have demonstrated significant benefits in terms of exercise capacity (Taylor, 1990), psychologic well-being (Sanne, 1977), risk factor levels, and rate of return to work and to previous social and recreational lifestyles (Coronary Prevention Group, 1989).

Clearly, in a relatively short space of time, there has been considerable development of cardiac prevention both in terms of service provision and measurable benefit to clients. However, surveys suggest that there is still a lack of standardization in program content among different centers and there is considerable need for additional programs (Greene et al, 1988; Kellerman, 1982; Taylor and Taylor, 1991). The purpose of this chapter is to describe the structure and organization of a comprehensive outpatient (phase II) cardiac prevention program based on the experience of the Exeter cardiac prevention program in the United Kingdom.

PROGRAM OVERVIEW

Content

Traditionally, outpatient cardiac prevention programs have principally been based on exercise therapy. However, the American College of Physicians, American College of Sports Medicine, and British Cardiac Prevention Group have recommended that cardiac prevention programs be comprehensive and also include components such as risk-factor education, vocational counseling, and psychologic support (American College of Physicians, 1980; American College of Sports Medicine, 1980; Coronary Prevention Group, 1989). The Exeter cardiac prevention program is based on three principle components:

1. Exercise and activity prescription
2. Education
3. Stress management

The theoretical basis and practical details of each of these three components are discussed later in this chapter.

Objectives

The overall aim of cardiac prevention is to optimize the physical, psychologic, and sociologic recovery of clients with CHD (World Health Organization, 1985). The specific objectives of the Exeter program are:

1. Physical: to enhance clients' levels of fitness and to teach clients to recognize their physical limitations
2. Educational: to provide information on CHD and its contributory factors and to encourage clients to recognize cardiac risk factors and modify their lifestyle accordingly
3. Psychologic: to provide emotional support and counseling and to teach clients to recognize stress and use relaxation therapy

Duration and Location

Outpatient cardiac prevention programs usually last 10 to 12 weeks. These programs generally meet on a supervised basis 2 to 3 times per week in a hospital outpatient facility or a free-standing setting with medical support, such as a university or clinic. This program duration has been based on evidence of exercise-related outcomes; a number of studies demonstrated an increase in exercise tolerance in programs lasting 10 to 12 weeks (Taylor, 1990). Nevertheless there is a need for flexibility and, in specific cases if judged appropriate by the program staff, a longer duration may be required for clients with particular difficulties.

Patient Referral

Entrance to phase II begins with a written referral usually from the client's attending hospital physician. Obtaining client background details from hospital records after referral can be extremely time consuming for the program staff. Therefore, a standard form should be considered for referring physicians that includes a summary of client's medical history, current clinical status, and medication details. A significant proportion of the Exeter program referrals came from the clients' general practitioners (i.e., community-based physicians). The referring physicians must be clearly informed of the program rationale, content, and objectives as well as details of client eligibility.

Client Eligibility

Clients are generally considered eligible for outpatient cardiac prevention if they have to meet one of following criteria:

1. Documented MI
2. Coronary artery bypass or angioplasty
3. Stable angina pectoris

A number of studies demonstrated that each of these CHD diagnosis groups benefits from a program of cardiac prevention (American Association of Cardiovascular and Pulmonary Rehabilitation, 1980). It is important that outpatient cardiac prevention starts as soon after hospital discharge as possible. However, all clients should be medically stable. Two to 4 days of recovery for post-MI clients and 1 to 2 days for coronary bypass surgery clients is advised. Clients can begin cardiac prevention virtually immediately after angioplasty. Surveys have shown that most cardiac prevention programs begin clients with CHD within 1 month of discharge (Davidson et al, 1989).

Patient Selection

Many individuals believe that performing exercise is associated with increased risk of cardiac arrest and death in both noncardiac and cardiac individuals. A comprehensive survey of 30 cardiac prevention programs found that the incidence of exercise complications among cardiac clients was relatively low (i.e., 1 arrest and 1 death per 33,000 and 120,000 patient-hours of activity, respectively) (Haskell, 1978). Nevertheless, this risk is considerably higher than for noncardiac exercise training (i.e., 1 death per 1,125,000 patient-hours of activity) (Haskell,

1978). Moreover, prevention programs have reduced the incidence of complications by excluding both clients with exercise contraindications and high-risk clients. A number of contraindications to exercise, both relative and absolute, have been published (American College of Sports Medicine, 1980). These contraindications include unstable angina, uncompensated heart failure, uncontrolled arrhythmias or hypertension, and severe aortic stenosis. Many cardiac clients are normally required to perform a graded exercise test either just before or shortly after their hospital discharge or as part of their general medical management. The results of these tests greatly assist in identification of high-risk cardiac clients. Using the recommendations of the American Health Association Committee on Exercise (American Heart Association, 1975), the Exeter program considers clients to be at high risk if they have one or more of the following exercise test features:

1. Functional capacity of less than 5 metabolic equivalents
2. Marked, exercise-induced ischemia as indicated by appearance of 2 mm (or more) ST depression by electrocardiogram
3. Decrease in systolic blood pressure of 15 mm Hg or more with exercise
4. Ventricular arrhythmias appearing or increasing with exercise

Although high-risk clients are often excluded from the exercise-training component of a cardiac prevention program, some centers do allow them to participate in the nonexercise components of their program. It is equally important to note that an increasing number of prevention centers, with well-developed electrocardiogram-monitoring capabilities, are prepared to admit high-risk clients into the exercise training component of their program.

Some programs also use other noncardiac reasons for excluding clients, such as a history of orthopedic problems, age, lack of transport, and poor motivation (Davidson et al, 1989). It is important to develop a set of client-selection guidelines that meets the needs of a particular center.

EXERCISE PRESCRIPTION

One of the most significant effects of CHD is a reduction in physical functional capacity. The gold-standard measure of functional capacity is maximum oxygen uptake (VO$_2$max). Studies have found that the VO$_2$max of cardiac clients is considerably lower than that of sedentary, aged-matched subjects (Blomquist, 1974). Reasons for this diminution in VO$_2$max include myocardial muscle damage after infarction, anginal pain on exertion, and deconditioning as the result of both immobilization and a reduction in daily physical activity (Nagle, 1989).

A reduction in client's functional capacity will considerably lower their exercise and physical activity tolerance, decrease general self-confidence, and therefore significantly compromise quality of life. The basis of the exercise program of cardiac prevention programs is to improve functional capacity by a program of individualized training prescription.

Aerobic Exercise Training

An exercise-training program can be designed for increasing muscle strength, muscular endurance, and functional capacity. Isometric (or resistance) exercise results in an increase in muscular strength. It involves developing muscular tension against resistance without movement. Although this results in an increase in muscular mass along with strength, there is limited evidence to indicate similar benefits to the circulatory system. Isometric exercise places considerable pressure load on the heart and has a marked effect on mean arterial blood pressure (Lind and McNicol, 1975). Dynamic exercise involves a rhythmic movement of large muscle groups and requires increased oxygen consumption; examples include walking, jogging, swimming, and cycling. Such exercise is also called aerobic because it must be performed with sufficient oxygen present. Aerobic training is associated with circulatory adaptations. Because of the circulatory benefits of regular aerobic exercise and pressure risk associated with resistance exercise, cardiac prevention programs have traditionally been based on aerobic training.

Benefits of Aerobic Training

Extensive investigation has shown beyond reasonable doubt that aerobic training can improve the VO$_2$max of clients with CHD and thereby increase functional capacity (Clausen, 1976).

Whereas in noncardiac individuals the improvement in functional capacity is associated with enhanced cardiac function, in clients with CHD much of the improvement is due to changes in the peripheral circulation that make better use of the cardiac function available (Thompson, 1988). In addition, aerobic training studies also consistently observed reductions in heart rate and blood pressure at any given submaximal level of work (Taylor, 1990). Myocardial oxygen requirements depend mainly on heart rate and systolic blood pressure. A reduction of these variables by physical training can thus enhance the exercise and physical activity capacity of people who have angina pectoris by increasing the threshold for chest pain. In addition to these effects on the circulation, exercise training can have a number of other beneficial effects for cardiac clients, such as a reduction in blood lipid levels, improvements in body composition, and enhanced psychosocial well-being (Coronary Prevention Group, 1989).

Patient Monitoring

Although, as previously described, the risk of complications in cardiac exercise-training programs has been shown to be relatively low, client monitoring is considered to be an important adjunct to program safety (American College of Sports Medicine, 1980; American Heart Association, 1975). Considerable variability in monitoring procedures is known to exist across various cardiac prevention programs. Some outpatient programs provide continuous electrocardiographic monitoring. Such a degree of monitoring has been questioned in terms of both high cost and unproved efficacy. A survey of the monitoring methods of various prevention programs found that the use of continuous electrocardiographic monitoring did not improve the rate of cardiac complication (Van Camp and Petersen, 1986). Thus, the arbitrary continuous electrocardiographic monitoring of all cardiac clients does not appear to be warranted. Indeed, it has been suggested that only a small proportion of high-risk clients require such monitoring (Greenland and Pomilla, 1989).

Although in the case of low-risk cardiac clients the need for continuous electrocardiographic monitoring is questionable, some degree of monitoring still remains appropriate. The maintenance of an appropriate training intensity of cardiac training programs depends on the monitoring of heart rate. In addition, arterial blood pressure measurement enables the hemodynamic response to exercise to be assessed. The development of inexpensive heart-rate and blood-pressure monitors has made such monitoring both practical and cost-effective. Client involvement and commitment to an exercise-training program can be substantially enhanced by directing clients to record their heart-rate and blood-pressure values in an exercise log. An exercise log is also extremely valuable in assessing training progress.

Emergency equipment should be readily available throughout the program, including a defibrillator, monitor, drug supplies, oxygen, and other general resuscitation equipment (American College of Sports Medicine, 1980).

Training Prescription

Training prescription is generally defined in terms of four elements: mode of exercise and the duration, frequency, and intensity of each exercise session. Training prescription should be individualized for each client.

Mode of Exercise. Aerobic exercise includes dynamic activities such as running, walking, cycling, and swimming. When the exercise duration, frequency, and intensity are comparable, these activities appear to be equally effective modes of training (Pollock et al, 1975). Because of the relatively high-intensity and high-impact nature of jogging, it has been recommended that this activity be initially avoided by cardiac prevention programs (Pollock and Wilmore, 1990). The relative consistency of oxygen expenditure in walking and static cycling lends these activities particularly well to exercise prescription for cardiac clients.

Duration. A minimum exercise duration of 10 to 15 minutes is generally required for improvements in functional capacity. Studies have shown that 30-minute sessions are even more effective, but there is little additional benefit beyond this point. Moreover, longer training sessions (45 minutes or more) are associated with a disproportionate incidence of orthopedic injury (Pollock et al, 1977). To prevent injury and overfatigue, session duration should be increased gradually over the period of the program.

Frequency. Although deconditioned cardiac clients may demonstrate circulatory benefits with only twice-weekly exercise, three to five sessions per week appear to present the optimal training frequency. Additional benefits of more than five sessions per week appear to be minimal, whereas the incidence of injury increases markedly (Pollock et al, 1977). Exercise should be scheduled so that no more than 2 days elapse between successive sessions.

Intensity. Probably the most important element of exercise prescription is training intensity. The risk of cardiovascular complication is considerably greater with high-intensity exercise in comparison with moderate- or low-intensity exercise (Hellerstein and Franklin, 1984). It is therefore widely accepted that the prescription of training intensity (and adherence to this prescription) is an important determinant of the safety of cardiac prevention programs. Nevertheless, it is important to emphasize that training intensity requires one to be above a certain minimal level to achieve cardiovascular adaptation.

During the initial period of a training program, it is recommended that a relatively low exercise intensity be prescribed. The most common guideline for estimating the upper limit of training intensity is 20 to 30 beats/min above standing resting heart rate (Pollock and Schmidt, 1986). After this initial period, cardiac training intensity can follow the American College of Sports Medicine exercise-training recommendation for healthy adults of 60 to 85% of heart rate reserve (American College of Sports Medicine, 1980). Training intensity should progress so that 85% is achieved only in the later stages of training.

The exercise prescription guidelines of the Exeter cardiac prevention program, which are based on these principles, are shown in Table 11–1.

Determining Client Training Intensity

As previously described, aerobic training intensity is often assessed in terms of percentage of heart rate reserve (%HRR), also known as the Karvonen method after the author who first described it (Karvonen et al, 1957). The HRR method takes into account clients' resting and maximal heart rates. It has the advantage of being nearly identical to the same percentage of maximal VO_2max used during exercise testing. The following example illustrates the calculation of training heart rate prescription of 60 to 70%HRR for a 45-year-old client with a maximal heart rate of 175 and a resting heart rate of 60 beats/min.

Table 11–1. Exercise Prescription Guidelines of Exeter Program

Training Stage	Session Duration	Session Frequency	Session Intensity	
Weeks 1–2	15 min	3/wk	RHR* + 30	beats/min
Weeks 3–5	20 min	3/wk	60–70	%HRR†
Weeks 6–8	30 min	4/wk	60–70	%HRR†
Weeks 9–12	40 min	4/wk	70–85	%HRR†

*RHR = resting heart rate.
†%HRR = percentage of heart rate reserve.

Heart rate reserve formulas:
Training HR = resting HR + (%effort ×
(maximum HR − resting HR)).

That is,

60 + (60% × (175 − 60)) = 129 beats/min.
60 + (70% × (175 − 60)) = 140 beats/min.

This client would therefore be directed to maintain the exercise heart rate above 129 beats/min but below 140 beats/min throughout training. If a value of maximal heart rate is not available from exercise testing, it can be predicted on the basis of a client's age (maximal heart rate = 220 − age in years).

Exercise and resting heart rates are usually monitored using either the carotid pulse or radial pulse. Often clients need considerable practice before they can assess exercise pulse accurately. A number of accurate, relatively inexpensive, and easy-to-use monitors are now commercially available. In the first weeks of exercise training, it is often useful to provide clients with such monitors until they become confident in taking their pulse.

Certain cardiac medications markedly influence heart rate. For instance, beta blockers reduce both resting and exercise heart rates. Clients on such medication are therefore not able to readily use the heart rate method to determine training intensity. The rating of perceived exertion is a useful and important alternative to heart rate as an intensity guide to exercise training. The rate of perceived exertion scale, first introduced by Borg (1967), consists of 15 grades from 6 (very, very light) to 20 (very, very hard). In the early stages of entry in the cardiac prevention program, it is recommended that clients exercise at a rating of 12 to 13 (somewhat hard). At later stages of training, ratings of 13 to 15 (hard) are appropriate, which has been shown to be equivalent to 60 to 80% HRR (Hage, 1981).

Circuit Training

Many adult fitness and cardiac prevention programs are solely based on leg training, such as walking, jogging, or cycling. Such programs are limited in scope and fail to consider that daily living activities use both upper and lower muscle groups. Many occupations require mostly arm work. Traditionally, upper extremity exercises were not included in cardiac prevention programs because it was believed that they produced ischemic changes and increased myocardial irritability, a belief that has been unsubstantiated in recent investigations (Fardy et al, 1977). There is little transfer of training adaptation between upper and lower extremity muscle groups (Saltin, 1973). Therefore, to improve upper and lower limb efficiency necessary for everyday life, cardiac prevention programs must include exercises that use muscle groups in both limbs.

Circuit training by definition involves the use of multiple exercise stations. An individual exercises at a station for a particular period of time and then moves on to the next station. Circuit training has the advantage of allowing both upper and lower limb dynamic exercise. Upper and lower limb exercise stations should be scheduled in sequence to minimize local muscular fatigue. An aerobic training effect depends on a sustained increase in heart rate during dynamic exercise. Because heart rate can fall considerably in moving from one exercise station to the next, the duration of this recovery should be kept to a minimum and clients should walk between stations. The organization of an exercise-training circuit of the Exeter program is shown in Figure 11–1.

In addition to allowing both upper and lower exercises, circuit training can have benefits in terms of both training compliance and program safety. The various exercise stations of circuit training provide variety and prevent the boredom and poor compliance often associated with

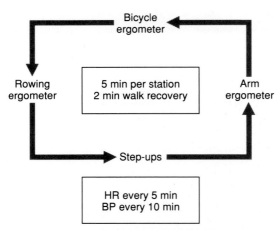

Figure 11–1. Exercise circuit of Exeter program.

single-mode exercise sessions. The recovery period between successive exercise stations provides a time during which monitoring, such as blood pressure and electrocardiogram, can be performed. As outlined earlier, the maintenance of client monitoring during exercise is an important element of program safety.

Warm-Up and Cool-Down

Warming up before and cooling down after an exercise session are normal features of any training program. Although the risk of cardiac complication in cardiac prevention programs is relatively low, evaluation of the timing of these complications has shown that they tend to occur most commonly during the warm-up and cool-down phases of exercise (Haskell, 1978). These results strongly suggest that the cool-down and warm-up periods are particularly important elements to be considered in the safety of a cardiac prevention program.

A warm-up normally consists of both stretching and cardiorespiratory elements. Stretching exercises develop and maintain flexibility as well as prepare muscles, joints, and ligaments for the additional stress of aerobic exercise. It is also believed that stretching is important in reducing the risk of orthopedic injury such as muscle strain, low back discomfort, and muscle soreness to some extent. Stretching exercises are relatively standard and are described in detail elsewhere (Fardy et al, 1988). The cardiorespiratory element of a warm-up increases circulation, prepares the cardiovascular system for exercise, and, most

important, reduces the potential for exercise-induced ischemic responses such as angina or even MI. A gradual progression of effort probably increases coronary circulation and oxygen supply in line with the increased myocardial demand (Bernard et al, 1973). A circulatory warm-up should include aerobic activity performed at lower intensity than prescribed for training, for example, slow walking or cycling at an intensity. Heart rate should be checked just before beginning aerobic training to ensure adequate warm-up.

The cool-down period is equal to the warm-up in importance. Abrupt cessation of activity after the completion of an aerobic training session will result in a pooling of blood and a decrease in venous return, possibly reducing coronary blood flow when heart rate and myocardial oxygen demands may still be high (Dimsdale et al, 1984). Thus, symptoms may include angina, palpitations (as a result of ventricular dysrhythmias), syncope, and nausea. Continued movement after aerobic exercise will enhance venous return and prevent these related consequences. Exercises such as slow walking and easy cycling are also appropriate for the cool-down phase. Postexercise activity can also help to prevent extreme muscle soreness. This is particularly true if the cool-down period includes selected stretching exercises. After a training session, clients should be advised to take a warm, not hot, shower, because hot showers after aerobic exercise can add to any postexercise complications as a result of peripheral vasodilation.

Home-Based Exercise

A number of outpatient programs involve clients performing unsupervised exercise sessions at home; some centers offer a complete program of home-based exercise training. However, most centers offer a specific number of home-based training sessions in conjunction with a supervised exercise program. These latter cardiac prevention programs normally exercise as a supervised group only once or twice per week. Additional home-based sessions are therefore required to achieve an adequate training stimulus. It is well established that cardiac clients can increase functional capacity by participating in home-based exercise training as they can in supervised sessions (Houston-Miller et al, 1984). To maintain the safety of home exercise, it is recommended that it be limited to low-risk clients. In addition, emphasis should be placed on the importance of adherence to the exercise prescription, especially exercise intensity. Clients must be taught how to monitor their heart rate accurately and to recognize untoward signs and symptoms. Records of exercise heart rate and problems should be maintained by clients and reviewed regularly by staff.

The lack of availability of specific exercise equipment often limits home-based exercise sessions to swimming, cycling, walking, or jogging. Allowing clients to choose their own mode of exercise can be an important factor in exercise compliance. However, before selection is made, the relative advantages and disadvantages of these exercise methods should be discussed. Swimming is an excellent exercise for aerobic conditioning, incorporating both the upper and lower extremities. Swimming has a relatively high oxygen cost. This means that for many clients the intensity of effort associated with swimming would exceed prescribed levels. Cycling offers the flexibility of outdoor and indoor training. In an urban environment, however, it is often difficult to find a cycling route that allows for a relatively continuous effort. Some centers allow clients to rent static exercise bicycles for the duration of the program. Walking is probably the easiest of all forms of aerobic activity. It requires little in terms of skill, facilities, and equipment, although a good pair of shoes is recommended. Walking training programs have the advantage of an easily tolerable intensity, high compliance, and few skeletomuscular injuries. Whether progress to higher intensity jogging exercise is achieved depends on the needs and rate of progress of the clients.

Environmental Conditions

Ideal temperature for exercise is between 40° F and 70° F (4° C to 24° C), and ideal humidity is below 65% (deVries, 1986). Clearly, it is important that the room conditions are controlled within these limits during supervised indoor group sessions.

The outdoors can often provide a pleasant and motivating surrounding for exercise training and should therefore be recommended wherever possible. Outdoor environmental conditions are often not ideal. Nevertheless, exercise should not be ruled out automatically but approached intel-

ligently by clients. The combination of high temperature and humidity increases the demand on the thermal regulatory systems; elicits peripheral vasodilation, which in turn may reduce central blood volume and peak cardiac output, thereby reducing physical work capacity; and provokes the onset of angina symptoms (Brannon et al, 1988). Cold climatic conditions can also present problems for exercise. Cold temperatures cause an increase in peripheral resistance and an increase in arterial blood pressure, which when coupled with the increased myocardial oxygen demands of exercise may cause clients to reach their anginal threshold more rapidly (deVries, 1986). All clients should be advised of the dangers associated with exposure to extremes in temperature. They should be instructed as to the best time of day to exercise, the appropriate clothing, and signs and symptoms of temperature intolerance. Instructors should also emphasize that the effects of temperature extremes should be avoided in daily life, such as bathing and showering, going from an air-conditioned building into extremes of heat or vice versa, and drinking very cold or extremely hot beverages.

STRESS MANAGEMENT

The second core component of cardiac prevention programs is stress management.

Stress and Coronary Heart Disease

Stress has been defined as a stressor (physical, psychologic, or social) reacting with an individual's unique personality to form a perception of stress (Brannon et al, 1988). Stress, like smoking and lack of exercise, is believed to be a causative factor in the development of CHD. The physiologic changes caused by stress exposure include increased blood pressure, which in turn can have pathophysiologic consequences through increased shearing forces on the arterial wall; increased catecholamine levels, which can damage the myocardium; and increased incidence of ventricular arrhythmias, a known risk factor for sudden death. In addition, stress can lead to increased levels of free fatty acid and serum cholesterol related to sympathetic activation of the liver, as well as increased platelet adhesion and aggregation in the arteries because of elevated catecholamine levels (Glass, 1977). Such a combination could set the stage for the development of atheromatous plaques in coronary arteries, which in turn may potentiate CHD.

As mentioned, personality is considered an important factor when discussing the concept of stress. Type A behavior has often been defined in terms of coronary-prone personality. Friedman and Rosenman (1974) described a type A behavior pattern as one with "an action-emotion complex that can be observed in any person who is aggressively involved in a chronic incessant struggle to achieve more and more in less and less time . . . against the opposing efforts of other things and other persons." Research has linked type A behavior to the development of CHD (Blumenthal et al, 1978) and increased rates of reinfarction (Williams et al, 1980).

Finally, it hardly requires saying that having a heart attack or undergoing heart surgery is associated with a substantial amount of stress in itself. These psychologic reactions may include anxiety, depression, and denial. For most clients, these reactions usually do not last long and they return to essentially normal lives within weeks. Between 20 and 30% of clients have severe and persistent psychosocial problems, which can include emotional distress and difficulty in returning to work, leisure, social, and family life (Mayou, 1979). However, not all the difficulties reported after a heart attack are due to the illness; some are the result of a previous life crisis such as divorce, death of a relative, or becoming unemployed.

Stress-Intervention Methods

Numerous investigators initiated evaluations of different treatment methods to reduce stress and modify type A behavior. Before discussing some of these methods, it is important to recognize the psychologic benefits associated with aerobic exercise training. Virtually all clinical trials of exercise-training programs that have measured psychologic variables have shown an improvement in clients' outlook and morale. For instance, a randomized controlled study reported a reduction in anxiety and depression levels of cardiac clients who were assigned to either home-based or hospital-supervised aerobic exercise programs (Kugler et al, 1990). Blumenthal and colleagues (Blumenthal et al, 1980) found that cardiac clients had a significantly lower type A rating after a 10-week supervised aerobic exercise program.

Relaxation methods are widely regarded as a central element of the stress-management component of a cardiac prevention program (Southard and Broyden, 1990). Studies showed that relaxation decreases heart rate, blood pressure, plasma catecholamine, and cholesterol levels (Cooper and Aygen, 1979). In addition, relaxation and imagery have been found to decrease the incidence of chest pain in angina clients (Amarosa-Tupler et al, 1989). These cardiac benefits are thought to be the result of relaxation reversing the sympathetically mediated responses associated with stress.

Relaxation Therapy

A number of different relaxation methods have been described (Sime and McKinney, 1988), including visual imagery, muscle tone awareness, biofeedback, and breathing strategies. Relaxation sessions often involve combining the basis of more than one of these methodologies. Contraindications for relaxation therapy are few, but routine precautions are advisable for high-risk clients. Prescriptive recommendations suggest that relaxation should be performed at least three times per week and preferably daily (Sime and McKinney, 1988). In an outpatient cardiac prevention program meeting twice per week, it is important that clients be expected to perform sessions on their own. The following sections describe relaxation therapy in both individual and supervised group sessions.

Supervised Sessions. *Location.* A relaxation session should be performed in an area that is as conducive as possible to the relaxation experience; noise level and other distractions should be minimized. The temperature of the room should be between 72° F and 78° F or be adjusted to the comfort level of the clients given their dress and previous activity levels. The clients should be able to lie down on a comfortable rubber mat. Placing a foam cushion or pillow under their lower legs can help to relieve the strain on the lower back when lying supine. Clients with some degree of cardiac failure or respiratory disease involvement often find that sitting upright in an easy chair is more comfortable.

Scheduling. It is strongly recommended that each relaxation session be performed as soon as possible after the cool-down period following aerobic exercise. After exercise, individuals are often aware of their muscle tone, have a pleasant sensation of fatigue, and are mentally ready to relax. These sessions are particularly important for persons who find it difficult, if not impossible, to relax adequately. Too often, persons maintain their hectic pace throughout the day and try to squeeze the exercise session into an already busy schedule. Typically, they rush into the exercise session, often late, try to hurry through their circuit, and then rush to the shower and to their next appointment without taking a moment to slow down. It is questionable whether those who approach exercise in this manner derive full benefits from it. Relaxation may ensure at least a brief respite from the frantic activity of the day. Finally, scheduling relaxation sessions after exercise training can have the additional advantage of safety. Because a large proportion of exercise-related cardiac complications occur in the postexercise period (during the shower or on the way home), the longer the staff can monitor clients after exercise, the more efficacious the safety element in the program. In addition, studies have demonstrated that relaxation can also reduce the risk of cardiac problems postexercise by reducing heart rate, blood pressure, and incidence of cardiac arrhythmias.

Duration. The duration of a relaxation session can vary according to clients' experience. Initially, clients find it difficult to concentrate for more than 10 to 15 minutes. Over time, sessions can increase in duration to 20 to 40 minutes. Moreover, some clients in the early stages are inclined to fall asleep during the relaxation session. These individuals are probably short on sleep and should be encouraged to improve the quality or quantity of their sleep.

Unsupervised Sessions. To obtain maximum benefit, relaxation should be practiced on a regular basis, preferably at least once per day. It is therefore important that clients should be encouraged to perform relaxation by themselves. To promote the transfer of group-based relaxation sessions to home, it is helpful to organize some of the group relaxation sessions so that clients are sitting as opposed to lying down.

Individual relaxation practice can be facilitated by providing clients with an audiotape that talks them through a session (Fig. 11–2). Such tapes are available commercially but can be recorded by the program staff themselves. Using this tape on a personal stereo with headphones can further facilitate the ease in which a relaxation session can be performed. Indeed, many clients choose

"Lie down on the mat provided. Spend a little time making yourself as comfortable as you can. Move around if necessary and loosen any tight clothing . . .
Close your eyes. Breathe easily and normally; don't force your breathing. Concentrate on your breathing for a few moments
Take a deep breath. Breathe out slowly and easily. Take a second breath. Slowly breathe out. As you do, feel yourself floating down . . .
. . . after some minutes
Slowly become aware of the sounds around you. When you are ready, open your eyes and get up slowly, gradually stretching as you do so."

Figure 11–2. Extract from Relaxation Session Instructions.

to perform some of their sessions at their place of employment. This can be particularly useful because work is often a major stressor. As with exercise training, promoting spouse participation in home-based relaxation sessions can be an important method of improving client compliance over time.

Counseling. The acceptance of all cardiac clients into a stress-management program is usually appropriate. However, as described previously, a small proportion of clients may have more significant psychosocial problems, such as the client with severe anxiety associated with a particularly stressful previous life event. These individuals generally require specific counseling support in addition to relaxation therapy. A counselor can often provide the emotional support and understanding required for clients to be able to talk through their fears and anxieties. Failure to provide counseling for these clients can result in their being unable to come to terms with their difficulties and, furthermore, the greater likelihood of a poor outcome (Cay, 1986). Counseling is believed to favorably alter the clients' perception of their health and thus potentially reduce the psychologic impact of illness (Steinhart, 1984). That counseling should be considered as an adjunct to stress management is supported by a randomized study of clients with infarction by Friedman (1985). In this study, type A counseling was more effective in reducing the reinfarction rate than a traditionally (i.e., no counseling) based cardiac prevention program. Although a review of psychosocial services in 202 North American cardiac prevention programs reported the prevalence of relaxation therapy to be relatively high (60% of respondents), the proportion of programs that reported individual counseling type sessions was low (32% of respondents) (Southard and Broyden, 1990). Clearly, more development is required in this area.

EDUCATION

The third and final core component of cardiac prevention is that of client education. Education-based cardiac prevention programs have produced promising results and benefits. For example, clients who took part in a structured teaching program after their MI had less anxiety on discharge compared with the control group. In addition, 70% of the clients who took part in the teaching program resumed their former activities, whereas only 48% of controls did so (Raleigh and Odotohan, 1985). Oldeberg and colleagues (1985) found that, among cardiac clients who took part in educational groups, psychologic health, physical activity, and symptoms of heart disease were improved significantly in the year after MI compared with controls.

Despite this supportive body of research and the belief that education should form an integral part of cardiac prevention programs, it has been stated that "health teaching . . . is often overlooked" or fragmented (Miller et al, 1984). Although many units provide some element of client education before discharge, it is important to remember that in the acute stages of recovery the cardiac client is frequently in a situation of considerable psychologic upheaval. Therefore, clients are often not receptive to the educational process at this stage. As the length of hospital stay for cardiac clients becomes shorter (e.g., 4 to 5 days for uncomplicated acute MIs), thus the time available for education before discharge becomes more limited. Surveys of cardiac prevention programs in the United Kingdom have shown that client education in many cases is limited to the provision of information pamphlets, with little or no opportunity for discussion of this material with staff (Davidson et al, 1989; Groden et al, 1981).

Clearly, there is a need for client education in outpatient cardiac prevention programs. Specific aims of cardiac teaching programs include:

1. Providing an understanding of the process of heart disease, its contributory factors, and its methods of treatment

2. Encouraging clients to recognize risk factors in their life and take responsibility for altering their lifestyle accordingly.

Organization

Group Discussion. Many cardiac prevention programs present their educational information as group sessions. Presentation of educational information in a group setting not only provides for economy of professional time but, in addition, affords clients an opportunity to interact with a peer group suffering similar problems. Moreover, clients appear less anxious in a group setting than with individual teaching, with a peer group facilitating adaptation to stress, decreasing frustration, and thus enhancing and reinforcing learning. It is important that these group sessions are kept relatively small (i.e., up to 10 to 15 clients) and informally structured in order to allow for any questions and facilitate client involvement.

Reinforcement of information by audiovisual techniques has been demonstrated to be extremely effective (Babarowicz et al, 1980). Cassette recordings, slide-tape packages, and videotapes can provide a varied educational presentation. In addition, take-home educational handouts are particularly valuable in facilitating client review of the material presented in classes.

Because the educational syllabus of cardiac prevention programs often involves a range of different topics, it is recommended not only to assign one member of the program staff to coordinate the running of the education program but also to involve other health-care professionals, such as a dietitian, re-employment officer (or equivalent), and pharmacist, to be responsible for particular sessions.

When possible, the family members, particularly the spouse or significant other, should be involved in this educational process. Involvement of the whole family unit in lifestyle changes can improve client compliance considerably. Families should also be made aware of the problem of overprotection that they can impose on the client after their cardiac event. It is, therefore, important that they are adequately informed so that they realize the client's true physical and mental capabilities. If it is not possible or practical for family members to actually attend educational sessions, clients should be encouraged to discuss the content of each session on their return home.

Timing and Length of Sessions. Education is an on-going process, and it is therefore important to schedule classes regularly throughout the program. In a 12-week outpatient program, it may be appropriate to include a new educational topic each week. Each session, including time for clients' questions, should last about 45 to 60 minutes. In a program that meets twice per week, it is possible to organize the education program so that the first session of the week can be used as a talk that introduces a particular educational topic, while the second session is devoted to clients' questions and discussion.

It is often practical to schedule the education class to take place after the exercise-training and relaxation sessions have been completed, thus allowing clients the opportunity to first take a shower and change back into their everyday clothing so that they feel alert and comfortable.

Syllabus

A core curriculum is a key element of any educational program. The educational syllabus outline of the Exeter program is given in Table 11–2. This list is in no way intended to be all inclusive or fixed. The syllabus of a cardiac program is determined by a variety of factors, such as the length of the program, availability of local staff expertise, changes that may be occurring in cardiac care (e.g., introduction of a new drug) and, most important, the educational needs of the clients themselves.

A brief overview of cardiac anatomy and physiology, as well as information about the atherosclerotic process causing coronary obstruction, can enable clients to understand the alterations that have occurred as the result of their MI. Such

Table 11–2. Exeter Program Educational Syllabus

1. Orientation to program
2. Cardiac anatomy/physiology
3. Coronary heart disease process
4. Medication
5. Diet
6. Body composition
7. Stress
8. Risk factors
9. Returning to work
10. Social benefit
11. Exercise and activity
12. Advances in cardiac medicine

explanatory background can assist clients in appreciating their symptoms, such as palpitations, shortness of breath, chest pain, and so on, thus reducing anxiety and improving the appropriateness of their response when such symptoms occur. Clients who understand the course and prognosis of their illness and the components of its management have an improved ability and motivation to adhere to medical regimes (Hogan and Neill, 1982) and to cope with the problems of illness. Central to the discussion of the coronary disease process is the emphasis on the role of risk factors. Detailed and practical suggestions for the modification of coronary risk factors should be provided. In terms of cardiac risk factor advice, it has been recommended that two of the most important aspects to be covered in a cardiac education syllabus are smoking and diet (Coronary Prevention Group, 1989).

For participants who are still smoking, cessation or reduction should be strongly advised and the basis for this recommendation presented, identifying the increased risk of reinfarction and cardiac death among clients of all ages who continue to smoke cigarettes after infarction. If the facility is available, smokers should be referred to a hospital or community antismoking program. Information should be provided about prescribed dietary alterations; changes in fat, sugar, and salt content; and caloric intake, with the rationale for these changes. Specific advice can be given on buying particularly food stuffs, reading food labels, and alternative methods of cooking. Spouse participation in dietary sessions is particularly important because many of these changes need to be directed specifically at the family member responsible for food preparation. The exchange of healthy recipes can be very helpful. Related to diet is the maintenance of a sensible body weight or fat content. In this respect, the concept of energy balance should be presented clearly so that clients can understand the importance of caloric intake versus caloric expenditure; and they therefore appreciate the importance of maintaining a reasonable physical activity level.

The most common medications cardiac clients are required to take should be discussed to ensure that they know the name, purpose, dosage and schedule, expected response, and any side effects or adverse response that should be reported. For example, over time some clients on beta blocker therapy reported increasing fatigue and noticed their resting pulse had fallen to 50 beats/min or less, suggesting that exercise training-induced bradycardia resulted in an overblocking; a simple reduction in the drug dosage is invariably sufficient to resolve this problem.

The concept of prescriptive, individualized, and progressive physical activity and exercise should be explained, together with detailed instruction on home-based aerobic exercise. Specific mention should be made of the adverse cardiovascular effects of static (or isometric) physical work as well as advice in modifying the daily activity pattern to minimize the amount of such work. Clients are often specifically fearful of resuming sexual activity. It can be of great psychologic reassurance to advise clients on the basis of the general guideline that sexual intercourse is appropriate and safe if other usual physical activities are reinstated. Specific cases of client impotence may require individualized client and spouse education and counseling.

Clients should be informed of the concept of stress, its physiologic sequelae, its potential pathologic role in coronary disease, and how to recognize stress in one's everyday life. This background information can assist clients in putting their relaxation and stress-management strategies into context.

Finally, instruction should be provided with regard to the vocational and social aspects of cardiac disease. This session can involve advice and information on government benefits and how to claim them, problems with returning to work, and legal and financial problems, including advice on housing problems. It can be valuable to invite former clients or members of local self-help groups along because they can offer much useful, practical advice to participants.

Assessment

In assessing the efficacy of an educational program, it is important to differentiate between the informal objectives of the teaching and the behavioral objectives. The acquisition of new knowledge (e.g., the health risks of smoking) has limited advantage if there is no desired alteration in behavior (e.g., cessation of smoking). This difficulty was highlighted by Steele and Ruzicki (1987). They found that, although introducing an educational program for clients awaiting coronary artery bypass surgery allowed clients to become measurably more knowledge-

able, they did not retain this knowledge and failed to make behavior changes such as stress modification and diet.

Because the end point of a cardiac education program is behavioral change associated with lifestyle modification, not whether the client tests well on information retention, a number of programs have added behavioral principles to the education process. These behavioral principles include goal setting, self-monitoring, rewards, and social support (Acierno, 1985). Details of these principles are given in other texts (Fardy et al, 1988).

ADMINISTRATIVE CONSIDERATIONS

Sensible administrative organization is vital to the establishment and daily operation of a successful cardiac prevention program.

Personnel

In view of the comprehensive philosophy of cardiac prevention programs, the personnel team is often multidisciplinary; a variety of professionals with different backgrounds and skills contribute to and work together in cardiac prevention programs.

Outpatient cardiac prevention programs are usually primarily staffed by a relatively small core of individuals with particular professional backgrounds, who are supported by a number of other individuals. The professional membership of this core is not absolute and can vary to some extent depending on the availability of local staff. The core staff of the Exeter cardiac prevention program is comprised of a physical therapist (or physiotherapist) who, assisted by an exercise physiologist, is primarily responsible for the organization of individual client exercise prescriptions and the supervision of the exercise classes; a nurse (with coronary care unit or general cardiac background) who is primarily responsible for the safety of the program and therefore qualified in resuscitation, the administration of drugs, and electrocardiogram interpretation; an occupational therapist who is primarily responsible for the coordination of the educational program and, assisted by a psychologist, is also responsible for leading the relaxation classes; and finally

Table 11–3. Types of Equipment and Approximate Costs*

Equipment	Cost ($)	Equipment	Cost ($)
Bicycle ergometer	300–3,000	Electrocardiogram recorder	6,000–20,000
Treadmill	3,000–12,000	Defibrillator	5,000–7,000
Step-up bench	100–300	Blood pressure monitor	150–500
Rowing ergometer	300–1,000	Slide projector	300–600
Arm ergometer	800–3,000	Screen	50–250
Exercise mat	20–100	Flip chart	100–250
Heart rate monitor	100–300		

*Calculated from U.K. costs.

the physician (consultant in cardiac medicine) who provides medical supervision of the program.

For the multidisciplinary team to be effective, it is important to emphasize that these responsibilities are not limited specifically to one professional but can be shared; the most important factor for the client is not who performs these specific responsibilities but that the responsibilities are met. It is often useful to have a particular member of this core group who is specifically responsible for the overall running of the program. This program coordinator or program leader should demonstrate the qualities of management and leadership.

The support personnel of a cardiac prevention program includes professionals who may contribute to specific educational talks such as a dietitian, pharmacist, or social worker, as well as administrative staff that assists in the organization and coordination of the activities of the program.

An important staffing consideration for cardiac prevention programs is staff certification. The American Heart Association organizes both basic and advanced life-support courses (American Heart Association, 1985). The American College of Sports Medicine organizes specific certification courses for individuals working in cardiac rehabilitation. These latter courses have specific behavioral objectives, which are listed in the American College Sport Medicine guidelines text (American College of Sports Medicine, 1980).

Facilities and Equipment

Surveys showed that tremendous variation exists in the facilities and equipment used by different cardiac prevention programs. Although no rigid regulations exist on the facility and equipment

provision of cardiac prevention programs, minimum guidelines have been suggested (American College of Sports Medicine, 1980; American Heart Association, Committee on Exercise, 1975; Coronary Prevention Group, 1989).

When setting up a program, it is important to consider first what facilities and equipment are already locally available. The minimum requirement for an outpatient cardiac program is the availability of a large, multipurpose room such as a gymnasium. However, access to changing rooms and showers as well as an additional room for client counseling or staff meetings is highly desirable. With some degree of reorganization, it is often possible to use the large room for the exercise, relaxation, and education classes. This room, therefore, should be relatively quiet, well lit, pleasantly decorated, and temperature controlled. It is also important that this room have sufficient space for 10 to 15 clients and their exercise equipment. Some authors recommended approximately 100 M^2 per client (Pollock and Schmidt, 1986).

The equipment requirements of cardiac prevention programs include not only upper and lower limb exercise devices, such as bicycle ergometers, stepping benches, and rowing machines, but also a number of important additional items such as heart-rate and blood-pressure recorders for client monitoring during exercise training and testing, emergency and resuscitation equipment, mats and a tape recorder for use during the relaxation program, and audiovisual aids for teaching, such as a flip chart and overhead display unit. A more comprehensive list of the items required for an outpatient cardiac program and their cost is given in Table 11–3.

Budget and Finance

The ultimate success of any cardiac prevention program depends on a well-developed and well-administered budget. In terms of the costs of a program, there are two main areas of expenditure: initial expenditure and operational costs.

Initial expenditure usually includes the purchase of new equipment, although it may involve renovation or construction costs if an adequate facility is not already available; this expenditure is often high but is generally one-off (see Table 11–3).

The most substantial component of operational costs is invariably staff salaries. It may be possible to reduce the magnitude of this expenditure by using otherwise fully employed staff on a per-session basis rather than employ them full time on the program. Such an arrangement is often negotiable with hospital and university staff. Operational costs also include materials such as stress-test supplies (e.g., electrodes and biochemical reagents), educational materials such as videos, models, slides, and printed materials, as well as other overhead such as facility rental, telephone costs, and client travel.

In addition to initial expenditure and operational costs, many programs also budget for additional expenses incurred by staff through travel or attendance at courses, thus facilitating staff development, which is so important to the continuance of any cardiac prevention program. Because of the diversity of staff involvement and the amount of equipment required for setup, the outpatient phase of cardiac prevention is considered the most expensive of the three phases of cardiac prevention. It has been estimated that the cost of a 12-week cardiac prevention outpatient exercise program can run anywhere between $720 and $2,160 per client.

Traditionally, an important source of financial income for cardiac programs in North America has been medical insurance reimbursement. Although no specific criteria have been published for programs wishing to receive the recognition of insurance carriers, many third-party carriers fund outpatient phase II exercise programs lasting 6 to 12 weeks. However, some considerable debate continues as to the continuance of such income. In the United Kingdom (UK), insurance does not cover cardiac prevention programs. Current changes in the UK National Health Service may lead to the greater development of North American type of insurance schemes.

An increasingly important source of income generation is fund-raising. Without the support of such income, many programs would have failed to develop to their current extent. However, programs often need to be established for a certain period of time and become locally recognized before fund-raising is successful. Potential fund-raising events include current and former clients taking part in sponsored walks or organizing profit-making events such as bring-and-buy sales or cheese and wine evenings. Clients are often pleased to organize such fund-raising events because they regard it as a means of showing their gratitude to the cardiac prevention program for their enhanced recovery. Another useful source of fund-raising is to contact local charities or local industries, particularly if they have had one or more of their employees enrolled in the program.

Legal and Safety Considerations

As has been outlined, clients with CHD enrolled in medically supervised group- or home-exercise programs are at increased risk of cardiac events such as MI or cardiac arrest. Therefore, cardiac prevention programs are morally obliged to provide a safe environment for all participants. The safety factors already described include client selection, individualized exercise prescription, warm-up and cool-down periods, exercise monitoring, and availability of emergency equipment and emergency procedures.

Certain legal considerations need to be taken into account whenever exercise testing or exercise prescription is provided. There is always a possibility that a legal claim and suit could be filed as the result of an untoward event during exercise; such events can and do happen. Although variations exist, some broad legal principles should be considered. Informed client consent should be sought before their participation in any form of exercise testing or training. Informed consent is normally obtained through a standard form that clearly states the material, risks, and benefits associated with a given procedure. Consent is given by the client signing this form and is countersigned by one or more of the program staff, one of whom is generally the program physician. Examples of informed-consent forms are published elsewhere (Brannon et al, 1988).

Standards of safety and legal practice have been promulgated by several professional associations (American College of Sports Medicine, 1980; American Heart Association, Committee on

Exercise, 1975). Although not completely uniform, these standards should be regarded as benchmarks of competency for cardiac prevention programs.

Evaluation and Research

A commitment to evaluation is a crucial element in any preventive program. Evaluation not only allows the efficacy of an intervention to be assessed, but also enables the composition of prevention program to be modified. Because previous evaluative research studies failed to show marked improvements in mortality with cardiac prevention programs, there is considerable need to collect research data on other outcome measures.

Although ideal, complete evaluation need not be accomplished from the outset; rather, it can be broadened or elaborated on as time and resources permit.

Initially, the program evaluation can be organized on a relatively simple basis that involves clients completing questionnaires. Standardized questionnaires that have been previously validated can often be used for this purpose. Factors that can be assessed in this way include psychologic well-being, educational knowledge, client satisfaction, and lifestyle (e.g., smoking, diet, and activity). Generally, assessment is performed both before and at the end of a prevention program so that the magnitude of change in a particular parameter can be assessed. More sophisticated forms of evaluation that involve specialized equipment and techniques are functional capacity (i.e., VO_2max), blood lipids, and precise dietary intake (using a weighed method). Another consideration usually taken into account in research programs evaluating an intervention is the importance of introducing a valid control group (Taylor and Taylor, 1990). A number of previous cardiac prevention studies have failed to include a control group, thus reducing the impact and generalizability of their results.

Many previous studies that evaluated the effectiveness of cardiac prevention programs have been performed only over a relatively short time. The problem with such short-term studies is illustrated by the measurement of compliance (or adherence). Studies demonstrated that clients generally maintain excellent rates of compliance during the 10 to 12 weeks of the program. However, programs that have extended this evaluation to 1 year or more have often found that compliance is considerably reduced (Oldridge, 1982).

An increasingly accepted measure of outcome for prevention programs is quality of life, and a number of standardized and validated questionnaires have now been designed to assess this concept. Few studies to date have examined the effectiveness of cardiac prevention programs in terms of specific quality-of-life assessment. A research study, based on these measures, is currently being performed to evaluate the quality-of-life outcome of the Exeter prevention program clients. It is hoped that the results of this study will be published in the near future.

References

Acierno LJ (ed): Comprehensive Cardiac Rehabilitation and Prevention: A Model Program. New York, Immergut & Siolek, 1985.

Amarosa-Tupler B, et al: Stress management through relaxation and imagery in the treatment of angina pectoris. J Cardiopulm Rehabil 9:348–355, 1989.

American Association of Cardiovascular and Pulmonary Rehabilitation: Cardiac Rehabilitation Services: A Scientific Evaluation. Middleton, WI, American Association of Cardiovascular and Pulmonary Rehabilitation, 1980.

American College of Physicians, Health and Public Policy Committee: Position Paper: Cardiac rehabilitation services. Ann Intern Med pp. 671–673, 1980.

American College of Sports Medicine: Guidelines for Graded Exercise Testing and Prescription, 2nd ed. Philadelphia, Lea & Febiger, 1980.

American Heart Association: Heart Facts. Dallas, American Heart Association, 1987.

American Heart Association, Committee on Exercise: Exercise Testing and Training of Individuals with Heart Disease or at High Risk for Its Development. Dallas, American Heart Association, 1975.

Barbarowicz P, et al: A comparison on in-hospital education approaches for coronary bypass patients. Heart Lung 9:127–166, 1980.

Bernard RJ, et al: Ischemic responses to strenuous exercise in healthy men. Circulation 55:396–400, 1973.

Blomquist G: Exercise physiology related to the diagnosis of coronary artery disease. In Fox SM (ed): Coronary Heart Disease Prevention, Detection, Rehabilitation with Emphasis on Exercise Testing. Denver, CO, Department of Professional Education, International Medical Corporation, 1974.

Blumenthal JA, et al: Effects of exercise on type A (coronary prone) behavior pattern. Psychosom Med 42:289–296, 1980.

Blumenthal JA, et al: Type A behavior pattern and coronary atherosclerosis. Circulation 58:634–639, 1978.

Borg G (ed): Physical Performance and Perceived Exertion. Lund, Sweden, Gleerup, 1967.

Brannon FJ, et al (eds): Cardiac Rehabilitation. Philadelphia, FA Davis, 1988.

Cay EL: Psychological aspects of cardiac rehabilitation. Update 32:377–386, 1986.

Clausen JP: Circulatory adjustments to exercise and the effect of physical training in normal individuals and patients with coronary heart disease. Prog Cardiovasc Dis 18:459–494, 1976.

Cooper MH and Aygen MM: A relaxation technique in the management of hypercholesterolemia. J Human Stress 5:24–27, 1979.

Coronary Prevention Group: Coronary Heart Disease: Statistics Fact Sheet. London, Coronary Prevention Group, 1990.

Coronary Prevention Group: Recovering from a heart attack. In Proceeding from the Coronary Prevention Group Conference, Regent's College, London. London, Coronary Prevention Group, 1989.

Davidson C, et al: Cardiac rehabilitation in the United Kingdom 1985/86. A questionnaire survey. In Proceedings from the Coronary Prevention Group Conference, Regent's College, London. London, Coronary Prevention Group, 1989.

deVries HA (ed): Physiology of Exercise, 4th ed. Dubuque, IA, WB Brown, 1986.

Dimsdale JE, et al: Post exercise peril: Plasma catecholamines and exercise. JAMA 51:630–632, 1984.

Fardy PS, et al (eds): Cardiac Rehabilitation, Adult Fitness, and Exercise Testing, 2nd ed. Philadelphia, Lea & Febiger, 1988.

Fardy PS, et al: Cardiorespiratory adaptation to submaximal and maximal arm and leg exercise. Physician Sports Med 5:32–38, 1977.

Friedman M: Behavior modification and myocardial infarction recurrence. Prim Cardiol 11:37–49, 1985.

Friedman M, Rosenman RH (eds): Type A Behavior and Your Heart. Greenwich, CT, Fawcett, 1974.

Glass DC: Stress behavior patterns and coronary disease. Sci Am 65:177–187, 1977.

Green V, et al: Cardiac rehabilitation in the United Kingdom 1985/86: A questionnaire survey. Physiotherapy 74:363–365, 1988.

Greenland P and Pomilla PV: Electrocardiographic monitoring in cardiac rehabilitation: An assessment. Physician Sports Med 17:75–82, 1989.

Groden BM, et al: Cardiac rehabilitation in Britain (1970). Br Heart J 33:425–427, 1971.

Hage P: Perceived exertion: One measure of exercise intensity. Physician Sports Med 94:43–56, 1981.

Haskell WL: Cardiovascular complications during training of cardiac patients. Circulation 57:920–924, 1978.

Hellerstein HK and Franklin BA: Exercise testing and prescription. In Wenger NK and Hallerstein HK (eds): Rehabilitation of the Cardiac Patient, 2nd ed. New York, Wiley, 1984.

Hogan CA and Neill WA: Effects of knowledge, physical activity and socialization of patients disabled by stable angina pectoris. J Cardiopul Rehabil 2:379–385, 1982.

Houston-Miller NH, et al: Home versus group exercise training for increasing functional capacity after a myocardial infarction. Circulation 70:645–649, 1984.

Karvonen M, et al: The effect of training heart rate: A longitudinal study. Ann Med Exp Biol Fennial 35:307–315, 1957.

Kellerman JJ: Rehabilitation survey: An international survey. In Kellerman JJ and Denholm H (eds): Critical Evaluation of Cardiac Rehabilitation. Basel, Switzerland, Karger, 1982.

Kugler J, et al: Hospital supervised vs home exercise in cardiac rehabilitation: Effects on aerobic fitness, anxiety and depression. Arch Phys Med Rehabil 71:322–325, 1990.

Lind AR and McNicol GW: Muscular factors which determine the cardiovascular response to sustained and rhythmic exercise. Can Med Assoc J 96:706–713, 1975.

May GS, et al: Secondary prevention after myocardial infarction: A review of long term trials. Prog Cardiovasc Dis 24:331–352, 1982.

Mayou RA: Psychological reactions to myocardial infarction. J R Coll Physicians Lond 13:103–105, 1979.

Miller MD: Health teaching in cardiac rehabilitation. In Hall LD, et al (eds): Cardiac Rehabilitation: Exercise Testing and Prescription. Champaign, IL, Life Enhancement Inc, 1984.

Multiple Risk Factor Intervention Trial Research Group: Multiple risk changes and mortality. JAMA 248:1465–1477, 1982.

Nagle R: The physical benefits of cardiac rehabilitation. In Proceeding of the Coronary Prevention Group Conference, Regent's College, London. London, Coronary Prevention Group, 1989.

Oldeberg B, et al: Controlled trial of psychological intervention in myocardial infarction. J Counsel Clin Psychol 53:852–859, 1985.

Oldridge NB: Compliance and exercise in primary and secondary prevention of coronary heart disease: A review. Prev Med 11:56–70, 1982.

Pollock ML and Schmidt DH (eds): Heart Disease and Rehabilitation, 2nd ed. New York, Churchill Livingstone, 1986.

Pollock ML and Wilmore JH (eds): Exercise in Health and Disease. Evaluation and Prescription for Prevention and Rehabilitation. Philadelphia, WB Saunders, 1990.

Pollock ML, et al: Effect of mode of exercise training on cardiovascular function and body composition of adult men. Med Exerc Sci Sport 7:139–145, 1975.

Pollock ML, et al: Effects of frequency and duration of training on attrition and incidence of injury. Med Exerc Sci Sport 9:31–37, 1977.

Raleigh EH and Odotohan BC: The effect of a cardiac teaching program on patient rehabilitation. Heart Lung 16:311–317, 1985.

Saltin B: Metabolic fundamentals in exercise. Med Exerc Sci Sport 5:137–146, 1973.

Sanne HS: Selection of patients for cardiac rehabilitation. In James WE and Amsterdam EA (eds): Coronary Artery Disease, Exercise Testing and Cardiac Rehabilitation. Miami, Symposium Specialists, 1977.

Sime WE and McKinney ME: Stress management applications in the prevention and rehabilitation of coronary heart disease. In American College of Sports Medicine. Resource Manual for Guidelines for Exercise Testing and Prescription. Philadelphia, Lea & Febiger, 1988.

Southard DR and Broyden R: Psychosocial services in cardiac rehabilitation: A status report. J Cardiopulm Rehabil 10:255–263, 1990.

Steele JM and Ruzicki D: An evaluation of the effectiveness of cardiac teaching during hospitalization. Heart Lung 16:306–311, 1987.

Steinhart MJ (ed): Emotional Aspects of Coronary Artery Disease. Baltimore, MD, Upjohn, 1984.

Taylor RS: Physiological Effects of Cardiac Rehabilitation. Paper presented at the XXIV World Congress of Sports Medicine, Amsterdam, May 27–June 1, 1990.

Taylor RS and Taylor CE: Cardiac Rehabilitation: A British Model of Practice. Paper presented at the American Occupational Therapy Association Annual Conference, Cincinnati, OH, June 1991.

Thompson PD: The benefits and risks of exercise training in

patients with coronary artery disease. JAMA *259*:1337–1440, 1988.

Van Camp SP and Petersen RA: Cardiovascular complications of outpatient cardiac rehabilitation programs. JAMA *256*:1799–1801, 1986.

Wenger N: *In* Pollock ML and Schmidt DH (eds): Heart Disease and Rehabilitation, 2nd ed. New York, Churchill Livingstone, 1986.

Williams RB, et al: Type A behavior, hostility and coronary atherosclerosis. Psychosom Med *42*:539–541, 1980.

World Health Organization: Prevention of Coronary Heart Disease, tech. rep. series no. 678. Geneva, World Health Organization, 1982.

World Health Organization: Rehabilitation After Myocardial Infarction. Copenhagen, World Health Organization, 1985.

CHAPTER

12

Julie Mount

Designing Exercise Programs for the Elderly

One danger of the growing field of gerontology is the implication that one can state generalizations about the elderly. Variability among individuals actually increases with age as a result of physical environmental influences, social and cultural influences, and increased opportunity for injury or disease processes to have altered the individual, along with the interaction effects of all of these factors. Any health-promotion program for the elderly has to be responsive to that variability. Some of the factors that must be considered when designing an exercise program for an elderly client or a group of elderly individuals are discussed here. Some methods of addressing special needs are also described.

CHANGES THAT TYPICALLY OCCUR WITH AGING

Changes that typically occur with age may be due to biologic aging, increased prevalence of chronic or degenerative disease processes, or decreased activity, which may be secondary to the previously mentioned causes or may be caused by psychosocial factors, or some combination of these. Because of the prevalence of a number of degenerative or chronic diseases among the elderly, it is often difficult to determine what constitutes a "normal change." If 49%

of individuals over 60 years of age have arthritis, is it normal for an older person to have arthritis? What percentage of older people must have a particular change for that change to be considered part of normal biologic aging? The average blood pressure of a group of older people will be higher than the average blood pressure of a group of younger people. Is this because there are large numbers of older people with some pathologic process causing hypertension whose high blood pressures are being averaged in with the lower blood pressures of the healthy older people? Even if a researcher eliminates all subjects with a diagnosed disease process, there are likely to be many subjects included in the study with undiagnosed diseases. Thus, although it would be useful to distinguish what changes are normal biologic changes and what changes are due to disease, it is difficult, in reality, to do so. Because of the interaction of disease and disuse, it is also difficult to distinguish what changes are caused primarily by decreased activity, and what ones are caused by biologic aging or disease, which then cause decreased activity. Despite these caveats, in the following review, an attempt is made to distinguish changes that are considered inevitable consequences of aging, changes caused by the more common disease processes, and changes that may be due to decreased activity.

Cardiovascular System

An individual's maximum ability to consume oxygen ($\dot{V}O_2$max) typically peaks at age 27 and decreases with age. At age 65, $\dot{V}O_2$max is about 60% of its peak value (Smith and Kampine, 1980). This decrease is largely due to decreased cardiac output, which is a function of heart rate and stroke volume.

$$\text{Cardiac output} = \text{heart rate} \times \text{stroke volume}$$

Maximum heart rate decreases with age because of a reduction in sympathetic activity and visco-elastic changes in the cardiac muscle resulting in mechanical resistance to movement. For a rough estimate of an individual's maximum heart rate, the formula 220 − age in years is typically used. Stroke volume also decreases with age. Stroke volume is affected by the amount of blood filling the left ventricle before contraction, cardiac muscle contractility, and the amount of pressure in the arterial system resisting the ejected blood. In the elderly, loss of elastin in veins, destruction of venous valves, and loss of skeletal muscle-pumping action result in poorer venous return. Increased myocardial rigidity with age may also reduce the pre-ejection filling of the left ventricle. The cardiac muscle's ability to generate force is also impaired with age, possibly because of a reduction of mitochondrial enzyme activity, infiltration of muscle by collagen fibers, or loss of coordinated contraction (Habasevich, 1985). Increased arterial pressure as a result of replacement of elastin with collagen and the buildup of atherosclerotic plaques results in increased arterial resistance to ejection of blood from the heart. All of these factors contribute to the decreased $\dot{V}O_2$max with age. $\dot{V}O_2$max is a good indicator of an individual's maximum aerobic work capacity.

Decreased sensitivity of the arterial baroreceptors with age contributes to orthostatic hypotension. It also may result in decreased blood pressure after eating, which could result in syncope or myocardial ischemia (Lipsitz et al, 1983). Therefore, the elderly should be advised not to exercise or engage in any activity stressful to the heart for at least an hour after eating a meal. Cardiac response to changes in activity level is slowed; thus, it takes longer to increase heart rate to accommodate increased activity, and the recovery time after an intense activity is greater. Therefore, warm-up and cool-down periods before and after exercise should be longer for the elderly.

Neuromuscular Changes

Larsson, Sjodin, and Karlsson (1978), in a cross-sectional study of sedentary men, found that strength peaked at the third decade of life, stayed relatively constant through the fifth decade, and then started to deteriorate. Power, which is the amount of tension produced within a given period of time, also decreases with age as a result of decreased strength along with decreased nerve conduction velocity, increased synapse conduction time, and increased muscle contraction time (Brown, 1987).

Because muscle and nerve cells are fixed post-mitotic cells, once destroyed they do not regenerate. Consequently, the number of muscle cells and motor units is likely to diminish with age as a result of normal wear and tear. Research has shown that fast-twitch fibers tend to atrophy with age, whereas slow-twitch fibers tend to remain relatively stable (Larsson et al, 1979; Orlander et al, 1978). According to Henneman's size principle (Brooks, 1986), slow-twitch fibers are always recruited first, therefore the slow-twitch fibers are stimulated more frequently by activities of daily living. In contrast to the effect of aging, total immobilization across a joint results in relatively more atrophy of slow-twitch than fast-twitch fibers, probably because there is a greater decrease in level of activity compared with normal in the slow-twitch fibers than in the fast-twitch fibers (Knortz, 1987). Older clients who have suffered an injury resulting in immobilization (e.g., a hip fracture) will have atrophy of both slow- and fast-twitch fibers. Because activation of slow-twitch fibers is essential to postural control and smooth control of movement, it makes sense for these clients to focus initially on low-intensity, long-duration activities to strengthen the slow-twitch fibers; as control and endurance improve, these clients should add high-intensity, brief-duration activities to strengthen the fast-twitch fibers.

Loss of strength with age is greater in the back and proximal muscles of the lower extremities and less in the upper extremities (Knortz, 1987). Unfortunately, deficits in these muscles may be missed in a typical quick evaluation in which strength testing is performed in a chair. It is essential to get the older client out of the chair to evaluate these muscles, which are critical for postural control.

Soft-Tissue Changes

Collagen is a major component of connective tissue, cartilage, tendon, and skin. In younger people, collagen tends to lie in parallel strands, but with age the alignment becomes more haphazard and the cross-links between proteins that make up collagen become more difficult to break. Also the number of elastin fibers, which are normally present in tissues that require elasticity such as lungs, blood vessels, skin, ligaments, and connective tissue, tend to decrease with age and are replaced with a tissue that is more rigid like collagen. These factors lead to increased stiffness in the involved tissues. Although more force is required to stretch these tissues, these tissues will stretch if exposed to a constant load over a period of time. Because of these structural changes, to increase range of motion (ROM) or length of muscles in older clients, it is important to provide prolonged stretches or use positioning to maintain a stretch (Lewis, 1985).

Decreased activity contributes to decreased flexibility. As Lewis (1985) pointed out, older clients often have decreased ROM that is within "functional" limits. Individuals retain ROM that they use daily. If certain clients have no need to flex the shoulder above 120 degrees, they are likely to lose that range. Clients who spend most of their time in a sitting position develop tightness in the hip and knee flexors. One could argue that there is no reason to try to retain or regain ROM that is not needed by the client, but loss of ROM limits possibilities.

Bone Mass Changes

Bone mass typically peaks in the fourth decade of life and declines at a rate of approximately 0.5% per year after that. During menopause and for 5 to 7 years afterward, the annual rate of bone loss increases to about 2%. Bone mass at any point in one's life is a function of the peak bone mass achieved and the subsequent loss of bone mass. Because women have a lower peak of bone mass and their rate of loss accelerates around menopause, older women are at a much higher risk for fracture as a result of decreased bone mass. It is predicted that more than 50% of women in the United States will, later in life, incur a fracture as a result of osteoporosis (Christiansen et al, 1987). The three most common sites of fractures resulting from osteoporosis are the hip, wrist, and vertebrae. One of the risk factors that increases age-related bone loss is inactivity. Studies showed that prolonged immobility results in osteoporosis (Dietrick et al, 1948; Donaldson et al, 1970).

When cervical vertebrae collapse as a result of osteoporosis or if osteophytes form, the pathway of the vertebral artery may be disrupted. Vertebral artery syndrome occurs when blood flow through the artery is impaired. The symptoms include dizziness, blurred vision, or blackouts when extending, laterally flexing, or rotating the neck. Before encouraging elderly clients to perform neck exercises, one should determine if these neck movements cause any vertebral artery symptoms.

Sensory Changes

One hearing deficit common among the elderly is difficulty distinguishing sounds from background noise. If verbal instructions are needed during an exercise program, it may be necessary to avoid background music or at least avoid music with words (unless the lyrics are the instructions). Also it is best to find a location that does not have a lot of other background noise (street noises, meeting next door, television noise, and so on). Give instructions in a moderately loud, deep voice. Higher pitched sounds are more difficult for the elderly to hear, and shouting tends to raise the pitch of one's voice. If clients have hearing problems, someone who is correctly demonstrating the exercises should be within their view.

Remember that vision may also be impaired. The lens becomes more opaque with age, causing increased sensitivity to glare, darkening of the visual field, and loss of acuity. If you are providing demonstration, be sure that the lighting is bright, that there are no shiny surfaces that might cause glare, and that the background behind the demonstrator contrasts with the demonstrator and is not busy. If you provide printed materials, use large letters, nonglossy paper, and high-contrast colors.

Balance

Balance is the ability to maintain a center of gravity over a base of support. To maintain balance in a dynamic environment, one must accurately perceive any displacement of balance through the vestibular, somatosensory, and visual systems, and one must have the flexibility of joints, the muscular strength, the response speed, and the motor planning ability to return the body to a stable position. Many of these components may be impaired in older persons. Bohannon and colleagues (1984) found an age-related decrease in balance in one-legged stance, with balance more impaired with eyes closed than with eyes open. Overstall and associates (1977) found a linear increase in postural sway with age.

Chronic Diseases

The U.S. Department of Health and Human Services (1989) reported the prevalence of the following chronic conditions for people 60 years or over in 1984:

Condition	% of Older Population
Arthritis	49.0
Hypertension	41.8
Cataracts	19.9
Heart disease	14.0
Varicose veins	9.9
Diabetes	9.5
Cancer (except nonmela- noma skin cancer)	6.6
Osteoporosis or hip fracture	5.5
Stroke	5.4

The department also reported that only 21.2% of individuals 60 or older had none of the chronic conditions listed, and 48.7% had more than one of these nine chronic conditions. These figures are based on subjects' responses to questions by census takers. Clinical studies suggest that over half of individuals in the United States over 65 years may have heart disease (Kennedy et al, 1977; Kitchin et al, 1973), and Hahn (1983) reported that 50% of people in their 60s and 78% of people in their 80s have osteoarthritis. Comparison of these clinical figures to those based on subjects' report suggests that subjects are likely to under-report their medical conditions. This may be because (1) many medical conditions are undiagnosed, (2) communication between the doctor and the client is inadequate, (3) clients may be in denial, or (4) clients may be unwilling to report their deficiencies to others. Whatever

the reason, if a therapist is providing a prevention program in a community setting, without the benefit of the clients' medical records it is very likely that some of the clients will have a chronic condition of which the therapist is unaware.

Traditionally, arthritics have been advised to avoid weight-bearing and resistive kinetic exercise and to perform nonresisted ROM to maintain flexibility and isometrics to maintain strength. As a consequence, arthritics tend to become deconditioned. However, a number of studies demonstrated that aerobic conditioning exercises are safe for individuals with rheumatoid or osteoarthritis (Dial and Windsor, 1985; Ekblom, 1982; Harkcom et al, 1985; Nordemar, 1981; Nordemar et al, 1981; Suwalska, 1982). The studies used a variety of types of exercise, including swimming, cycling, walking, and calisthenics, and found that (1) the arthritics benefited in terms of cardiovascular conditioning, muscle strength, ROM, and increased functional ability and (2) there was no aggravation of the arthritic disease process. Ekblom (1982), in fact, found a significant slowing of the rheumatic disease process in his subjects over a 5.5-year period of exercising an average of 339 minutes per week compared with a control group that exercised an average of 96 minutes per week. Bland (1983) advocated weight-bearing activities for treatment of osteoarthritis to stimulate the cartilage. So, for the approximately 50% of older clients who have some type of arthritis, although high-impact activities should be avoided, there is no reason to avoid a low-impact aerobic program or a calisthenics program. Remind the clients to use the 2-hour rule: If they still have pain as a result of exercising more than 2 hours after they stopped, or if the symptoms are worse the next day, then the exercise routine was too vigorous and should be cut back. They should also, of course, rest and protect any joints that are having an acute flare-up. All older clients should be advised to wear shoes with shock-absorbing soles to reduce the force imparted to the joints on impact.

Sedentary Lifestyle

It is commonly believed that there is both a moral and a physiologic imperative to slow down and take it easy as one becomes older. Older clients often express the philosophy that after working all their lives they deserve to rest during their retirement. People also believe that physical decline is inevitable with age. All members of society, even health professionals, tend to support them in these beliefs. Younger people offer to carry things or perform heavy chores for older people. Older people are expected not to participate in strenuous leisure activities. Health professionals may comment to older clients that they are functioning well for their age, suggesting lower expectations. Unfortunately, lowered expectations of activity level are a self-fulfilling prophecy. According to the National Health Survey, 68% of men and 72% of women over age 65 reported that they did not exercise regularly. In 1982, the American Medical Association issued the following statement: "At least a portion of the changes that are commonly attributed to aging are in reality caused by disuse and, as such, are subject to correction" (Bortz, 1982, p. 1205).

One could argue, for all situations in which a function is lost as a result of disuse, that if clients were not using it, what do they need it for anyway? However, it is one's reserve capacity that permits variety in one's life: to cope with crises, experience new pleasures, or take on new challenges. If an elderly woman fractures her hip, will she have the cardiopulmonary endurance and the strength and ROM in her arms to use a walker or will she be confined to a wheelchair? If there is a fire, will she be able to get out of the house? If her granddaughter has a baby, will she be able to pick up her great grandchild? If she wins a free trip to the Caribbean, will she have the endurance to enjoy the trip? If she meets someone who enjoys playing tennis, will she be able to play? If clients say that they have no need to increase physical capacity, change the subject. After fantasizing about nice things that could happen to them in the next 5 years, ask them if they would have the capacity to take advantage of the opportunities.

BENEFITS OF EXERCISE FOR THE ELDERLY

When one thinks of the preventive benefits of exercise, one tends to think of preventing cardiovascular disease. For a population such as the elderly who tends to have a decrease in physical challenges in their daily routine, exercise must be considered in its entirety as a means not only of challenging the cardiovascular system, but also of maintaining flexibility, strength, coordination, balance, and motor problem solving ability. An exercise program may prevent the downward-spiral cycle of decreased activity leading to physical losses and further immobility. The losses that result from a sedentary lifestyle not only place one at risk for cardiovascular disease, but they also increase one's risk for a variety of other problems including fractures and possibly death as a result of falls; malnutrition resulting from inadequate mobility to purchase, prepare, or eat healthy food; death by fire because of the inability to drop to the floor and roll or to leave a burning building; unnecessary dependence on others for physical needs; and depression.

There is evidence in the literature that many of the changes that typically accompany aging can be ameliorated by exercise. Although extreme stress may cause injury, the body responds to moderate stress by building up reserve capacity. This reserve capacity not only comes in handy in emergencies, but it makes daily activities feel relatively easy. Humans typically do not stress their bodies to maximum capacity. Therefore, even though there is some inevitable loss of cells and efficiency of various systems with aging, in many cases (sensory systems being the major exception) this loss can be partially compensated for by using more fully one's reserve capacity. The majority of the research demonstrating the benefits of exercise is performed on young adult subjects, and the generalizability of this research to older subjects is questionable. However, there is now a substantial body of literature demonstrating the effects of exercise on elderly subjects.

Cardiovascular Fitness

There is ample evidence that cardiovascular fitness can be improved in the elderly through exercise (Adams and deVries, 1973; Amundsen et al, 1989; Benestad, 1965; deVries, 1970; Schurer and Tipton, 1977). Some argued that the elderly do not tolerate aerobic exercise at an intensity adequate to achieve a training effect. However, Shepard (1990) noted that some conditioning can occur even if training at only 30 to 40% of maximum oxygen uptake; the training effect just takes longer. Generally improvement in aerobic fitness in the elderly is measured the same way as in younger people with one exception. When younger people become more physically fit, there is a decreased resting heart rate. Resting heart rate does not decrease among the elderly with training, but rather resting systolic and diastolic blood pressures decrease (Sidney, 1981). For older persons, whose maximum work load will be lower than that of younger persons, increasing physical fitness causes submaximal work loads, such as activities of daily living, to become easier. Some argue that, although older people benefit from aerobic exercise by finding functional activities less effortful, it is too late to expect any decrease in risk of heart disease. However, Posner and colleagues (1990) found a decrease in incidence of cardiac disease symptoms and an increased time to onset of symptoms in elderly subjects who were placed on an exercise program compared with control subjects.

Strength, Flexibility, and Bone Density

Older people can also make significant gains in strength with exercise (Adams and deVries, 1973; deVries, 1970; Larsson, 1982; Moritani and de-Vries, 1980; Tzankoff et al, 1972). More recent studies demonstrated not only that older individuals can gain strength with training, but that the strength gains are accompanied by functional gains (Fiatarone et al, 1990; Frontera et al, 1988).

Several studies demonstrated that exercise can help regain some of the joint flexibility that is lost with age (Germain and Blair, 1983; Munns, 1981; Raab et al, 1988).

Several studies demonstrated a significant difference in bone density between older people who participate in an exercise program and matched controls who do not (Ayalon et al, 1987; Dalen and Olsson, 1974; Smith et al, 1981). Other studies suggested that a walking program of 30 to 60 minutes 3 times a week can slow the rate of bone loss in postmenopausal women (Cummings et al, 1985; Sandler et al, 1987). Smith and colleagues (1981) found significant improvement in bone density of the radius among older women who participated in upper extremity activities for 45 minutes 3 days a week over a 3-year period. Jacobson (1984) and Krolner (1983) and their colleagues found that exercise programs for the elderly could increase vertebral bone mass.

Balance

Exercise may decrease the risk of falls among the elderly. According to Speechley and Tinetti (1990), fewer than 10% of falls among the elderly are due to one overwhelming circumstance, such as loss of consciousness or being hit by a car. Instead, most falls result from multiple factors, usually a combination of a mild irregularity in the environment with some personal risk factors such as impaired sensation, strength, or flexibility or the consumption of sedatives or antihypertensive drugs. Several studies demonstrated significant differences in balance between elderly individuals with and without a history of falling (Chandler et al, 1990; Ring et al, 1988; Wolfson et al, 1986). Fansler, Poff, and Shepard (1985) were able to improve one-legged balance in elderly women with a combination of mental imagery and physical practice. Insofar as balance reactions are limited by flexibility or strength, improvements in these components may also decrease the incidence of falls. Exercise may also decrease the need for drugs that may increase the risk of falls.

Psychologic Benefits

There may also be psychologic benefits of exercise for the elderly. Studies suggested improvements in mood (Stacey et al, 1985), body image (Riddick and Freitag, 1984), locus of control (Perri and Templer, 1985), and self-esteem (Parent and Whall, 1984). Millar (1987) found that, after a 3-month program of walking or jogging, subjects had decreased tension, anger, depression, and fatigue.

EXERCISE PROGRAMS

Aerobic Exercise

Because of the prevalence of heart disease among the elderly, it is recommended that older individuals have a medical exam and stress test before initiating an exercise program. However, when one is providing exercise programs as a preventive measure, this may not be feasible. Many clients may be fearful of medical examinations or may find it too great an economic burden. Medicare and other third-party payers typically do not cover stress tests as a screening tool. A stress test is covered only when a diagnosis warrants it, such as angina. In some cases, doctors listed hypertension or hypercholesterolemia as the diagnosis and had the test covered. In situations in which it is not possible to obtain a medical exam and stress test for an individual, it would be a disservice to recommend that the individual avoid exercise. Instead, one should recommend starting at a low intensity and increasing the intensity slowly. Payton and Poland (1983) recommended that Graf's (1981) guidelines for inpatients with cardiac disease would be safe (Table 12–1).

Habasevich (1985) recommended that before elderly persons start exercising the resting pulse should be between 60 and 100 and the rhythm should be regular; if the resting systolic blood pressure is over 150 mm Hg, one should proceed with caution. In the elderly, systolic blood pressure over 160 mm Hg or diastolic blood pressure over 100 mm Hg is considered hypertensive.

It is generally recognized that to achieve a cardiovascular training effect individuals must train at least 60% (American College of Sports Medicine, 1978) of their maximum heart rate for at least 20 minutes 3 times a week. However, for very deconditioned older persons, it may be more appropriate to start at 40 to 60% of maximum (Lewis, 1984). Clients who are unable to endure a full 20 minutes of exercise might be encouraged to exercise 10 minutes twice a day until their endurance improves.

Intensity of an aerobic exercise is usually monitored through heart rate, which may be difficult for some older individuals. Among 60 clients who participated in a program at senior centers in Philadelphia, only 40% learned to monitor their own pulses (Mount, in press). Some clients were unable to feel their pulses, and some were unable to count the beats accurately. These problems may have been due to peripheral neuropathies, impaired circulation, or slowed processing time. If impaired peripheral circulation is the problem, clients may be able to feel the apical pulse just under the left breast or the carotid

artery. If clients are instructed to monitor their pulse at the carotid artery, therapists must be certain that they will not press so hard as to restrict blood flow and not massage the artery, which may set off a vagal response. If clients have a peripheral neuropathy or slow processing time, a monitor may be needed, but pulse monitors that attach to the finger may not be accurate means of measuring heart rate for clients with impaired peripheral circulation, and they are not accurate while clients are moving. A more accurate tool that is available for about $200 is a heart-rate monitor consisting of two electrodes strapped around the chest and telemetered to a receiver on the wrist that displays the heart rate in large, easy-to-read digits. This monitor is less sensitive to client movement. For clients who cannot take their own pulse and do not have access to an alternative means of monitoring heart rate, it may be useful to assess whether Borg's perceived exertion scale (Borg, 1974) is a relatively accurate way to monitor their exercise intensity (see Chapter 2).

Clients must be educated about indicators that they need to stop exercising or to decrease the exercise intensity. Some indicators that circulation is not adequate for the intensity of exercise being performed are:

Decreasing heart rate with increasing activity level
Pain in the chest, arm, or jaw
Irregular heart beats
Excessive dyspnea
Cool and clammy skin
Nausea
Decreased coordination
Confusion
Dizziness
Headache

Clients should also be reminded that if they stop exercising suddenly, the blood will pool in the muscles that had been exercising, and there will be inadequate venous return, causing hypotension and myocardial ischemia. They should decrease their activity to minimal intensity, with just enough contraction of the active muscles to facilitate venous return (e.g., walking slowly in place or pedaling without resistance), and they should notify their physician immediately. If it is necessary to stop suddenly, one should lie down or elevate the legs.

Exercising in extreme temperatures is more

Table 12–1. Graf's Exercise Guidelines for Inpatients with Cardiac Disease

Avoid activities that:
    Increase heart rate greater than 20–30 beats/min above resting
    Increase systolic blood pressure greater than 40 mm Hg above resting
    Decrease systolic blood pressure greater than 20 mm Hg below resting
    Decrease diastolic blood pressure greater than 15 mm Hg below resting
    Increase diastolic blood pressure greater than 110 mm Hg

problematic as one ages. Sweating is less efficient with age; therefore, older individuals may not be able to dissipate the heat being produced by exercise and may suffer heat stroke or heart failure from trying to use the circulatory system to cool the body. Extremely cold weather is also dangerous because poor peripheral circulation may result in frostbite, and the cutaneous vasoconstriction results in a rise in blood pressure and a reflex coronary artery vasoconstriction, which could result in myocardial ischemia (Shepard, 1990).

A walking program is ideal for older individuals. One can vary the pace of walking to achieve an appropriate target heart rate. For relatively sedentary individuals, walking usually increases the heart rate adequately to achieve cardiovascular benefits, and walking is useful for its functional carryover. Walking with cushioned-sole shoes does not traumatize the bones and joints. Aside from good shoes, which people should wear even if not participating in an exercise program, walking requires no expensive equipment. In moderate climates outdoor routes may be used, but in areas of inclement weather it is useful to identify appropriate indoor routes (e.g., a mall, museum, visitor's center, community center, or any building with long halls or large, open areas). Buildings such as malls and museums that also provide visual stimulation are preferable. Many malls have been persuaded to open their doors early in the morning to accommodate walking programs. However, this time of day may be an economic problem in cities where the elderly rely on cheaper rates or free travel on public transportation between the hours of 10:00 A.M. and 3:00 P.M. For whatever area is selected for the walking program, one should create a map with distances between various landmarks labeled. Make the walking program a social activity to motivate clients to stick with it.

Nonaerobic Exercise

Nonaerobic exercises may be undertaken to increase strength, flexibility, balance, or coordination. Strength can be gained through the repetition of isometric, isotonic, or isokinetic exercises against adequate resistance. Isometric exercises may be dangerous for older individuals because they increase the amount of work by the heart. During exercise, the blood vessels in the exercising muscles dilate, whereas other blood vessels

throughout the body constrict to shunt the majority of the blood to the needed area. However, during isometric exercise, the dilated vessels are compressed by the contracted muscle so that peripheral resistance is increased, which is reflected in the increased diastolic blood pressure. This increases the pressure that the heart has to push against to eject blood, thus increasing the work of the heart to produce the needed cardiac output. In individuals who have limited cardiac reserve, this could result in inadequate cardiac output to meet the increased needs of the heart muscle. The stronger the muscular contraction and the longer the contraction is held, the greater will be the increase in systolic and diastolic blood pressure. Holding a quad set for 5 counts might not be too stressful, but maintaining knee extension with a 5-lb cuff weight for a count of 10 may be. If in doubt, monitor blood pressure during the contraction. Smith and Kampine (1980) reported that the blood pressure response to isometric contraction is independent of the mass of the muscle. This means that sustained contraction of the abductor digiti minimi at 50% of maximum contraction is as stressful to the cardiovascular system as a sustained contraction of the hamstrings at 50% of maximum.

A Valsalva maneuver (i.e., tightening of the abdominal muscles while holding the breath) causes an initial rise in blood pressure as the increased intrathoracic pressure is transmitted to the aorta. However, the increased intrathoracic pressure also restricts venous return, thus after the first heartbeat the blood pressure starts decreasing to below resting level. Normally the baroreceptors respond to this decreased blood pressure by increasing heart rate to maintain cardiac output. However, in situations where the baroreceptor reflex is not working adequately, the decreased blood pressure may result in syncope. Because the elderly have decreased sensitivity of the baroreceptors as well as slowing of other components of the autonomic nervous system, they are more prone to fainting if they perform a Valsalva maneuver. If a therapist notices older clients holding their breath during exercise, they should be advised to count aloud, exhale, sing, or talk during the exercise to prevent the Valsalva maneuver.

To maintain ROM, frequency of movement is more important than number of repetitions (Lewis, 1985). This means that clients must remember to move through the range on their own, not just when they see a therapist. The best way to ensure frequency of a particular movement is to incorporate the movement into some activity of daily living. For example, to maintain shoulder flexion, have clients store a light object, such as napkins, on a shelf just barely within reach (Fig. 12–1). For each of three meals a day, then, clients will flex the shoulder through the full range while reaching for napkins. To maintain hip rotations, clients might be advised to put on and take off socks by placing the foot on the opposite knee and put on and take off slip-on shoes by rotating the foot outward and using the ipsilateral hand.

Balance and coordination are perceptual motor skills that rely on strength, flexibility, and the ability to develop an appropriate motor plan to respond to the environment as experienced through the senses. Gains in balance or coordination, therefore, may result from gains in strength or flexibility or, if these were not limiting factors, may require a learning process. In some cases, clients must learn to attend to the more useful sensory input and ignore or correct for distorted input. Among the elderly, visual changes, decreased nerve conduction velocity, and frequently peripheral neuropathies resulting in impaired tactile sensation may interfere with coordinated movement or balance. The environment can be adapted to make it easier to perceive accurately, or clients may learn to attend to

sensory input that is more accurate or to slow their movements to give more time to respond to any unexpected changes in the environment. In any case in which the clients are lacking an appropriate motor response to an environmental situation, they must participate in adequate practice with feedback to develop appropriate motor programs to address these types of situations.

Because the elderly have less bone mass than younger adults, high-impact exercises and activities that place sudden torque on the bones could cause fractures. However, stress is necessary to maintain the structural integrity of the bone. Stress can be applied through weight bearing (e.g., walking or leaning forward on the arms) or through resistance. Exercises will increase skeletal mass but only in the areas where the forces are applied; therefore, a good walking program may decrease the chances of hip or vertebral fracture, but arm exercises are necessary to increase bone mass of the radius to decrease the risk of Colles' fracture. There is evidence that trunk-flexion exercises may cause vertebral compression fractures (Goodman, 1985; Sinaki, 1982), whereas trunk-extension exercises may decrease the risk of vertebral fractures (Sinaki and Mikkelsen, 1984). In a study of older women with osteoporosis, Sinaki and Mikkelsen provided some subjects with a trunk-extension exercise program, some with a trunk-flexion ex-

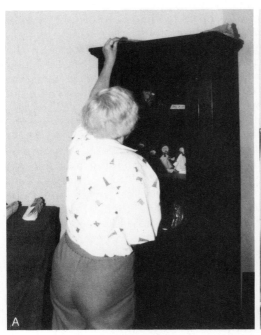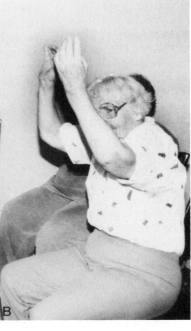

Figure 12–1. Functional activities *(A)* may elicit more range of motion than an exercise program *(B)*.

ercise program, some with a program of both extension and flexion, and some with no exercise. Additional vertebral compression fractures occurred in 67% of the nonexercising group, but in only 16% of the extension exercise group. Among the flexion group, 89% had additional fractures, and in the group that did both flexion and extension exercises 53% had additional fractures. On the basis of these results, extension exercises should be encouraged among older clients who already have osteoporosis, and abdominal muscles should be strengthened isometrically rather than by trunk flexion.

FACILITATING PARTICIPATION IN EXERCISE

Kohler (1988) argued that the elderly typically have already experienced loss of control in many aspects of their lives and are likely to view health-care advice as a further impingement on their autonomy. They may also believe that there is not a strong relation between their behavior and what happens to them. To optimize compliance with health-care advice, clients should be involved in the decision-making process and should also be shown the effects of their behavior. Kohler gave the example of charting a person's blood pressure and correlating it with the client's inconsistency in taking blood-pressure medications. Teitelman (1982) reported that older clients who believed they had more control over themselves and their environment were more cooperative with rehabilitation. Low (1987) observed that the elderly are likely to be locked in the present and have difficulty in participating in interventions that require an orientation toward the future. She recommended that therapists working with the elderly deal with small, quickly attainable goals that may lead toward the larger goals that are too far in the future to appreciate. Mobily (1982) cited evidence that the elderly believe that exercise is dangerous for them and that family, friends, and even health professionals encourage them to take it easy. Herbert and Teague (1989) noted that, although the reason for starting an exercise program is often health benefits, the reason for continued participation is more likely to be enjoyment, convenience, socialization, and social support.

This literature on compliance among the elderly suggests that what motivates the elderly is not different from what motivates everyone else.

We all want to be in control of our lives. If someone suggests that we change our lifestyle to be healthier, we have to believe that the change will actually make a difference and we want to see immediate effects. If the change is inconvenient or no fun, we will not keep it up unless the effects are adequately rewarding or there is adequate social pressure.

The demeanor of the health professional with respect to clients should be that of advisor, not parent. The health professional can tell clients what is possible and how the possible can be achieved, but clients must decide what goals to aim for and the client must do what is necessary to accomplish the goals. The health professional can provide encouraging feedback for clients by frequently measuring and pointing out changes produced by their behavior.

Exercise for prevention is critically different from exercise for remediation in that the latter can be terminated when the goal is reached, with the expectation that returning to a normal lifestyle retains the regained function. Unlike a remedial exercise program, a preventive program cannot be tolerated as merely a temporary inconvenience because it is not temporary. In order for a preventive measure to be followed for the rest of one's life, it must either become a habit, a pleasure, or a challenge.

Lifestyle modifications described under the section on ROM are examples of integrating preventive measures into lifestyles so that they can become habits. One can also create rituals such as walking to the store for a daily newspaper or walking to the neighborhood church to light a candle. Selecting activities that have social rewards or inherent interest for clients are examples of turning preventive measures into pleasures. Square dancing, golfing, swimming, and walking through the woods alone or with friends may be pleasures that happen to preserve physical function also. Group exercise classes should use enjoyable music, dance-like movements, games such as balloon volleyball, or parachute activities to make the exercise session fun. For individuals who desire a higher level of function, the role of the therapist may be to develop appropriate challenges. The next section addresses how to make challenges appropriate.

PROBLEM-SOLVING APPROACH

For physical and occupational therapists, problem solving is the implicit modus operandi. Therapists evaluate clients, determine what problems need to be addressed, determine means of addressing the problems, and prescribe appropriate activities. However, because clients are often not involved in the process of problem solving, they may perceive the activity as a sort of penance. If clients suffer through their penance, the gods may look favorably on him. If clients do not have faith in their therapist, they are unlikely to do their penance. Clients who have suffered an acute injury expect that they can return to their previous level of functioning and will perform what they must to achieve that level. Older clients who have gradually lost functions and have observed many of their aging friends losing the same functions are unlikely to believe that performing a few exercises will enable them to improve. Therapists will have to prove to clients that improvement is possible. To do this, the problem-solving process needs to be made explicit, and a quickly achievable goal needs to be identified. Discuss with clients what they would like to be able to do and help them select a small goal (e.g., to get out of their favorite soft chair independently or to be able to pick up their grandchild). Help clients identify the limiting factors (e.g., decreased ROM into knee flexion, decreased strength of the quadriceps, poor body mechanics). Judge whether a focused exercise program will solve the problem or whether a modification of the environment is necessary. Determine as many intermediate goals as possible, so that progress can be demonstrated. If an exercise program involves increasing ROM, measure with a goniometer so that improvement can be demonstrated. If an intermediate goal is strengthening a certain muscle and you have access to a machine that gives a force readout, use that to identify small gains. Use photography or videotape where possible to document improvements in body mechanics. This method of engaging clients in the problem-solving process gives them control and demonstrates to them that their actions have consequences. Identifying multiple subgoals addresses the problem of living in the present and provides swift, positive reinforcement. Focusing on the functional goal rather than on exercise per se may bypass the clients' concern that exercise is too dangerous for older persons.

Explicit problem solving may appear to be practical only in a one-to-one situation, but in some ways it may be more valuable in a group setting. Humans need to be problem solvers to adapt their motor programs to meet the changing demands produced by the interaction of their changing bodies with their changing environment. In a group setting, clients may be better able to generalize the problem-solving process because their focus is not always on their immediate needs. The focus may rotate among the clients. Those clients who are not the current focus of attention should be encouraged to assist in the problem-solving process. Therapists may be surprised to learn how other clients have solved similar functional problems for themselves, their spouses, or friends. Clients who provide suggestions will gain self-esteem and self-confidence.

Introduce each exercise period with a problem-solving session. Initially you may want to identify in advance a client who is willing to discuss a problem in front of the group for group problem solving. Identify a specific activity that a client would like to be able to do but has difficulty with. For example, a client might express a desire to be able to walk up four stairs so he or she can go to church, to pick up a grandchild, to walk to the corner store and carry groceries home, or to reach cabinets over the kitchen counter. The client should enact his or her attempt to perform the activity so that the therapist can analyze whether the problem is loss of ROM, weakness, poor balance, poor motor planning, poor cardiovascular or pulmonary condition, pain, or some combination of factors. On the basis of the analysis, the therapist should determine if some type of exercise program would make the activity achievable or if there is an alternate method of accomplishing the task. Problem solving aloud and receiving input from the other clients will provide insight on how to address similar problems that they, their family, or their friends may have, will teach clients the problem-solving method, and will give them a sense that one can exert control over one's own life to bring about positive change. It will also cause them to perceive exercise as a useful activity, and guide them to see the results of an exercise routine (i.e., make the association between the exercises and the improvement in function). The problem-solving sessions are also useful forums for teaching clients to recognize when they are overstressing a system and what activities or situations may be best avoided for individuals with some of the conditions common to the elderly.

After a group problem-solving session, a group exercise program may be provided that incorporates the recommended exercises. If the proposed solution to the problem was an aerobic program, the group exercise session could be an aerobic workout that guides each participant to determine their safe intensity and duration, monitor the intensity throughout the exercise, and include an appropriate warm-up and cool-down. If the problem addressed involved a biomechanical solution, the exercise program should include that solution. The exercise routine can be designed to set clients up for biomechanically efficient movement patterns, thus training them in good movement strategy. For example, if a client's problem was getting up out of a soft chair, the therapist may have recommended a combination of strengthening and flexibility exercises with a change in technique. All of these activities could be choreographed into a group exercise class that moves from exercises while sitting to exercises while standing. Figure 12–2 shows a sequence of exercises that might be done to music in a sitting position to lead to a biomechanically efficient sit to stand exercise.

When providing an exercise program, it must be clear that exercise must not be confined to the class. It is unlikely that any class has adequate funding to provide frequent enough exercise sessions to get results. Exercise programs are also unlikely to last the lifetime of the individuals. Clients must be guided to incorporate the appropriate activities into their daily lives, and during the class they should be rewarded for having done so. The reward may consist of social recognition or an evaluation demonstrating that their efforts have produced results in the right direction. For lonely individuals, an appropriate motivator may be a buddy system in which the buddy keeps records of the individual's progress. The individual's reward for performing the recommended activity is that he or she may then call the buddy to report that the activity was accomplished and to report any relevant parameters such as changes in distance, number of repetitions, or subjective response.

Occupational and physical therapists are the ideal team members to lead the problem-solving sessions. Both disciplines have training in analyzing movement and identifying appropriate exercise or movement strategies to remediate the problems. Often physical therapists are better trained to analyze the physiologic basis for disabilities, and occupational therapists are better trained to analyze how movement patterns can be adapted to fit each client's lifestyle. Occupa-

tional and physical therapists are also skilled educators and will be able to assist clients in learning not only the specific exercises and activities, but also the method of solving problems.

FUNDING

Although some health-maintenance organizations may contribute to membership in a health club, Medicare and other third-party payers do not cover preventive exercise. However, among the elderly, often a decrease in function can be at least partially attributed to a diagnosis for which a doctor can prescribe therapy. To be reimbursed for treatment by Medicare, there must be a doctor's prescription and documentation of improvement. In documenting improvement, it is important to find an objective measure that contributes to a functional improvement (e.g., walking endurance increased from 15 feet to 30 feet, which enables the client to ambulate from the bedroom to the bathroom; shoulder ROM increased from 60 to 70 degrees, enabling the client to brush his or her hair and teeth independently).

For funding a group exercise program for the elderly, one can apply for a grant from one of the many governmental and private agencies that support programs for the elderly. Holstein (1986) is a good resource for ideas. Aside from the standard grant sources, she suggested finding local companies in whose best interest it may be to fund such a program. An example might be a company that targets the elderly as potential customers, who might find this type of project to be simultaneously a good tax write-off and good public relations. She also recommended finding creative ways to have different sources contribute to various aspects of the program. For instance, a mall may be willing to open early 3 days a week to accommodate a walking program. A company with a van may lend the van for transportation 3 times a week. An area agency on aging may reimburse therapists for their time for supervising the program.

CONCLUSIONS

There is ample evidence that exercise can improve the quality of life for the elderly, decrease dependence on mechanical and human assistance, and prevent injury and disease. It is im-

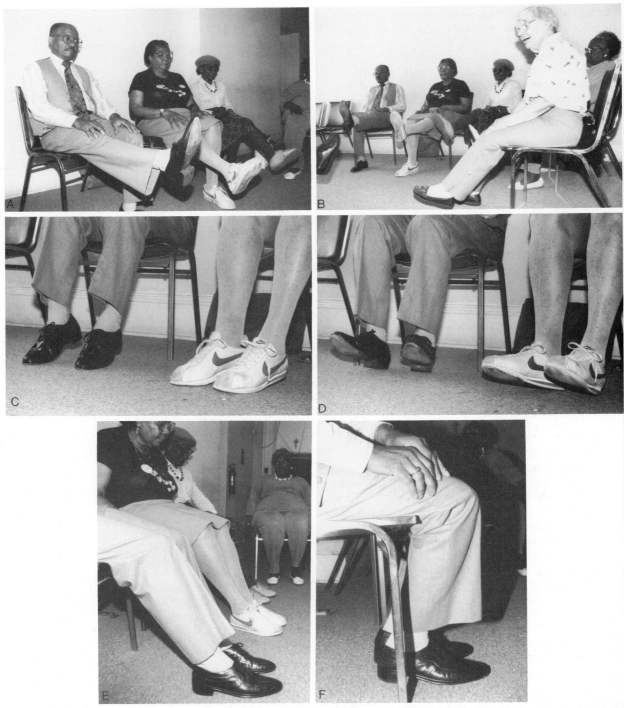

Figure 12–2. The problem-solving approach was used to design this exercise sequence for clients who have trouble getting up out of a soft chair. *A* and *B*, Knee extension, alternate legs. *C* and *D*, Heels up, toes up. *E* and *F*, Keeping heels on the floor, slide feet forward and back.

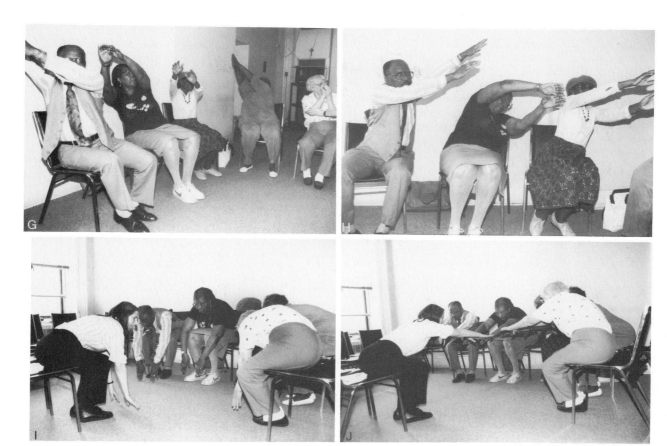

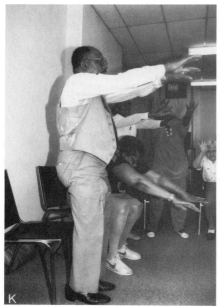

Figure 12–2 *Continued G* and *H*, Raise both arms over one shoulder, then over the other. While raising both arms over one shoulder, advance the opposite hip. Alternate to scoot forward in chair. *I*, Bend forward at the hips, keeping the back relatively straight, and touch the floor. *J*. Reach forward to shift the body weight toward the feet in preparation for standing. *K*, Come to a standing position.

perative that we act to improve the health of the elderly, not just because the proportion of the elderly in the population is increasing and will have greater financial consequences for the nation but also because if we live long enough we will all become members of that group. What we are doing now is making our beds that we will have to lie in. Let us try not to have to lie in it for too long.

References

Adams GM and deVries HA: Physiological effects of an exercise training regimen upon women aged 59–74. J Gerontol 28:50–55, 1973.

American College of Sports Medicine: The recommended quantity and quality of exercise for developing and maintaining fitness in healthy adults. Med Sci Sports Exerc 10:vii–x, 1978.

Amundsen LR, DeVahl JM, and Ellington CT: Evaluation of a group exercise program for elderly women. Phys Ther 69:475–483, 1989.

Ayalon J, et al: Dynamic bone loading exercises for postmenopausal women: Effect on the density of the distal radius. Arch Phys Med Rehab 68(S pt. 1):280–283, 1987.

Benestad AM: Trainability of old men. Acta Med Scand 178:321, 1965.

Bohannon RW, Larkin PA, Cook AC, et al: Decrease in timed balance test scores with aging. Phys Ther 64:1067–1070, 1984.

Bland J: The reversibility of osteoarthritis: A review. Am J Med 74(6A):16–26, 1983.

Borg GAV and Noble BG: Perceived exertion. Exerc Sport Sci Rev 2:131–153, 1974.

Bortz W: Disuse and aging. JAMA 248:1203–1206, 1982.

Brooks V: The Neural Basis of Motor Control. Oxford, England, Oxford University Press, 1986.

Brown M: Selected physical performance changes with aging. Top Geriatr Rehabil 2(4):68–76, 1987.

Chandler JM, Duncan PW, and Studenski SA: Balance performance on the postural stress test: Comparison of young adults, healthy elderly, and fallers. Phys Ther 70:410–415, 1990.

Christiansen C, Riis BJ, and Rodbro P: Prediction of rapid bone loss in postmenopausal women. Lancet 5:16, 1987.

Cummings SR, Nevitt MC, and Haber RJ: Prevention of osteoporosis and osteoporotic fractures. West J Med 143:684–687, 1985.

Dalen N and Olsson KE: Bone mineral content and physical activity. Acta Orthop Scand 45:170, 1974.

deVries HA: Physiological effects of an exercise training regimen upon men aged 52–88. J Gerontol 25:235–336, 1970.

Dial C and Windsor RA: A formative evaluation of a health education–water exercise program for class II and III adult rheumatoid arthritis patients. Patient Educ Counsel 7:33–42, 1985.

Dietrick JE, Whedon GD, and Schorr E: Effects of immobilization upon various metabolic and physiologic functions of normal men. Am J Med 4:3–36, 1948.

Donaldson CL, Hulley SB, Vogel JM et al: Effect of prolonged bed rest on bone mineral. Metabolism 19:1071–1084, 1970.

Ekblom B: Short- and long-term physical training in patients with rheumatoid arthritis. Ann Clin Res 14(Suppl 34):109–110, 1982.

Fansler CL, Poff CL, and Shepard KF: Effects of mental practice on balance in elderly women. Phys Ther 65:1332–1336, 1985.

Fiatarone MA, Marks EC, Ryan ND, et al: High intensity strength training in nonagenarians: Effects on skeletal muscle. JAMA 263:3029–3034, 1990.

Frontera WR, Meredith CN, O'Reilly KP, et al: Strength conditioning in older men: Skeletal muscle hypertrophy and improved function. J Appl Physiol 64:1038–1044, 1988.

Germain NW and Blair SN: Variability of shoulder flexion with age, activity and sex. Am Correc Ther J 37:156–160, 1983.

Goodman CE: Osteoporosis: Protective measures of nutrition and exercise. Geriatrics 40:59–70, 1985.

Graf RS: Rehabilitation during the acute and convalescent stages following myocardial infarction. In Amundsen LR (ed): Cardiac Rehabilitation. New York, Churchill Livingstone, 1981.

Habasevich RA: Implications of cardiovascular aging. In Lewis CB (ed): Aging: The Health Care Challenge. Philadelphia, FA Davis, 1985.

Hahn BH: Arthritis, connective tissue disorders and extraarticular rheumatism. In Steinberg FU (ed): Care of the Geriatric Patient. St. Louis, CV Mosby, 1983.

Harkcom TM, Lampman RM, Banwell BF, et al: Therapeutic value of graded aerobic exercise training in rheumatoid arthritis. Arthritis Rheum 28:32–39, 1985.

Herbert L and Teague ML: Exercise adherence and older adults: A theoretical perspective. Activ Adapt Aging 13(1/2):91–105, 1989.

Holstein M: Funding health promotion for elders. In Dychtwald K (ed): Wellness and Health Promotion for the Elderly. Rockville, MD, Aspen, 1986.

Jacobson PC, Beaver W, Grubb SA, et al: Bone density in women: College athletes and older athletic women. J Orthop Res 2:328–332, 1984.

Kennedy RD, Andrews GR, and Caird FI: Ischemic heart disease in the elderly. Br Heart J 39:1127, 1977.

Kitchin AH, Lowther CD, and Milne JS: Prevalence of clinical and electrocardiographic evidence of ischemic heart disease in the older population. Br Heart J 35:946, 1973.

Knortz KA: Muscle physiology applied to geriatric rehabilitation. Top Geriatr Rehabil 2(4):1–12, 1987.

Kohler P: Model of shared control. J Gerontol Nurs 14(7):21–25, 1988.

Krolner B, Toft B Nielsen SP, et al: Physical exercise as prophylaxis against involutional vertebral bone loss: A controlled trial. Clin Sci 64:541–546, 1983.

Larsson L: Physical training effects on muscle morphology in sedentary males at different ages. Med Sci Sports Exerc 14:203–206, 1982.

Larsson L, Grimby G, and Karlsson J: Muscle strength and speed of movement in relation to age and muscle morphology. J Appl Physiol 46(3):451–456, 1979.

Larsson L, Sjodin B, and Karlsson J: Histochemical and biochemical changes in human skeletal muscle with age in sedentary males, age 22–65 years. Acta Physiol Scand 103:31–39, 1978.

Lewis CB: Clinical implications of musculoskeletal changes with age. In Lewis CB (ed), Aging: The Health Care Challenge. Philadelphia, FA Davis, 1985.

Lewis CB: Effects of aging on the cardiovascular system. Clin Manag 4(4):24–29, 1984.

Lipsitz LA, Nyquist RP, Wei JY, et al: Postprandial reduction in blood pressure in the elderly. N Engl J Med *309*:81–83, 1983.

Low JF: Time perception and rehabilitation of the elderly. Phys Occupat Ther Geriatr *5*(4):17–30, 1987.

Millar PM: Realistic exercise goals for the elderly: Is feeling good enough? Geriatrics *42*(3):25–29, 1987.

Mobily KE: Motivational aspects of exercise for the elderly: Barriers and solutions. Phys Occupat Ther Geriatr *1*(4):43–54, 1982.

Moritani T and deVries H: Potential for gross muscle hypertrophy in older men. J Gerontol *35*:672–682, 1980.

Mount J: Evaluation of a health promotion program provided at senior centers by physical therapy students. Phys Occup Ther Geriatr. (in press)

Munns K: Effects of exercise on the range of joint motion in elderly subjects. *In* Smith EL and Serfass RC (eds): Exercise and Aging: The Scientific Basis. Hillside, NJ, Enslow, 1981.

Nordemar R: Physical training in rheumatoid arthritis: A controlled study, Vol II. Scand J Rheumatol *10*:25–30, 1981.

Nordemar R, Ekblom B, Zachrisson L, et al: Physical training in rheumatoid arthritis: A controlled study, Vol I. Scand J Rheumatol *10*:17–23, 1981.

Orlander J, Kiessling K, Larsson L, et al: Skeletal muscle metabolism ultrastructure in relation to age in sedentary men. Acta Physiol Scand *104*:249–261, 1978.

Overstall PW, Exton-Smith AN, Imms FJ, et al: Falls in the elderly related to postural imbalance. Br Med J *1*:261–264, 1977.

Parent CJ and Whall AL: Are physical activity, self-esteem, and depression related? J Gerontol Nurs *10*:8–11, 1984.

Payton OD and Poland JL: Aging process, implications for clinical practice. Phys Ther *63*(1):41–48, 1983.

Perri S and Templer D: The effects of an aerobic exercise program on psychological variables in older adults. Int J Aging Hum Dev *20*:162–172, 1985.

Posner JD, Gorman KM, Gitlin LN, et al: Effects of exercise training in the elderly on the occurrence and time to onset of cardiovascular diagnosis. J Am Geriatr Soc *38*:205–210, 1990.

Raab DM, Agre JC, McAdams M, et al: Light resistance and stretching exercise in elderly women: Effect upon flexibility. Arch Phys Med Rehab *69*:268–272, 1988.

Riddick CC and Freitag R: The impact of an aerobic fitness program on the body image of older women. Res Aging *6*:59–70, 1984.

Ring C, Nayak USL, and Isaacs B: Balance function in elderly people who have and who have not fallen. Arch Phys Med Rehabil *69*:261–264, 1988.

Sandler RB, Canley JA, Hom DL, et al: The effects of walking on the cross-sectional dimensions of the radius in postmenopausal women. Calcif Tissue Int *41*:65–69, 1987.

Schurer J and Tipton CM: Cardiovascular adaptation to physical training. Ann Rev Physiol *39*:221, 1977.

Shepard RJ: The scientific basis of exercise prescribing for the very old. J Am Geriatr Soc *38*:62–70, 1990.

Sidney KH: Cardiovascular benefits of physical activity in the exercising aged. *In* Smith EL and Surfass RC (eds): Exercise and aging: The scientific basis. Hillside, NJ, Enslow, 1981.

Sinaki M: Postmenopausal spinal osteoporosis: Physical therapy and rehabilitation principles. Mayo Clin Proc *57*:699–703, 1982.

Sinaki M and Mikkelsen BA: Postmenopausal spinal osteoporosis: Flexion versus extension exercises. Arch Phys Med Rehabil *65*:593–596, 1984.

Smith EL, et al: Physical activity and calcium modalities for bone mineral increase in aged women. Med Sci Sports Exerc *13*:60, 1981.

Smith JJ and Kampine JP: Circulatory Physiology—The Essentials. Baltimore, Williams & Wilkins, 1980.

Speechley M and Tinetti M: Assessment of risk and prevention of falls among elderly persons: Role of the physiotherapist. Physiother Can *42*:75–78, 1990.

Stacey C, Kozma S, and Stones MJ: Simple cognitive and behavioral changes resulting from improved physical fitness in persons over 50 years of age. Can J Aging *4*:67–74, 1985.

Suwalska M: Importance of physical training of rheumatic patients. Ann Clin Res *14*(Suppl 34):107–109, 1982.

Teitelman JL: Eliminating learned helplessness in older rehabilitation patients. Phys Occup Ther Geriatr *1*:3–10, 1982.

Tzankoff SP, Robinson S, Pyke FS, et al: Physiological adjustment to work in older men as affected by physical training. J Appl Physiol *33*:346–350, 1972.

U.S. Department of Health and Human Services: Health Promotion and Disease Prevention. Data from the National Health Survey, Series 10, No. 163 (DHHS Publication No. [PHS] 88-1591) Washington, DC, U.S. Government Printing Office, 1985.

Wolfson LI, Whipple R, Amerman P, et al: Stressing the postural response: A quantitative method for testing balance. J Am Geriatr Soc *34*:845–850, 1986.

Bibliography

Aisenbrey JA: Exercise in the prevention and management of osteoporosis. Phys Ther *67*:1100–1104, 1987.

CHAPTER

13

Pamela J. Holliday
Cheryl A. Cott
Wendy D. Torresin

Preventing Accidental Falls by the Elderly

OVERVIEW OF THE PROBLEM

The population over 65 years of age, and in particular those over 85 years of age, are the fastest growing segment of the population in North America. Falls represent a major threat to health status and independence of these older individuals.

Approximately one third to one half of all persons over 65 years of age fall at least once per year (Kellogg International Work Group, 1987). Fortunately, most falls do not result in serious injury and are therefore not reported (Gryfe et al, 1977, Holliday et al, 1985, Kellogg International Work Group, 1987). The absence of injury probably accounts for the poor reporting of falls and underestimation of the magnitude of the problem. Many older individuals who fall do not seek medical attention. Society, in general, tends to accept these falls by the elderly as an unavoidable part of aging (Wolf-Klein et al, 1988). However, a less recognized but serious consequence of falling is the fear of falling; this fear, which may be present with or without actual falling events, limits mobility and promotes social isolation and loss of confidence (Kellogg International Work Group, 1987).

Falls are the leading cause of accidental death in persons 75 years of age and over and the second leading cause of death from accidents for all ages (National Safety Council, 1990). Falls are the leading cause of death from accidents in the home, and one third of the persons killed in home accidents are 75 years of age and older. For every fall that is the underlying cause of death, almost 20 cases result in hip fracture (Baker and Harvey, 1985). The diagnosis of hip fracture is the most common among all injuries leading to hospital admission in the United States. Of the approximately 200,000 hip fractures each year, 84% involve persons 65 years of age or older. The health-care costs of new hip fractures exceed 2 billion dollars annually. The incidence of falls in clients admitted to institutions ranges from 25 to 89% of all hospital incidents; the elderly represent a significant proportion of hospital admissions (Raz and Baretich, 1987).

The published research on incidence and management of falls in community or institutionalized elderly is inadequate. The descriptive and evaluative assessments await studies of reliability and validity and longitudinal examination of the effects of interventions. Early detection of fall risk factors and intervention may prevent the cycle of increasing frailty as a result of increasing inactivity and disability, but this has not yet been proved by rigorous clinical trials. Several reports identify the effectiveness of exercise programs in the elderly for improving joint range, muscle strength, balance, and endurance, but these have not been related to fall prevention in the elderly.

Clinical research on the effectiveness of specific techniques used with homogeneous subgroups based on diagnoses and age is required for clinicians to predict those clients who can benefit from treatment and to determine appropriate procedure variations that improve impairments and impact on disabilities.

MODEL OF ASSESSMENT

An assessment of the elderly person includes multiple components. The theoretic model outlined in Figure 13–1 provides a useful base on which the organization of the information may be collected. This model, adapted from Engel (1981) and modified by Torresin (1989) for assessment of the older person, is individual-centered and identifies the three major areas of interaction as the attributes of the individual, her or his personal environment, and societal conditions that exist. The content areas of this model may be defined as follows:

1. Individual: the individual's unique internal physiologic, emotional, cultural, perceptual, cognitive, and spiritual aspects. These aspects are interrelated and interdependent and have multiple subdivisions (e.g., the physiologic aspect of the individual includes chemical, molecular, cellular, and systematic subdivisions). The individual's behavior is the observable reaction to his or her internal aspects and external environment.

2. Environment: the individual's personal external physical and social surroundings. The physical environment includes the physical living conditions at home, work, and recreation. The individual's immediate social environment includes all people with whom he or she interacts, such as family, friends, colleagues, and caregivers.

3. Society: the external environment that indirectly affects the individual (e.g., the political, cultural, and economic conditions that exist). The social environment is the societal system within which the individual exists, such as consumer groups, social groups and organizations, other groups and organizations, and government services and policies.

This model can be expanded to incorporate the prevention of falls at the primary, secondary, and tertiary stages (Fig. 13–2). A brief summary of the model applied to the assessment and

Figure 13–1. The individual-centered model for assessment of the elderly.

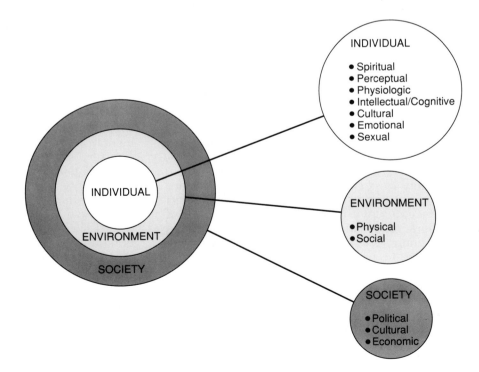

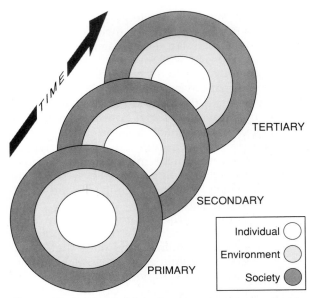

Figure 13–2. The individual-centered model applied to stages of health promotion.

treatment of falls in the elderly is outlined in Table 13–1.

Primary prevention is targeted at those older persons who have not fallen or who do not consider falling to be a problem and who are generally healthy. Secondary prevention is targeted at screening individuals who are at risk of falling and at preventing serious injury and loss of confidence. Tertiary prevention focuses on those for whom falling is a problem.

The continuum of stages relating to balance can also be described by commonly used terminology from the World Health Organization (WHO). WHO recognized the lack of a framework for the classification of chronic diseases and suggested several definitions (WHO, 1980; Wood, 1980). An *impairment* is "any loss or abnormality of psychological, physiological or anatomical structure or function"; because impairments represent physiologic disturbances, loss of or alteration of balance can be thought of as an impairment. A *disability* is "any restriction or lack of ability to perform an activity in a manner within the range considered normal." Disabilities represent functional disturbances at the individual level, and falling and gait disorders are disabilities. A *handicap* is "a disadvantage for a given individual, resulting from an impairment or a disability, that limits or prevents the fulfillment of a role that is normal for that individual (de-

pending on age, sex, social, and cultural factors)." Handicaps represent disturbances in the interaction with the individual's surroundings. Balance impairments, falling, and gait disabilities may result in an inability to move around freely. Individuals restricted in their social or physical environment have a handicap.

At the stage of primary prevention, no impairment is present. At the secondary stage, impairment is present and the goal is to prevent disability or handicap. At the tertiary stage, disability is present and the goal is to prevent handicap.

Balance includes the ability to maintain a position, to adjust to voluntary or self-initiated movement, and to react to external disturbances or perturbations (Berg, 1989). A fall may be defined as "an event which results in a person coming to rest inadvertently on the ground or other lower level" (Kellogg International Work Group, 1987). A fall occurs when a perturbation or disturbance, either external, sensory, or physiologic (internal), causes a transition from stability to instability. Either failure to compensate for a perturbation or failure of the postural control system itself can lead to a fall. Before designing measures to prevent falls, it is essential to understand why older people fall so that appropriate measures can be specifically targeted at the relevant contributing factors.

PRIMARY PREVENTION

Capsule Summary

Primary prevention averts the occurrence of disease and includes health promotion, environmental intervention, and prophylactic therapies (Warren, 1985). It is anticipatory and directed at promoting health in general or at disease, injury, or disability that might occur; many of the individuals who are in the target population may never have the disorder. Primary prevention includes such issues as health promotion, nutrition, housing, control of environmental hazards, physical activity, consumer protection, and prevention of injury.

The goals of primary prevention are to encourage maintenance of a healthy, active lifestyle, promotion of the awareness of the high accident rate in the elderly, and introduction of measures to reduce accidental fall risk. As yet, no data support the efficacy of health promotion meas-

Table 13–1. Brief Summary of the Model for Prevention of Falls

Stage	Area	Action
Primary	Individual	Lifestyle emphasis on physical activity, fitness, nutrition
	Environment	Safe environment for everyone; aging in place at home
	Society	Public awareness and individual responsibility for accident prevention; safety and support in the community; positive attitude toward aging
Secondary	Individual	Falls screening and risk identification; rehabilitation based on assessment; improve balance; preventive programs
	Environment	Assess/modify home for maximum safety and independence
	Society	Increase knowledge and promote positive attitudes toward devices to enhance independent living; educate professionals and lay people regarding resources and fall risk factors
Tertiary	Individual	Multidisciplinary approach to multiple issues; treatment programs based on function (i.e., activities of daily living); recognize fear of falling
	Environment	Modify and support to make up for the deficits and to encourage safety and independence
	Society	Importance of continuing role of the family; promote positive attitude of health-care workers to long-term illness

ures on the occurrence of falls and subsequent mortality and morbidity in the elderly. However, some specific research studies demonstrated that positive changes can be made in the elderly, such as an increase in muscle strength (Vandervoort et al, 1986).

The Individual

In the model of assessment, a number of factors were identified for consideration (spiritual, perceptual, physiologic, intellectual/cognitive, cultural, emotional, and sexual). However, in this chapter, physiologic factors (e.g., balance, sensory, motor, cardiovascular, and musculoskeletal) are discussed.

Many normal aging changes have a minimal effect on activities of daily living (ADL) but may place an individual at risk for falling and subsequent injury.

Stelmach and Worringham (1985) described a scheme of processing stages that control responses to postural control and stability.

1. Sensory input or feedforward: In this stage, a potential fall is imminent. Sensory processes alert the centers in the nervous system responsible for response selection.
2. Response selection: In this stage, the sensory information is interpreted and a corrective or protective response is selected.
3. Response execution: The actual corrective response or movement is carried out. It involves muscular action and is therefore affected by

the speed, strength, and phasing of the muscles involved.

Deterioration in balance and impaired postural control have been cited as major contributing factors to falls among the elderly. Posturography may be used to identify subtle balance impairments that may not be observed during clinical and functional balance test protocols (Tinetti et al, 1986).

Balance

To maintain balance, the postural control system keeps the body center of gravity over the base of support. Horak (1987) described how subjects use a limited repertoire of rapidly initiated, stereotyped responses (strategies) to external perturbations of balance. The ankle strategy is the most common response to small perturbations and involves shifts of the center of body mass as a rotation about the ankle joint with little or no movement of the hips. The hip strategy shifts the center of body mass by flexing or extending at the hips. Larger perturbations or narrowing of the base of support (i.e., walking on a narrow rail) normally evoke a hip strategy response. The ankle and hip strategies may be used separately or in combination. A larger displacement may require a stepping response. Studies showed that the elderly tend to routinely use the hip strategy as opposed to the ankle strategy in response to even small displacements of balance (Horak, 1987). This may result in overbalancing and perhaps a greater risk of falling.

A decline in the ability of older individuals to control both static (spontaneous) and dynamic balance and postural control exists (Isaacs, 1978). Spontaneous postural sway with aging increases (Black et al, 1977; Fernie and Holliday, 1978; Hayes et al, 1985; Kirshen et al, 1984; Maki et al, 1990; Sheldon, 1963). In addition, balancing synergies deteriorate, which results in delayed muscle contractions and a reverse of the muscle activation sequence in response to postural perturbations (Woollacott et al., 1986). The response to impulsive (posterior) force perturbations are more extreme and less effective in older persons (Wolfson et al, 1986). Holliday and Fernie (1985) observed an increase in postural sway in response to rotational platform perturbations in nondisabled older subjects compared with a younger control group. Age-related differences in postural control are more pronounced when postural response is examined on a perturbation platform that can simulate a trip or a slip (Maki et al, 1990). The platform stimulus during testing was a small acceleration, pseudorandom motion; the data were then fitted with a model that was used to determine the response to a sudden (transient) platform movement, thus simulating an actual fall. Maki and associates (1990) compared measures of spontaneous postural sway with the results of induced sway in community-based elderly subjects. Sway was measured in terms of the displacement of the center of pressure on the feet. Both induced- and spontaneous-sway tests showed significant age-related declines in stability; however, the induced-sway tests produced a more pronounced age-related effect. Alternatively, spontaneous-sway measures were more successful in distinguishing between fallers and nonfallers in a small sample of five elderly fallers. There was no correlation, or an inverse relationship, between spontaneous-sway and induced-sway measures in the older subjects.

Since Sheldon (1963) first described the relationship between postural sway and falling, numerous attempts to examine this correlation have been made (Brocklehurst et al, 1982; Fernie et al, 1982; Overstall et al, 1977). Overstall and associates (1977) tried to relate postural sway to falls and reported that fallers sway more than nonfallers when the cause of the fall is other than a trip or a slip. Brocklehurst and colleagues (1982) found a significant correlation between history of falling and spontaneous sway with the eyes closed only in subjects 75 to 84 years of age.

Fernie and associates (1982) demonstrated an increase in the mean speed of postural sway in a group of elderly fallers compared with an elderly control group.

As a result of age-related changes in postural control, older persons may be more prone to falls in response to slight routine losses of balance during everyday activities (Wild et al, 1987). A disruption in balance that in younger persons would lead to a misstep or trip might cause a fall in older individuals. Environmental considerations in these at-risk individuals assume even greater importance (Tinetti et al, 1988).

The motor, sensory, and central integrative systems are involved in maintaining balance and postural control; integration occurs at multiple levels in the central nervous system (e.g., the cortex, thalamus, basal ganglia, cerebellum, brain stem, and spinal cord) (Wolfson et al, 1985). The cardiovascular, skeletal, and cognitive systems also contribute to the maintenance of balance and postural control.

Sensory

Normal age-related sensory changes result in diminished proprioception, cutaneous sensation, and a loss or decrease in vibration sense (Imms and Edholm, 1981; Wolfson et al, 1985). Impaired proprioception may result in the requirement of greater joint angle movements for movement detection. Loss of sensory function, particularly cutaneous sensation, proprioception, and vibration in the foot and ankle, may contribute to impaired gait and instability as a result of improper foot placement (Guimares and Isaacs, 1980) and may contribute to an increased incidence of slips, trips, and missteps. In addition, chronic disease, such as osteoarthritis, may contribute to error in foot placement. Proprioceptive alterations in the cervical region may also provide misleading information about the position of the head in space (Wyke, 1979). Reliance on remaining sensory cues, particularly vision, are necessary to compensate for decreases in the other sensory domains.

Visual information is important for balance. Even in young, healthy subjects, there is an increase in postural sway when visual cues are removed (Dornan et al, 1978; Fernie and Holliday, 1978; Maki, 1987). Age-related changes in vision decrease the ability of the older person to use visual reference information about the environment. Decline in visual acuity, restriction of the visual field, increased susceptibility to glare, deficient gaze stability, decline in color vision, and decreased depth perception occur with advancing age and have implications for the older person's ability to interact with their physical environment to guide locomotion and avoid obstacles (Andreasen, 1980; Kokman et al, 1977; Owen, 1985; Spooner et al, 1980). The resulting misinterpretation of spatial information can lead to impaired judgment and disorientation.

Age-related changes in the vestibular system that affect function have not been widely studied. The number and size of vestibular neurons decrease with age (Babin and Harker, 1982; Kenshalo, 1979; Oosterveld, 1983), which, in combination with declines in the visual system and reflexes such as the righting reflex, may result in failure to protect oneself from a fall. The central processing of information from the three primary systems that contribute to balance (i.e., visual, somatosensory, and vestibular) may also be disrupted by age (Kellogg International Work Group, 1987).

Safety of the older person in general may be compromised by age-related declines in the auditory system (presbycusis) and other sensory domains such as taste and smell. Failure to hear warning signals such as in pedestrian travel or the doorbell at home may reduce the time remaining to avoid an accident; delayed failure to detect odors such as smoke or gas could similarly put older persons at risk for an accident.

Motor

Decreased muscle strength and speed of contraction may also be associated with increased falling in the elderly. Although controversy exists over the exact physiologic explanation, limb muscles in older individuals tend to be weaker, atrophied, slower, and more susceptible to fatigue and have decreased numbers of motoneurons (Davies and White, 1983; Grimby and Saltin, 1983; Vandervoort et al, 1990). There may be a 20 to 40% decline in isometric strength in both proximal and distal musculature in healthy older individuals in their 60s and 70s. This decline continues into the older decades. Simple duration of movement has also been shown to increase with age (Shumway-Cook and Horak, 1986). These changes in muscle function, in combination with other age-related deficits, result in a slowing of response that presents as delayed movement initiation, particularly when time

stress allows little opportunity for advance response preparation (Shumway-Cook and Horak, 1986).

Changes in muscle strength in relation to falls may be particularly related to the ankle musculature. Whipple and co-workers (1987) conducted isokinetic studies of muscle strength comparing fallers and nonfallers among nursing home residents. The knee flexors and extensors and the ankle dorsiflexors and plantarflexors were examined. Significant decline was found in the muscle strength of the ankle musculature, particularly in the dorsiflexors, of the fallers compared with nonfallers. This weakness might be implicated in observed declines in the use of the ankle strategy in the elderly as well as the increased predisposition to backward falls. Foot clearance and trajectory may also be decreased by changes in ankle musculature. Certain daily activities such as rising from a chair and negotiating stairs may similarly be affected.

Changes in gait may also be implicated in falls, particularly slips, trips, and missteps. The elderly tend to have decreased steppage height, shorter stride length, and slower walking speed (Imms and Edholm, 1981). Senile gait disorder—described by Koller and associates (1985) as being of gradual onset after age 60 and including a broad-based gait with small steps and gait dysrhythmia, flexion at the hips and knees, decreased associated movements, poor tandem gait, and truncal instability—may be applied to older individuals. However, it is uncertain whether this disorder is related to age alone or to other factors. Koller and associates (1985) postulated that senile gait disorder is a separate clinical entity related to degeneration of specific parts of the nervous system and not to chronologic age per se.

Degenerative age-related changes in the motor cortex neurons and spinal motoneurons may interfere with relaxation of the antigravity muscles, producing decrements in motor performance and agility (Scheibel, 1979). The speed of balance response may also decrease with aging as a result of a reduction in the conduction velocity (Dorfman and Bosley, 1979). A decline in postural reflexes has also been reported (Stelmach et al, 1989).

Cardiovascular

Alterations in the regulation of blood pressure are thought to contribute to some of the falls in the elderly (Lipsitz, 1985). Declines in barorecep-tor sensitivity, cerebral blood flow, and extracel-lular volume regulation have been reported. The overall impact on balance in the older person may mean that minor changes in homeostasis such as a change in posture, acute illness, or medication changes may affect blood pressure and precipitate a fall.

Musculoskeletal

Musculoskeletal changes such as calcification of tendons and ligaments and loss of bone min-eral content may result in postural changes such as kyphosis, which in turn may alter the body biomechanics and lead to instability and poor recovery from loss of balance (Tideiksaar, 1989).

Although not implicated as a cause of falls, osteoporosis is significant in terms of the injury resulting from falls. Osteoporosis, the most com-mon skeletal disorder in North America, is an age-related decrease in bone mass and subse-quent increased susceptibility to fractures (Martin and Houston, 1987; National Institutes of Health [NIH], 1984). A fall or twisting activity that would not affect the average person may result in bone fracture in an individual with osteoporosis. By 65 years of age, 50% of women are likely to have osteoporosis. Up to 1.3 million fractures annually (in the United States) are attributable to osteo-porosis in individuals 45 years and older, and most older individuals fail to recover normal activity (NIH, 1984). There is a high proportion of women (32%) and men (17%) over 90 years of age who suffer osteoporosis-related hip fractures. The annual health-care costs related to osteopo-rosis in the United States are estimated at $3.8 billion (NIH, 1984).

No laboratory tests exist to define persons at risk or to detect those with mild osteoporosis (NIH, 1984). The primary goal of intervention is the prevention of bone loss and subsequent frac-tures (Bornor et al, 1988). The treatment options include hormone therapy, diet, and exercise. Estrogen therapy is of established benefit in the prevention of postmenopausal osteoporosis but is not without risk (NIH, 1984); calcium supple-mentation and fluoride may have limited benefit (Bornor et al, 1988). The significance of nutrition on the development of osteoporosis is obscure, and diet modifications such as liberal intake of calcium may be considered prophylactic rather than therapeutic. More recently, emphasis has been placed on the role of exercise as a nonin-vasive approach to prevent bone loss, falling accidents, and fall-related trauma. Exercise in-volving weight bearing, such as walking, may be recommended; however, the optimal type and amount of physical activity required to retard the bone-loss process and prevent osteoporosis have not been established (NIH, 1984).

Treatment/Management

Important health goals for all older persons in-clude maintenance of function, delay of chronic disease, and minimization of disability (Larson and Bruce, 1987). With the increasing concern regarding health and utilization of health re-sources, interest in exercise has increased as a mechanism to enhance active life expectancy (the portion of remaining life with independence) and achieve the aforementioned goals. Prevention of the development of age-related disorders leading to falling and instability may be enhanced by a lifestyle that includes proper nutrition and phys-ical activity (Astrand, 1987; Larson and Bruce, 1987). The benefits of regular physical activity (training) are vast, including cardiovascular, musculoskeletal, and metabolic effects. Exercise, however, is not without hazards, including sud-den death and nonfatal myocardial infarction, musculoskeletal injuries, cardiologic changes, and fatigue and exhaustion (Larson and Bruce, 1987).

Physical activity may be considered a health-promoting behavior for older adults potentially at risk of falling but who are currently not expe-riencing any difficulties. Although no studies exist in the literature to support this assumption, it is known that by maintaining physical activity levels one maintains strength, range of move-ment, and endurance, all of which improve the ability to balance. In addition, studies on reaction times suggest that healthier adults have faster reaction times than less healthy adults of com-parable age and that adults who engage in physical exercise have faster reaction times than age-matched sedentary adults (Stelmach and Worringham, 1985). Speedy response to an over-balancing event may prevent a fall.

Activities that increase strength and endurance and challenge posture and balance are suitable suggestions for the primary prevention stage. Not all such activities have to be exercise. Social dancing is an excellent physical activity that may not be perceived as such by those who do not enjoy exercise. Bowling, gardening, tai chi (a form of Chinese exercise), community exercise groups, and walking are all physical activities that should be encouraged.

Individuals should be able to evaluate their fitness level and know what criteria are used to determine changes in the program. Qualified medical and fitness instructors are resources who can be involved in regular physical activity programs for seniors.

Wellness also includes nutrition, social supports (friends, family, acquaintances), lifestyle behaviors (moderate alcohol intake, no smoking, exercise), clean environment (air, water, soil), health care (regular medical checkups), and awareness of genetic factors (e.g., predisposition to heart attack and stroke). In general, poor nutrition may exacerbate or directly affect disorders related to falling, such as peripheral neuropathy. Proper nutrition discourages excessive use of salt and sugar, which may be ingested to compensate for decreased taste sensitivity. The presence of these substances may exacerbate conditions such as diabetes, which, in turn, may lead to falling.

No controlled trials have been published that evaluate the effect of exercise and specific exercise programs on balance and postural control and falling in healthy, elderly persons. The optimal type, intensity, duration, and frequency of exercise required to achieve beneficial training effects and minimize hazards have not yet been established (Larson and Bruce, 1987).

Environment and Society

Most persons over 65 years of age consider themselves to be in good health, even though 80% of them suffer from at least one chronic condition (Heckler, 1985). Each year they report 39 days of restricted activity and 14 days of confinement to bed.

Societal attitudes toward aging and activity and toward women and activity must be considered when advocating physical activity as a health-promoting behavior in older adults. Most cross-sectional studies of activity patterns throughout the life cycle indicate that, although physical activity declines with age, factors such as social status, education, income, marital status, and gender also affect activity patterns within age cohorts (McPherson and Kozlik, 1987). It does not appear that declines in physical activity levels

with aging can be wholly attributed to inevitable physiologic declines (Serfass, 1981). The current elderly population was not reared to place high value on leisure time and activities (McPherson and Kozlik, 1987). In addition, negative attitudes toward women and activity exist (Snyder and Spreitzer, 1983). Declines in physical activity with aging, particularly for women, may therefore be a cohort effect. It could be argued that as the baby boomer cohort ages, they may not demonstrate similar declines in activity levels.

In addition to the attitudes of the elderly themselves, the larger societal attitudes bear consideration. Age discrimination may operate to restrict opportunities for the elderly to be active as well as to define acceptable activity levels for them (McPherson and Kozlik, 1987, p. 225):

> "There is little social reinforcement in the older adult world for the individual who 'thinks and acts young,' or who wants to be 'physically active,' although some changes are taking place concerning adult leisure norms and opportunities within some segments of the elderly and middle age population."

The need for preventive measures to combat the risks of aging is not only a medical issue but also a societal responsibility. In some societies the elderly are considered a burden, whereas in others they are viewed and used as valuable resources (International Association of Gerontology, 1980).

Community-based education programs aimed at increasing the public's awareness of falls, the potential serious consequences, and environmental safety measures are required. Program initiatives may come from volunteer agencies, for example, the American Association of Retired Persons, self-help groups, safety councils (local, state, and national, such as the National Safety Council), and health and social facilities (Kellogg International Work Group, 1987). Many of the aforementioned agencies and groups provide information (often free of charge) for seniors related to falls and general accident prevention in and around the home. Pamphlets and checklists are available for the general public that focus on safety and accident prevention in the home; however, the rationale for the suggestions is rarely included (Lok, 1990; Tideiksaar, 1986). Table 13–2 provides a list of some of the available print resources for accident prevention in the home. A manual has been developed for community-based seniors that is comprehensive and provides a self-awareness quiz for the user as

Table 13–2. Available Print Resources for the General Public Aimed Toward Accident Prevention in the Home

Source	Title
American Association of Retired Persons 1909 K St, NW Washington, DC 20049	Dangerous Products, Dangerous Places
Canada Safety Council 1765 St. Laurent Blvd, Ottawa, Ontario K1G 3V4 Canada	How to Avoid Falls
Health and Welfare Canada, Supply and Services Canada, 1984	Let's Talk About . . . Falls and the Elderly
Krames Communications, 312 90th St, Daly City, CA 94015–1898	Home Safe Home
National Easter Seal Society 2023 Ogden Ave, Chicago, IL 60612	Home Safety Round-Up. A Family Checklist
National Safety Council 444 North Michigan Ave, Chicago, IL 60611 and The American Association of Retired Persons (see above)	FALLING! The Unexpected Trip
Saskatchewan Consumer and Commercial Affairs Consumer Information Centre, Box 3000, Regina, Saskatchewan, S4P 3V7 Canada	Proceed with Caution: Consumer Safety in the Home
Scriptographic Commun. 150 Consumers Rd, Ste 404 Willowdale, Ontario M2J 1P9 Canada	1. Accident Prevention and Older People 2. Slips, Trips, and Falls
U.S. Consumer Product Safety Commission, Washington, DC 20207	Safety for Older Consumers: Home Safety Checklist
University of Southern California Geriatric Research, Education & Clinical Center Sepulveda VA Medical Center Sepulveda, CA	80 Do's and 58 Don'ts for Your Safety: A Practical Guide for Eldercare

well as the rationale for suggested home-safety modifications; also included is a separate manual directed toward health-care professionals that provides background on the age-related changes that contribute to accidents, particularly falls, in the elderly (Lok, 1990). A handbook has been prepared for general accident prevention in the home that also includes some background information about accidents and some rationale for preventive measures (Egger and Taves, 1986).

Public-awareness campaigns should focus on safety in the home and providing a safe environment for all users, not only the older family members. Personal responsibility for accident prevention should be encouraged. Architects,

planners, and safety authorities are recognizing the need for barrier-free design for the disabled, as evidenced by articles in widely circulated home-renovation magazines ("Barrier-free living," 1990) but are not yet required by law to institute environmental designs that enable, not disable, individuals. For example, in addition to towel bars in the bathroom, grab bars should be properly placed and installed on a routine basis; these facilitate safe bathroom use by all family members, not just the older person.

The attitude of homeowners and society in general toward home modifications to facilitate independent living requires focus and redirection. Many environmental safety modifications are considered signs of disability; therefore, healthy older persons are unwilling to institute these measures because they represent signs of decreasing function and loss of independence (Kellogg International Work Group, 1987). By targeting the marketing of products and services to provide a safe environment for *all* users, societal attitudes may be gradually changed.

SECONDARY PREVENTION

Capsule Summary

Secondary prevention halts or retards the progression of a disease by early detection (Warren, 1985). Impairment is present, and the emphasis is on falls screening and preventive programming.

The Individual

The older person is either at risk of falling or has recently experienced one or more falls. The goal at this stage is to either identify those older persons at risk of falling or to determine why a particular individual may be falling. To perform a comprehensive assessment or screening, a basic understanding of the reasons why older people fall is needed.

We can only speculate about causal relationships in falling accidents. It is difficult to establish a single cause for a fall, because many factors usually come into play (Holliday et al, 1990; Speechley and Tinetti, 1990). In addition, with the exception of one study reported by Holliday and associates (1990), data are available only after the fall has occurred. Falls are often classified as intrinsic or extrinsic (Wild et al, 1981). Intrinsic factors include the effects of age-related changes in postural control or disease that predispose individuals to fall, such as visual impairment, muscle weakness, or cervical spondylosis, whereas extrinsic factors comprise environmental hazards. Furthermore, Wild and associates (1981) distinguished between ordinary and extraordinary displacements. The latter includes instances that would cause a healthy, young adult to fall, such as missing a step while climbing a ladder. Ordinary displacements occur during daily activities such as rising from a chair. Speechley and Tinetti (1990) observed that very few falls are caused solely by either an overwhelming intrinsic

or extrinsic cause; instead, the causes of most falls are multifactorial. At present, there is no classification scheme that allows systematic determination of the contributing factors for each fall; however, Maki and associates (1989) proposed a control systems classification scheme based on observations of spontaneous falls of elderly people during their occurrence. Preliminary findings suggest that mechanical perturbations, which can be imposed by the environment (i.e., a push) or self-induced (i.e., movement of the center of gravity outside of the base of support) and which change the external forces acting on the body, can be identified in almost all of the falls. The videotapes are less useful for observing internal physiologic factors associated with falling because these conditions do not produce visible evidence of their occurrence.

An accurate history is important as part of a falls screening or assessment. Concurrent pathologies and medications need to be considered because many diseases or drugs may cause falling in the elderly. Falling is one of the features of the elderly sick syndrome, a nonspecific pattern of presentation of illness peculiar to the elderly (Isaacs, 1981). In addition, there are specific disease states and conditions particularly associated with an increase in falling. These include Parkinson's disease, rheumatologic disorders, cardiovascular disorders, and "drop attacks." Lipsitz (1983) stated that the drop attack is a common, potentially dangerous, and poorly understood symptom in the elderly population. It represents a sudden, transient interruption of postural tone. The typical drop attack is a sudden, unexpected fall, usually while standing or walking, and often following head or neck turning, with no loss of consciousness, in an otherwise well elderly individual. The individual often experiences difficulty standing up after the fall and may be on the floor for several hours.

Dementia and depression are also associated with an increased risk of falling. Both conditions present with impaired judgment, distraction, and psychomotor retardation, which may be implicated in the increased risk of falling (Mossey, 1985). However, Buchner and Larson (1987), in a study of Alzheimer-type dementia, found that the combined features of toxic reaction to drugs and wandering were associated with increased incidence of falls and fractures. Buchner and Larson (1987) cautioned against merely attributing falls to dementia without checking for reversible conditions affecting cognition. Masdeu and associates (1989) compared gait, balance, and cognition with brain computed tomography in fallers and nonfaller controls. The findings indicated that fallers had significantly worse scores on gait and balance testing and more white-matter hypodensity than the control groups. White-matter hypodensity correlated with impaired gait and balance but not with impaired performance on cognitive testing.

Consumption of three or more drugs is associated with falling (Granek et al, 1987). The elderly are susceptible to the effects of medications for two main reasons: (1) As the body ages it becomes less efficient in metabolizing drugs, and (2) the elderly tend to have more diseases than the young and therefore are at greater risk of polypharmacy (MacDonald, 1985). Drugs implicated in toxic falls include alcohol, tranquilizers, hypotensive agents, sedatives, hypnotics, antidepressants, and diuretics (Granek et al, 1987; MacDonald, 1985).

The history of falls is also useful to consider. If the older individual has recently and suddenly begun experiencing falls, disease or drugs may well be implicated (Gryfe et al, 1977). Thorough medical review is indicated because physical therapy intervention will have limited success if the older person has an underlying illness or is overmedicated. However, it is important to consider that the reliability of data surrounding falling incidents is poor and often ambiguous (Raz, 1986; Maki et al, 1989). Most studies of falling, as well as interviews of fallers, rely on self-reports. The first direct observations of spontaneous falls of elderly people have been provided in a study in which video cameras were used to record spontaneous falls of elderly residents in a geriatric center (Holliday et al, 1988 and 1990; Maki et al, 1989). The videotaped falls were compared with self-reports of the falling events; in only 3 of 12 falls in which we could compare self-reports with the videotaped information of the fall were the self-reported descriptions validated by the videotaped observations.

Age-related changes in blood pressure homeostasis also increase an older person's vulnerability to falls (Lipsitz, 1985). Orthostatic hypotension may be defined as a decline in blood pressure of over 20 mm Hg systolic or 10 mm Hg diastolic when upright posture is assumed. Age-related changes may lead to decreased cardiovascular responses to changes in position or posture, eating, or Valsalva maneuvers. A clear history of when the fall is occurring might implicate impaired blood pressure homeostasis.

Other medical conditions may put individuals at risk of falling. Visual conditions such as macular degeneration, cataracts, and glaucoma are common in the elderly and increase the risk of falling (Tinetti et al, 1986). Gait dysfunction secondary to parkinsonism, hemiparesis, peripheral neuropathy, or arthritic changes in the foot, ankle, knee, and hip are conditions that may contribute to loss of balance. Common musculoskeletal disorders include osteoarthritis and osteoporosis.

A number of investigators attempted to determine the risk of falling using clinically based measures and multivariate analysis to examine the factors and their interactions in community-based elderly (Campbell et al, 1989; Robbins et al, 1989; Tinetti et al, 1988), and institutionalized elderly (Morse et al, 1989a and b; Raz and Baretich, 1987; Robbins et al, 1989). In the community elderly, risk factors included the use of sedatives, cognitive impairment, lower extremity disability, palmomental reflex, and gait and balance abnormalities; the risk of falling increases with the number of risk factors present from 8% when no risk factors are present to 78% when four factors or more are present (Tinetti et al, 1988). Robbins and associates (1989) observed that poor balance, hip weakness, postural hypotension, and cognitive impairment were associated with falls in noninstitutionalized elderly, with an overall predictive accuracy of 75%. Raz and Baretich (1987) examined fall risk factors in hospitalized clients in four different institutions. The client characteristics that consistently were associated with increased risk of falls included admission to a rehabilitation service, age 75 years and older, increased number of diagnoses and surgical procedures, and government source of payment for hospital services. The Morse Fall Scale (Morse et al, 1987 and 1989a) was developed from the examination of falls in hospitalized elderly clients. Risk factors included history of a previous fall, presence of a secondary diagnosis, intravenous therapy, impaired gait, use of walking aids, and poor mental status. A scoring scheme was developed using the aforementioned factors to determine the level of risk. Predictive value of the scale and prospective studies using the scale have been reported (Morse et al, 1989a and b). Campbell and associates (1989), in examining risk of falls in community-based older individuals, noted that the contribution of each individual factor to the risk of falling is small. Falls are multifactorial in nature and more commonly result from an accumulation of factors rather than a single major contributing cause. Many factors are potentially remediable and, once identified, clinicians should attempt to correct as many of the potential additive factors as possible.

In tandem with clinical-based multivariate studies to determine risk of falling in community-based and institutionalized elderly (Campbell et al, 1989; Morse et al, 1989a and, b; Raz and Baretich, 1987; Robbins et al, 1989; Tinetti et al, 1988), laboratory testing of balance and postural control has been undertaken to identify the response characteristics to experimental conditions that simulate falls and predict falling liability (Maki et al, 1987; Nashner, 1981).

Few laboratory studies attempted to assess the ability of the balance measure to predict falling liability. Bartlett and colleagues (1986) examined the ability of the measure, mean speed of spontaneous postural sway, to predict the likelihood of falling in an individual. In a sample of 119 fallers and 86 nonfallers, the misclassification rate was 43% for both groups. Kirshen and associates (1984) also used spontaneous postural sway to determine falling liability. Fifty-three per cent of the fallers (9 of 17) and 76% of the nonfallers (37 of 49) were classified correctly. These findings, however, do not indicate that spontaneous postural sway is a clinically useful measure to predict falling liability in an individual. Falling liability was currently being assessed in 100 elderly residential-care individuals by Maki (1990). Quantitative balance measures were compared with clinical measures including visual and neurologic examination, balance and gait tests, and physical activity questionnaires. One-year prospective recording of falling was conducted using a weekly reporting schedule and fall follow-up modified from Cummings and associates (1988). The results showed significant differences among fallers and nonfallers in spontaneous and induced-sway amplitude measures in the mediolateral direction. Other measures such as one-leg stance, anticipatory postural control, and clinical balance assessments were unsuccessful in demonstrating faller/nonfaller differences. In fact, the eyes open one-leg stance was much more closely associated with fear of falling than with actual risk of falling. Stepwise discriminant analysis showed that a single spontaneous-sway measure, blindfold mediolateral sway amplitude, was able to predict prospectively the risk of experiencing one or more falls during a 1-year period at success rates of up to 71%.

Treatment/Management

Assessment and management of the elderly are interactive and multifaceted and require a holistic approach by the multidisciplinary team. Quality treatment for the prevention of falls depends on a thorough and accurate assessment of the individual (see Fig. 13–1). A falls clinic has been suggested as a mechanism to provide specialized multidisciplinary care for the individual who falls (Wolf-Klein et al, 1988). The specialized clinic setting has been found to be useful in recognizing undiagnosed factors such as neurologic disease (i.e., parkinsonism) or to adjust for medication problems such as oversedation.

In the elderly, the primary goal is to prevent permanent disability and irreversible deficits. This is achieved by preventing problems and declining functional abilities, improving status when possible, and compensating for abilities that cannot be improved. Management depends on whether or not the underlying problem is treatable. If the problem is treatable and clinically important change is possible, the course of action is intervention and rehabilitation; if change is not expected, the course of action is compensation for the impairment and disability (Sackett et al, 1985). With the elderly, management is often a combination of prevention, rehabilitation, and compensation.

A number of researchers have taken into consideration the multifactorial nature of falls and developed indices of risk factors for falling. These scales include a fall risk index designed to identify prospectively the individual characteristics associated with falling among elderly persons admitted to intermediate-care facilities (Tinetti et al, 1986), a physical therapy checklist for identification of at-risk older individuals (Speechley and Tinetti, 1990), and a screening tool for at-risk older individuals in acute-care hospital settings (Morse et al, 1987). Reliability and validity testing is completed on only some of the instruments. These tools may be useful for screening or identifying at-risk individuals, but physical and occupational therapists should also be interested in more in-depth assessment tools.

Physical therapists commonly assess balance in the clinic in a subjective manner (Berg, 1989). Balance is usually described as either static or dynamic and rated as poor, fair, or good. Some attempts have been made in the literature to identify more quantitative, clinical measures of balance. Berg (1989) reviewed balance measures in the elderly. One measure that is commonly reported is bilateral and unipedal stance. One-leg stance represents 50% of the gait cycle and therefore is of importance to consider in balance. Falls are reported to be more common in those who cannot stand on one leg (Berg, 1989). Unipedal stance has standardized values for normals. Nelson (1974) found that 30 seconds in a unilateral stance is a sufficient time period to demonstrate stability without including isometric endurance. Potvin and Tourtellotte (1975) showed that the ability to stand on one leg declined with age. These findings suggest that a time period shorter than 30 seconds be used when testing elderly subjects. Most authors concur that 30 seconds in bilateral stance and 5 seconds in unilateral stance are normative values for the elderly population (Berg, 1989; Maki et al, 1991).

Nelson (1974) reported on a measure used clinically that he referred to as dynamic weight transfer. A functional ambulation profile was developed by identifying components of gait: maintaining a stable base of support, transferring weight from one leg to another, and transferring weight while walking forward. The time to complete each task rather than a cumulative score was recorded. The assessment of balance was not the intended purpose of the scale; however, the scale does provide suggestions for quantifying weight shifting, a task requiring postural adjustments and one often used in physical therapy (Daleiden, 1990).

Wolfson and colleagues (1986) reported on a clinical postural stress test in which a pulley-weight system commonly found in physical therapy departments is used to deliver a reproducible destabilizing force to subjects. The displacement involved is in a backward direction. A nine-level grading scale was developed to evaluate the subject's response. The interrater reliability of scoring of balance using the scale was high. Although the scale is straightforward and simple to apply, the use of such an assessment should be approached with caution, particularly with fearful elderly individuals. In addition, because the scale only examines backward displacement, it may not account for all of the types of falls encountered. The advantage of the scale clinically is that it might be used to evaluate backward displacement applied manually at the pelvis by the therapist during regular testing procedures.

Shumway-Cook and Horak (1986) and Horak (1987) attempted to incorporate laboratory methods of evaluating balance into a systematic clinical evaluation. Subjects are tested with normal vision, using a blindfold, and using a dome to give inaccurate visual information. The support surface input is changed by placing foam underfoot. The subject's movement strategy (i.e., ankle rotation strategy, hip strategy, combination, or step strategy described earlier in the Primary Prevention, The Individual section) and ability to hold a position for 30 seconds is recorded. Using this systematic assessment, it may be possible to differentiate whether balance impairment is primarily related to visual input, proprioceptive input, or vestibular impairment. The observations and data from this test may bring clinical practice more parallel to laboratory research.

All of the studies discussed to this point examined balance in standing but not balance and equilibrium during gait.

McDowell and Newell (1987) described several scales developed to measure ADL that include crude but possibly useful measures of gait disability. These scales, such as the PULSES profile (Moskowitz and McCann, cited in McDowell and Newell, 1987), the Barthel Index (Mahoney and Barthel, cited in McDowell and Newell, 1987), the Index of Independence in ADL (Katz, cited in McDowell and Newell, 1987), the Kenny Self-Care Evaluation (Schoening, cited in McDowell and Newell, 1987), and the Functional Status Index (Jette, cited in McDowell and Newell, 1987) are all global measures of ADL that are valid measures of overall functional levels. As such, they are probably not sensitive enough to provide the therapist with accurate measures of gait, but they do provide useful overall information. The Barthel Index is the most commonly used of these scales, but it only examines the single category of ambulation in a very broad, nonspecific manner. The PULSES profile is less useful with the elderly because it has no standards for 80-year-olds. The Functional Independence Measure developed by Granger (1987) is a relatively new global assessment scale that may be more useful clinically than the previously mentioned scales. It is a seven-level scale that is more sensitive in the measurement of transfers, walking on the level, or using stairs.

Mathias and colleagues (1986) devised the functionally based "get up and go" test. The individual is asked to rise from a chair, stand still momentarily, walk a fixed distance, turn around, and return to the chair. The quality of movements is scored. This is a practical and simple test but has limited use because of its global scoring system ranging from 1 (normal) to 5 (abnormal). It may be useful as a screening tool but not for monitoring change over time. A variation in scoring might include recording of the time taken to perform the maneuver; this score may be repeated to examine change over time.

Berg and co-workers (1989) developed a scale to measure balance in the elderly that consists of 14 movements common in everyday life, such as rising from a chair, bending, and reaching forward. It is easy to administer and score, and reliability testing has shown high levels of inter-rater- and intrarater reliability. Validity testing has been completed but not yet published.

Tinetti (1986), Tinetti and Ginter (1988), and Tinetti and colleagues (1988) described a clinical gait test to examine the characteristics of gait that increase the risk of falling. Three gait factors, of the total of nine that represented the highest risk, included increased trunk sway, inability to increase walking pace, and increased path deviation.

Therapists use a variety of techniques to improve balance. Unfortunately, clinical research supporting the effectiveness of these activities is limited. Daleiden (1990) reviewed the literature on one such activity: weight shifting. She concluded that little published support exists for the effectiveness of this activity, although laboratory-based research on control of posture may indirectly support its use. Clinical research on the effectiveness of specific techniques used with homogeneous subgroups is required for clinicians to predict who will benefit from treatment and to determine appropriate procedure variations that improve impairments and impact on disabilities.

Overall, treatment should be geared to improving balance, but attention also needs to be paid to adequate joint range, muscle strength, and endurance, which are important factors in maintaining balance. Clinical measures used should be evaluated for their reliability and validity if these data are not already available. Validity testing for balance and gait measures represents a challenge because there is no accepted gold standard for balance measurement; however, some laboratory testing of balance may provide a measure against which to assess the effectiveness of clinical balance and postural control tests (Maki and Fernie, 1988; Maki et al, 1987; Nashner, 1981 and 1987).

The Environment

Thorough screening of the individual includes medical and rehabilitation work-up and home assessment. In some locations, a falls clinic has been instituted to coordinate the multidisciplinary assessment of the individual who is falling or who is at risk of falling (Wolf-Klein et al, 1988). One of the most important factors in the prevention of falls is education of the fallers, the elderly, and their caregivers, including environmental awareness information (Kellogg International Work Group, 1987; Wolf-Klein et al, 1988).

Environmental hazards have been observed in videotapes of spontaneous falls of elderly people and are present in up to 64% of falls; these included frictional changes in flooring, elevator doors, and thresholds; improper use of wheelchairs; nonuniform lighting; and crowding and congestion (Holliday et al, 1990). Although causal studies have not been conducted to establish the relationship of environmental factors to falls, there is often an interaction between the environment and the individual that leads to the falling event, such as during a trip or a slip (Maki et al, 1989). Because the risk of falling may increase with increasing number of risk factors, modification of even a few factors may help reduce falling incidence and associated morbidity and mortality (Campbell et al, 1989; Tinetti et al, 1988). Campbell and associates (1989) found that in only about 20% of falls in community-based elderly could the fall be attributed to a single major factor. Environmental factors may be more easily modifiable than other risk factors such as cognitive impairment or presence of neurologic disease.

Environmental hazards should be assessed on site and corrected. A simultaneous functional assessment provides the most accurate information of need because the interaction between the individual and the environment is a vital component of the assessment. One of the number of home-safety checklists that are available may be used or modified for the home-safety component of the assessment (Snipes, 1982; Tideiksaar, 1986, U.S. Consumer Product Safety Commission, 1986). A sample of some items that may be included in a home visit to review safety and accident prevention are listed in Table 13–3. The resources previously listed in Table 13–2 may also be useful with this group of elderly individuals who are sustaining falls or who are at risk of falling.

Table 13–3. Sample Items to be Included in an Environmental Assessment of Safety and Accident Prevention in the Home*†

Consider	Examine/Inquire
Self-care measures	Diet/nutrition
	Physical activity
	Personal care (i.e., feet, eyes)
	Care of footwear
	Medications: proper use and periodic review
Personal precautions	Proper lifting/carrying
	Placement of most frequently used items in comfortable reach
	Change position slowly
	Knowledge of emergency procedure should injury occur
Exterior	Clear walkways and stairs of snow and ice
	Ensure adequate lighting for nighttime use
	Sidewalks and stairs in good repair
	Handrail for stairs
Hallway and stairs	Lighting sufficient and available at top and bottom of stairs; no glare from lights or adjacent windows
	Secure handrails bilaterally
	Handrail diameter should be 38 mm (1.5 in)
	Handrail extending 29.4 cm (12 in) beyond top and bottom of stairs
	Clear of visual distractions
	Clear of stored objects
	If carpeted, secure and without thick underpad
	Removal of loose rugs
	Contrasting marker to indicate top and bottom steps
Bathroom	Nonskid strips or mats in tub and shower
	Grab bars available for bathing and toileting
	Appropriate toilet seat height
Kitchen	Storage areas accessible without excessive reaching or bending
	Safe use of stove and oven, including turning off when cooking completed
	Stove controls clearly marked
Bedroom	Clear, lit path to bathroom for nocturnal visits
	Bed height adequate for safe transfer
General safety	Adequate lighting; fixtures with multiple bulbs
	Night lights available
	Telephones accessible in several locations to facilitate emergency calls
	Removal of extension cords and other cords that cross paths of travel
	Floors and carpets in good repair and secured; nonslip surfaces on floors
	Environment free from obstructions to allow ease of movement
	Furnishings with armrests and of appropriate height for ease of ingress and egress
	Appropriate heating and cooling

*Compiled from Kellogg International Work Group (1987), Lok (1990), Snipes (1982), Tideiksaar (1986), and the U.S. Consumer Product Safety Commission (1986).
†This list is not exhaustive.

The majority of falling accidents by older persons occur during their usual daily activities such as walking or changing position and can occur anywhere in the home. Of accidents in the home that are associated with consumer products, the largest number involve stairs and steps (Czaja et al, 1982). The severity of injuries associated with stairs and steps increases with age (Czaja et al, 1982). Stairs are second to fires in causing the highest frequency of death in persons over 65 years of age. Research on stairway accidents indicates that proper design and installation of handrails may contribute to the prevention of falls on stairways.

Most of the serious stair injuries occur during descent (Archea, 1985; Cohen et al, 1985). Properly designed handrails should reduce the incidence and severity of stairway falls (Maki et al, 1984 and 1985). However, existing handrail design standards have been proposed with little regard to basic biomechanical principles. Maki and associates (1984 and 1985) modeled the beginning of a stairway fall as a simple mechanical event. The test rig was designed to measure maximum forces and moments that subjects were able to exert on handrails of different heights, stairway pitches, shapes, and textures (Holliday et al, 1985) while standing stationary. The handrail support was cantilevered and mounted on a force platform. The results showed that existing standards for handrail height are too low; handrail height for use by the adult population should be at least 0.91 m (36 in), measured from the nose to the top of the handrail in the plane of the riser. If small children are present, a second lower handrail should be installed. Handrails should be constructed from varnished wood, or enamel or vinyl on steel; the diameter should be 38 mm (1½ in).

Floors and flooring materials are products that are also often associated with falls and high injury frequency in the elderly (Czaja et al, 1982). Research studies are underway to examine impact forces during falls on different floor surfaces to determine appropriate floor coverings for at-risk individuals. Maki and Fernie (1990) conducted an experimental study to examine whether the magnitudes of the impact forces generated in falling accidents on level surfaces are affected by the type of the floor covering. A simple inverted pendulum simulating the fall of an average elderly woman was used to assess and compare 13 different floor coverings. When peak decelerations were measured for impacts at the hip and at the hand, it was found that floor coverings differ significantly in terms of the peak impact force occurring during a fall. For hip impacts, padded carpets provided the best impact attenuation, and the mean differences between the floor coverings ranged up to 23%. In hand impacts, the impact forces were independent of the nature of the flooring. More research is required to validate these results. Whether a fracture may be prevented depends on many other factors, such as bone strength and dynamics of the fall.

Technologies such as assistive devices have the potential to enhance safety in the home and reduce dependence of older persons. The potential usefulness of technologies to assist in independent living in the elderly was assessed by a survey of 356 community-dwelling individuals over 65 years of age (Holliday and Fernie, 1986). Assistive devices and technologies found to have the potential to reduce dependence of individuals considered at risk for institutionalization were (in order of priority): bathroom aids (related to bathtub entry and safety), emergency alarm systems, mobility devices (for reaching, carrying, and seating), toileting aids, stair handrails and ramps, kitchen alterations and safe cooking, adequate lighting systems, and reminding devices

(e.g., for medications, appointments). Many safety and assistive devices such as emergency response systems are readily available (Associated Planning Consultants, 1989a and b; Ontario Ministry of Community and Social Services, 1986). Useful assistive devices need not be "high tech." Research is still required to develop appropriate selection of assistive devices and to examine criteria that determine whether provided devices or strategies are incorporated into everyday activities.

Society

Family and community supports, especially the presence of a spouse, make a difference in the priority placed on an exercise regimen and compliance with the program and professional suggestions. Use of community resources for the elderly should be encouraged, such as swimming, local exercise classes for the elderly, activity groups, and mall-walking classes. The community programs tend to increase individual visibility, motivation and commitment, and provide socialization in the process.

Health professionals should be aware of the resources available for falls screening and environmental assessment and should continue to educate other health professionals and the general public regarding management of falls and safety issues. It is easy for a health-care worker to forget to ask the older person if falls have occurred because injury is often not present (Kellogg International Work Group, 1987). Knowledge of local resources that may be needed to provide home modifications is beneficial. In general, there is no central registry that provides such information. The Canadian Council for the Disabled is currently establishing a national central data bank on safety initiatives undertaken in Canada pertaining to the home and immediate environment as it relates to senior citizens (Canadian Rehabilitation Council for the Disabled, 1990). The registry includes information on educational programs, media campaigns, and other initiatives directed toward the safety needs and issues of seniors.

TERTIARY PREVENTION

Capsule Summary

Tertiary prevention minimizes the disabilities and handicaps that result from irreversible disease or injury (Warren, 1985). Permanent disability and irreversible deficit are present at this stage. Fear of falling is an important consideration for maintenance and rehabilitation.

The Individual

Age alone is not predictive of the need for geriatric care (Winograd, 1989). Fraility is a term reflecting risk for injury in combination with ill health or decreasing function in daily activities, medical condition, and social or psychologic status.

Treatment/Management

At this stage, older persons may be considered to be handicapped because of their falling problem. They may be bed- or wheelchair-bound. Management may be geared to increasing mobility and reversing the effects of immobility. Identification of institutionalized individuals who are at risk of falling is a first step. Risk factors may vary among institutions (Kellogg International Work Group, 1987) but may include admission to a rehabilitation service, age over 75 years, increased number of diagnoses and surgical procedures, government source of payment for hospital services, history of falls, intravenous therapy, impaired gait, use of walking aids, and poor mental status (Morse et al, 1987 and 1989a; Raz and Baretich, 1987). Periodic review of risk assessment and prevention is required as situations and patterns change (Raz and Baretich, 1987).

Many individuals at this stage manifest fear of falling. Murphy and Isaacs (1982) described postfall syndrome as one in which, after a fall and in the absence of any neurologic or orthopedic abnormality that would adversely affect gait or balance, the client is unable to stand or walk unsupported. Murphy and Isaacs (1982) suggested that this is actually a phobic reaction to standing and walking. Bhala and colleagues (1982) also described phobic fear of falling and suggested that post-fall syndrome can be treated very effectively by gradually exposing the client to the feared situation (standing or walking) without adverse consequences. This syndrome is not well documented, and its incidence is not known. If unrecognized as having post-fall syndrome or fear of falling, the older person could easily be labelled as unmotivated or noncompliant.

The fear of falling is being recognized as a potentially confounding and significant factor in the investigation of falling in the elderly (Isaacs, 1983; Maki et al, 1991). Fear of falling may ultimately result in a loss of independence and may be a more pervasive problem than previously anticipated. Fear of falling can develop in individuals who have not yet experienced a falling event. A cross-sectional study was performed to investigate the association between fear of falling and postural performance in the elderly (Maki et al, 1991). One hundred independent ambulatory volunteers (aged 62 to 96 years) underwent five types of balance tests: spontaneous postural sway; induced anteroposterior sway; induced mediolateral sway; one-leg stance; and a clinical balance-assessment scale. The induced sway tests used consisted of pseudorandom platform motions. The subjects were classified into faller/nonfaller (self-reported history in the previous year) and fear/no-fear (response to an ordered-choice, closed-ended question) categories. The results indicated that the subjects who expressed fear of falling had significantly poorer balance performance in blindfolded spontaneous sway tests and in eyes-open, one-leg stance tests. The clinical balance scale was the only balance measure that showed significant association with retrospective, self-reported history of falling. The results of the study indicate that balance measures must be interpreted with caution when dealing with apprehensive individuals. The following case history illustrates fear of falling that may be seen in individuals referred for rehabilitation.

CASE HISTORY

Mrs. M.C. was a 94-year-old widow who was living in an apartment with her youngest son. Her activity was limited, but she did get about quite well using a walker. In November 1984, she began to complain of hip pain and loss of balance that gradually limited her mobility to the point where she was bed-bound. She was investigated for a hip fracture, but x-ray results were negative. It was found that she was suffering from a urinary tract infection. This was treated successfully, but she never regained the ability to walk. Her mental functions remained intact. Although Mrs. M.C. did receive some assistance from a housekeeper and another son, the main onus for her care fell on the younger son. A hospital bed was purchased, and for the next 3 months she remained in bed. Applications for chronic care were submitted.

Mrs. M.C. was seen on a home visit conducted by a physician from a nearby geriatric assessment unit. She was admitted to the unit in March 1985 where she was given a full neurologic and orthopedic work-up. There were no neurologic problems associated with the decreased mobility, and although she did have some arthritic changes and some weakness in her legs, these were not sufficient to account for the inability to ambulate. As assessment proceeded, it was evident that her difficulties with walking were mainly related to a great fear of falling. She would cooperate quite happily with any activities while sitting or lying down, but as soon as she had to perform any activity involving standing or walking, she became anxious and would need considerable encouragement. She stated that she had fallen once and was fearful of falling again.

The clinical picture was very similar to that described by Murphy and Isaacs (1982). When asked to stand or walk unsupported, Mrs. M.C. became fearful and anxious, but the provision of support modified the behavior and allowed a fairly normal pattern of stepping. The literature suggests that post-fall syndrome can be treated very effectively by gradually exposing the client to the feared situation (standing or walking) without adverse consequences. It is very important for the therapist to provide reassurance both verbally and physically (by putting a hand on the client's waist or by holding her hand). A progressive ambulation program began with walking using a stable walker and two assistants. Gradually support was withdrawn until she was walking short distances with a walker and just the therapist's hand on her arm. She required considerable encouragement but, if given a specific distance to walk, she always cooperated. As her walking improved in physical therapy, the nursing staff began walking with her on the ward, to the bathroom, and to sit in a regular chair in the lounge. This carryover onto the ward was essential to allow Mrs. M.C. to accept that walking was an everyday part of her life.

After a trial visit, Mrs. M.C. was discharged home April 26, 1985. Her mobility continued to improve to the point at which she no longer required physical reassurance, just supervision. She remained at home with her son for a further 2 years until her death at the age of 96 from a myocardial infarction.

In general, goals of treatment are similar to those of secondary stage (to increase joint range and to improve muscle strength, endurance, and balance) combined with environmental modification. Achievement of the latter goals should be accomplished by conducting functionally related activities. Often it is difficult to separate treatment into individual and environmental components because, in practice, these are dealt with simultaneously, as is seen in some of the following discussion.

If the older person is falling at the bedside, a number of strategies can be considered. First, it is important to determine if a problem exists with orthostatic hypotension. Orthostatic hypotension is defined as a decline in blood pressure of over 20 mm Hg systolic or 10 mm Hg diastolic upon assuming an upright posture (Lipsitz, 1985). Blood pressure should be taken when lying, sitting, standing, and 2 minutes after standing. Clients with long-standing hypotension probably have learned to accommodate; however, if hypotension remains a significant problem, medications should be reviewed, and the older person should be taught management techniques. In addition to the recommendation of changing positions slowly, it may be useful to teach the older person to perform a few active or isometric exercises when lying down so that the blood pressure rises. When the upright position is assumed, the drop in blood pressure may be less significant.

To prevent falls, older residents are often confined to bed by raising bed rails; this is not satisfactory because inevitably older persons may try to climb over them, placing themselves at greater risk of injury by falling from a greater height (Cape et al, 1983). The incidence of falls from bed and of subsequent injury increases with the use of bed rails (Tideiksaar and Kay, 1986). Lowering the bed is more effective. In addition, mats placed beside the bed will soften potential falls. Nonskid rubber bath mats and nonskid strips on the floor by the bed may also help the person having difficulties at bedside. Multidisciplinary assessment and management can be effective in developing alternative strategies to restraints (Brockenshire, 1985).

Falls may occur at night when the older person gets up to void. A night-light left on to help the client find the way to the bathroom might be useful. A commode by the bedside might lessen the risk of falls on the way to the bathroom. Strategies to lessen nocturnal voiding might be appropriate in some cases. These include limiting fluids before bedtime, reviewing medications, and regular toileting at night.

Rocking chairs are very useful for the restless, possibly cognitively impaired older individual. A walker-chair (i.e., GO-CHAIR, Canhart Industries Inc, 140 Renfrew Dr, Ste 205, Markham, Ontario, Canada L3R 6B3), which allows mobility while sitting, is a compromise for the individual who will try to get up even though they are unsafe. A walker-chair is a combination wheelchair and walker. It has six casters, four of which are pivotal, and a pivotal seat, which allows transfer of weight to the feet for easy propulsion. Although technically the person is restrained by a lap tray and a safety belt, the ease of propulsion of the chair allows the older person to remain mobile despite being in a seated position.

Attention to appropriately designed furnishings that passively restrain, such as by the seat rake (angle to horizontal) and presence of a lap tray, may alleviate wandering and falls from chairs by older people who cannot transfer or ambulate safely by themselves. Difficulty getting out of a chair has been cited as the most important consideration for choice of seating by the elderly and the disabled (Munton et al, 1981). The recommended seat height (front) for institutionalized elderly users is 470 mm (19 in) (Holden and Fernie, 1989). All chairs should have armrests that protrude beyond the edge of the seat approximately 120 mm (½ inch) to facilitate egress (Holden and Fernie, 1989).

Teaching methods of recovery after a fall may increase the confidence, reduce the fear, and facilitate mobility in these individuals who are known to fall. One method of recovery may include rolling onto the stomach, raising onto all fours, and crawling to a nearby stable object to use for assistance in rising. If an injury is suspected, the faller should summon assistance rather than attempt to rise (Kellogg International Work Group, 1987). Emergency response systems, which may provide additional security for identified fallers, are available for institutionalized individuals as well as community-living elderly (see Environment, Secondary Prevention Section). New electronic monitoring systems to track wanderers (Brett, 1990) have the potential to be technically advanced in the near future enough to sense events such as falls.

Environment

The goal of an environmental evaluation is the same as for primary and secondary fall prevention: to determine the safety and adequacy of the environment for the individual.

Data from institutional environments, which are generally designed to be safe, show that falls represent the leading type of accident (Raz and Baretich, 1987). Residents of institutions are more frail than the elderly living in the community and sustain a higher frequency of falls than their community-based counterparts (Tinetti and Speechley, 1989). Although institutions are designed for the frail and infirm, modifications are often required to enhance safety while promoting mobility. Often the dilemma at this stage is whether restricted movement should be enforced or whether residents should be allowed the freedom to be mobile; in the latter case, falls should be anticipated, and personal and environmental modifications should be enforced.

The contribution of individual factors to the risk of falling is small but additive (Campbell et al, 1989); therefore, identification and correction of as many risk factors as possible is recommended. Environmental needs of the resident faller may conflict with those of the institution and the other residents (Kellogg International Work Group, 1987). Minimally, environmental alterations may include the provision of an assistive walking device and the use of grab bars, nonskid mats, or cushioning surfaces. A thorough assessment of when and why falls are occurring may provide information crucial to modifying the environment to allow as much mobility as possible. However, often few details about previous falls are available; the data that are available are often inaccurate (Maki et al, 1989). The bathroom and the bedroom are high-risk areas for falls because this is where residents spend most of their time (Kellogg International Work Group, 1987).

Many health professionals' understanding and conceptualization of the environment are influenced by the biomedical model to the extent that the environment is often simply thought of as the physical environment in which a person functions. What the model fails to take into account are the other components of the environment that can either promote or discourage an older person's independence. The other components are the socioemotional aspects of the environment. Does the environment encourage the older person to be passive and dependent? Although institutionalization is frequently precipitated by a decline in functional capacity, the behaviors of dependency, passivity, and apathy are out of proportion to the physical incapacity and are related more to the physical and interpersonal environment than to institutionalization per se (Soloman, 1982). Dependency behaviors may be reinforced inadvertently by the caregiver. This may be particularly true for the older faller who may be fearful of another, possibly damaging fall and who, unless encouraged, may find it easier to take the path of least of resistance and give up their independence in mobility. Staff requirements and time are reduced when residents are less mobile and do not require careful watching a great deal of the time.

The goal for design of any physical environment in which an older person lives is to maximize function in terms of safety and security, ADL, personal choice and independence, and opportunities for social interaction and privacy (Pastalan and Pawlson, 1985). The environmental design in institutions can facilitate independence and finding one's way if proper attention is paid to designing for the common deficits and conditions of residents, such as limited mobility, visual impairment, and cognitive disorders and disorientation. Specific examples include use of increased ambient temperature to accommodate the sedentary lifestyle and poor regulation of homeostasis that accompanies aging (Reichel, 1989); barrier-free design (elimination of barriers such as stairs, uneven sidewalks, ramps); appropriate height, color, size, and arrows for signs giving directions; the use of color, texture, and contrast to allow residents to distinguish the floor and the walls and to make furnishings visible (Hiatt, 1982; Windley and Scheidt, 1980). Placement of call bells, color coding for different locations and for finding one's way, and use of electronic devices to track wandering residents should be considered. Placement of furniture, lighting and glare, and floor coverings should be modified to accommodate for age-related and pathologic conditions of vision and mobility. Unlike modifications made to private homes, alterations made to the institutional environment also affect others who share the space.

Residents must be assisted in learning how to use the signs and cues in their environment; a consistent education policy for staff describing effective ways to communicate with residents is essential. Confusion and disorientation can contribute to falls.

Society

Fall-prevention programs should be instituted to educate the health-care professional, caregivers (such as family members), and the faller; this goal does not differ from the other two stages of fall prevention.

Becker and Kaufman (1988) stated that American cultural beliefs about old age that are reflected throughout the health-care system may in part prevent effective rehabilitation. Attitudes as to the effectiveness of rehabilitation in this population are reflected in the tendency to warehouse the elderly instead of providing rehabilitation. Low expectations about older persons' adaptive capacities, coupled with low expectations about what the level of functioning should be in old age, determine the treatment elderly persons receive. The whole issue of restraints, used with the older person at risk of falling, is an example of societal attitudes condoning a morally questionable activity. Despite evidence to the contrary, the practice of restraining older persons for their own protection and safety continues.

A comprehensive evaluation and charting of a client's support system may be useful (Winograd, 1989). Caregivers are prone to physical and emotional stress, and recent data suggested that almost one third of caregivers of frail elderly in the community suffer depressive disorders (Gallagher et al, 1988 cited in Winograd, 1989). Hospitalization is often a transition point between independent living and nursing home care. Frequently prehospitalization situations need to be drastically altered or changed altogether. A nursing home may be the final residence of an elder. Family involvement in nursing home programs and care of their relative can benefit both the well-being of the resident and the function of the nursing home and its programs. Availability of a range of activities is essential for residents at all levels of care.

Elimination of unnecessary institutionalization and enhancement of alternatives to institutionalization are processes that involve families, health-care agencies, and medical funding bodies. A multivariate study conducted to identify the key determinants of long-term care (LTC) institutionalization found five variables predictive of institutionalization: advancing age (over 80 years), use of ambulatory aids, mental disorientation, living alone, and increasing functional disability (Branch and Jette, 1982). These factors accounted for only 10% of the variance in LTC institutionalization. Community programs designed to assist the elderly in remaining at home may benefit from the study results by more specifically addressing the design of services and alternatives to LTC institutionalization.

HOW CURRENT RESEARCH OFFERS HELP IN PREVENTION OF FALLS

Current research findings have been integrated into this entire discussion of fall prevention in the elderly.

Future environmental studies should focus on causal relationships among falling events and assessment of environmental interventions, such as investigations of footwear, visual capacity, lighting levels, floor covering, and so on, and the ability to balance and prevent falls. Specific visual conditions such as level of lighting, glare, color, contrast, and figure-ground effect have not been studied in controlled settings with respect to the specific effects on balance and postural control of the elderly. These studies have awaited quantitative and sensitive measures of balance and postural control.

Current research is beginning to provide insights into the nature of balance and postural control of the elderly. Predictions of individuals at risk and appropriate tests to identify these individuals will be available for clinical use. Transfer of technology from the laboratory into the clinical setting can facilitate quantitative assessment of balance and monitoring of therapies for balance and falling disorders.

References

Andreasen MEK: Color vision defects in the elderly. Gerontol Nurs 6:383–384, 1980.

Archea JC: Environmental factors associated with stair accidents by the elderly. Clin Geriatr Med 1:555–570, 1985.

Associated Planning Consultants: Final Report. Emergency Response Systems. Vol 1, Executive Summary. Prepared for The Ministry of Housing, Government of Ontario. Toronto, Ontario, Canada, Associated Planning Consultants, 1989a.

Associated Planning Consultants: Final Report. Emergency Response Systems. Vol 2, Technical Report. Prepared for The Ministry of Housing, Government of Ontario. Toronto, Ontario, Canada, Associated Planning Consultants, 1989b.

Astrand P: Exercise physiology and its role in disease prevention and in rehabilitation. Arch Phys Med Rehabil 68:305–309, 1987.

Babin RW and Harker LA: The vestibular system in the elderly. Otolaryngol Clin North Am 15:387–393, 1982.

Baker SP and Harvey AH: Fall injuries in the elderly. Clin Geriatr Med 1:501–512, 1985.

Barrier-free living: Better Homes and Gardens Building Ideas. Home Products Guide, pp. 87–89, February 1990.

Bartlett SA, Holliday PJ, Maki BE, et al: On the classification of a geriatric subject as a faller or non-faller. Med Biol Eng Comput 24:219–222, 1986.

Becker G and Kaufman S: Old age, rehabilitation, and research: A review of the issues. Gerontologist 28:459–468, 1988.

Berg K: Balance and its measure in the elderly: A review. Physiother Canada 41:240–246, 1989.

Berg K, Wood-Dauphinee S, Williams JI, et al: Measuring balance in the elderly: Preliminary development of an instrument. Physiother Canada 41:304–311, 1989.

Bhala RP, O'Donnel J, and Thoppil E: Ptophobia-phobic fear of falling and its clinical management. Phys Ther 62:187–190, 1982.

Black FO, O'Leary DP, Wall C, et al: The vestibulo-spinal stability test: Normal limits. Trans Am Acad Ophthalmol Otol 84:549–560, 1977.

Bornor JA, Dilworth BB, and Sullivan KM: Exercise and osteoporosis: A critique of the literature. Physiother Canada 40:146–155, 1988.

Branch LG and Jette AM: A prospective study of long-term care institutionalization among the aged. Am J Public Health 72:1373–1379, 1982.

Brett G: Device tracks wander-prone. Toronto Star, p. C3, May 19, 1990.

Brockenshire A: Restraints: Whose needs do they serve? Can Fam Physician 31:2301–2303, 1985.

Brocklehurst JC, Robertson D, and James-Groom P: Clinical correlates of sway in old age - sensory modalities. Age Ageing 11:1–10, 1982.

Buchner DM and Larson EB: Falls and fractures in patients with Alzheimer-type dementia. JAMA 257:1492–1495, 1987.

Campbell AJ, Borrie MJ, and Spears GF: Risk factors for falls in a community-based prospective study of people 70 years and older. J Gerontol Med Sci 44:M112–117, 1989.

Canadian Rehabilitation Council for the Disabled: National Central Data Bank on Safety Initiatives for Senior Citizens. Toronto, Canada, Canadian Rehabilitation Council for the Disabled, 1990.

Cape RDT: Freedom from restraint (Abstract). The Gerontologist 23:Special Issue 217, 1983.

Cohen HH, Templer J, and Archea J: An analysis of occupational stair accident patterns. J Safety Res 16:171–181, 1985.

Cummings SR, Nevitt MC, and Kidd S: Forgetting falls. The limited accuracy of recall of falls in the elderly. J Am Geriatr Soc 36:613–616, 1988.

Czaja SJ, Hammond K, and Drury CC: Accidents and Aging. A Final Report. Buffalo, NY, Buffalo Organization for Social and Technological Innovation, 1982.

Daleiden S: Weight shifting as a treatment for balance deficits: A literature review. Physiother Canada 42:81–87, 1990.

Davies CTM and White MJ: Contractile properties of elderly human triceps surae. Gerontology 29:19–25, 1983.

Dorfman LJ and Bosley TM: Age-related changes in peripheral and central nerve conduction in man. J Gerontol 35:185–193, 1979.

Dornan J, Fernie GR, and Holliday PJ: Visual input: Its importance in the control of postural sway. Arch Phys Med Rehabil 59:586–591, 1978.

Egger K and Taves A: The Homesafe Handbook. A Family and Child Safety Manual. Toronto, Ontario, Canada, The Homesafe Company, 1986.

Engel GL: The clinical application of the biopsychosocial model. In Haug MR (ed): Elderly Patients and Their Doctors. New York, Springer, 1981.

Fernie GR, Gryfe CI, Holliday PJ, et al: The relationship of postural sway in standing to the incidence of falls in geriatric subjects. Age Ageing *11*:11–16, 1982.

Fernie GR and Holliday PJ: Postural sway in amputees and normal subjects. J Bone Joint Surg (Am) *60A*:895–898, 1978.

Granek E, Baker SP, Abbey H, et al: Medications and diagnoses in relation to falls in a long-term care facility. J Am Geriatr Soc *35*:503–511, 1987.

Granger CV: Functional Independence Measure. New York, State University of New York Research Foundation, 1987.

Grimby G and Saltin B: The aging muscle. Clin Physiol *3*:209–218, 1983.

Gryfe CI, Amies A, and Ashley MJ: A longitudinal study of falls in an elderly population: I: Incidence and morbidity. Age Ageing *6*:201–210, 1977.

Guimares RM and Isaacs B: Characteristics of gait in old people who fall. Int Rehabil Med *2*:177–180, 1980.

Hayes KC, Spencer JD, Lucy SD, et al: Age-related changes in postural sway. *In* Winter DA, Norman RW, Wells RP, Hayes KC, and Patla AE (eds): Biomechanics IX-A. Champaign, IL, Human Kinetics, 1985.

Heckler MM: Health promotion for older Americans. Public Health Rep *100*:225–230, 1985.

Hiatt L: Care and design. Ontario Nursing Homes *13*:4–8, 1982.

Holden JM and Fernie GR: Specifications for a mass producible static lounge chair for the elderly. Appl Ergonomics *20*:39–45, 1989.

Holliday PJ and Fernie GR: Postural sway during low frequency floor oscillation in young and elderly subjects. *In* Igarashi M and Black FO (eds): Vestibular and Visual Control in Posture and Locomotor Equilibrium. Basel, Karger, 1985.

Holliday PJ, and Fernie GR: A Study of Technological Applications to Promote Independent Living for the Elderly. Toronto, Ontario, Canada, Government of Ontario, Ministry of Community and Social Services, 1986.

Holliday PJ, Fernie GR, Gryfe CI, et al: Video recording of falling in the elderly. *In* Proceedings of the International Conference for the Advancement of Rehabilitation Technology. Montreal, Quebec, Canada, Resna, Association for the Advancement of Rehabilitation Technology, 1988.

Holliday PJ, Fernie GR, Gryfe CI, et al: Video recording of spontaneous falls of the elderly. *In* Gray BE (ed): ASTM Special Technical Publication: Slips, Stumbles and Falls: Pedestrian Footwear and Surfaces. Philadelphia, ASTM Special Technical Publication (STP) *1103*:7–16, 1990.

Holliday PJ, Fernie GR, Maki BE, et al: Some bioengineering approaches to the falling problem. Geriatr Med *1*:161–164, 1985.

Horak FB: Clinical measurement of postural control in adults. Phys Ther *67*:1881–1885, 1987.

Imms FJ and Edholm OG: Studies of gait and mobility in the elderly. Age Ageing *10*:145–156, 1981.

International Association of Gerontology: Foundations of a policy for the aged in the 1980s and beyond. Gerontology *28*:271–280, 1980.

Isaacs B: Are falls a manifestation of brain failure? Age Ageing *7*(Suppl):79–111, 1978.

Isaacs B: Falls in old age. *In* Hinchcliffe R (ed): Hearing and Balance in the Elderly. New York, Churchill Livingstone, 1983.

Isaacs B: Why do the elderly fall? Geriatr Med *11*:17–23, 1981.

Kellogg International Work Group: The prevention of falls in later life. Dan Med Bull *34* (Suppl 4):1–24, 1987.

Kenshalo DR: Changes in the vestibular and somesthetic systems as a function of age. *In* Ordy JM and Brizzee K (eds): Sensory Systems and Communication in the Elderly. New York, Raven Press, 1979.

Kirshen AJ, Cape RDT, Hayes KC, et al: Postural sway and cardiovascular parameters associated with falls in the elderly. J Clin Exp Gerontol *6*:291–307, 1984.

Kokman E, Bossmeyer RW, Barney J, et al: Neurological manifestations of aging. Gerontol *32*:411–419, 1977.

Koller WC, Glatt SL, and Fox JH: Senile gait: A distinct neurologic entity. Clin Geriatr Med *1*:661–669, 1985.

Larson EB and Bruce RA: Health benefits of exercise in an aging society. Arch Intern Med *147*:353–356, 1987.

Lipsitz LA: Abnormalities in blood pressure homeostasis that contribute to falls in the elderly. Clin Geriatr Med *1*:637–648, 1985.

Lipsitz LA: The drop attack. J Am Geriatr Soc *10*:617–620, 1983.

Lok C: The Safety Challenge Manual and Supplement. Unpublished manuscript, University of Toronto, Division of Physical Therapy, 1990.

MacDonald JB: The role of drugs in falls in the elderly. Clin Geriatr Med *1*:637–648, 1985.

Maki BE: A balance test to predict falling in the elderly: Final progress report. National Institute on Aging, Grant #R01AG 06357, 1990.

Maki BE: A Posture Control Model and Balance Test for the Prediction of Relative Postural Stability. Unpublished doctoral dissertation, University of Strathclyde, Glasgow, Scotland, 1987.

Maki BE, Bartlett SA, and Fernie GR: Effect of stairway pitch on optimal handrail height. Hum Factors *27*:355–359, 1985.

Maki BE, Bartlett SA, and Fernie GR: Influence of stairway handrail height on the ability to generate stabilizing forces and moments. Hum Factors *26*:705–714, 1984.

Maki BE and Fernie GR: Impact attentuation of floor coverings in simulated falling accidents. Appl Ergonomics, *21*:107–114, 1990.

Maki BE and Fernie GR: A system identification approach to balance testing. Prog Brain Res *76*:297–306, 1988.

Maki BE, Holliday PJ, and Fernie GR: Aging and postural control. A comparison of spontaneous- and induced-sway balance tests. J Am Geriatr Soc *38*:1–9, 1991.

Maki BE, Holliday PJ, and Fernie GR: A posture control model and balance test for the prediction of relative postural stability. IEEE Trans Biomed Eng *BME-34*:797–810, 1987.

Maki BE, Holliday PJ, Fernie GR, et al: Observations of Fallers in the Act: An Analysis of Postural Perturbations and Contributing Situational Factors. Paper presented at the meeting of The Gerontological Society of North America, Minneapolis, MN, November 1989.

Maki BE, Holliday PJ, and Topper AK: Fear of Falling and Postural Performance in the Elderly. J Gerontol: Medical Sciences *46*:M123–M131, 1991.

Martin AD and Houston CS: Osteoporosis, calcium and physical activity. Can Med Assoc J *136*:587–593, 1987.

Masdeu JC, Wolfson L, Lantos G, et al: Brain white-matter changes in the elderly prone to falling. Arch Neurol *46*:1292–1296, 1989.

Mathias S, Nayak USL, and Isaacs B: Balance in elderly patients: The "get up and go" test. Arch Phys Med Rehabil *67*:387–389, 1986.

McDowell I and Newell C: Measuring health: A guide to rating scales and questionnaires. New York, Oxford University Press, 1987.

McPherson BD and Kozlik CA: Age patterns in leisure participation: The Canadian case. *In* Marshall VW (ed): Aging in Canada: Social perspectives, (2nd ed). Markham, Ontario, Canada, Fitzhenry and Whiteside, 1987.

Morse JM, Black C, Oberle K, et al: A prospective study to identify the fall-prone patient. Soc Sci Med 28:81–86, 1989b.

Morse JM, Morse RM, and Tylko SJ: Development of a scale to identify the fall-prone patient. Can J Aging 8:366–377, 1989a.

Morse JM, Tylko SJ, and Dixon HA: Characteristics of the fall-prone patient. Gerontologist 27:516–522, 1987.

Mossey JM: Social and psychologic factors related to falls among the elderly. Clin Geriatr Med 1:525–539, 1985.

Munton JS, Chamberlain NA, and Wright V: An investigation into the problems of easy chairs used by the arthritic and the elderly. Rheumatol and Rehabil 20:164–173, 1981.

Murphy J and Isaacs B: The post-fall syndrome: A study of 36 elderly patients. Gerontology 28:265–275, 1982.

Nashner LM: Analysis of stance posture in humans. In Towe AL and Luschei ES (eds): Handbook of Behavioral Neurobiology, Vol 5: Motor Coordination. New York, Plenum Press, 1981.

Nashner LM: A Systems Approach to Understanding and Assessing Orientation and Balance Disorders. Clackamas, OR, NeuroCom International, 1987.

National Institutes of Health: Osteoporosis. Consensus conference. JAMA, 252:799–802, 1984.

National Safety Council: 1990 Accident Facts. Chicago, IL: National Safety Council, 1990.

Nelson AJ: Functional ambulation profile. Phy Ther 54:1059–1065, 1974.

Ontario Ministry of Community and Social Services: Information on Emergency Response Systems. Toronto, Ontario, Canada, Ontario Government, 1986.

Oosterveld WJ: Changes in vestibular function with increasing age. In Hinchcliffe R (ed): Hearing and Balance in the Elderly. Edinburgh, Churchill Livingstone, 1983.

Overstall PW, Exton-Smith AN, Imms FJ, et al: Falls in the elderly related to postural imbalance. Br Med J, 1:261–264, 1977.

Owen DH: Maintaining posture and avoiding tripping. Optical information for selecting and controlling orientation and locomotion. Clin Geriatr Med 1:581–599, 1985.

Pastalan LA and Pawlson LG: Importance of physical environment for older people. J Am Geriatr Soc 33:874, 1985.

Potvin AR and Tourtellotte WW: The neurological examination: Advancements in its quantification. Arch Phys Med Rehabil 56:425–437, 1975.

Raz T: An information theoretic method for classifying patients according to the risk of adverse hospital incidents. J Med Syst 10:195–208, 1986.

Raz T and Baretich MF: Factors affecting the incidence of patient falls in hospitals. Med Care 25:185–195, 1987.

Reichel W: Clinical aspects of aging: Accidents in the elderly population, 3rd ed. Baltimore, Williams & Wilkins, 1989.

Robbins AS, Rubenstein LZ, Josephson KR, et al: Predictors of falls among elderly people. Results of two population-based studies. Arch Intern Med 149:1628–1633, 1989.

Sackett DL, Haynes RB, and Tugwell P: Clinical epidemiology: A basic science for clinical medicine. Boston, Little, Brown, 1985.

Scheibel AB: Aging in human motor control systems. In Ordy JM and Brizzee K (eds): Sensory Systems and Communication in the Elderly. New York, Raven Press, 1979.

Serfass RC: Exercise for the elderly: What are the benefits and how do we get started? In Smith EL and Serfass RC (eds): Exercise and Aging. The Scientific Basis. Hillside, NJ, Enslow Publishers, 1981.

Sheldon JH: The effect of age on the control of sway. Gerontolog Clin 5:129–138, 1963.

Shumway-Cook A and Horak FB: Assessing the influence of sensory interaction on balance. Suggestion from the field. Phys Ther 66:1548–1550, 1986.

Snipes GE: Accidents in the elderly. Am Fam Physician 26:117–122, 1982.

Snyder EE and Spreitzer EA: Social Aspects of Sport. Englewood Cliffs, NJ, Prentice-Hall, 1983.

Soloman K: Social antecedents of learned helplessness in the health care setting. Gerontologist 22:282–285, 1982.

Speechley M and Tinetti M: Assessment of risk and prevention of falls among elderly persons: Role of the physiotherapist. Physiother Canada 42:75–79, 1990.

Spooner JW, Sakala SM, and Baloh RW: Effect of aging on eye tracking. Arch Neurol 37:575–576, 1980.

Stelmach GE, Phillips J, DiFabio RP, et al: Age, functional postural reflexes, and voluntary sway. J Gerontol 44:B100–106, 1989.

Stelmach GE and Worringham CJ: Sensorimotor deficits related to postural instability: Implications for falling in the elderly. Clin Geriatr Med 1:679–694, 1985.

Tideiksaar R: Falling in Old Age: Its prevention and Treatment. New York, Springer, 1989.

Tideiksaar R: Preventing falls: Home hazard checklists to help older patients protect themselves. Geriatrics 41:26–28, 1986.

Tideiksaar R and Kay AD: What causes falls? A logical diagnostic procedure. Geriatrics 41:32–50, 1986.

Tinetti ME: Performance-oriented assessment of mobility problems in elderly patients. J Am Geriatr Soc 34:119–126, 1986.

Tinetti ME and Ginter SF: Identifying mobility dysfunctions in elderly patients. JAMA 259:1190–1193, 1988.

Tinetti ME, Speechley M, and Ginter SF: Risk factors for falls among elderly persons living in the community. N Engl J Med 319:1701–1707, 1988.

Tinetti ME and Speechley M: Prevention of falls among the elderly. N Engl J Med 320:1055–1059, 1989.

Tinetti ME, Williams TF, and Mayewski R: Fall risk index for elderly patients based on number of chronic disabilities. Am J Med 80:429–434, 1986.

Torresin W: Model for Assessment of Geriatric Patients for Physical Therapists. Unpublished manuscript, 1989. (Available from Chedoke McMaster Hospitals, Box 2000, Station A, 1200 Main St, W, Hamilton, Ontario L8M 3Z5, Canada.)

U.S. Consumer Product Safety Commission. Safety for Older Consumers: Home Safety Checklist. Washington, DC: U.S. Consumer Product Safety Commission, 1986.

Vandervoort A, Hayes KC, and Belanger AY: Strength and endurance of skeletal muscle in the elderly. Physiother Canada 38:167–173, 1986.

Vandervoort A, Hill K, Sandrin M, et al: Mobility impairment and falling in the elderly. Physiother Canada 42:99–107, 1990.

Warren M: Promoting health and prevention disease and disability—an introduction to concepts, opportunities and practice. A review—part 1. Physiother Pract 1:57–63, 1985.

Whipple RH, Wolfson LI, and Amerman PM: The relationship of knee and ankle weakness to falls in nursing home residents: An isokinetic study. J Am Geriatr Soc 35:13–20, 1987.

Wild D, Nayak USL, and Isaacs B: Description, classification and prevention of falls in old people at home. Rheumatol Rehabil 20:153–159, 1981.

Windley PG and Scheidt RJ: Person-environment dialectics: Implications for competent functioning in old age. *In* Poon LW (ed): Aging in the 1980's: Psychological Issues. Washington, DC, American Psychological Association, 1980.

Winograd CH: Geriatric assessment and concepts: Components and settings. Paper presented at the meeting of the Gerontological Society of America, Minneapolis, November 17, 1989.

Wolf-Klein GP, Silverstone FA, Basavaraju N, et al: Prevention of falls in the elderly population. Arch Phys Med Rehabil 69:689–691, 1988.

Wolfson LI, Whipple R, Amerman P, et al: Gait and balance in the elderly: Two functional capacities that link sensory and motor ability to falls. Clin Geriatr Med 1:649–655, 1985.

Wolfson LI, Whipple R, Amerman P, et al: Stressing the postural response: A quantitative method for testing balance. J Am Geriatr Soc 34:845–850, 1986.

Wood PH: The language of disablement: A glossary relating to disease, and its consequences. Int Rehabil Med 2:86–92, 1980.

Woollacott MP, Shumway-Cook AT, and Nashner LM: Aging and postural control: Changes in sensory organization and muscular coordination. Int J Aging Hum Devel 23:81–98, 1986.

World Health Organization: International Classification of Impairments, Disabilities, and Handicaps. Geneva, World Health Organization, 1980.

Wyke B: Cervical articular contributions to posture and gait: Their relation to senile disequilibrium. Age Ageing 8:251–258, 1979.

CHAPTER

14

Sally H. Bennett

Low Vision: Clinical Aspects and Interventions

An elderly woman with cataracts has difficulty dialing the telephone and locating desired items on a grocery shelf. A younger man with glaucoma faces daily challenges in cooking his meals and the inability to read his bills and maintain a checkbook. Once an avid reader and quilter, a woman with diabetic retinopathy can no longer read printed matter unassisted or thread a needle independently. Are these people merely isolated cases, examples of clients rarely seen by occupational and physical therapists? On the contrary, in each instance, the person could benefit from direct intervention in the area of visual rehabilitation. Additionally, therapists could find themselves working with such clients when they are treated for visual and nonvisual conditions in acute-care, rehabilitation, or psychiatric settings.

Far from being isolated cases, each of these persons is a member of a large and ever-growing segment of American society: the low-vision population. This chapter defines and explains low vision and explores its implications for treatment in the clinical setting as well as environmental adaptations in the home and world beyond the clinic.

DEFINITION AND DEMOGRAPHICS

The clients mentioned in the opening paragraph are only three examples of people with low

vision. Approximately 14 million Americans have congenital or adventitious vision loss that cannot be fully corrected with surgery or conventional optical aids. Of this population, 80,000 are totally blind and 800,000 are legally blind (Seligmann, 1990). The remaining millions find themselves in the position of having some degree of residual vision but having experienced enough visual change to function initially at a decreased level of independence and often with a continued perceived lower skill level (Cullinan, 1986).

Low vision may appear to be a new phenomenon, but visual changes resulting from the natural aging process (Cristarella, 1977; Henig, 1989) and the ability to treat conditions that, in the past, progressed to total blindness (Seligmann, 1990) have, during the past 2 decades, brought low-vision treatment out of relative obscurity into the respected subspecialty of ophthalmology (Greenblatt, 1989). As people live longer with medical conditions that previously proved fatal and as the graying of the American public continues, clients with low vision continue to increase in number (Ballard, 1988; Greenblatt, 1989). However, a number of low-vision clients, although diagnosed, are often untreated because of physicians' lack of awareness of services available (Faye, 1984; Greenblatt, 1989). Medical and societal attitudes concerning visual impairment and the ability to function independently with various conditions may also lead to interrupted treatment and rehabilitation (Greenblatt, 1988; Parrish, 1988; Stetten, 1981).

To treat low vision, it is first necessary to understand exactly what it is and is not. The majority of health professionals who have taken part in disability-simulation activities during their training no doubt are familiar with performing a task with simulated total blindness while wearing a blindfold. Many therapists who have visual deficits find them to be corrected through prescription glasses or lenses. However, unless one has experienced it firsthand, low vision is not so easily understood. Low vision lies somewhere between total blindness and correctable vision, but the territory it occupies is vast and can mean many things to the people who inhabit that territory. Eleanor Faye, an ophthalmologist pioneering low vision as a subspecialty, viewed low vision in a functional capacity rather than strictly derived from vision testing (Faye, 1984). Low vision, according to Faye, covers a wide spectrum of conditions, all of which have specific commonalities: bilateral visual impairment, either below-normal acuity or reduced visual fields, and the inability to correct the vision loss through standard lenses or medical intervention. In the case of restricted visual fields, the field loss must interfere with premorbid or customary functioning (Faye, 1984). Indeed, functioning is a primary concern in low-vision diagnosis and treatment. Functional changes are of two types, as Faye (1984) pointed out: those resulting from the visual condition and those resulting from the person's reactions to the visual change.

BIOLOGIC ASPECTS

To understand low vision and its impact on functional capability, an understanding of ocular anatomy and specific conditions resulting in vision change is necessary. Although the biologic aspects of low vision are perhaps the most observable from a medical viewpoint, they are by no means the only definition of low vision. The psychosocial implications of visual change, which are discussed later, combine with the biologic aspects of low vision to have a direct impact on one's sense of identity and functioning. However, because the biologic aspects lay the foundation for the diagnosis, it is helpful for allied health professionals to have a basic understanding of the eye's anatomy and how a change in the ocular system can have a profound impact on the client's daily routine and capabilities.

Although the eye is delicate and small, a major portion of human sensory input is obtained visually. When any part of the eye is damaged through trauma or disease, that input is altered, which can in turn result in a marked change in functioning (Jose, 1983). A brief introduction to specific structures within the eye is followed by discussion of a number of pathologic conditions of those structures that can lead to or be indicative of low vision.

Structures Within the Eye

The *cornea* is the clear, avascular covering of the eye. Along with its protective qualities, the cornea, with the lens, focuses what one sees on the retina. Because the cornea is extremely sensitive as a result of its numerous nerve fibers, even a small abrasion can result in pain. A damaged cornea can ultimately cause infection in other ocular structures.

Directly behind the cornea lies the *aqueous,* a fluid continually in flux. Through its cycle of production and drainage, it both nourishes and cleanses the cornea and lens as well as aids in controlling the eye's shape. The colored portion of one's eye, the *iris,* regulates the amount of light entering the eye through pupil regulation.

In back of the iris, the *lens* focuses rays of light on the retina. The *ciliary body* has two main functions: production of aqueous fluid and lens focusing. The gelatinous substance accounting for two thirds of the eye's mass, the *vitreous,* is almost totally water; it gives the eye transparency and shape. The *sclera* is the outermost protective covering of the eye. It encapsulates the eyeball, with the exception of the cornea. Located between the sclera and the retina, the *choroid* is responsible for ocular blood supply.

Behind the choroid lies the *retina,* the neural layers in which the process of actual visual perception begins. Rods and cones within the retina are stimulated by differing degrees of light. Cones are more predominant in central vision; they are more reactive to bright light and play an important role in color perception. Cones are present only in two specialized areas of the retina: the *macula* and the *fovea.* Located on the macula, the tiny fovea provides the most detailed, acute vision. Rods, alternatively, predominate in the retinal periphery and are more functional in decreased light. Through stimulation of the retina, nerve impulses are relayed to the visual cortex by the *optic nerve.* In relaying the nerve impulse to the brain, the optic nerve is the link between the eye and the brain, where visual perception actually occurs.

Pathologies of the Eye

Although specific pathologic conditions such as cataracts and glaucoma occur more frequently in the elderly (National Institute on Aging, 1988), the physiologic aspects of the natural aging process itself can present a number of visual changes common to most individuals (Bennett, 1988; Cristarella, 1977). Accommodation for near vision has been found to begin to decrease by 10 years of age, whereas ongoing changes in visual acuity by the age of 18 years are not uncommon (Cristarella, 1977).

Additional changes in vision throughout the life span have two causes: neural and non-neural (Cristarella, 1977; Marmor, 1986). The retina, as it gradually loses neurons with aging, is responsible for the major neural changes. Depending on which retinal neurons die, central and peripheral vision may be affected. The rate of retinal neuronal deterioration and the resultant field losses can have a marked effect on functional capacity. In the case of macular degeneration, occurring through neuronal atrophy secondary to a compromised blood supply, color perception, fine-detail discrimination, and dark/light accommodation are also influenced.

The aging process and its effects on the lens account for the majority of non-neural visual changes (Marmor, 1986). With the loss of elasticity, an aging lens has an accompanying decrease in focal ability. This decline in focal ability, known as presbyopia, affects one's near vision, with an increased difficulty in reading print or performing tasks requiring close vision (National Institute on Aging, 1988). More common in people past the age of 40 years, presbyopia is progressive throughout the next 2 decades with a subsequent decline in progression past the fifth decade of life.

In addition to becoming less elastic with age, the lens may also undergo a protein degeneration resulting in its becoming opaque. This opacification, or clouding, is commonly known as a cataract. Specific characteristics of cataracts and their functional implication are covered in greater depth in the following section. Although cataracts are not universal in the elderly, many older individuals discover some loss of acuity from opacification (Crombie, 1986).

Although visual changes do occur frequently with age, most clients with low vision have decreased acuity and function secondary to a specific disease process or condition. Low vision accompanying such a disease process is generally more acute than that resulting from natural aging; in addition to the severity of the visual change, the client must often cope with other medical concerns while learning to function capably again (Cullinan, 1986).

Of the many causes of low vision, four are primarily responsible for vision loss in the elderly individual: cataracts, glaucoma, diabetic retinopathy, and macular degeneration (Weinreb et al, 1990).

Cataracts

As previously stated, a *cataract* is an opacification of the lens. This clouding prevents light from reaching the retina. Although cataracts associated with aging comprise the majority of low-vision cases related to cataracts, three other types of cataracts also exist: congenital, secondary, and traumatic (Yeadon and Grayson, 1979). Congenital cataracts result from a multitude of causes including metabolic defects, rubella, nystagmus, and strabismus. Although secondary cataracts, as the name implies, are related to another ocular condition (e.g., glaucoma), traumatic cataracts are associated with injury. Cataracts are often bilateral, although they usually develop at varying rates (Yeadon and Grayson, 1979). The progression, although gradual, varies; some people find their vision severely compromised by a wide area of opacification, whereas others find that their cataracts never develop to the point of severe impairment. The amount of functional impairment one may undergo with a cataract depends on its size, density, and location within the lens (National Eye Institute, 1986). Cataracts are treated surgically to remove the opacified lens; after surgery, the natural lens is replaced by one of three options: eyeglasses, contact lenses, or intraocular lens transplants (National Eye Institute, 1986).

Functionally, individuals with cataracts have hazy or blurred vision. Although some people report double vision in the early stages, it generally is resolved as opacification increases. Difficulty with glare and light is also a problem;

night driving becomes problematic, as does finding the correct type and distance of lighting necessary for close work such as reading and sewing. A simulation of functional vision with cataracts is shown in Figure 14–1.

Glaucoma

Glaucoma is a relatively insidious disease, because in its most common form, open-angle glaucoma, it is relatively asymptomatic until visual fields have been lost. Initially, glaucoma occurs as pressure in the aqueous increases; this increase, brought on by a change in the fluid flux, can eventually result in a hardening of the eye, causing permanent damage to the optic nerve (Whitmore, 1986; Yeadon and Grayson, 1979). Glaucoma is found in all age and ethnic groups, but it is more common in individuals over 35 years, diabetics, relatives of glaucoma clients, near-sighted people, and blacks (Whitmore, 1986).

Two major types of glaucoma exist. Open-angle glaucoma, the more common form, is found in 2.5 million Americans (Whitmore, 1986). Symptoms of this type of glaucoma are not noticeable in the early stages; the angle between the iris and cornea is open and wide. Although it is a chronic, lifelong condition, progression is slow. People with open-angle glaucoma generally respond favorably to medication and, if necessary, surgery (Whitmore, 1986). Closed- or narrow-angle glaucoma, alternatively, is less common. Symptoms are immediately apparent and require prompt attention, because the condition progresses rapidly. The angle between the cornea and iris is narrow or closed. With prompt microsurgery or laser surgery, the prognosis for narrow-angle glaucoma is good (Whitmore, 1986). Other types of glaucoma are secondary, low-tension, and developmental; each of these conditions can be found in one or both eyes and is, to varying degrees, a form of the two major types (Whitmore, 1986).

Functionally, people with glaucoma vary greatly in their ability to perform daily tasks and routines. If detected early through regular eye examinations, glaucoma may be treated. Depending on the progression, many people may have little need to adjust their lifestyles. If the condition is not discovered in its early stages and if the progression is not slowed down, peripheral fields are lost; in some cases, the outcome of glaucoma is total blindness. Individuals with glaucoma may notice the following symptoms: decreased peripheral vision, difficulty adjusting to changing light, fluctuating and blurred vision, and shadow-like halos around lights (Yeadon and Grayson, 1979). A simulation of functional vision with glaucoma is shown in Figure 14–2.

Diabetic Retinopathy

Diabetic retinopathy is found in over 90% of people with diabetes (Faye, 1984). However, not all people with diabetes have a significant vision loss because diabetic retinopathy exists in two stages: background and proliferative. In background retinopathy, the initial phase, visual acuity fluctuates but is better than 20/200. Microaneurysms form but are reabsorbed by the retina. With the second phase, proliferative retinopathy, visual acuity is less than 20/200 and may eventually be only light perception or total blindness, especially if glaucoma is also present (Faye, 1984). The term proliferative retinopathy is derived from the new blood vessels growing throughout the retina. Easily ruptured, these vessels bleed into the eye, producing scotoma, or blind spots, in central visual fields. Retinal detachment may also occur when scar tissue forms near the retina and detaches it from the eye (National Eye Institute, 1985).

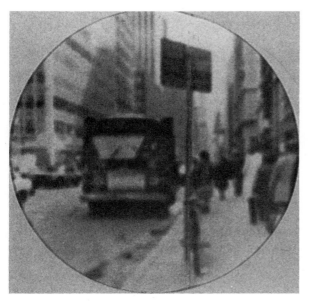

Figure 14–1. Cataracts produce an overall blurred vision, especially in bright light. (Photograph courtesy of The Lighthouse, Inc.)

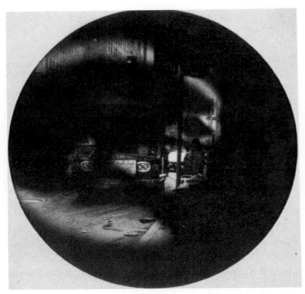

Figure 14–2. Glaucoma results in a loss of peripheral visual fields and can, in some cases, lead to total blindness. (Photograph courtesy of The Lighthouse, Inc.)

Relatively asymptomatic in its early stages, diabetic retinopathy is more common in people who have had diabetes for a number of years (National Eye Institute, 1985). Fluctuating vision and a change in focal power may be the first noticeable symptoms; people with diabetes require regular eye examinations to detect early signs of retinopathy (National Eye Institute, 1985). It is important for health professionals to realize that blurred vision in a client recently diagnosed with diabetes is often the result of a change in blood sugar level and is not always indicative of retinopathy (Yeadon and Grayson, 1979). Diabetic retinopathy is treated either by photocoagulation with a laser or through a vitrectomy. In photocoagulation, a laser is aimed at the retinal hemorrhages, often stopping the hemorrhages and preventing new retinal bleeding. Photocoagulation is not always an option, however. In some cases, the retinal bleeding is too profuse, obscuring the exact retinal areas to be lasered. There may also be some decrease in central and peripheral vision with laser treatments (National Eye Institute, 1985). When laser treatments are not an option or when successive photocoagulations do not stop the bleeding, blood and scar tissue are removed from the vitreous in a delicate surgical procedure known

as a vitrectomy (National Eye Institute, 1985; Yeadon and Grayson, 1979).

Functionally, people with diabetic retinopathy are similar to those with glaucoma in that they may not have any need to adapt their lifestyles because of a mild degree of retinopathy or they may need to make continued or major adaptations as their vision changes or is lost completely. Fluctuating vision in the background stage may be especially frustrating. Figure 14–3 is a simulation of vision with diabetic retinopathy.

Macular Degeneration

The final major cause of low vision in the elderly is *macular degeneration,* also known as age-related macular degeneration. With macular degeneration, central vision of 5 to 15 degrees is lost (Weinreb et al, 1990), but total blindness resulting from the condition is rare. The macula degenerates, through decreased circulation, as a result of human aging (Yeadon and Grayson, 1979). Clients with this condition often report decreased central vision, changes in color perception, and loss of fine-detail discrimination (Yeadon and Grayson, 1979). However, if the condition is found in one eye only, the client usually compensates with the other eye, finding little need to change daily routines (Weinreb et al, 1990). Many individuals find that they have enough residual vision in the affected eye to function

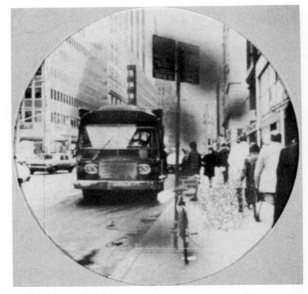

Figure 14–3. Diabetic retinopathy produces blind spots throughout the visual fields. (Photograph courtesy of The Lighthouse, Inc.)

independently or with a minimum of low-vision aids (Yeadon and Grayson, 1979). Argon laser treatments have proved effective as a preventive measure against additional field loss. A simulation of functional vision with macular degeneration is shown in Figure 14–4.

In addition to the previously discussed pathologic conditions, low vision is also the outcome of other diseases and conditions. Among them are cerebrovascular accidents, multiple sclerosis, detached retinas, retinitis pigmentosa, and retinopathy of prematurity (formerly called retrolental fibroplasia). The psychosocial stressors are similar for all low-vision clients no matter what the diagnosis, whereas the activities of daily living (ADL) interventions and environmental adaptations discussed are, to varying degrees, necessitated by the particular condition.

PSYCHOSOCIAL ASPECTS

Following AIDS and cancer, loss of vision is the most dreaded medical condition in America today (Seligmann, 1990). However, when most people think of vision loss, they think of total blindness. Rarely do they consider low vision the type of vision loss more likely to happen to them (Seligmann, 1990). Society and culture have historically divided individuals into two seg-

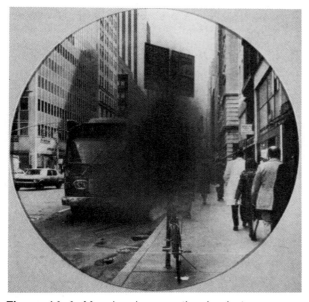

Figure 14–4. Macular degeneration leads to compromised central vision. (Photograph courtesy of The Lighthouse, Inc.)

ments of the population: sighted and blind. Whether sighted or blind, the role one assumes is based on both society's and one's own perception of the condition. The parameters for each role are well defined medically and culturally (Morse, 1983).

Many individuals with low vision believe themselves to be more blind than sighted because of either their physician's telling them that there was nothing else they could do for them (Fletcher, 1989; Ruben, 1990a) or a legal definition of blindness set forth half a century ago to determine eligibility for federal government benefits (Weinreb et al, 1990). Although legal blindness is defined as visual acuity of 20/200 or visual fields of 20 degrees or less, people with any amount of residual vision are now considered to benefit from low-vision rehabilitation (Neal, 1987; Weinreb et al, 1990). This shift in treating clients with low vision and training them to use rehabilitative techniques differs from previous sight-saving measures in which clients were discouraged from using remaining vision (Yeadon and Grayson, 1979).

Although rehabilitation specialists may have come to consider clients with low vision as partially sighted rather than as partially blind, individuals who undergo visual change often initially believe that they are more blind than sighted. Depression, anger, denial, and acceptance are interrelated emotions accompanying vision loss (Yeadon and Grayson, 1979). People who adventitiously lose vision must not only cope with their own visual loss but also acknowledge and reconsider societal expectations of and discrimination against people with visual impairments (Morse, 1983; Yeadon and Grayson, 1979). The stigma of blindness (Yeadon and Grayson, 1979), coupled with the general public's misunderstanding of low vision (Seligmann, 1990; Wainapel, 1989), does not make for an easy transition. Fluctuating vision and acute visual changes also are problematic, as can be the reactions of family, friends, colleagues, and strangers (Ruben, 1990b; Seligmann, 1990; Wainapel, 1989; Warnke, 1989). However, as individuals learn to function independently, they often perceive themselves to be more sighted than blind, although fully sighted people may still view them as blind (Morse, 1983). An additional stressor for many clients with low vision is an accompanying or underlying medical condition (Bennett, 1988) or the lack of acknowledgment of visual deficits and functional abilities by many health professionals (Ruben, 1990b).

ROLE OF THE THERAPIST

Although occupational and physical therapists have not traditionally worked exclusively with a visually impaired population, clients with low vision often are seen for related or other conditions in a variety of settings. In many of these settings, vision difficulties may not be treated because of more pressing medical concerns (Bennett, 1988) or a lack of knowledge or acknowledgment on the part of the therapist (Ruben, 1990b). However, therapists have begun to address the issue of vision impairment and the role of therapy in the rehabilitative process (Bennett, 1988; Reichley, 1987; Ruben, 1990b). Physicians, too, have begun to understand and value therapy intervention with their low-vision clients (Fletcher, 1989; Ruben, 1990a). This section deals with occupational therapy's place in visual rehabilitation, as part of a team, within the clinic. Environmental adaptations beyond the clinic walls are also discussed. The role of physical therapy, although not specifically related to ADLs or environmental adaptations, can be integral if the client in question is also in need of a specific physical therapy intervention from either a rehabilitative or preventive stance.

As part of a visual rehabilitative team, the occupational therapist works as an integral member with the physician, social worker, rehabilitation teacher, and orientation and mobility instructor (Ruben, 1990b). Depending on the type or amount of functional vision lost, a client may require the services of all or a few members of the team at any given time. As occupational therapists begin to evaluate and treat clients with low vision, few professional guidelines exist for working exclusively with this population (Ruben, 1990b). Evaluation and treatment are best performed from a holistic perspective (Fletcher, 1989; Ruben, 1990b). Occupational therapy personnel who have described their specific programs in recent professional literature (Reichley, 1988; Ruben, 1990b) focus mainly on evaluation and treatment in the area of ADL, often with the use of low-vision equipment.

Before exploring the aspects of ADL relevant to low-vision rehabilitation and some of the low-vision equipment available, two areas of clinical importance are discussed: mobility within the clinic and language as it relates to cultural attitudes toward vision change. Although both of these areas may not be considered specific to occupational therapy, they are, nonetheless, important clinical considerations.

Mobility for the newly diagnosed client with low vision is a skill best taught by the orientation and mobility instructor on the team. Should the client have an accompanying medical diagnosis or ambulation difficulty under treatment with a physical therapist, collaboration between the physical therapist and the orientation and mobility instructor enhances the client's skill and safety. Among the numerous areas orientation and mobility instruction covers are traveling indoors and outside (with or without the use of a white cane or low-vision aids) and using public transportation. However, therapists work with clients in clinical or home settings and need to be aware of some basic mobility techniques and common courtesies to be observed in such settings.

Functional vision differs for virtually every individual with low vision (Seligmann, 1990) and may fluctuate or change abruptly for many (Ruben, 1990b). However, some rules of thumb and specific techniques work well with a variety of clients. Clinical treatment and mobility are enhanced by observing the following guidelines:

1. Do not raise your voice when talking to a person with low vision unless he or she is also hearing impaired.
2. Observe before instructing. Many individuals with low vision may have already incorporated specific techniques through life experience and ingenuity.
3. Be specific when giving directions rather than pointing or providing vague directions such as "the table is over there."
4. Tactile cueing may be appropriate but always preface it with a request.
5. The "clock" method of locating items on a surface may be helpful (i.e., on a dinner plate, the meat is located at 6:00 and the vegetables at 9:00).
6. Do not attempt to second-guess the appropriateness of assistance. If you are unsure of the need for or amount of assistance, ask the individual directly.
7. When speaking to the client with low vision and family or care givers, direct your questions to the appropriate person. Many sighted people find themselves initially more comfortable talking to other sighted people, and family members may tend to be overly protective by answering for the client.

8. Identify yourself upon meeting until the individual recognizes your voice.
9. If you must leave the immediate area during treatment, let the client know this so that he or she will know your whereabouts and will not continue to talk to you.
10. If mobility is problematic, use a sighted-guide technique, allowing the client to take your arm and follow a step or two behind you.
11. Do not leave newly diagnosed persons alone in an area without aiding them in locating landmarks.

Language, because it is reflective of attitude, is also an important but often unconsidered aspect of clinical treatment. Sighted people often try to avoid visually loaded words such as "see" or phrases such as "Do you watch television?" when speaking to persons who are visually impaired, believing it is upsetting for them. This type of language is perfectly acceptable. Making obvious changes or retracting statements in embarrassment could prove to be a distancing technique. Common, everyday language need not be restructured (Yeadon and Grayson, 1979). When referring to the actual visual impairment, however, realistic yet positive language is in order (Baron, 1985). The terms "low vision" and "partially sighted" rather than "blind," "legally blind," and "partially blind" reflect a positive attitude, and yet they do not deny the impairment and may serve to promote competence and a more positive self-image.

EVALUATION AND TREATMENT

The role of occupational and physical therapy with visual rehabilitation is 2-fold: evaluation and treatment. Functional vision, tactile skills, olfactory and auditory systems, and cognition are often used in combination to perform daily tasks. Physical abilities and other medical conditions also need to be addressed in treatment planning. Because each client with low vision may present differently, the evaluative approach should be individualized to each. The main thrust of current occupational therapy treatment is in ADL skills (Reichley, 1988; Ruben, 1990b).

ADL skills in the client with low vision are enhanced in several ways. Two areas that are relevant to all low-vision conditions are lighting and color contrast. *Lighting* is considered an important clinical and environmental adaptation as well as one of the least expensive (Dickman, 1983). Although the type and amount of light necessary is determined by the condition and the task, several general lighting rules hold for a variety of individuals. Ceiling lighting is not as effective as a shaded lamp that illuminates one particular area. Although fluorescent lighting provides more light in a large area than does incandescent lighting, it can be problematic for many clients with low vision. In general, fluorescent light is harsher; fluorescent lights also flicker, which may, with the aging eye's sensitivity, lead to tearing and headaches. The amount of incandescent light necessary depends on the task involved. Reading, for example, generally requires half the amount of light needed for sewing. Glare, whether caused by natural sunlight streaming through a window, wax on a kitchen floor, or inappropriate lighting, should be avoided to maximize safe mobility (Dickman, 1983).

Color contrast is also an effective technique to enhance ADL performance and independence. Whether the contrast is used in an individual project in a task group, in writing utensils and paper, or in specific environmental adaptations, it generally promotes and facilitates independent functioning.

Many clients with low vision find *low-vision aids* of use in ADL areas. Although some aids are expensive and dispensed by other team members, some, such as simple magnifiers, are often found during an occupational therapy evaluation to be beneficial. Occupational therapists may also be called on to incorporate the use of a variety of low-vision aids into specific ADL skills. Familiarity with the categories of aids is helpful to the clinician.

Although using low-vision aids can indeed enhance ADL performance, they cannot restore lost vision (Bennett, 1989; Silver, 1986). However, the wide range of aids available affords the client with low vision a variety of options. Although some individuals find one or two aids useful, others discover the benefits of using several different aids for specific tasks.

Low-vision aids are divided into three categories: convex lenses, telescopic systems, and electronic systems (Faye, 1984). Convex lenses, including monocular and binocular spectacles, hand-held magnifiers, stand magnifiers, and illuminated magnifiers, are often used in close work such as reading, sewing, and writing (Fig. 14–5). The price and magnification vary depend-

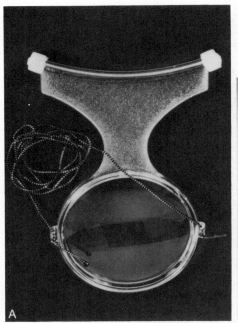

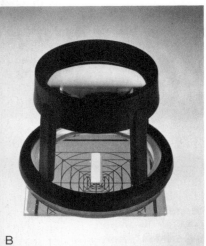

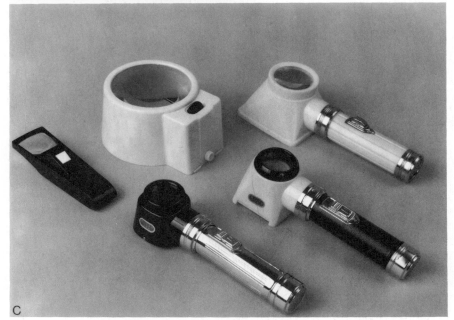

Figure 14–5. *A,* Hand-held magnifiers are sometimes worn on a neck chain for easy access. *B,* Although many people find stand magnifiers useful, if used for a prolonged time, they can become fatiguing. *C,* Illuminated magnifiers enhance ADL skills (*A, B,* and *C,* Photographs courtesy of Science Products.)

ing on the particular type of lens. Telescopic systems (Fig. 14–6) can also be used for close work requiring a longer working distance than that provided by a convex lens. However, they are used most efficiently for distance viewing such as reading street signs and viewing objects across a room (Bennett, 1989; Faye, 1984). Electronic aids such as large-print computers and closed-circuit televisions (CCTVs) (Fig. 14–7) further enhance reading and written communication skills.

Although low-vision aids enable many persons to read printed matter with assistance, other options exist for the person who wishes to read aurally. The National Library Service for the Blind and Physically Handicapped provides free discs and four-track cassette books playable on special equipment that it loans. Adaptive equipment companies have also produced smaller, more portable players for four-track books (Fig. 14–8). Standard two-track recorded cassette books are now a popular option as well. Recording for the Blind, Inc., records and loans four-track cassettes (mainly textbooks and professional material) to qualified borrowers.

Occupational therapists, in addition to working with these low-visions aids, also need to be

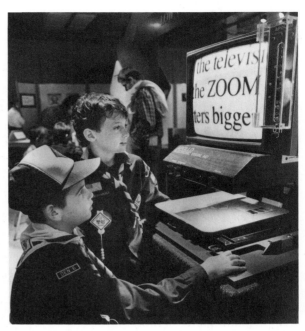

Figure 14–7. CCTVs promote independence in reading printed matter. (Photograph courtesy of Pennsylvania College of Optometry.)

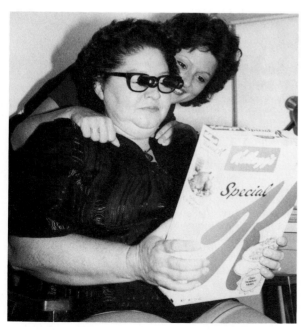

Figure 14–6. Telescopes facilitate ADL independence. (Photograph courtesy of Pennsylvania College of Optometry.)

familiar with adaptive equipment specific to the low-vision population. This equipment ranges from simple items such as signature, check, and envelope guides to complex health-maintenance equipment such as talking scales and auditory/tactile diabetes-monitoring items. Therapists wishing additional information should refer to the Appendix.

In addition to considering low vision in the clinical setting, therapists need to be aware of *environmental adaptations* beyond the clinic walls. When working in the area of ADLs with low-vision individuals, therapists (both occupational therapists enhancing ADL skills and physical therapists promoting maximum safe mobility within the home) find the following adaptations, specific to a room in the client's home, useful.

In the kitchen, safety is of prime importance. Independence in cooking can be facilitated through large-print cookbooks and recipes, large-print timers, and tactile markings on stove dials, microwaves, and so on. Using long-armed oven mitts and contrasting colors in pans and stoves further promotes safety. Organization aids the individual in locating required items; utensils hung on the wall are easier to find than those stuffed in a drawer. Large-print labels or tactile

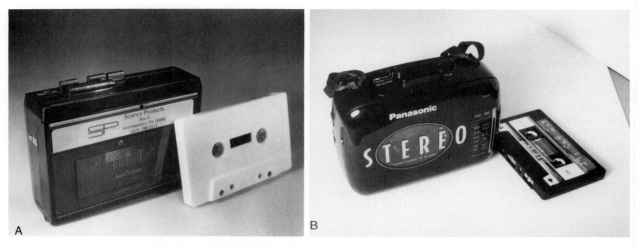

Figure 14–8. Adaptive equipment companies have modified standard cassette players for use with four-track cassette books. (Photographs courtesy of Science Products.)

markers on canned goods are also methods of identification many people find useful.

In the bathroom, safety is, again, important. Color contrast is effective in promoting safety. A darker bath mat in a white tub is a safety measure, as is contrasting heavy-duty tape on grab bars and tub sides. Soap color should be in contrast to the fixtures; towels and toilet paper are located more readily if they are in contrast to the walls.

In the living room and bedroom, color contrast is also important. Upholstered furniture and bedspreads should contrast with the carpeting to facilitate safe mobility and ease of seating. Overly patterned rugs or upholstery may also cause mobility difficulty, as can scatter rugs or highly polished floors. Lighting can also be a problem because blinds and curtains tend to obscure natural light.

It is important, especially when working in the client's home, to work as a team with the client. Ultimately, it is his or her home; he or she has to live in it long after the therapist leaves. Safety, although of primary importance, should always be promoted through adaptations the client and care givers are involved with and understand.

SUMMARY

This chapter, although not meant to be inclusive, provides therapists with basic, introductory material concerning low vision. Whether one is working as part of a visual rehabilitation team or in another clinical setting, therapists find themselves evaluating and treating clients with visual impairments. As the population with low vision grows, therapists discover that a larger percentage of their clients have one or more visual impairments. Therapists, with their ability to view a person holistically and to problem solve effectively through the clinical reasoning process, are in a unique position to both teach and learn from the individual with low vision.

References

Ballard MT: Leaders in low vision optometry see visual impairments reaching "epidemic" proportions. Braille Forum 26(4):23–24, 1988.

Baron LS: The Adult Low Vision Population: A Treatment Guide for Allied Health Professionals. Houston, Author, 1985.

Bennett SH: Low vision technology: An overview for occupational therapy personnel. Gerontology Special Interest Section Newsletter of the American Occupational Therapy Association, pp. 4–5, December 1989.

Bennett SH: Occupational therapy can effect change in the lives of visually impaired individuals. O.T. Week, pp. 4–5, July 21, 1988.

Cristarella MC: Visual functions of the elderly. Am J Occup Ther 31:432–440, 1977.

Crombie AL: Cataract. In Caird FI and Williamson J (eds): The Eye and Its Disorders in the Elderly. Bristol, England, Wright, 1986.

Cullinan T (ed): Visual Disability in the Elderly. London, Croom Helm, 1986.

Dickman IR: Making Life More Livable: Simple Adaptations for the Homes of Blind and Visually Impaired Older People. New York, American Foundation for the Blind, 1983.

Faye EE: Clinical Low Vision. Boston, Little, Brown, 1984.

Fletcher DC: Vision loss: An ophthalmologist's perspective. *In* Greenblatt SL (ed): Providing Services for People with Vision Loss: A Multidisciplinary Perspective. Lexington, MA, Resources for Rehabilitation, 1989.

Greenblatt SL: Physicians and chronic impairment: A study of ophthalmologists' interactions with visually impaired and blind patients. Soc Sci Med 26(4):393–399, 1988.

Greenblatt SL (ed): Providing Services for People with Vision Loss: A Multidisciplinary Perspective. Lexington, MA, Resources for Rehabilitation, 1989.

Henig RM: The aging eye. New York Times Magazine, pp. 47–48, March 26, 1989.

Jose RT: The eye and functional vision. *In* Jose RT (ed): Understanding Low Vision. New York, American Foundation for the Blind, 1983.

Marmor MF: Visual changes with age. *In* Caird FI and Williamson J (eds): The Eye and Its Disorders in the Elderly. Bristol, England, Wright, 1986.

Morse JL: Psychosocial aspects of low vision. *In* Jose RT (ed): Understanding Low Vision. New York, American Foundation for the Blind, 1983.

National Eye Institute: Cataracts (DHHS publication no. 86–201). Washington, DC, U.S. Government Printing Office, 1986.

National Eye Institute: Diabetic Retinopathy (DHHS publication no. 85–2171). Washington, DC, U.S. Government Printing Office, 1985.

National Institute on Aging: Aging and Your Eyes (DHHS publication no. 88–195). Washington, DC, U.S. Government Printing Office, 1988.

Neal H: Low Vision. New York, Simon & Schuster, 1987.

Parrish RK: How we deal with our own feelings about blindness. Arch Ophthalmol 106:31–33, 1988.

Reichley TL: Occupational therapy and low vision rehabilitation. Occup Ther Health Care 5(2/3):99–109, 1988.

Reichley TL: Program for low vision patients brings independence into focus. O.T. Advance, pp. 3–4, July 27, 1987.

Ruben B: Ophthalmologist looks to OT for vision rehab. O.T. Week, pp. 4, 10, June 28, 1990a.

Ruben B: OT brings insight to the field of visual impairment. O.T. Week, pp. 4–5, June 28, 1990b.

Seligmann J: Making the most of sight: A brighter future for the millions of Americans with "low" vision. Newsweek, pp. 92–93, April 6, 1990.

Silver J: Optical aids in low vision. *In* Cullinan T (ed): Visual Disability in the Elderly. London, Croom Helm, 1986.

Stetten D: Coping with blindness. N Engl J Med 305(8):458–460, 1981.

Wainapel SF: Vision loss: A patient's perspective. *In* Greenblatt SL (ed): Providing Services for People with Vision Loss: A Multidisciplinary Perspective. Lexington, MA, Resources for Rehabilitation, 1989.

Warnke JL: Mental health services: The missing link. *In* Greenblatt SL (ed): Providing Services for People with Vision Loss: A Multidisciplinary Perspective. Lexington, MA, Resources for Rehabilitation, 1989.

Weinreb RN, Freeman WR, and Selezinka W: Vision impairments in geriatrics. *In* Kemp B, Brummel-Smith K, and Ramsdell JW (eds): Geriatric Rehabilitation. Boston, College Hill, 1990.

Whitmore LA: Living with and Understanding Glaucoma: A Reference Guide for Patients and Their Families. San Francisco, Foundation for Glaucoma Research, 1986.

Yeadon A and Grayson D: Living with Impaired Vision: An Introduction. New York, American Foundation for the Blind, 1979.

APPENDIX I: RESOURCE LIST

National Library Service for the Blind and Physically Handicapped Library of Congress 1291 Taylor St, NW Washington, DC 20542 (202) 707–5100 or (800) 424–8567

Recording for the Blind, Inc. 20 Roszel Rd Princeton, NJ 08540 (609) 452–0606

American Foundation for the Blind 15 West 16th St New York, NY 10011 (212) 620–2000

Science Products P.O. Box 888 Southeastern, PA 19399 (800) 888–7400

Council of Citizens with Low Vision c/o American Council for the Blind 1010 Vermont Ave, NW Suite 1100 Washington, DC 20005 (202) 393–3666

Vision Foundation, Inc. 818 Mt. Auburn St Watertown, MA 02171 (617) 926–4232

National Eye Institute National Institutes of Health Building 31, Room 6A32 Bethesda, MD 20892 (301) 496–5248

National Association for the Visually Handicapped 22 West 21st St New York, NY 10010 (212) 889–3141

Resources for Rehabilitation 33 Bedford St Suite 19A Lexington, MA 02173 (617) 862–6455

CHAPTER
15
Roseann C. Schaaf
Wendy S. Davis

Promoting Health and Wellness in the Pediatric Disabled and "At Risk" Population

The goal of any wellness program is to promote optimal, independent functioning so the individual may lead a more satisfying life and become an accepted and contributing member of society. In terms of occupational and physical therapy, preventive health care includes life-enhancing services directed toward maintenance, restoration, and development of a sense of physical well-being, social productivity, and self-actualization. This goal is realized for pediatric therapists by working not only with the child but also with the families, caregivers, and team members involved with the child. Effective therapy for the pediatric therapist is not merely a "doing to" the child but rather a collaborative teaching process in which the child, family, and caregivers are encouraged to establish beneficial goals, skills, and habits so the need for continual rehabilitation services is eliminated. In short, preventive health care uses a team approach to promote competence in both the child and the family/caregiver. The information in this chapter assists therapists in refocusing traditional medical and educational models of therapy and encourages their collaboration in a holistic, team-oriented, family-centered approach to pediatric wellness. Therapists

are encouraged to constantly evaluate the effectiveness of intervention in terms of the children's and families' competence and life satisfaction. To do this, therapists must move beyond technical knowledge and skills into understanding the families' culture, including their values, interests, and goals. All of these factors shape the children's success. The adage "an ounce of prevention is worth a pound of cure" is the basis for this chapter. By promoting strategies for wellness and prevention of disability (or its expansion), occupational and physical therapists are aiming to decrease the need for lifelong rehabilitation.

This chapter targets two major pediatric populations to exemplify the aforementioned philosophy for preventive health care:

1. The "at-risk population, which includes children and families who may be:
   a. at risk biologically for delayed or abnormal development as a result of neurologic disorders, learning disabilities, sensory-processing disorders
   b. at risk environmentally as a result of child abuse, sociocultural deprivation, or abnormal parent-child attachment relationships

2. Children with known established risk such as congenital or acquired physical and mental handicaps or diagnosed medical disorders.

The therapists' roles as neurodevelopmental experts, facilitators of competence in care-givers, and environmental adapters in the promotion of wellness in these pediatric populations are explored by focusing on three areas that are essential in preventive pediatric health care: early identification, early intervention, and direct intervention. These are summarized now and elaborated on throughout the chapter.

Early identification includes a list of assessments designed to identify the child, family, and environmental situations in need of intervention, referral, or consultation. This section also includes an overview of risk factors and situations that may require further follow-up and intervention.

Intervention programs highlight and discuss progressive, therapeutic early intervention by occupational and physical therapists as a preventive measure. Therapeutic roles such as consultant, direct-service provider, early identifier, and referral source are explored. A team approach in a variety of possible work settings and roles is emphasized, and referral information for secondary or related difficulties is presented. A discussion on mainstreaming into the community provides suggestions and references for promoting health and wellness through social, recreational, and personal awareness activities for the developing child, his or her family, and peers.

Direct intervention describes the potential roles and functions of the therapist in primary care. A family-centered framework for promoting family competence is presented as an example of occupational and physical therapy intervention using a collaborative, holistic approach. The chapter concludes with a case example, which exemplifies the principles of prevention and demonstrates potential roles for therapists in preventive health careers. Prospectives for future therapists' roles in prevention and wellness are suggested.

EARLY IDENTIFICATION

Early identification is a primary factor associated with prevention. Children and families identified

as at risk or children disabled from an early age can be referred for early intervention services. These services are offered to a child and their family before the preschool or school-age years. As part of the early identification process, it is important for therapists to note the initial signs of disability and to be sensitive to indicators that may reflect a child or family who is at risk. Timely referral may interrupt a potentially dysfunctional cycle and prevent further complications from a disability (Reynolds et al, 1983). An overview of vulnerability and risk factors is presented to help familiarize therapists with common factors and their potential for resultant atypical/abnormal behaviors.

Vulnerability and Risk Factors

Continual advances in medical technology have resulted in the survival of many gestationally younger, smaller, and medically fragile infants (Bauchner et al, 1988; Mitchell, 1985; Weiner and Koppelman, 1987). Much research has been focused on determining the early indicators of later neuromuscular, learning, and adjustment difficulties (Ayres, 1972; Bates, 1980; Brown, 1983; Fewell et al, 1983; Field, 1980; Fish and Dixon, 1978; Greenspan and Porges, 1984; Hobel, 1985; Hutchins et al, 1983; Pasamanick and Knobloch, 1960; Sell et al, 1985; Thomas and Chess, 1981). These researchers concluded that risk factors are not mutually exclusive because they can occur singularly or in multiple combinations, with their interaction resulting in a greater potential for delayed or abnormal behavior (Enshner and Clark, 1986; Klaus et al, 1982; Simmer, 1983). Significant historic factors that may result in neuromuscular, learning, and adjustment difficulties include prematurity and low birth weight, respiratory difficulties, interventricular hemorrhage or intercranial bleeds, metabolic disorders, ophthalmologic disorders, audiologic disorders, environmental factors, and exposure in utero to excessive drugs and alcohol (Pratt and Allen, 1989). A brief overview of each of these risk factors and their potential sequel follows.

Prematurity and low birth weight (defined by Semmler, 1989, as less than 36 weeks' gestation or less than 5 pounds, 8 ounces) require prolonged hospitalization. The neonatal intensive care unit (NICU) environment exposes the immature, vulnerable nervous system of the infant to the negative effects of deprivation, disorganization, and inappropriate or excessive stimuli of various types. It also places the family at risk for poor bonding experiences, which may lead to later adjustment and coping difficulties (Brazelton, et al, 1974; Clarke-Stewart, 1983; Klaus et al, 1982).

Respiratory difficulties (such as brachiopulmonary dysplasia, meconium aspiration, or apnea) requiring prolonged ventilation may result in decreased movement, decreased stimulation, decreased parent-infant interaction, increased incidence of abnormal muscle tone, movement patterns and oral feeding difficulties, asthmaticlike conditions, and repeated hospitalizations as a result of respiratory infections.

Interventricular hemorrhage or cranial bleeds cause neurologic insults and subsequent neurodevelopmental deficits.

Metabolic disorders (e.g., hyperbilirubinemia, hypocalcemia, and hypoglycemia) may cause neurologic defects, excessive irritability, and seizures.

Ophthalmologic disorders may result in retinal detachment, impaired acuity, strabismus, and problems with perception.

Audiologic disorders (such as recurrent otitis media and primary hearing problems) may result in delays in language development and delays in the acquisition of motor skills (Price and Techman, 1979; Schaaf 1985).

Environmental factors (including parental neglect or abuse, social deprivation, and poverty) may negatively influence the child's cognitive, socioemotional, motor, and language development. The enrichment/deprivation literature (Bishop, 1982; Cotman and Nieto-Stampedro, 1982; Elardo et al, 1977; Lund, 1978) indicates that positive, enriched environments are potentially growth-perpetuating to the young child, whereas deprived, understimulating environments may limit the child from developing to his or her fullest potential. In view of this literature, it is important to ensure an optimal amount of appropriate stimulation for the developing child. This includes sensory and motor stimulation as well as socioemotional support from caregivers. Occupational and physical therapists often identify children and families who need enrichment experiences and involve them in education that entails sensory, motor, and socioemotional support for the infant.

Recent literature on in utero exposure to excessive drugs and alcohol indicates that babies exposed to cocaine and alcohol in utero are often born prematurely and of small gestational weight. Because of this exposure, these infants are at a greater risk for developmental difficulties. Intrauterine exposure to cocaine has been associated with several atypical infant behaviors such as abnormal or delayed state behavior, atypical state organization, mother-infant attachment disorders, and impairment of orientation and motor control. Prolonged and excessive intrauterine exposure to alcohol has been associated with a variety of developmental anomalies and delays including mental retardation and fetal alcohol syndrome (Chasnoff et al, 1989; Hadeed and Seigel, 1989; Destefano-Lewis et al, 1989; Hume et al, 1989; Schneider et al, 1989).

In terms of these vulnerability and risk factors in general, the predictive value of any one neurologic or neurobehavioral factor has not been well established. Instead, it appears that the long-term outcome depends on the number of risk factors and the interactions between those risk factors. The following diagram exemplifies the impact of increasing number of untreated risk factors on the individual's potential for dysfunctional or maladaptive behavior (Fig. 15–1).

The literature suggests that as the child ages prenatal factors become considerably less important, whereas environmental factors become more significant. "There is reason to believe that the detrimental effects of prematurity are exacerbated in nonsupportive environments and ameliorated in supportive, caregiving environments" (Pratt and Allen, 1989, p. 363). Figure 15–2 demonstrates how risk factors at birth may be exacerbated by unfavorable environmental conditions and result in incompetence, unhappiness, and an individual who is a problem for society.

Assessment

In view of the complex and interactional nature of risk factors on the outcome of the child, assessment and intervention must be focused not only on the child but the family and primary environments as well. In terms of assessment, child-centered evaluations have traditionally been developmental in nature, measuring the child's skill levels in comparison to "the norm." More current thinking encourages assessment and intervention plans that also include a holistic view of preventive, compensatory, maturational abilities, and the needs of the child and his or

Figure 15–1. Potential interactions between untreated risk factors. Risk factors can and generally do occur in combinations. Their numbers and interactions result in a greater degree of probability for delayed or abnormal behavior.

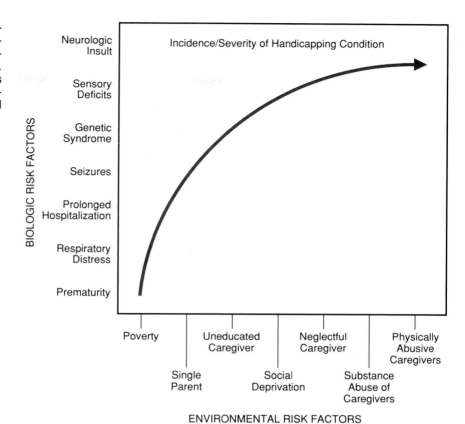

her family (Bailey et al, 1988; Bailey et al, 1989; Dunst et al, 1988b). Table 15–1 presents an overview of screening and assessment tools currently in use that are designed to evaluate the strengths and weaknesses of the child, the family system, and the environments in which the child and family interact. These assessments can be used to assist therapists in determining primary areas of strength and need. Therapists can then design intervention to address these needs and support the areas of strength, thus interrupting or preventing a dysfunctional life cycle.

INTERVENTION PROGRAMS

Overview

Early intervention programs started in the 1950s and 1960s and focused primarily on each child's cognitive and motor development. Over time, a more holistic view of child development was adopted. This approach incorporated language, cognitive, and social abilities with physical stimulation. Currently, in the 1990s, early intervention programs include the parents' involvement as a critical component and aim to not only enhance the child's potential for development but also promote family competence and coping strategies (Hanft, 1988). This focus has partially been shaped by PL 99–457, The Education of the Handicapped Act Amendment of 1986, which places a major emphasis on family services. A family-centered approach allows the strengths and needs of the family to shape and direct the focus of intervention and seeks to develop strategies that enhance the families' competence in raising a child with special needs. This focus on the family has been further elaborated on by current research (American Occupational Therapy Association, 1989; Bailey, 1987; Bailey et al, 1989; Dunst et al, 1988a and b; Foley, 1987; Hanft, 1988 and 1989; Hinojosa and Anderson, 1987; Hinojosa et al, 1988; Kochnek and Friedman,

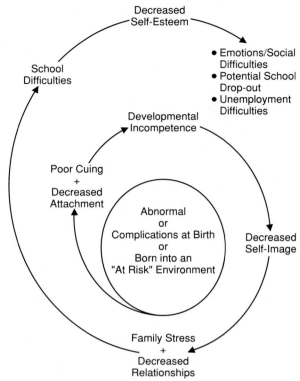

Figure 15–2. Potential ontogenetic evolution of an individual born at risk.

1988; Pierce, 1989; Pratt and Allen, 1989; Schaaf and Gitlin, 1989; Schaaf and Mulrooney, 1989; Dunn, 1989).

Individual Family Service Plans

One means by which the family is incorporated into the early intervention process in education-related facilities is through the individual family service plan (IFSP). The IFSP is a listing of goals and services that are needed for the child and family for the upcoming year. Through the IFSP, parents are encouraged to take an active role in the planning, coordinating, and decision-making process for their child's education. This interactive process between professionals and family members is designed to determine the strengths, needs, and priorities of the family. The goals for the child and family and the services provided to them are stipulated in the IFSP. The services and goals facilitate the capacity of the family to enhance the development and meet the special needs of their child, for example: (1) expanded

therapeutic skills, (2) decreased dependence on professionals, (3) increased competence in caregiving abilities, and (4) increased confidence in their role as a parent (Foley, 1987; Kochnek and Friedman, 1988).

Settings and Roles

Therapists may find themselves in a variety of settings when working with children and families. These include the NICU, the pediatric inpatient floor of an acute-care hospital, neonatal follow-up clinics, outpatient department of a medical facility, home- or center-based early intervention program, and public or private school-based programs. Within these settings they may also have a variety of roles in interacting with families and children: They may serve as *consultants* to a team that addresses the child's and the family's needs; as a *direct-service providers* working with children and families in the hospital, home, or early intervention center; as a source of *identification* of special needs and at-risk children and families; and as a source of *referral* for appropriate services.

Common to all these roles in any setting is the philosophy of promoting wellness by striving toward the following goals:

1. Preventing or reducing the primary problems resulting directly from risk conditions that may impair or interfere with the child's emotional, perceptual, cognitive, language, or motor development and maximizing the child's potential capabilities in these areas
2. Preventing secondary problems by aiding the child in the development of appropriate adaptive skills or mechanisms to compensate for a primary disability, which may prevent a later need for extensive rehabilitation
3. Encouraging parenting that reinforces positive developmental patterns and encourages changes toward more healthy lifestyles
4. Strengthening family development by lessening parental guilt, anger, frustration, and ignorance and enhancing parent-child interactions and bonding
5. Facilitating the child's own adjustment to outside environments (school and community groups) through environmental adaptations, teacher training, and community advocacy.

A brief overview of the therapists' role as con-

Table 15–1. Screening and Assessment Tools

Assessment/Author	Method	Target Population	Yield/Description
Assessment Area: Child			
Brazelton Neonatal Behavioral Assessment Scale (Brazelton, 1984)	Standardized, not normed 9-pt. scale	Infants 38 weeks'gestational age	Designed to measure the interactive capacity and individual behavioral style of the infant: (1) capacity to habituate to stimuli, (2) regulate changes in state of consciousness, (3) respond to animate and inanimate objects, (4) Neuromotor integrity, (5) physiologic stability
Neurological Assessment of the Pre-Term and Full-Term Newborn Infant (Dubowitz and Dubowitz, 1981)	Standardized, not normed 5-pt. scale	Preterm and full-term infant	Measures: (1) various stages of neurologic maturation, (2) interactive capacity of the newborn
Neurological Examination of the Full-Term Newborn Infant (Prectl and Heinz, 1977)	Standardized, not normed performance 4-pt. rating scale	Infants	Designed to assess (1) muscle tone, (2) reflexes, (3) postures, (4) movements
Gesell Developmental Schedules (Haines et al, 1980)	Performance scale	4 weeks–36 months	Designed to determine developmental levels in the following behaviors: (1) adaptive, (2) gross motor, (3) fine motor, (4) language, (5) personal and social
Bayley Scales of Infant Development (Bayley, 1969)	Performance scales	2–30 months	Motor and mental scales
Early Intervention Developmental Profile (Rogers et al, 1981)	Curriculum-based developmental checklist	Birth to 6 years	Designed to determine developmental levels in: (1) gross motor, (2) fine motor, (3) cognitive, (4) social, (5) language, and (6) self-help
Hawaii Early Learning Profile (Furuno et al, 1979)	Curriculum-based developmental checklist	Birth to 6 years	Designed to determine developmental levels in the following behaviors: (1) gross motor, (2) fine motor, (3) cognitive, (4) social, (5) language, and (6) self-help
Peabody Developmental Motor Scales (Folio and Fewell, 1983)	3-pt. performance scale	1–83 months	Designed to assess and program for children with deficits in: (1) gross motor, (2) fine motor skills
Mullen Scales of Early Learning (Mullen, 1988)	Performance scales Infant scales space	0–36 months 15–68 months	Four scales assess areas of strength/weakness and learning style: (1) visual receptive organization visual discrimination, sequencing, organization, and memory; (2) visual expressive organization, unilateral and bilateral hand skills; (3) language receptive organization language, comprehension, verbal/spatial awareness, short-term and long-term memory; (4) language expressive organization verbal ability
Miller Assessment for Preschoolers (Miller, 1982)	Screening	2 years–9 months 5 years–8 months	Designed to identify children with later school-related problems; screens: (1) cognitive, (2) language, (3) perceptual, (4) motor
DeGangi-Berk Test of Sensory Integration (Berk and DeGangi, Western Psychological Services, Los Angeles, CA)	Screening 3-pt. scale	3–5 years	Screens sensory-motor functions: (1) postural control, (2) bilateral motor integration, (3) reflex integration
Bruininks–Oseretsky Test of Motor Proficiency (Bruininks, 1978)	Standardized test	4.5–14.5 years	Assesses gross and fine motor skills yields developmental age
Preschool Play Scale (Knox, 1974; Bledsoe and Shephard, 1982)	Observation rating scale	Preschool 0–5 years of age	Overall play age score for 4 domains: material management, space management, imitation, participation
Play History (Takata, 1969)	Semistructured interview	Children and adolescents	Qualitative information on play history, play environments. Implications for treatment
Standardized Clinical Play Observation (Kalverboer, 1977)	Standardized setting: observation and video recordings	Children (no age range specified)	Frequency and types of play and nonplay activities
Social Play Scale (Parten, 1933)	Time sampling Observation tool	Preschoolers	Developmental level of social play and related information on play groups, roles, language use, and types of games and toys
Organization of Play Behavior (Hulme and Lunzer, 1966)	Observation rating scale based on diary of observations	Children 2–6 years	Single numerical score representing degree of organization in play
Playfulness Scale (Lieberman, 1977)	Observation rating tool	Children and adolescents	Give score indicating overall playfulness
Parent/Teacher Play Questionnaire (Schaaf et al, 1987)	Questionnaire or interview	Children 0–18 years	Qualitative information regarding play interests, play times, play behaviors, play routines

Table continued on following page

Table 15–1. Screening and Assessment Tools *Continued*

Assessment/Author	Method	Target Population	Yield/Description
Assessment Area: Family			
Parenting Stress Index (Abidin, 1986)	Questionnaire/rating scale, self report	Families with disabled/special needs 0- to 3-year-olds, parent-child systems under stress or in high-risk situations	Information to determine specific stress factors related to dysfunctional parenting; helps parents understand importance of creating positive environment; At-risk screening tool for parent-child relationship
Parent Needs Survey (Darling, 1989)	Self-report survey	Families with special-needs children	Information regarding the needs of families in areas such as treatment needs for the child, formal and informal support for the family, eliminating competing family needs, and needs for information
Family Environment Scale (Moos and Moos, 1988)	Questionnaire (true/false) 90 questions	Families including single parent and step-families	Score indicates each family member's view of their environment; measures the social-environmental characteristics of all types of families; measures family relationships (i.e., support, expression of feelings, and conflict), personal growth of family and family members, and system maintenance (i.e., organization and control of family life)
Early Coping Inventory (Zeitlin et al, 1988)	Systematic observation and 5-pt. rating scale	Infants 4 to 36 months of age	5-point rating scale measures a range of coping effectiveness in the 4- to 36-month-old child. Fifty-four items in three categories: Sensorimotor organization, reactive behavior, self-initiated behavior
Impact on Family Scale (Stein and Reissman, 1980)	Structured interview, 24-item questionnaire	Mother of children with chronic illness (ages of children not specified)	A measure of the variability of impact of chronic illness in a child on the family
Questionnaire on resources and stress for families with a chronically ill or handicapped member (Friedrich et al, 1983; Holroyd, 1974)	Self-administerd 285 item true/false questionnaire	Families with a member who is ill or disabled	Measures stress and coping in families caring for ill relatives and examines events/factors influencing the family; using 15 scales, covers 3 domains; personal problems for respondent; family problems; problems for client and family member
Family Needs Scale (Dunst et al, 1988)	Self-rating scale, 41 times	Families with special-needs children	Provides information regarding family identified needs; also assists families to clarify their concerns and to define the nature of their needs
The McMaster Family Assessment Device (Epstein et al, 1983)	60-item self-report scale	Family members over the age of 12 with family member in medical and psychiatric facilities	Provides a score of healthy versus nonhealthy family functioning; requires 15–20 minutes to complete; based on family function over the past 2 months; Assesses seven dimensions of family functioning: problem solving, communication, roles, affective responsiveness, affective involvement, behavior control, general functioning.
Assessment Area: Environment			
Home Observation for Measurement of the Environment (Bradley and Caldwell, 1984)	Observation and interview allow rater to complete a checklist	Home environment of families with children aged 0–6 (two versions, one for infants to age 3 and one for children aged 3 to 6)	Total and subscale scores describing household environment; measures environmental influences that facilitate or inhibit various behaviors; examines quality and quantity of social, emotional, and cognitive support available to children in the home environment and factors that facilitate or limit play
Checklist of Environmental Factors (Burke and King-Thomas, 1989)	Guided observation checklist	Designed for but not limited to environments of children aged 0–5	Qualitative data about the physical and emotional social aspects of the environment
Environmental Questionnaire (Dunning, 1972)	Semistructured interview	Environment of adult psychiatric outpatients; revision available for mentally retarded adults in the community; also may be useful for families with young children when requiring more information about parents' and caregivers' environmental interactions	Descriptive information about the individual's preferences and the environment; contains questions about the physical, social, and task environments; information yielded may suggest possibilities for modification

sultant and team member, direct-service provider, early identifier, and referral source follows.

Consultant Role and Team Approach

The therapist's role as consultant involves interaction and collaboration with a variety of team members. The success of an early intervention program depends largely on the integration of the child's individual program components into a comprehensive system carried out by a cooperative team of professionals. The emphasis of intervention should be the child within the family unit, school, or community rather than the child alone. Teamwork is critical because of the interrelated nature of the problems of the developing child and the need for skills and resources from many professionals to meet the needs of not only the child but also the family and significant others. This interprofessional collaboration takes on a variety of configurations and can be called by various names. Whether the team is large or small and multidisciplinary, interdisciplinary, or transdisciplinary, the key concepts to a successful team are (Logigian and Ward, 1989):

1. Cooperation and collaboration between members
2. Understanding and respect for others' roles
3. Willingness to share expertise and knowledge
4. Role-release when appropriate
5. Sharing a similar philosophic framework and value system
6. Inclusion and respect for the role of the parents on the team

Darling and Ogg (1984) identified four major requirements for effective interdisciplinary service delivery as listed in Table 15–2. They believed that team effectiveness is dependent on several factors, most critically, the ability of members to interact effectively. Effective interactions include

---

Table 15–2. Requirements for an Effective Team*

Common values supporting the interdisciplinary process
Interpersonal communication skills
Similarity between disciplines
Minimal level of perceived threat between disciplines or individuals

---

*From Darling LA and Ogg HL: Basic requirements for initiating an interdisciplinary process. Phys Ther *64*(11):1684–1686, 1986.

support among team members, shared values, ability to manage conflict in a productive manner, and role clarity. Hemming (1988, p. 16) defined a team as "a group of individuals who must work interdependently in order to attain individual and organizational objectives. True teamwork maximizes performance through the open sharing of talent, cooperative action and goal achievement in the interest of the team's common cause." In terms of a family-centered approach to early intervention, all members of the team work together with the family to establish priorities and collectively make decisions regarding the most effective means to meet the needs of the family. Darling and Ogg (1984) stressed that "an interdisciplinary process of service delivery leads to improvement in the quality of service; to communication between professionals; and ultimately to communication between professionals, patients and their families" (p. 1689). The team approach has been demonstrated to be an effective mechanism for enhancing family competence and developing the strengths of the child (Hanft, 1988 and 1989; Maple, 1987).

As a consultant and team member, therapists must share information with parents and all other staff involved with the child. Consultation tasks for the therapist may include the following:

Suggestions for facilitating adaptive responses while inhibiting abnormal behaviors (most effective when designed as a consistent part of the natural caretaking environment)
Consultation with nurses on techniques for normalizing the amount of sensory stimulation imposed on the child while hospitalized
Demonstration of proper positioning for feeding and activities for oral-motor development for speech therapists
Training in positioning and handling during daily care, bathing, feeding, and play activities for parents
Training in sensory techniques that improve attention, postural stability, visuomotor control, and other academic-related tasks for teachers.

The team needs to work together with the family to determine which areas are of primary importance and which members of the team can be most effective in working with the family to meet these needs.

Referral

Equally important as being skilled in working with teams and families is being skilled at recognizing children and families who may be at risk for developmental, social, and learning delays and making appropriate referrals. Early identification and referral may prevent the need for lifelong rehabilitative services. Therapists may initially see a child for a variety of reasons such as fabricating a splint, addressing a gait abnormality, assessing a developmental delay, or evaluating incoordination and difficulty with hand skills. The therapist must learn to recognize related signs and symptoms that may indicate a more global or potential delay or difficulty. It is the therapist's responsibility to be aware of risk factors that may be indicators of present or future disability and to be aware of appropriate referral sources for families and their child with special needs. Some examples include referral to:

Medical professionals for further assessment
Structured developmental programs for early intervention services
Special education programs for comprehensive, educationally oriented services
Private therapists for direct speech, physical, or occupational therapy

Therapists can also direct families to services that are available through their community or school districts. For example, a boy who is having difficulty in school because of mild incoordination may be referred to the local Young Men's Christian Association for a developmentally appropriate movement or gymnastics program. A child who needs to develop social skill might be referred to a scouting troop. Some useful community services that therapists typically refer to are listed in Table 15–3. Linkages within the community are also an important aspect of family

---

Table 15–3. Potential Community Referrals
Developmental optometry or visual training
Gymboree or preschool movement programs
Adaptive swimming programs
Therapeutic horseback riding
Art and music programs
Specialized camp programs
Scout troops
4H clubs
Church-related groups

---

coping and acceptance (Boukydis, 1987). The interaction of children with special needs children and families with community members helps the families gain support networks, self-esteem, confidence, and a sense of worth and well-being. Community interaction also helps to lessen the bias of nonhandicapped persons, promoting a better understanding, awareness, and attention to persons' capabilities rather than to disabilities.

The role of the therapist is frequently to identify and bridge the gap between the special-needs family and the community. This may be accomplished through modification of the task, individual adaptations, or modification of the environment to ensure success. This may require some of the following therapeutic skills: (1) identification of equipment needs (such as proper seating, flotation devices, splints, or mobility equipment); (2) teaching of specific rehabilitative or compensatory strategies; (3) removal of architectural barriers; or (4) education toward community awareness through teaching and simulation activities.

Therapists can also direct parents to a variety of national and local groups to solicit support and information. These include organizations such as The Association for Children with Learning Disabilities or The Association for Retarded Citizens. Many parents report that a primary need and coping strategy is to obtain information regarding their child's disability and networking with other parents who have undergone similar experiences (Boukydis et al, 1983; Bristol, 1984; Lipsky, 1985; Peterson and Wikoff, 1987; Roberts, 1986). A list of national organizations that provide information and linkages for families and professionals can be found in Hanft (1989) and Hanson and Lynch (1989, Appendix 3). The goal of these organizations is to assist with timely and appropriate referrals, which may prevent further delays and problems with the child and family.

DIRECT INTERVENTION

Direct intervention, which involves the therapist working with the child on a hands-on, individual, and on-going basis, continues to have an important and necessary place in preventive care. If intervention priorities, which require direct intervention, are identified by the family as the primary need of the child, a variety of techniques may be used, some of which are listed in Table 15–4.

Table 15–4. Common Direct-Intervention Techniques
Facilitation of normal movement patterns to promote motor skills
Positioning to encourage movement and independence and to prevent deformity
Handling techniques to facilitate normalization of movement patterns
Splinting or casting to decrease spasticity and prevent contractures
Training in self-care techniques such as feeding and dressing to increase independence
Sensory integration and sensory stimulation techniques to enhance sensory processing and integration of sensory input and facilitate adaptive interactions with the environment

The goal of direct intervention is to enhance the child's ability to interact in the environment in a more adaptive and functional manner, and it should always be in keeping with the family priorities. For example, the major aim of a handling program that facilitates movement patterns for the school-aged child should be to improve the child's ability to function in the classroom more effectively, to encourage more independence in self-care activities, and to facilitate movement patterns that will allow more age-appropriate social and play interactions. Another important consideration of direct intervention is collaboration with other professionals and family to ensure that all team members are in agreement regarding goals and intervention strategies for the child. Finally, when using direct-intervention strategies, it is essential to evaluate constantly the effectiveness of such intervention by monitoring and measuring progress with solid quantitative and qualitative assessment measurements.

FAMILY-CENTERED FRAMEWORK

A framework that addresses the therapists' role as a direct-service provider, consultant, and team member is the family-centered framework for early intervention (Schaaf and Mulrooney, 1989). This framework places the child and family within the context of their environment and presents a systematic method for assessment and intervention. Human (family and caregiver) and nonhuman environmental factors are considered as they influence the child's competence. Assessment of and intervention strategies for three major areas—the child, the family and care-

givers, and the primary environments—are derived from structured observations and interviews in the home and other primary environments. From these data, strategies for enhancing family and child competence are determined.

A major mechanism for assessment and intervention using the family-centered framework is observation and assessment of the family and child during play activities. Play is viewed as the primary occupation of childhood and an arena for the development of competence. Intervention may be focused on the child, the family, the environment, or a combination of these depending on the areas of need determined through assessment. For example, if the play observation, family interview, and other assessment data yield information regarding the inadequacy of the play environment (lack of developmentally appropriate toys and lack of parent-child interactions during play), intervention can be focused on enhancing the play environments to facilitate child development; working with the parents and caregivers in the play situation to encourage more appropriate interactions; and referral to a community play group for the child. The ultimate goal of this framework is to promote optimal competence in families for dealing with, recognizing, and seeking assistance for their child with special needs. The reader is referred to Schaaf and Mulrooney (1989) for a more in-depth description of the family-centered framework.

CASE EXAMPLE: PREVENTIVE CARE IN ACTION*

The following case example* demonstrates how many of the aforementioned principles can be applied to promote competence in the child and family, to decrease the need for lifelong rehabilitative intervention, and to assist a child in realizing his or her fullest potential. It also illustrates utilization of the family in the intervention process because it is the family who ultimately sets the direction and makes the decisions regarding the child's care and services, cares for the child on a daily basis, and works with the community and educational systems, which are designed to service the needs of the child and family. This case illustrates that therapists can work as part-

---

*This case is used with permission of the family. The child's name has been changed, and additional information has been added to illustrate pertinent concepts.

ners with parents in the preventive and rehabilitative process in several different environments and through several different phases of the child's life.

Case Description: David is the first of two children of a middle-class suburban family. He was born after an unremarkable pregnancy and a prolonged and difficult labor and delivery. After several attempts at forceps delivery, fetal bradycardia developed and a cesarean section was performed. Apgar scores were 0 at 1 minute, 0 at 5 minutes, and 2 at 10 minutes. As a result of the forceps-delivery attempts, David sustained a skull fracture on the right side and further complications. His discharge diagnoses were: (1) prenatal asphyxia with shock, respiratory failure, and encephalopathy with seizures; (2) bilateral pneumothoraces; and (3) right-sided depressed skull fracture.

Hospital Environment. David spent 2 weeks in the NICU of the hospital during which he underwent surgery for his right skull fracture and was administered Dilantin for tonic-clonic seizure activity. He demonstrated increased muscle tone and deep tendon reflexes. During his hospital stay, David received nursing, medical, and therapy services. Family-centered care was used by the occupational and physical therapists in the NICU. Specifically, the therapists assisted the family in bonding and feeling comfortable with David by helping them with handling, feeding, and sensory stimulation techniques. David was weaned from a respirator after 3 days and was discharged 2 weeks after delivery. He had made significant improvements in responsiveness, and seizures had ceased; therefore, Dilantin was discontinued.

Posthospital Period. At 1 month of age, David was referred to the local United Cerebral Palsy Association for evaluation. A neurologic examination indicated low muscle tone in the trunk area, increased flexor tone in the left upper extremity, and increased muscle tone in the lower extremities. Speech and social development were reported as age appropriate. Private physical and occupational therapy in the home was recommended to address his sensory-motor delays.

Home Environment. The therapists worked collaboratively with the parents in the home to help make the daily care and interactions with David a positive and enjoyable experience. The therapists also worked with the family to integrate stimulation activities into daily care and play times. For example, techniques for carrying and transporting David were demonstrated. These served to decrease atypical muscle tone and posturing. Other activity suggestions included developmentally appropriate toys hanging over the changing table, stimulation and play activities during bath time, and the use of a mirror in the crib. The therapists also served as support and resource persons for the family by providing them with needed information regarding David's development. The therapists took their cues from the parents and shaped intervention around their needs.

Early Intervention Program. During the next few months, David's mother expressed a need for a more global program for him. The therapists encouraged the family to explore early intervention programs in their local area and provided them with a list of local centers. David was evaluated and placed in an early intervention program by 8 months of age. The early intervention program was able to address several areas of need for David and his family. It provided a well-rounded developmental program including educational programming, speech, and occupational and physical therapy, which addressed David's motor, social, and self-help delays and facilitated his cognitive development. The program also served as a support system for the family by providing them with information, support groups, and referral sources that addressed their family needs.

David remained in the early intervention program until 3 years of age. The early intervention team, which included David's parents, felt that at this point David's needs could best be met in a nonspecialized nursery school program with supplemental support services.

Nursery School Period. David was enrolled in a private nursery school, which also offered a developmental movement program. Occupational and physical therapy services were delivered privately, and the therapists collaborated often to ensure coordinated care. During this time, the focus of physical therapy was on developing balance and gross motor coordination and refining movement patterns. Occupational therapy concentrated on body awareness, postural stability, and fine motor skills as necessary prerequisites for independence in self-care, preacademic and classroom activities, and play activities. Home and school visits by the therapists were used to make suggestions and adaptations to increase David's independence and success. For example, David's swing set was adapted with a wider seat, thus enabling David to become more independent in outdoor activities. His tricycle was adapted with foot blocks, which enabled David to reach the pedals and propel the tricycle independently. Zipper pulls were added to his jacket and pants to enhance independence in dressing. Chunky crayons and loop scissors were suggested to increase independence in the classroom. Over the next 2 years (from age 3 to

5), David continued to make steady gains in self-care, socialization, and motor skills.

Kindergarten. At 5 years of age, David was accepted into a public school kindergarten program. He continued to receive private occupational therapy services, which assisted him in refining his fine visual motor and self-help skills. These skills are necessary for optimal functioning in kindergarten and to prepare him for first grade. The physical therapist recommended a therapeutic horseback-riding program in lieu of private physical therapy. This program continued to address his mild balance and coordination difficulties. During this year, David became independent in all his self-care skills and was able to keep pace with his peers in pencil and paper and other academic and social activities. He was able to play and interact with the other children in an age-appropriate manner and developed several healthy peer relationships. He seemed to feel competent in his environment, and the family was pleased with David's school placement and academic and social progress.

Happy Ending. David entered first grade at 6 years of age. He presently receives no supportive services and functions quite competently in his classroom. His parents continue to monitor his progress and to seek support services on a consultative basis. The family has since had another child who is developing quite typically. They appear to be a well-adapted, typical family who has quite competently managed the challenges of raising a child with special needs.

Summary. This case illustrates early intervention and family-centered care as preventive health care. To summarize, the occupational and physical therapist worked with the child and his family using a preventive, collaborative approach in the following capacities:

In the hospital NICU as a consultant and support person to parents and nurses regarding positioning, handling, feeding, and appropriate stimulation levels

In a center-based program as part of the early intervention team, which stimulated the child's development and worked with his parents

On a private, on-going basis during the nursery and kindergarten-age period to prepare the child for success in the social and academic challenges of first grade

As a resource and support person for the family after discharge from direct-therapy services

References

Abidin RR: Parenting stress index, 2nd ed. Charlottesville, VA, Pediatric Psychology Press, 1986.

American Occupational Therapy Association: Guidelines for Occupational Therapy Services in School Systems, 2nd ed. Rockville, MD, American Occupational Therapy Association, 1989b.

Bailey D: Collaborative goal-setting with families: Resolving differences in values and priorities for services. Top Early Childhood Spec Ed 7(2):59–71, 1987.

Bailey D, Dunst C, Kramer S, et al: Identifying child and family strengths and needs. *In* Hanft B (ed): Family-Centered Care: An Early Intervention Resource Manual. Rockville, MD, American Occupational Therapy Association, 1989.

Bailey DB and Worley M: Assessing Infants and Preschoolers with Handicaps. Columbus, OH, Merrill, 1988.

Bayley N: Manual for the Bayley Scales of Infant Development. New York, Psychological Corp., 1969.

Bishop B: Neural plasticity in the developing nervous system. Phys Ther 62(8):1122–1131, 1982.

Bishop B: Neural plasticity: Post maturational and functionally induced plasticity. Phys Ther 62(8):1132–1143, 1982.

Bledsoe NP and Shephard JT: A study of reliability and validity of a preschool play scale. Am J Occup Ther 36:783–794, 1982.

Boukydis Z: Research on Support for Parents and Infants in the Prenatal Period. Noorwood, NJ, Albex, 1987.

Boyer CB (ed): Occupational therapy in the schools (special issue). Am J Occup Ther 42(11), 1988.

Bradley BM and Caldwell RH: Home Observation for Measurement of the Environment. Seattle, University of Washington, School of Nursing, 1984.

Brazelton TB: Neonatal behavioral assessment scale, 2nd ed. Clinics in developmental medicine, No. 50. Philadelphia, JB Lippincott, 1984.

Bristol MM: Family resources and successful adaptation to autistic children. *In* Schoper PL and Mesibor G (eds): The Effects of Autism on the Family. New York, Penton Press, 1984.

Bruininks RH: Bruininks-Oseretsky Test of Motor Proficiency. Circle Pines, MN, American Guidance Service, 1978.

Burke JP and King-Thomas L: Checklist of Environmental Factors, AOTA Practice Symposium. Rockville, MD, American Occupational Therapy Association, 1989.

Cotman C and Nieto-Stampedro X: Brain function, synapse renewal and plasticity. Annu Rev Psychol 33:371–401, 1982.

Darling LA and Ogg HL: Basic requirements for initiating an interdisciplinary process. Phys Ther 64(11):1684–1686, 1984.

Darling R: Parent Needs Survey. *In* Seligman M and Darling R: Ordinary families, special children: A systems approach to childhood disability. New York, NY, Guilford Press, 1989.

Dunn W: Occupational therapy in early intervention (special issue). Am J Occup Ther 43(11), 1989.

DeGangi G and Berk R: DeGangi-Berk Test of Sensory Integration. Los Angeles, CA, Western Psychological Services, 1983.

Dubowitz L and Dubowitz V: The neurological assessment of the preterm and fullterm newborn infant. Clinics in developmental medicine, No. 79. Philadelphia, JB Lippincott, 1981.

Dunning HD: Environmental occupational therapy. Am J Occup Ther 26, 292–298, 1972.

Dunst C, Carol T, and Deal A: A family system assessment and intervention model. *In* Dunst C, Trivette C, and Deal A (eds): Enabling and Empowering Families. Cambridge, MA, Brookline Books, 1988a.

Dunst C, Trivette C, and Deal A: Enabling and Empowering

Families: Principles and Guidelines for Practice. Tucson, AZ, Therapy Skill Builders, 1988b.

Dunst CJ, Cooper CJ, Weeldreyer JC, Snyder KD, and Chase JH: Family Needs Scale. *In* Dunst CJ, Trivette CM, and Deal AG (eds): Enabling and empowering families: Principles and guidelines for practice. Cambridge, MA, Brookline Books, 1988, p. 151.

Epstein NB, Baldwin LM, and Bishop DS: The McMaster family assessment device. J Marital and Family Therapy 9:174–180, 1983.

Foley GM: Three Frames of Reference for Family Service with a Guide to Developing Individual Family Service Plans. Reading, PA, Albright College Psychological Services Center, 1987.

Folio MR and Fewell RR: Peabody Developmental Motor Scales and Activity Cards. Allen, TX, DLM Teaching Resources, 1983.

Friedrich WN, Greenberg MT, and Crnic K: A short form of the questionnaire on resources and stress. Am J Ment Deficiency 88, 41–48, 1983.

Furuno S, O'Rielly A, Hosaka C, et al: The Hawaii Early Learning Profile. Palo Alto, CA, VORT, 1979.

Gallagher JJ, Beckman P, and Cross AH: Families of handicapped children: Sources of stress and its amelioration. Except Child 50(1):10–19, 1983.

Haines J, Ames LB, and Gillespie C: The Gessell Preschool Test Manual. Lumberville, PA, Modern Learning Press, 1980.

Hanft B: The changing environment of early intervention services: Implications for practice. Am J Occup Ther 42(11):26–33, 1988.

Hanft B: Family Centered Care: An Early Intervention Resource Manual. Rockville, MD, American Occupational Therapy Association, 1989.

Hanson M and Lynch E: Early Intervention: Implementing Child and Family Services for Infants and Toddlers Who Are At Risk or Disabled. Austin, TX, Pro-Ed, 1989.

Hemming D: The titanic triumvirate: Teams, teamwork and teambuilding. Can J Occup Ther 55(1):15–20, 1988.

Hinojosa J and Anderson J: Working relationships between therapist and parents of children with cerebral palsy: A survey of Attitudes. Occup Ther J Res 7(2):123–125, 1987.

Hinojosa J, Anderson J, and Ranum G: Relationship between therapists and parents of preschool children with cerebral palsy: A survey. Occup Ther J Res 8(5):285–298, 1988.

Holroyd J: The questionnaire on resources and stress: An instrument to measure family response to a handicapped member. J Community Psychol 2:92–94, 1974.

Hulme I and Lunzer E: Play, language, and reasoning in subnormal children. J Child Psychol 7:107–123, 1966.

Kalverboer AF: Measurement of play: Clinical applicants. *In* Tizard B and Harvey D (eds): Biology of Play, p. 100–122. Philadelphia, JB Lippincott, 1977.

Knox SH: A play scale. *In* Reilly M (ed): Play as Exploratory Learning: Studies of Curiosity Behavior. Beverly Hills, CA, Sage Publications, 1974, pp 247–266

Kochnek T and Friedman D: Incorporating Family Assessment and Individualized Family Service Plans into Early Intervention Programs: A Developmental Decision Making Process. Rhode Island College Press, 1988.

Lieberman J: Playfulness: Its relationship to imagination and creativity. New York, Academic Press, 1977.

Lipsky DK: A parental perspective on stress and coping. Am J Orthopsychiatry 55:614–617, 1985.

Logigian MK and Ward JD: Pediatric Rehabilitation: A Team Approach for Therapists. Boston, Little, Brown, 1989.

Lund RD: Development and Plasticity of the Brain: An Introduction. New York, Oxford University Press, 1978.

Maple G: Early intervention: Some issues in co-operative teamwork. Aust Occup Ther J 34(4):145–151, 1987.

Miller LJ: Miller Assessment for Preschoolers. Littleton, CO, The Foundation for Knowledge in Development, 1982.

Mitchell RG: Objectives and outcomes of prenatal care. Lancet 2(8461):931–934, 1985.

Moos RH and Moss BS: Family Environment Scale Manual. Palo Alto, CA, Consulting Psychologists Press, 1988.

Mullen E: Mullen Scales of Early Learning. Cranston, RI, T.O.T.A.L. Child, Inc., 1988.

Parten M: Social play among preschool children. J Abnorm Social Psychol 28:136–147, 1933.

Peterson P and Wikoff RL: Home environment and adjustment in families with handicapped children: A canonical correlation study. Occup Ther J Res 7(2):67–82, 1987.

Pierce D (ed): Occupational therapy and the family, Parts 1 and 2 (special issues). Developmental Disabilities Special Interest Section Newsletter 12(1,2).

Pratt PN and Allen C: Occupational Therapy for Children. Baltimore, CV Mosby, 1989.

Prectl Heinz FR: Neurological Examination of the Full-term Newborn Infant. London, Spastics International Medical Pub; Philadelphia, JB Lippincott, 1977.

Reynolds L, Egan R, and Lerner J: Efficacy of early intervention on preacademic deficits: A review of literature. Top Early Childhood Special Education 3(3):47–55, 1983.

Roberts M: Three mothers: Life-span experiences. *In* Fewell R and Vadasy P (eds): Families of Handicapped Children: Needs and Supports Across the Life Span. Austin, TX, Pro-ED, 1986.

Rogers SJ, Donovan CM, D'Eugenio DB, et al: Early Intervention Developmental Profile. Ann Arbor, The University of Michigan Press, 1981.

Schaaf R and Gitlin L: Early intervention: New directions for occupational therapists. Occup Ther Health Care 6(2/3):75–89, 1989.

Schaaf R and Mulrooney L: Occupational therapy in early intervention: A family-centered approach. Am J Occup Ther 43(1):745–754, 1989.

Shaaf R, Merrill S, and Kinsella N: Parent/Teacher Play Questionnaire. Occupational Therapy in Health Care 4(2):61–75, 1987.

Simmer M: The warning signs of school failure: An updated profile of the at-risk kindergarten child. Top Early Child Special Education 3(3):17–28, 1983.

Stein REK and Reissman CK: The development of an impact-on-family scale: Preliminary findings. Med Care 18, 465–472, 1980.

Takata N: The play history. Am J Occup Ther 23, 314–318, 1969.

Weiner R and Koppelman J: Birth to 5: Serving the Youngest Handicapped Children. Alexandria, VA, Capital Publications, 1987.

Zeitlin S, Williamson GG, and Szczepanski M: Early coping inventory. Bensonville, IL, Scholastic Testing Service, 1988.

VULNERABILITY AND RISK FACTORS

Ayres AJ: Sensory Integration and Learning Disorders. Los Angeles, Western Psychological Services, 1972.

Bates JE: The concept of difficult temperament. Merrill-Palmer Q 26:299–319, 1980.

Bauchner H, Brown E, and Peskin J: Premature graduates of the newborn intensive care unit: A guide to follow-up. Pediatr Clin North Am 35(6):1207–1226, 1988.

Brazelton TB, Koslowski B, and Main M: The origins of reciprocity. *In* Lewis ML and Rosenblum LA (eds): The Effects of the Infant on Its Caregiver. New York, Wiley, 1974.

Brown CC (ed): Childhood Learning Disabilities and Prenatal Risk. Skillman, NJ, Johnson and Johnson Baby Products Co, 1983.

Chasnoff IJ, Griffith DR, MacGregor S, et al: Temporal patterns of cocaine use in pregnancy: Prenatal outcome. JAMA *261*(12):1741–1744, 1989.

Clark-Stewart KA: Interactions between mothers and their young children: Characteristics and consequences. Monogr Soc Res Child Dev *38*(6–7, serial no. 153, 1–109, 1983.

Destefano-Lewis K, Bennet B, and Schmeder NH: The care of infants menaced by cocaine abuse. Am J Matern Child Nurse *14*:324–329, 1989.

Elardo R, Bradley R, and Caldwell BM: A longitudinal study of the relation of infants' home environments to language development at age three. Child Dev *48*:595–603, 1977.

Enshner G and Clark D: Newborns at Risk. Rockville, MD, Aspen, 1986.

Fewell RR, Garwood SG, More AA, et al: (eds): Children at risk for academic failure. Top Early Childhood Special Ed *3*(3):7–16, 1983.

Field T: Interactions of high risk infants: Quantitative and qualitative differences. *In* Sawin D, Hawkins DF, Walker I, and Penticuff J (eds): Current Perspectives on Psychological Risks During Pregnancy and Early Infancy. New York, Brunner/Mazel, 1980.

Fish B and Dixon WJ: Vestibular hyperactive in infants at risk for schizophrenias. Arch Gen Psychiatry *35*:963–971, 1978.

Greenspan SI and Porges SW: Psychopathology in infancy and early childhood: Clinical perspective on the organization of sensory and effective-thermatic experiences. Child Dev *55*:49–70, 1984.

Hadeed AJ and Seigel SR: Maternal cocaine use during pregnancy: Effects on the newborn infant. Pediatrics *84*(2):205–210, 1989.

Hobel CJ: Factors before pregnancy that influence brain development. *In* Prenatal and Prenatal Factors Associated with Brain Disorders (U.S. Dept. of HHS, NIH pub. no. #85–1149). Washington, DC, U.S. Government Printing Office, 1985.

Hume RF, O'Donnell KJ, Stanger CL, et al: *In* utero cocaine exposure: Observations of fetal behavioral state may predict neonatal outcome. Am J Obstet Gynecol *161*(3):685–690, 1989.

Hutchins V, Placek P, and Walker A: Trend on Maternal and Infant Health Factors Associated with Low Infant Birth Weight. United States 1972 and 1980. Paper presented to the Institute of Medicine, October 17, 1983.

Klaus MH, Leger T, and Trause MA (eds): Maternal Attachment and Mothering Disorders: A Round Table. Skillman, NJ, Johnson and Johnson Baby Product Co., 1982.

Pasamanick B and Knobloch H: Brain damage and reproductive casualty. Am J Orthopsychiatry *3*:298–305, 1960.

Price A and Techman J: Otitis media, allergy and vestibular function. Center for the Study of Sensory Integrative Dysfunction News Letter *VI*(1):1–2, 1979.

Schaaf RC: The frequency of vestibular disorders in developmentally delayed preschoolers with otitis media. Am J Occup Ther *39*(1):247–252, 1985.

Schneider JW, Griffith DR, and Chasnoff IJ: Infants exposed to cocaine in utero: Implications for developmental assessment and intervention. Infants Young Children *2*(1):25–36, 1989.

Sell EJ, Gaines JA, Gluckman C, et al: Early identification of learning problems in neonatal intensive care graduates. Am J Dis Child *139*(5):460–463, 1985.

Semmler CJ (ed): A Guide to Care and Management of Very Low Birth Weight Infants: A Team Approach. Tucson, AZ, Therapy Skill Builders, 1989.

Thomas A and Chess S: The role of temperament in the contributions of individuals to development. *In* Lerner RM and Busch-Rossnagel NA (eds): Individuals as Products of Their Development: A Life-Span Perspective. New York, Academic Press, 1981.

CHAPTER

16

Kieron Sheehy

Preventing Disabilities in Children: Active Intervention in the Developmental Process

This chapter considers two innovative approaches to early intervention that have been highly influential in the United Kingdom during the last 5 years. Both methods originate outside the United Kingdom and have arisen from completely different historic and theoretic backgrounds. These methods are concerned with prevention of disability through active intervention in children's developmental process. The Portage approach to early education originated in the United States and is based firmly in the Western behaviorist tradition. It is a home-based service using parents as teachers. Conductive education developed in Hungary. Its theoretic basis, although independent, has a strong relation to the Russian school, particularly to the work of Vygotsky. It is performed primarily in a residential setting and is highly intensive. The Portage approach is considered for children with developmental delay in almost any area of their functioning. By contrast, conductive education is for a selected group of children with motor disorders.

PORTAGE APPROACH

Brief History

The Portage guide to early education (Shearer and Shearer, 1972) is an early intervention program designed to ameliorate or prevent developmental handicaps. The Portage approach originated in Wisconsin in 1969 and developed into a home-based teaching program involving weekly home visits to provide a quality service over a vast geographic and mainly rural area in southwest Wisconsin. Teaching is performed by parents with support from the Portage service workers. This approach aims to teach children the appropriate skills in the developmental repertoire.

In England the Wessex Health Care Evaluation Research Team based in Winchester, Hampshire, became interested in this approach and, after a training workshop run by the Wisconsin project, two Portage projects were initiated: the Wessex Portage Research Project (Smith et al, 1977) and a sister project in Cardiff, South Wales (Revill and Blunden, 1979). Cameron (1988) described the rapid expansion of services following this. Today there are more than 300 Portage services in the United Kingdom.

In 1985, the National Portage Association was established. This body has regulated the development of the Portage approach and its materials in England. In 1985, the Department of Education and Science began awarding a government grant (initially £1.2 million [approximately $2.1 million dollars]) to fund new Portage services (Sturmey and Crisp, 1986). This grant enabled local authorities to appoint staff to act as home visitors. New United Kingdom Portage materials were published in 1987. The Portage approach trains parents to teach their children behaviors that are appropriate developmentally through precision teaching. It can be described through the component parts, which combine to form a Portage service.

Client Group

The criteria for selection into the program are varied and differ among various services. Originally, any child with a significant developmental delay in any sphere of functioning was considered.

The South Glamorgan service narrowed the entry criteria to children who were younger than 4.5 years old, who attended nursery school fewer than 2.5 days per week, and who scored less than 78 on two or more subscales of the Griffiths Mental Development Scale (Griffiths, 1954). The Griffiths Mental Development Scale assesses young children on subscales: personal/social, hearing and speech, hand development, eye development, and performance. The test yields quotients for each subscale and a general quotient from the whole test (Bidder et al, 1982). Although this gives an indication of the children involved, it does not reflect practice in the United Kingdom today. Generally the practice is to focus on children with a recognized handicapping condition, such as Down's syndrome, and who have a delay of 1 year or more in at least two Portage checklist areas. However, this varies among services across the United Kingdom. It has been estimated that generally 15 to 19 children per 100,000 are eligible for the Portage approach (Revill and Blunden, 1980).

Service Structure

Personnel

Schemes are staffed in a variety of ways but are in essence multidisciplinary. Home visitors can be occupational therapists, physical therapists, psychologists, teachers, and other professionals (Lloyd, 1986).

The home visitor performs an initial develop-

mental assessment using the Portage Developmental Checklist. This allows assessment of levels of function and selection of teaching goals. The Portage model is based on the sequence of normal development. Goals, both long and short term, are derived from this. In line with Shearer and Shearer's original work (1972), goals are selected that the child will achieve within 1 week. The home visitor takes and records a baseline measurement. It is then the parents' role to teach the new skill. The service model is illustrated in Figure 16–1. Clients are visited at home by home teachers; home teachers have meetings with a supervisor; and the whole scheme is overseen by a management team.

The checklists cover early development from birth to 6 years in five areas: socialization, language, self-help, cognition, and motor skills (Shearer and Shearer, 1972). In addition, an Infant Stimulation Checklist describing neonatal and early infant behaviors has subsequently been developed.

Weekly Teaching Activities

The core of the Portage approach is the weekly teaching activities. A precision teaching model is used. Generally three behaviors are chosen so that the child (and then the parents) will achieve success within a defined period of time. Baseline data are recorded by the home visitor on each new task. After 1 week, post-teaching data are recorded to assess the effectiveness of the learning program.

During the week, the parents implement the teaching process, which includes rewarding desired behaviors and reducing inappropriate ones. This teaching is recorded and described by an activity chart.

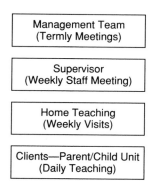

Figure 16–1. The Portage service model.

Activity Charts

Each chart includes a teaching target, criterion of success, materials, setting, presentation, reward, correction and prompting, and recording. The teaching target identifies the behavior to be taught within 1 week. The target might be "Jane will turn her head in the direction of sound" or "Simon picks up red toy on request." The context and interaction are specified in the rest of the chart. The criterion of success is the level of performance that is expected at the end of 1 week. For example, a criterion of success may be that the target behavior is produced "on 3 of 4 successive trials." The materials are the specific items used in the teaching session. For example, a particular toy may be used in teaching visual tracking, or the utensils necessary for developing feeding skills may be used.

The setting is the place where the teaching is to occur, such as the bathroom or the kitchen. This may be important in developing generalization of acquired skills between environments. Presentation describes how the teachers (parents) present the task. Their actions are described in clear behavioral terms. This allows fine-tuning of the teaching process to make it more effective.

A child's success is rewarded immediately. The type of reward used depends on each child. Guidance is given on selecting appropriate rewards for each individual. In the correction and prompting component, if children do not attain the selected behavior on a teaching trial they are helped to succeed. This correction procedure usually involves the minimum prompting necessary for children to complete the task and the graded use of verbal, gestural, and physical prompts. Thus, a verbal reminder may be used, or the child may require physical guidance. In the recording component, usually charts use a tick to show success and a 0 if a prompt is used. Sometimes other symbols are used to record the nature of any prompts used. Thus, it can be seen if a child has progressed from physical to verbal prompts.

On average, 30 minutes per day is needed for teaching activities. However, new or developing skills may be practiced throughout the day (White and Cameron, 1988).

Parent Support

Because of the diversity of possible goals, parent training and support are critical for the success of the intervention. Training usually occurs in the home environment through modeling. A parent behavior instrument monitors parent skills, but, in my experience, this is rarely used.

Parents are helped to remain effective through the actual process of planning weekly goals and designing activity charts. Bidder and colleagues (1982) found that parents rated activity charts as preferable to other methods.

Each developmental behavior from the checklist corresponds to a card contained in a box. This card contains "what to do" information and useful hints to help a child achieve that particular behavior. Thus, parents have ready access to appropriate information throughout the week.

Sturmey and Crisp (1986) reviewed the effectiveness of parent training and concluded that a wide range of strategies had evolved in this area other than teaching specific skills and that this variety enables the needs of parents (and therefore children) to be met more effectively.

Funding

In the United Kingdom, funding for Portage services has come from a variety of sources. The largest single source of support from professionals who are "seconded" (i.e., the professional is released to pursue study or develop skills while still being paid by his or her employer) from their roles within an education or health authority setting. Bendall and colleagues (1984a) examined funding for Portage services (Fig. 16–2). No special funding usually occurs when a professional is seconded on a part-time basis from their normal duties. Special funding is usually in the form of a grant from local or central government. Voluntary agencies refers to national charities such as the Church of England Children's Society. Bendall and colleagues noted a strong correlation between services with a management team and those attracting long-term funding.

CONDUCTIVE EDUCATION

Brief History

This approach was developed in Budapest, Hungary, by Dr. Andreas Peto over 40 years ago and is continued today by Maria Hari. Peto published little about his method; thus, it has been through Hari and others that the system has been described and evaluated. Conductive education aims to establish orthofunction in children and

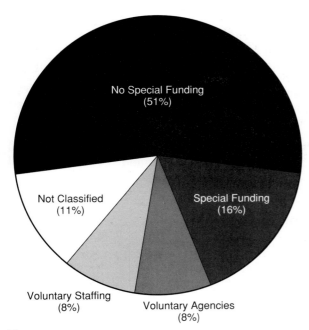

Figure 16–2. Funding for Portage services in the United Kingdom, as described by Bendall.

No Special Funding (51%)

Not Classified (11%)

Special Funding (16%)

Voluntary Staffing (8%)

Voluntary Agencies (8%)

adults with motor disorders. Orthofunction is achieved not by curing the underlying condition but by being able to live independently of artificial aids such as wheelchairs and ramps (Foundation for Conductive Education, 1990). Historically, this idea evolved because children in Hungary cannot attend mainstream schools if they are unable to walk.

In 1968 British physiotherapist Ester Cotton visited Budapest and the National Motor Therapy Institute, as it was then known, to see Peto's method first-hand. (In 1985 the institute was renamed the Andreas Peto Institute of Motor Disorder). On returning to England, Cotton began to introduce elements of the system into schools run by the Spastics Society for People with Cerebral Palsy. However, conductive education has developed a high profile within the United Kingdom only during the last 5 years. In 1986 the Foundation for Conductive Education was established as a national charity to introduce conductive education to England. In 1987 the foundation established the Birmingham Institute for Conductive Education. This occurred through close collaboration with the Peto Institute and was the first attempt to replicate the approach within the United Kingdom.

In 1990 the British government announced the provision of £5 million to support a new International Peto Institute over a 4-year period and allow training of British nationals in Hungary (Spastics Society for People with Cerebral Palsy, 1990).

At present, many physiotherapists and occupational therapists have incorporated elements of the approach in their work, often with other techniques such as those devised by Bobath and Bobath (1984).

Conductive Education and Bobath Approaches

Both approaches emphasize early treatment to prevent the establishment of abnormal patterns of behavior. However, there appear to be significant differences. Bobath considered that a child with cerebral palsy has both abnormal postural tone and abnormal postural activity. In addition, the child's range of selective movement patterns is limited by the persistence of infantile reflexive patterns (Sharpe Banus, 1979). Conductive education is based on Peto's belief that cerebral palsy is an impairment of the total function of the brain, which prevents the child from learning from the environment. Thus, conductive education takes an educational viewpoint. In contrast, the Bobath approach may be viewed as neurologic in nature. The Bobath procedure aims to modify abnormal postural tone by moving the child through sequences of movement that make up the motor skills used for antigravity mobility and functional purposes (Hong, 1985). Conductive education does contain a basic motor pattern, but its emphasis is more concerned with the child's conscious and nonautomatic levels of movement. It aims to unite language, function, and movement (Levitt, 1986) and to form a relationship between the body and the cortex and give opportunities to reinforce this learning.

Client Group

Children with cerebral palsy and spina bifida (and also adults with Parkinson's disease and post-traumatic hemiplegia) have entered Peto training. Because conductive education views the situation as an educational one where control problems (of the nervous system) require teaching (Sutton, 1987), it follows that intellectual potential is a better indicator of long-term progress rather than the degree of motor impairment. However, Cotton and Parnwell (1967) noted that the ability to participate is more important than an intelligence test score. Typically, the majority of children treated have intelligence quotients greater than 70. Robinson and colleagues (1989) studied the Peto Institute's assessment and selection procedure. They noted that children were not accepted if they had any of the following:

Learning difficulties making the pupil unresponsive to conductor requests
Impairment of vision or hearing
Poorly controlled epilepsy
Progressive disorders
Biochemical disorders
Major orthopedic problems

MacDonald (1990) described children with spina bifida who attended a kindergarten group at 3 years of age and later entered school groups. She noted the institute's aims to teach these children as follows:

1. Develop existing movement and coordination
2. Compensate for disability but not be permanently dependent on external equipment
3. Compensate for sensory loss through visual awareness
4. Protect themselves from temperature extremes
5. Develop meticulous hygiene

For children with cerebral palsy, referral to the institute as early as possible is recommended. Those with hypotonia have the goal of active fixation of any position. Where athetosis is concerned, controlled, rhythmic voluntary movement is the goal. Spasticity presents a greater challenge. A normal posture is achieved through relaxing, attempting a posture, modifying it, and then holding it (MacDonald, 1990). Conductive education can best be described through the components that contribute to the approach as a whole.

The Conductor

The conductor is the central conductive education professional (Spastics Society for People with Cerebral Palsy, 1990). It is the conductor's role to meet all the child's needs at any one time.

Most conductors are women who have undertaken 4 years of training at the Peto Institute.

Two of these years are in conjunction with a teacher-training college. The remaining time is allocated between theoretic work on basic medical sciences, principles of physiotherapy and speech therapy, and working alongside a trained conductor (Robinson et al, 1989). Thus, the conductor combines roles that are linked traditionally to other professions, is responsible for all aspects of pupil welfare, and teaches across all curriculum areas.

The Group

The teaching group "Czoport" consists of between 10 and 20 children (Cotton and Parnwell, 1967). It is seen as a pedogogic tool, a therapeutic force rather than a unit to be taught. A group of children may exhibit mixed physical abilities but similar developmental levels. In Hungary, children with spina bifida and paraplegia are taught in their own groups. The conductor educates the child through daily activities in a group situation. At the beginning of the group's work, the conductor must set a lively pleasant tone, and this tone should be maintained throughout the session (Hari, 1988). The ability to motivate a group and use its dynamics is vital.

Rhythmic Intention

Conductive education is in harmony with the neurophysiologic research of Pavlov and on the findings of Luria (1961) and Vygotsky (1978). This work discusses the relationship between speech and active movement. Vygotsky proposed that communication with the self is important for self-guidance and self-direction.

Tasks with a child's "zone of proximal development" (Vygotsky, 1962) are too difficult for the child to carry out alone but can be accomplished with the verbal guidance and assistance of adults. Children take this language (verbal instruction) and internalize it. This develops and becomes part of their own private speech. They use this speech to organize independent efforts in the same way (Berk, 1986). Speech acts as a conditioning stimulus.

Rhythmic intention enables the child to perform unaided active normal movements. The initial exercises that are used in conductive education are guided by the child's speech or efforts to speak. Training is intense and repetitive. The therapist "conducts" a group, encouraging them to verbalize their activities as they move through them (Cotton and Kinsman, 1983).

The needs of each member of the group are analyzed by the conductor, and required exercise movements are reduced to common component parts. The conductor puts each intended movement into words, and the children repeat it and perform the movement to a count of one. A count of five follows (with accompanying movement), and the movement is consolidated. This sequence is repeated until the total movement required is performed. Thus, the group repeats the intention and is led rhythmically into the activity by speech. The rhythm used is appropriate to the group, and song as well as counting is used. Wilson (1970) described a session at the Peto Institute and conveyed the mood of the approach very well.

That a child with a brain lesion learns by active sensorimotor experiences and that repetition is needed is well established (Kong, 1987). Rhythmic intention goes beyond this, emphasizing the power of intention. Hari (1988) wrote:

Conductive education seeks to change intention rather than performance. Intention is an activity special to the human being. It is a powerful initiative, a decision to act. It is an internal rhythmic harmony. It can be more or less concrete and becomes abstract when the function becomes automatic (p. 3).

Programs

Programs depend on the skills of each group but aim to achieve a number of functional skills within a set period of time. Goals are set and worked toward through smaller steps. Functional skills are broken down into component movements, and these are placed within activities throughout the daily timetable.

Overall programs develop from general training to specialization. The intensive use of rhythmic intention establishes new motor patterns of symmetry and selective independent movements. These form the building blocks of later specialized movements involved in the activities of daily living. This progression is common to the occupational therapy process in England. Cotton (1983) described a prewriting program that includes not only exercises but also

games, songs, and poems. The general prerequisite skills include:

Ability to sit on an armless chair
Independent head movement
Symmetric position
Independent hand movement

As the prerequisite skills develop, students progress to horizontal activities on a plinth. The goals used here might include:

"I join my hands together" to help achieve symmetry, balance, and group in the functional position.
"I stretch my elbows," an exercise for increased control in the holding position against gravity.

One complete activity may take months to complete correctly (Cotton, 1983). Programs follow a basic motor pattern developed by Peto. For children with spina bifida, toilet training is performed through daily conditioning using deep abdominal breathing, trunk flexion, and extension. Even in this, rhythmic intention and group motivation play an integral part.

Daily Routine

By British standards, residents' days are long. In the Peto Institute, the schedule may be from 6:30 A.M. to 8:30 P.M. (Kerslake, 1970). Children are ready to begin 2 hours of gross motor programs by 9:00 A.M. The daily agenda also includes academic and social activities. Walking is emphasized throughout the day (MacDonald 1990). Although the residential aspect of conductive education has been highlighted in England, the Hungarian Institute does run nonresidential groups (between 8:30 A.M. and 4:30 P.M.). Hari (1988) wrote on conductive education for children's and toddler's day groups, which work every other day for 1.5 to 2 hours. In these programs, the parents are taught how to manage short tasks designed to activate the child at home, typically during feeding and dressing.

Equipment

The room is sparse with equipment, and toys not in use are stored away. In Budapest, rooms are light and airy but warm (Cotton and Parnwell, 1967). Visual aids are produced at appropriate times but are never used solely for decoration. A recognized feature in many special schools in England, slatted plinths are used as tables and supports when moving around or to exercise or lie upon.

The ladderback chair is wooden with a flat seat and is used for a variety of exercises. Other equipment includes wooden boxes and ladders (Fig. 16–3).

In developing conductive education in the United Kingdom, the Birmingham Institute is attempting to replicate the Peto methods and results. Conductors are now being trained in the United Kingdom under the supervision of the Peto representatives.

Physiotherapists (physical therapists) and occupational therapists working in the National Health Service are including elements of the approach in their work.

The Spastics Society for People with Cerebral Palsy runs two schools along lines inspired by the Peto approach. They employ a multidisciplinary team including occupational therapists and physiotherapists rather than conductors.

Many special schools are developing their own programs drawing on conductive education but with a multidisciplinary approach. Usually this occurs on a sessional basis. An interesting development is the small number of schools for children with learning difficulties who are using rhythmic intention as a group approach to their work. This client group would typically be excluded from standard Peto teaching. No studies have yet examined the effectiveness of this.

Examining conductive education in Britain, Cottam and Sutton (1986) identified four common features among the variety of programs being run:

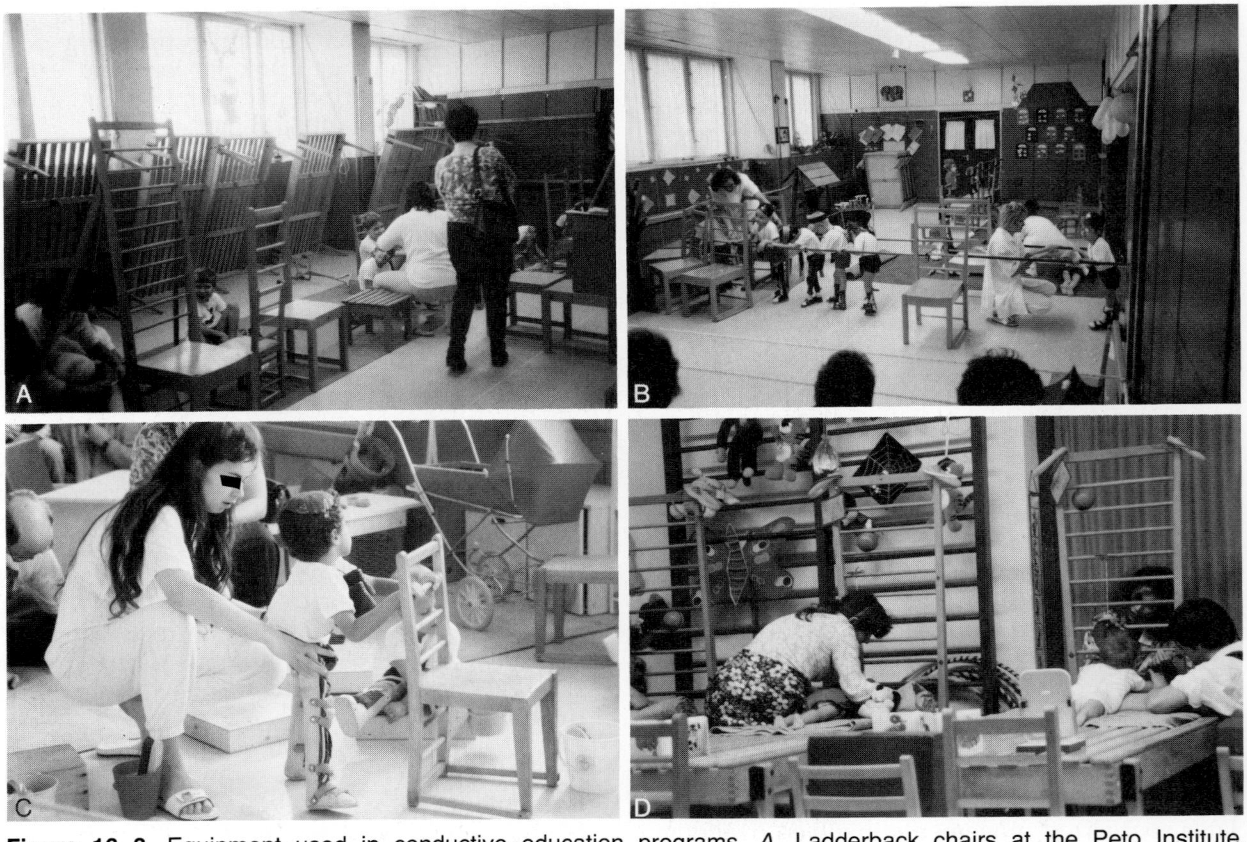

Figure 16–3. Equipment used in conductive education programs. *A,* Ladderback chairs at the Peto Institute, Budapest. *B,* Group of children working together at the Peto Institute. *C,* Ladderback chair being used as an aid to walking. *D,* Plinths being used at a mother and toddler group. (Photographs courtesy of Vranch House School, Exeter, Devon, England.)

1. Treatment of the whole child (achieved by uniting disciplines and relevant professionals or by training a conductor)
2. Rhythmic intention used as a teaching method
3. Programs that follow a basic motor pattern (Cotton, 1983)

Funding

The Foundation for Conductive Education is supported by local and central government. However, by establishing fund-raising groups throughout the United Kingdom, it has also received support from private industry and commerce. At present, most children are supported through local fund-raising.

The Spastics Society for People with Cerebral Palsy schools are funded by this large national charity and are committed to invest £2.3 million (approximately $4 million) in their Peto-inspired programs with £250,000 (approximately $440,000) in addition providing local outreach services (Spastics Society for People with Cerebral Palsy, 1990).

EFFECTIVENESS OF EARLY INTERVENTION—A DISCUSSION OF PORTAGE AND CONDUCTIVE EDUCATION

Both approaches emphasize early treatment and a sound understanding of developmental stages. This is common to many other programs (Levitt, 1986).

Bijou (1988) considered the requirements for early intervention in general. An effective program must have an underpinning of the psychology of learning, adjustment, and personality. If a program is to compensate for restrictions in development, then the instruction to teachers and children should be individualized to meet their own needs. Within the teaching format, Bijou listed six vital areas:

1. Assessing initial competency
2. Setting instructional goals
3. Teaching effectively
4. Monitoring progress
5. Evaluating progress to modify goals or programs
6. Preparing the child to transfer to the next training situation (transition)

Both systems satisfy these requirements; the Portage approach corresponds most directly. The crucial area to be considered is the effectiveness of the teaching techniques. When considering this, it is worth emphasizing the difference in client groups. The Portage system is in a sense open to all: it encompasses a wide range of children whose needs vary immensely. In conductive education, the dysfunction of the selected client group is primarily physical. This difference is reflected in the teaching methods.

The Portage approach is based on sound behavioral principles that function across the spectrum of human experience. Conductive education functions using aspects of personality and cognition not possessed by all children.

Some very impressive claims have been made for the effectiveness of conductive education. The criterion for its success is orthofunction. Monitoring this through handwriting ability, Aubrey and Sutton (1987) noted that most school-aged children at the Peto Institute had achieved orthofunction. Further examination of official Hungarian statistics found that 83.7% of students were identified as orthofunctional; 9.1% were unable to benefit because of profound learning difficulties (Sutton, 1987).

Still discussing this work in Hungary, Sutton wrote that a 2-year-old child with spasticity may become orthofunctional after a year or so, and a child with athetosis may become orthofunctional in 3 to 4 years. This time increases with the age of the child and the degree of learning difficulties. Robinson and associates (1989) concluded that children attending the Peto Institute certainly function better as a result of the program, but they emphasized that these children are a carefully selected minority of children with cerebral palsy and spina bifida. The question raised is, "Does this selection make the results apparently achieved less impressive?" Results from British programs have not yet achieved this level of success. Jernqvist (1980) evaluated the progress of a group of children at a Peto unit within a Spastics Society for People with Cerebral Palsy school: Ingfield Manor. During a 2-year period, children made significant improvements in all areas examined. These areas included social responsiveness, gross and fine motor skills, and self-help skills. However, orthofunction was not achieved, and the children had not progressed enough to enter mainstream schooling unaided.

In 1984 the conductive education interest group listed 22 schools using the approach. Sutton (1987) described the very wide range of practices, in particular the failure of many groups to use the group as a pedogogic instrument. Three of the schools did, however, claim that orthofunction had been achieved with a small number of students.

A survey performed in 1988 (Louton, 1989) of schools for physically handicapped children noted that 18 schools practiced conductive education with 198 children. Five per cent of these children were reported to have achieved orthofunction.

The wide range of approaches to conductive education and the lack of a rigorous examination of their methods make a clear evaluation of the approach difficult. As Barrera and colleagues (1972) pointed out, methods of evaluating interventions need to be rigorous because the cost in human terms of applying ineffective programs is immeasurable.

The Portage guide to early education has been evaluated many times, and research has produced some interesting data. Several studies reported a significant increase in intelligence quotient levels by children on Portage schemes (Cochran and Shearer, 1984; Shearer and Shearer, 1972). Furthermore, these results have been replicated in the United Kingdom. Sturmey and Crisp (1986), when examining such studies, noted that more modest results emerge from studies that include children with organic handicaps.

Because the Portage system sets clear goals and records progress, the rate of goals achieved can be measured (Cole, 1982; Daly, 1980; Sturmey and Crisp, 1986). The rate of goals achieved, as measured by these studies, averaged 82%. The use of this as a valid measure of outcome has been questioned because rapid acquisition of goals may be due in part to eliciting skills already within the child's repertoire (Sturmey and Crisp, 1986). Developing responsiveness and generalizing behaviors into a teaching situation could, however, be argued to be a new behavior in itself.

Short (1984) wrote that parental opinion is a crucial part of any evaluation for this type of intervention. Mundell (1988) found that parents who were involved with the Portage scheme had significantly more accepting attitudes toward their children than parents of comparable children who were not involved. Mundell pointed out that this alone may have far-reaching consequences in relation to the child's development.

WHY HAVE THESE APPROACHES BECOME INFLUENTIAL IN THE UNITED KINGDOM?

Portage has spread rapidly and attracted the time and interest of many professionals working in pediatrics. Cameron (1988) noted how the Warnock report (Warnock, 1978) produced by a national committee charged with investigating provision for children with special needs helped publicize the Portage approach at a national level among professionals.

Included in the Portage literature are guidelines on setting up a service and attracting funds (White and Cameron, 1987). As with all Portage materials, these are clearly presented and easily read. It has been estimated that the teaching materials are easily read by 80% of the population. This is in marked contrast with other comparable materials (Sturmey and Crisp, 1986). The support literature gives practical guidance on topics such as setting up a management team, office duties, and appointing personnel. Furthermore, administrators can easily cost a potential service, and its cost benefits are obvious.

As an effective, cost-efficient approach, the Portage method has won the support of professional and administrative services. It includes within itself the means to establish new services, and its strong theoretic basis and clear guidelines have allowed its achievements to be replicated and developed throughout the United Kingdom. Cameron (1988), in a discussion of the success of the Portage model, described its achievements as remarkable because they "rely mainly on parents, use a minimum of professional time, utilize no complex educational technology and materials and can often be provided at a fraction of the cost of traditional services for families" (p. 68).

Conductive education has attracted national interest to a large extent through media reports of the "miracles" being achieved in Budapest. Pressure groups such as Rapid Action for Conductive Education and the work of the Foundation for Conductive Education have influenced government policy and funding arrangements. Unlike the Portage method, its theoretic basis is not easily accessible, and its approach is often misinterpreted and misunderstood. Transferring conductive education to the United Kingdom and replicating its results has not proved to be straightforward due partly to cultural and philosophic differences. An evaluation of the recent work at the Foundation for Conductive Education is keenly awaited.

FUTURE DEVELOPMENTS

The Portage approach will continue to grow for reasons outlined previously, and its development in the United Kingdom is mirrored internationally (Yamaguchi, 1988). Recent developments include making use of strategies to facilitate group interaction and a proposed model of continuing professional development for parents, home teachers, and supervisors in the United Kingdom (Cameron, 1988).

Conductive education has influenced the practice of many therapists and has had a significant effect on the approaches used in early intervention. If, however, it is to expand internationally in a meaningful way, the critical elements of the system must be determined and clear guidelines must be developed for establishing the approach in a different culture. It is hoped that this will occur in the near future.

For those working in the area of prevention and rehabilitation, both these approaches offer exciting opportunities to make a qualitative difference to the lives of children and their families.

References

Barrera MEC, Routh DK, Carol AP, et al: Early intervention with biologically handicapped infants and young children: A preliminary study with each child as his own control. In Tjossem TD (ed): Intervention Strategies for High Risk Infants and Young Children. Baltimore, University Park Press, 1972.

Bendall S, Smith J, and Kushlick A: National Study of Portage-Type Home Teaching Services. Vol 1: Report. Southampton, England, University of Southampton, 1984a.

Bendall S, Smith J, and Kushlick A: National Study of Portage-Type Home Teaching Services. Vol 2: Methodology and Results. Southampton, England, University of Southampton, 1984b.

Bendall S, Smith J, and Kushlick A: National Study of Portage-Type Home Teaching Services. Vol 3: Detailed Reports of Nineteen Services Visited. Southampton, England, University of Southampton, 1984.

Berk L: Private speech learning: Out loud. Psychol Today 20(5):34–42, 1986.

Bidder RT, Hewitt RE, and Gray OP: Evaluation of teaching methods in a home-based training scheme for developmentally delayed children. Child Care Health Dev 9:1–12, 1982.

Bijou R: Practical implication of an interactional model of child development. Except Child 44:64–14, 1988.

Bobath K and Bobath B: The neuro-developmental treatment. In Scrutton D (ed): Management of the Motor Disorders of Children with Cerebral Palsy. Clinics in Development Medicine and Child Neurology. London, MacKeith Press, 1984.

Cameron RJ: Portage in the U.K. In Yamaguchi K (ed): Proceedings of the 1988 International Portage Conference, Tokyo: A Challenge to Potentiality. Japan, Japan Portage Association, 1988.

Cole D: Essential record keeping and administration. In Cameron RJ (ed): Working Together: Portage in the U.K. Windsor, NFER-Nelson, 1982.

Cottam PJ and Sutton A: Conductive Education: A System for Overcoming Motor Disorder. London, Croom Helm, 1986.

Cotton E: Conduct training in England. Conductive Education Interest Group Newsletter 3(Suppl), 1983.

Cotton E and Kinsman R: Conductive Education and Adult Hemiplegia. London, Churchill Livingstone, 1983.

Cotton E and Parnwell M: From Hungary the Peto method. Special Educ 56(1):50–56, 1967.

Daly B: Evaluation of portage home teaching. Pilot project for pre-school handicapped children. June 1979–80. A Summary Report, No. P/S 02. Dagenham, Essex, England, Barking and Dagenham School Psychological Service, 1980.

Foundation for Conductive Education. The conductor. The Newsletter of the Foundation for Conductive Education 2(6):50–57, 1989.

Griffiths RE: The Abilities of Babies. London, London University Press, 1954.

Hari M: The Human Principle in Conductive Education. (Elizabeth Appleyard, trans). Budapest, Hungary, Peto Conductive Education, International Institute, 1988.

Hong S: The Bobath approach and its application in occupational therapy for children with cerebral palsy. Br J Occup Ther 48(1):4–7, 1985.

Jernqvist L: Preliminary Evaluation of Conductive Education: The Progress of Twelve Children with Two Years Attendance at the Conductive Education Unit at Ingfield Manor School. Unpublished manuscript, 1980.

Kerslake C: Visit to the Institute for Conductive Pedagogy in Budapest. Unpublished manuscript, 1970.

Kong E: The importance of early treatment. In Galjaard J, Precht HFR, and Velickovic N (eds): Early Detection and Management of Cerebral Palsy. Dordrecht, The Netherlands, Martinus Nijhott, 1987.

Levitt S: Paediatric Developmental Therapy. Oxford, England, Blackwell Scientific, 1986.

Lloyd J: Jacob's Ladder—A Parent's Experience of Portage. Tunbridge Wells, Kent, England, Costello, 1986.

Louton AP: The Conductor. Oxford, England, Oxford University Press, 1989.

Luria LS: The Role of Speech in the Regulation of Normal and Abnormal Behaviour. Oxford, England, Pergamon Press, 1961.

MacDonald J: The International Course on Conductive Education at the Peto Andreas State Institute for Conductive Education, Budapest. Br J Occup Ther 53(7):295–300, 1990.

Mundell N: Changes in parental attitude following involvement in portage. In White M and Cameron RJ (eds): Portage, Problems and Possibilities. Windsor, NFER-Nelson, 1988.

Revill S and Blunden R: A home training service for preschool developmentally handicapped children. Behav Res Ther 17(3):207–214, 1979.

Revill S and Blunden R: A Manual for Implementing a Portage Home Training for Developmentally Handicapped Pre-School Children. Windsor, NFER-Nelson, 1980.

Robinson RO, McCarthy GT, and Little TM: Conductive education at the Peto Institute, Budapest. Br Med J 288:1145–1151, 1989.

Sharpe Banus B: The Developmental Therapist, 2nd ed. Thorofare, NJ, Slack Inc, 1979.

Shearer DE and Shearer MS: The portage project: A model for early childhood intervention. *In* Tjossem TD (ed): Intervention Strategies for High Risk Infants and Young Children. Baltimore, MD, University Park Press, 1972.

Short AB: Short term treatment outcome using parents as co-therapists for their own autistic children. J Psychol Psychiatr 25:443–458, 1984.

Smith J, Kushlick A, and Glossop C: "The Wessex Portage Project. A Home Teaching Service for Families with a pre-school mentally handicapped child", Research Report No. 125, Part 1; Report Part II. Southampton, England, University of Southampton, 1977.

Spastics Society for People with Cerebral Palsy: News release title. London, England, Spastics Society for People with Cerebral Palsy, February 28, 1990.

Sturmey P and Crisp AG: Portage guide to early education education: A review of research. Educ Psychol 6(2):1301–1357, 1986.

Sutton A: The challenge of conductive education. *In* Booth T and Swann W (eds): Including Pupils with Learning Difficulties. Philadelphia, Open University Press, 1987.

Vygotsky LS: Mind in Society. The Development of Higher Mental Processes. Cambridge, MA, Harvard University Press, 1978.

Vygotsky LS: Thought and Language. Cambridge, MA, MIT Press, 1962.

Warnock M (chair): The Warnock Report. Special Educational Needs. Official Report of the Council of Enquiry into the Education of Handicapped Children and Young Children. London, Her Majesty's Stationery Office, 1978.

White M and Cameron RJ: The Portage Early Education Programme: A Practical Manual. Windsor, NFER-Nelson, 1987.

White M and Cameron RJ: Portage: Progress, Problems and Possibilities. Proceedings of the Sixth National Portage Conference. Windsor, NFER-Nelson, 1988.

Wilson M: The Institute for the Treatment and Education of Patients with Motor Disability. Unpublished manuscript in Cottam PJ and Sutton A, 1970.

Yamaguchi K: Development of the portage teaching model in Japan. *In* Proceedings of the 1988 International Portage Conference, Tokyo: A Challenge to Potentiality. Japan, Japan Portage Association, 1988.

C H A P T E R

17

Caryn R. Johnson

Aquatics for Promoting Health in People with Physical Disabilities

Disability co-exists with ability, disease with freedom from disease. An individual has health and morbidity. A disabled man may possess good health. A disability-free man may enjoy poor health.

Ruth Weimer (1972)

According to *Healthy People: The Surgeon General's Report on Health Promotion and Disease Prevention* (U.S. Surgeon General's Office, 1979), *"medical care* begins with the sick and seeks to keep them alive, make them well, or minimize their disability; *health promotion* begins with people who are basically healthy, and seeks the development of community and individual measures which can help them to develop lifestyles that can maintain and enhance the state of well-being." *Wellness* is a way of being, the process of maintaining a balance between the body, the mind, the spirit, and the environment (Johnson, 1986).

Health promotion and wellness are important issues when considering the physical and psychologic well-being of those with long-term physical disability. The existence of a disability or chronic disease process need not commit an individual to the ranks of the "sick". Nor does it necessitate that the individual receive "medical" care to promote health. For example, a 20-year-old man 4 years after a spinal cord injury is not

"sick", although he continues to require the use of a wheelchair. A 63-year-old woman with amyotrophic lateral sclerosis may achieve wellness despite progressive loss of strength and function.

Recent trends in prevention, health promotion, and fitness have helped to separate medical care from health care, making the pursuit and promotion of health more accessible to Americans as a whole. However, as interest in physical and mental fitness soars, expanding into health clubs, hospital-based fitness centers, and industry, it often remains unavailable to individuals with physical disabilities because of cost, architectural barriers, or program design.

Aquatic programming offers a wide range of options to people with physical dysfunction who seek to achieve a state of wellness through health-promoting activities. The WETSwim program is an example of community-based, wellness-oriented aquatic programming. In this chapter, the WETSwim program is described in detail to illustrate ways in which an aquatic program may address a variety of health-promotion concepts including personal responsibility, active participation, accessibility, and quality of life.

LONG-TERM DISABILITY

The actual number of people in the United States who have long-term disability is not known.

According to the American Hospital Association, over 101,000 people were discharged from rehabilitation hospitals, units, and services in 1987. The Arthritis Foundation reported in 1989 that an estimated 37 million people have arthritis. National Heart Association estimates place the number of people who experience strokes each year at 500,000. The Multiple Sclerosis Society estimates the number of people with multiple sclerosis at approximately 250,000. Reflecting dramatic advances in medicine and technology, the number of people surviving serious illness or injury resulting in long-term disability is increasing each year.

Insurance does not usually cover health maintenance or health-promotion activities for people with chronic conditions such as arthritis and multiple sclerosis. Few community-based opportunities are available that provide fitness-oriented or recreational activities in barrier-free locations.

Most people with long-term disability reside in the community. In cases in which physical capacity is impaired, there are often large amounts of leisure time but no leisure activity.

BARRIERS TO PARTICIPATION

Health-promotion goals for the person with long-term disability are based on personal interests and values and are highly individualized. For some, the emphasis is on improving physical capacities or on preventing further physical deterioration. Others are interested in socialization or in achieving maximal independence.

However, access to health-promoting activities is often limited once the person with long-term disability has completed a hospital-based rehabilitation program. Home health services are available only to those who are homebound and who continue to demonstrate progress within a limited number of visits. Outpatient therapy is also reserved for those who are expected to make measurable gains in performance-related rehabilitation goals. For the individual with a long-term disability, maintenance of physical status and mental health is often a critical goal, and it is almost never reimbursable.

Therapeutic recreation and fitness programs are offered in many rehabilitation settings, but they are frequently restricted to that facility's own client population. In addition, many traditional recreation and fitness programs are often unavailable to this population because of architectural barriers and limited staff awareness.

Attitudinal barriers may be the most difficult to overcome, however. Managers and members of community health and fitness facilities often discourage people with disabilities from buying memberships, fearing it may affect their image. Fear of the unknown and concerns about increased liability also cause clubs to hesitate to accept disabled members.

AQUATIC PROGRAMS

Aquatic therapy has a long, established history. Physical therapists, occupational therapists, and recreational therapists have been providing this type of therapy in swimming pools, hubbard tanks, and therapeutic pools since injured soldiers began returning home after World War I.

Aquatic programs can be categorized as either social/recreational, therapeutic, or holistic. In recreational programs, the emphasis is placed on the development of play and leisure skills and having fun. Therapeutic aquatic programs focus more on an individual's physical attributes, such as strength, range of motion (ROM), and endurance, using water as a therapeutic medium. A holistic program combines the two to promote health on both physical and psychosocial levels. Water activities, including swimming, offer meaningful opportunities that can be structured to promote a wide range of occupational therapy and physical therapy goals, focusing on the individual's strengths and addressing performance skills as well as habits, values, and roles.

The President's Council on Physical Fitness ranked swimming as "one of the best physical activities." Water provides resistance, thus promoting balanced strengthening of muscles throughout the body. Swimming is an aerobic activity and, when performed appropriately, has a conditioning effect on the cardiovascular and pulmonary systems. Blood circulation increases automatically when the body is submerged. The pressure of the water on the body promotes deeper ventilation. With well-planned activity, circulation and ventilation can increase even more. The buoyancy of water, reducing the apparent weight of the body by 90%, may relieve pain and stress on weight-bearing joints (President's Council on Physical Fitness and Sports, 1977).

Although aquatic programming is frequently used with, and is thought to be beneficial for, people with short-term disability, such as an individual recovering from knee surgery, the emphasis of this chapter is on the use of aquatics for people with long-term disability.

Swimming, or water activity, is considered to be one of the best forms of exercise for persons with long-term disability for a variety of reasons (Hallpike, 1983; Johnson, 1988; Schapiro, 1987; Simons, 1984; Weinstein, 1986). The cooling effect of the water prevents the body from overheating. The pool provides an optimal setting for addressing the spectrum of occupational and physical therapy concerns. Strength, ROM, and endurance programs may be performed in the pool using the water to provide assistance or resistance, swimming strokes to encourage limb movements through a desired ROM, and aerobic activities to promote conditioning. Functional activities such as ambulation and balance are facilitated by the buoyancy of the water while fear of falling is reduced. Water games and group activities provide unlimited opportunities for socialization and recreation. Warm water can have a relaxing effect on tight or spastic muscles, and relaxation techniques can be successfully taught and performed in the water. The buoyancy of the water facilitates movements that can be difficult or impossible when not in the water, and activities not possible on land may become possible in the water (e.g., walking without a cane, playing volleyball). By eliminating stress on weight-bearing joints, reduced pain levels may be noted. Increased self-esteem and feelings of well-being may be achieved through carefully designed, goal-oriented programs structured for success (Johnson, 1988).

For many, aquatic programs provide an opportunity for positive social interaction with others in an environment in which the emphasis is on ability. People are able to overcome barriers to participation more readily in the swimming pool than in most other environments. Architectural barriers do not exist in the water, and mobility equipment, such as walkers and wheelchairs, are replaced with commercial flotation equipment or with no equipment at all. For those with communication disorders, it affords the opportunity to participate successfully in an activity that does not require verbal interaction. Submerged, disabling conditions are less apparent; mobility is facilitated by the buoyancy of the water; and independent self-fulfillment can be achieved.

One factor that often discourages an individual from even attempting to participate in therapeutic or recreational programming is the anticipation of pain or failure, which is usually based on personal experience. For those who have not been in a pool since the onset of their disability, however, expectations about what will happen in the water are not as likely to be influenced by recent experiences. The novelty of the aquatic environment introduces them to a new experience, free of preconceived notions, and positive suggestions by the therapist regarding performance and pain reduction are likely to be well received.

THE WETSWIM PROGRAM

The WETSwim program is a community-based, wellness-oriented aquatic program in which people with physical limitations combine therapeutic, social, and recreational goals. It originated in 1982 at the Jewish Community Center (JCC)-Kaiserman Branch in Philadelphia. The nonprofit community center sought to develop an aquatic program for adults with disabilities as part of its mandate to serve the community.

WETSwim is an acronym for "water exercise and therapeutic swimming." Using a supportive group format, the program encourages personal responsibility for wellness. Group members, or swimmers, are asked to identify their goals, and individualized programs are developed jointly by the swimmer and the therapist. The swimming pool is also a place where people without physical challenges participate in leisure and fitness activities. It represents health rather than illness, and the community location is distinctly separate and different from traditional rehabilitation settings. Community volunteers largely staff the program, providing a solid link to the community.

The WETSwim program "was developed to enable people with disabilities to develop and maintain a level of physical fitness, to continue working toward rehabilitation goals, to resume interrupted leisure and social roles, and to promote self-confidence and independence" (Johnson, 1988, p. 117). Additional goals of the WETSwim program are to provide opportunities for people with long-term physical dysfunction to take an active role in promoting their mental and physical health, to restore their quality of life, and to prevent the complications of long-term disability. In keeping with a wellness orientation, the WETSwim program seeks to return responsibility for setting goals and making decisions and choices to the individuals concerned. It was designed to integrate able-bodied and disabled members of the community by accessing "normal" leisure activities in an environment where many physical and psychologic barriers can be eliminated. Participants feel free to speak to the therapist about issues that concern them, such as deteriorating balance or deepening depression. Access to a health-care professional on a weekly basis encourages participants to address these concerns promptly.

Classes are held once a week at an indoor pool in a building where entry, showers, locker rooms, and hair dryers are all accessible by wheelchair. A private changing area is available for couples where one spouse (or an assistant of the opposite sex) can assist the other in dressing and undressing.

The pool is heated to 86° F, and steps with a handrail facilitate pool entry and exit for people who have adequate lower extremity strength. Volunteers learn how to assist swimmers safely up and down the stairs. Options for those who cannot use the steps include manual (two to three person) lifts or a mechanical pool lift (Fig. 17–1). The use of proper lifting techniques for back protection is essential, and all volunteers receive training.

The program is directed by an occupational therapist. In addition, the program is staffed by assistants—community volunteers, occupational and physical therapy students, lifeguards, and pool personnel—who are trained by the occupational therapist to assist in setting up individualized programs for the swimmers. The ratio of assistants to swimmers ranges from three assistants for one swimmer to one assistant for three swimmers based on swimmers' goals and needs. Class size is limited to 12, and diagnoses vary, covering a wide range of chronic and acute orthopedic and neurologic disorders. A variety of special equipment is available to the swimmers, including flotation vests, inflated inner tubes, snorkels and masks, and adaptive buoyancy equipment.

REFERRAL

Referrals to the WETSwim program come from physicians, physical and occupational therapists, insurance companies, friends, and neighbors. Publicity is largely word of mouth, but enrollment is stimulated by periodic coverage in local news media. A required physician's prescription for each swimmer supplies the Jewish Community Center with a higher degree of comfort. The perceived need for a medical prescription for a wellness program that addresses physical and psychosocial health is certainly worthy of further discussion.

EVALUATION AND GOAL SETTING

Evaluation of each swimmer is based on observation and self-report. It is informal and ongoing. On the registration form, swimmers indicate personal and medical information, past and present water-activity levels, and goals (Fig. 17–2). During the first few sessions, the therapist works with each swimmer to determine which technique is best for pool entry and exit, level of independence in the water, and which water skills, if any, the swimmer possesses.

Swimmers exhibit varying degrees of independence in the water. Activities are structured and graded to promote maximal independence and safety. Independence in ambulation, for example, can be promoted by using inner tubes or floating barbells while walking in the water at chest level. When assistence is needed, the swimmer may hold onto the hand of the volunteer, who gradually reduces the amount of support offered until the swimmer's confidence and skill levels have improved and independence is

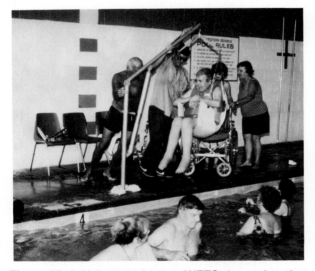

Figure 17–1. Volunteers lower a WETSwimmer into the pool using a mechanical pool lift.

Name ——————————————————— Date ———————
Address ——————————————————— Zip ———————
Phone ——————— Emergency phone ——————— Age —— Sex —— Birthdate ————
Referred by ————————————————————————
Physician's Name ————————————— Phone ———————
Address ——————————————————————————

1. Please state your primary medical condition

2. How long have you had this condition? ————————————————
   ☐ Less than 1 year
   ☐ 1-2 years
   ☐ 2-5 years
   ☐ 5-10 years
   ☐ More than 10 years

3. Please list any other medical conditions you have ————————————

4. Please indicate level of mobility
   ☐ wheelchair   ☐ walker   ☐ cane
   ☐ crutches   ☐ no aides   ☐ other ————————

5. How would you describe your ability to swim before the onset of your primary medical condition?
   ☐ I never went into the water
   ☐ I went into the water but did not know how to swim
   ☐ I swam in my own way but had no formal training
   ☐ I was able to swim but did not swim laps
   ☐ I was a lap swimmer
   ☐ I was a competitive swimmer

6. How would you describe your ability to swim now?
   ☐ I have not been in the water since the onset of my medical condition
   ☐ I have not yet tried to swim
   ☐ I cannot swim at all
   ☐ I can swim with the help of an assistant
   ☐ I can swim in an improvised fashion (no formal stroke)
   ☐ I am able to swim but I don't swim laps
   ☐ I can swim laps
   ☐ I am a competitive swimmer

7. What would you like to emphasize during class? Please indicate four choices, placing a "1" in the box in front of your first choice, a "2" in the box in front of your second choice, and so on.
   ☐ Exercises for strength and flexibility   ☐ Recreation and socialization
   ☐ Overall conditioning   ☐ Walking and balance
   ☐ Water safety skills   ☐ Independence in the water
   ☐ Other ————————   ☐ Swimming skills

Figure 17–2. Registration form for the WETSwim program.

achieved. When assessing independence, it is particularly important to note balance skills and righting reactions, as well as problem-solving, impulse control, and direction-following abilities.

People with chronic, degenerative illnesses usually experience progressive physical deterioration. It is not unusual, however, for people to continue to improve functionally in the areas of swimming skills and independence in the water, while losing function out of the water. This can be attributed to improved skill and efficiency in the water, areas not entirely dependent on strength and balance.

The components necessary for swimming are known as water skills. The therapist observes swimmers to determine if they are able to perform a back float, roll from a prone float position to a supine (back-float) position, and alternate breathing with putting the face in the water. Swimmers are also observed for their ability to perform swimming strokes, including the doggie paddle, front crawl, back crawl, breast stroke, side stroke, and elementary back stroke. Observers also note the swimming distance and quality of stroke.

Many swimmers choose to swim laps. To structure lap-swimming as a goal-oriented activity, it became necessary to devise a method for setting individual goals and for keeping track of progress. Two creative occupational therapy students on a field work placement developed a "Swim to Atlantic City" game, a terrific visual reinforcer. To "reach" Atlantic City, a swimmer needed to swim 1 mile (72 laps). Along the way, every 10 laps or so, the students established stopping points of interest, such as the Liberty Bell, a horse and carriage ride, and slot machines. These stopping points became end-goals in themselves for some swimmers. This game enabled lap-swimmers to set their goals according to personal ability.

THE SWIMMERS

WETSwim participants come from all over Philadelphia and its suburbs and present with a wide range of diagnoses including multiple sclerosis, muscular dystrophy, stroke, heart disease, cerebral palsy, arthritis, amyotrophic lateral sclerosis, brain injury, blindness, back pain, chronic pain, and postsurgery. Functional deficits present in the swimmers include limitations in strength, ROM, coordination, and endurance; muscle im-

balance; pain; poor self-image and self-confidence; impaired balance and mobility; impaired perceptual and cognitive status; and impaired communication skills (speech, visual, auditory). Problems may also be noted in the areas of sensation, circulation, and vital capacity.

STAFF

WETSwim personnel include an occupational therapist, volunteers (including occupational therapy and physical therapy students), and a lifeguard with advanced lifesaving and cardiopulmonary resuscitation certifications. Volunteers and swimmers are matched according to a variety of personal attributes such as personality, knowledge level, teaching ability, and size. Although the makeup of the class may not be constant week to week because of illness or scheduling conflicts, the same volunteers and swimmers usually work together. This consistency is essential to attain goals and to develop strong relationships.

Formal volunteer training takes place before the first class. Informal training is on-going. Volunteers receive instruction on the physical and psychosocial aspects of disability, transfers and pool entry, program planning and goal setting, and teaching methodology and safety.

Although the WETSwim program was designed and implemented by an occupational therapist, aquatic programming lends itself readily to direction by both occupational therapists and physical therapists. Of the aquatic programs currently in existence, some are directed by occupational therapists, some by physical therapists, and some jointly. The philosophies and theoretic foundations a therapist brings to a program generate influences on program design, but similarities in goals and outcomes are shared.

PRECAUTIONS

Precautions that may need to be observed include cardiac and seizure conditions as well as chilling in those swimmers with sensory, circulatory, or temperature regulation problems. Cooler water may encourage spasticity and muscle spasms, whereas water that is too warm may prove to be intolerable to those with multiple sclerosis. Overfatigue must be avoided in swimmers with cardiac conditions, multiple sclerosis, and amyotrophic lateral sclerosis. Insensate limbs may be susceptible to injury on the bottom or sides of the pool, and in some cases swimmers are advised to wear socks. People known to have poor judgment or impulsive behavior must be supervised closely. It is often necessary to observe positional orthopedic precautions with people with back injuries. Along those lines, proper lifting techniques and body mechanics must be emphasized among the staff.

CLASS FORMAT

Each class begins with a 20-minute group warm-up session, starting with a variety of ambulation styles (forward, backward, on toes, and so on), which facilitates adjustment to the water while working on balance, ambulation, lower extremity strength and ROM, and cardiovascular conditioning (Fig. 17–3). Warming up is important to raise deep muscle temperature and stretch ligaments, muscles, and connective tissues to pre-

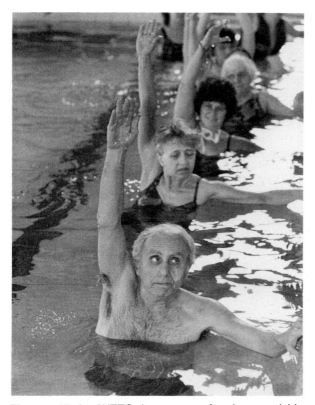

Figure 17–3. WETSwimmers performing poolside warm-ups.

pare the body for work and to help prevent injury. Constant movement in the water is necessary to maintain body temperature in people with circulatory problems. For the elderly, in whom the rate of metabolism is slower and the fatty tissue just under the skin has begun to diminish, chilling may also be a problem. Swimmers are encouraged to perform each activity as independently as possible within their psychologic and physical comfort ranges: flotation devices, assistants, and walls are frequently used to increase comfort and safety levels. As confidence and skill in the water increase, the swimmers require less and less assistance. Independent mobility in the water (with or without assistive devices) is generally a long-term goal for each swimmer.

A period of stretching (ROM) exercises for neck, trunk, and extremities follows the ambulation activities. Swimmers receive assistance or resistance as needed. Good posture is emphasized, and appropriate precautions are observed.

During the second half of the class, the group breaks up into smaller units of people with similar goals, and the swimmers have an opportunity for more individualized attention. Each group works with trained assistants. The swimmers and assistants follow the individualized program plan developed for each swimmer by the therapist based on the goals indicated by each swimmer. A good aquatic program can combine several goals into one activity. During this time, the focus is usually on water-safety skills, swimming skills, and exercise. Water-safety skills include prone float and recovery (return to standing position), back float and recovery, turning prone to supine, changing directions, and rhythmic breathing (American Red Cross, 1977). Each skill is broken down into steps small enough to allow each swimmer to achieve recognizable goals. Individualized instruction takes into account different rates of progress. It is important for each swimmer to be exposed to successful experiences regularly, and verbal reinforcement is applied generously.

Development of swimming skills includes the breakdown and reassembly of components of the various strokes. Swimmers are usually instructed in the arm movements and leg movements separately before putting the whole stroke together. Instruction may be performed in the form of demonstration, verbalization, or manual manipulation depending on the learning needs of the individual swimmer. Recommendations are usually made as to the most appropriate stroke for each swimmer based on the individual's strengths and precautions. The choice, however, is always made by the swimmer. This allows the swimmer to retain control and remain the deciding force behind his or her program. Specific swimming skills include the flutter kick, frog kick, elementary back stroke, crawl, breast stroke, and side stroke. Flotation devices are used as needed (Fig. 17–4).

Some people are more interested in performing exercises in the water than in functional activities, particularly those with acute problems. Exercises are prescribed according to each individual's needs and may include active, active-assisted, or passive ROM; resistive exercise; or walking and balance activities.

Many of the swimmers indicate that opportunities for recreation and socialization are important to them. These elements seem to be inherent to the class itself. Group activities such as water baseball or volleyball generally receive an enthusiastic response when used to conclude sessions (Fig. 17–5). Great care is taken to ensure that the activities are adult-oriented.

Although the locker room seems to be the ideal place to work on activities of daily living (ADL) independence, in reality by the time the swimmer with a long-term disability gets out of the water there is not much energy left to work on independent dressing skills. In fact, swimmers often need more assistance than they do for morning ADLs either because they are fatigued or because their transportation is waiting for

them and they need to get changed quickly. A therapist can still take advantage of the opportunity to address ADLs and may recommend equipment or techniques for use at home. Volunteers and staff provide assistance with dressing both before and after class. The number of swimmers who require assistance with dressing must be balanced with the number of staff and volunteers available to help.

TRANSPORTATION

Insufficient transportation options remain the single most significant barrier to participation in the WETSwim program. Many people obtain rides from friends or family members, whereas others use the local paratransit system. People residing outside of the county in which the JCC is located have no public transportation options, however.

FINANCIAL CONSIDERATIONS

The WETSwim program is inexpensive enough for people dependent on Social Security income (SSI) or Social Security disability income (SSDI) to easily afford. Scholarships are available from the JCC and the local chapter of the Multiple Sclerosis Society for those who require financial assistance. Third-party payers do not typically cover this type of program. As with many health-promotion programs, it could save them money in the long run.

Corporate sponsorship is largely responsible for funding the WETSwim program. The costs of staffing the program and using the facility exceed the revenues generated by registration fees.

The WETSwim program is marketed to the community, volunteers, occupational therapists, physical therapists, and physicians through periodic press releases, word of mouth, and mass mailings.

EQUIPMENT

Special equipment may be used to enable swimmers to reach their goals. Some items are available commercially, whereas others are custom made by students and staff. For a list of suppliers and prices, see Appendix I.

Flotation devices are used to increase safety or

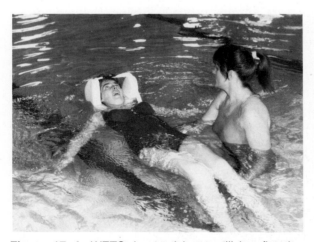

Figure 17–4. WETSwim participant utilizing flotation belt for head support with volunteer.

Figure 17–5. WETSwimmers playing a game of volleyball.

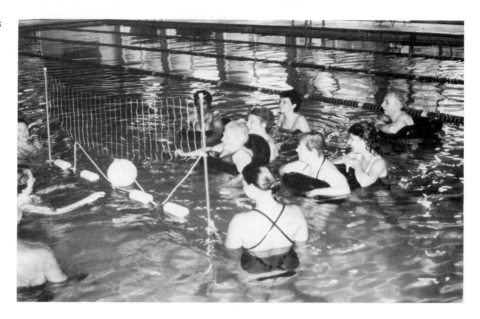

comfort in the water, allow the wearer to relax, eliminate fear, achieve a desired position, or facilitate independence (Heckathorn, 1980). Use of flotation devices allows swimmers to concentrate on propelling themselves through the water without having to devote all of their energy toward keeping their faces above water to breathe. They can be used to perform deep-water exercises and relaxation activities. They should not be used as a life-saving device.

When using a flotation device, it is important to remember that when a person is submerged in water up to the neck, the center of balance shifts from the hip area (where it lies when out of the water) to the lungs. Therefore, the flotation device, as an assist to balance, should be placed around the chest not the waist. Typically, a long-term goal for each swimmer is to reduce the use of flotation devices.

There are several different types of flotation

Figure 17–6. Swimmers using inflated inner tubes for flotation.

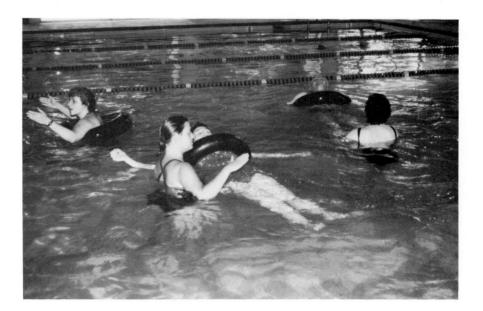

devices. Inner tubes (Fig. 17–6) are black, dough-nut-shaped rubber tubes used inside automobile and truck tires to keep them inflated. They are available in a variety of thicknesses and diameters and may be purchased for under $10 at local gas stations or tire stores.

The Wet Vest (Fig. 17–7) is a blue vest with a crotch strap lined with flotation material. It is the most comfortable and streamlined of all flotation vests. Originally designed for injured athletes undergoing aquatic rehabilitation, the Wet Vest allows the user to float in a supine, prone, or vertical position without restricting the upper extremities. It comes in several sizes and is very durable. The thick, foam-like material is also useful for insulating the torso, thus helping to retain warmth.

Flotation belts are designed to be strapped around the waist and secured in place with an easy-to-use clip. They are available in several sizes. They may be placed around the waist, head, feet, or where increased buoyancy is needed (see Fig. 17–4).

Barbells, or "swim trainers," are made up of two air-filled plastic balls connected by a plastic tube. They can be placed under the knees to prevent legs from sinking or to reduce spinal hyperextension and are also useful in preventing trunk rotation while swimming supine.

Goggles are often worn to protect the eyes from chemicals in the water. Snorkels and masks are useful for people who want to swim a prone stroke but who are unable to turn their heads to the side to breathe. Flippers and hand paddles can be used to increase resistance to the upper and lower extremities.

DOCUMENTATION

As a community-based wellness program, WET-Swim requires no formal documentation. As previously mentioned, physician and participant forms are completed by all swimmers and their physicians. These forms provide useful information about a swimmer's goals, functional capacities, and medical status. The participant's form also includes liability, research, and photography waivers. A swimmer evaluation form has been devised to help students organize information so that they can more successfully evaluate, plan, and implement health-promotion strategies. Upon request, progress reports can sent to physicians and insurance companies.

Attendance records for swimmers and volunteers are kept and have been useful for obtaining funding and for validating the program to the administration and other institutional bodies.

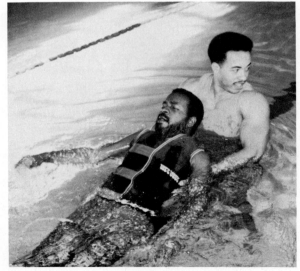

Figure 17–7. WETSwimmer wearing a "Wet Vest" for flotation, accompanied by a staff person.

Case History: Ralph S., a 36-year-old man with multiple sclerosis, lived with his wife and two school-aged children in a three-story South Philadelphia rowhouse. He had been working as an engineer for a local utility company for most of his adult life but was on a medical leave of absence after an exacerbation of multiple sclerosis. Referred by a nursing agency, Ralph first arrived at the WETSwim program via paratransit in January 1986. He was using a wheelchair and was accompanied by a full-time aide.

Ralph had been diagnosed as having multiple sclerosis in December 1979. When he joined the WETSwim program, he had no functional lower extremity strength or active ROM. He had severe spasticity and displayed hip, knee, shoulder, and elbow contractures. Fair to good shoulder, elbow, wrist, and hand strength enabled Ralph to use his upper extremities for many purposeful activities including a computer at work. However, he was dependent in transfers and many of his ADLs.

As a young adult, Ralph had been a competitive swimmer and a lifeguard. He had not been in a pool since the onset of his multiple sclerosis. Ralph had a close and supportive family and always sported a cheery disposition but verbalized that he felt limited in his ability to enact his worker role and in his ability to pursue leisure activities and to achieve personal satisfaction.

On the participant's form, Ralph indicated four goals (in order of importance): exercises for strength and flexibility, overall conditioning, walking and balance, and recreation.

A mechanical pool lift was used to get Ralph into and out of the pool. It required three to 4 staff people, and it took 15 minutes to get Ralph into the pool and another 10 minutes to get him out. In the water, Ralph initially required assistance to float in an inner tube. Without the tube, Ralph was able to abduct and adduct his left arm minimally, helping to propel himself through the water while a volunteer supported him under his neck and upper back.

The difference between what he had once been able to do and what he was currently able to do was difficult for Ralph to accept. He was adventuresome, motivated, and willing to take risks. After several sessions, Ralph was outfitted with a flotation vest and was able to propel himself several crooked feet using his left arm. Attempts at kicking were futile. His right arm remained tightly flexed at the elbow, but some movement was available at the shoulder joint. As his coordination in the water improved, Ralph was able to use his right arm more functionally but continued to swim a crooked course because of the difference in right and left upper extremity strength. It was apparent that to straighten out his stroke, he needed greater power from his right arm.

An occupational therapy student working with the WETSwim program volunteered to design and fabricate a splint for Ralph, which would give him the increased power he needed. The first attempt, an elbow extension splint, failed, because of the force of Ralph's spasticity. After months of revision and adjustment, a new thermal-plastic splint was finally perfected (Fig. 17–8). The proximal portion was designed to fit onto Ralph's upper arm like a cuff and was secured with two Velcro straps. The double-reinforced distal end extended 8 inches beyond Ralph's flexed elbow, in line with his upper arm, and acted as a flipper-shaped extension of his upper arm. It was curved to maximize force as it pushed through the water.

Wearing his splint and flotation vest, Ralph was able to propel himself the length of the pool, using a modified elementary back stroke, with minimal assistance from a volunteer for direction and head support (Fig. 17–9). As his skill and efficiency improved, he increased the distance of his lap-swimming.

In February 1987, Ralph revised his goals, having decided that independence in the water was a high priority. To prepare him for greater independence, he and his volunteer began working on his ability to turn from prone to supine in the water (an important water safety skill). This would eventually enable him to regain a safe, back-floating position in the water in case he ever found himself face down and unable to breathe. It also prepared him for times when he might get water in his face while swimming.

Figure 17–8. Occupational therapy student assists Ralph S. with donning his "Wet Vest." Next to him is the custom-made splint used for lap swimming.

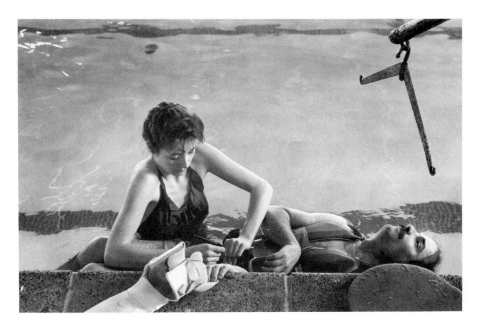

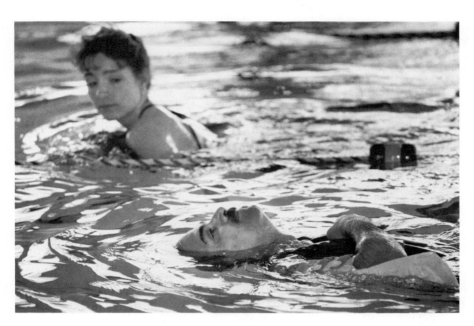

Figure 17–9. Ralph S. swims laps accompanied by occupational therapy student. Note the customized splint on Ralph's right arm.

Ralph was eventually able to perform a prone to supine roll independently.

With the addition of a "water wing" (a small, air-filled, plastic tube) to one ankle to prevent his legs from sinking, Ralph was finally able to swim laps, requiring only distant supervision from a volunteer. Ralph was eventually able to swim 8 to 10 laps per session without becoming unduly fatigued by the time class was over. He gradually developed enough skill to swim without the flotation vest, which contributed drag in the water and slowed him down. However, the insulation and warmth provided by the vest proved to be advantageous; the warmer he felt, the less severe his spasticity. Ralph chose to continue wearing the vest to stay as warm as possible.

Ralph enjoyed standing for the last 10 minutes of each session. Using a walker or holding onto the side of the pool, Ralph was able to enjoy independently maintaining an upright posture, which was impossible out of the pool.

In the summer of 1988, Ralph returned to work at the utility company. He confided in us that he was only able to do so because of the increased confidence in his abilities he had obtained from participating in the WETSwim program.

BENEFITS OF THE WETSwim PROGRAM

Participants, their families, and society as a whole stand to benefit from programs like WET-Swim.

The proper level of physical activity is particularly important to the person with long-term disability. Participation in fitness programming may result in increased strength, endurance, balance, coordination, and flexibility. A group format facilitates socialization, and participation in challenging and successful experiences promotes self-confidence and individuality. Psychologic benefits of exercise, socialization, and recreation can include enhanced self-esteem, greater self-reliance, decreased anxiety, relief from mild depression, and adoption of a healthier lifestyle.

Aquatic programs can be designed to meet a wide variety of therapeutic goals. Applications for visual and auditory discrimination, creativity and self-expression, eye–hand coordination, following directions, sequential thinking, spatial awareness, kinesthetic awareness, and body awareness abound (Priest, 1976). Programs can offer opportunities for competition and independent self-fulfillment.

Family members and caregivers may also benefit from participation in the WETSwim program. For some, it offers a period of free time while their swimmer is in the water. For those who choose to participate in the WETSwim program, it may offer an opportunity to interact with their family member on a unique level.

Community-based fitness programming can be a wellness-oriented and proactive form of health care. Weekly access to a skilled health-care provider through participation in an inexpensive water-exercise program can make community-based fitness programming a cost-effective method for preventing complications that can lead to secondary disability in the person with long-term disability. It is well recognized that improvements in physical fitness and improvements in health status are interrelated (Paffenbarger et al, 1978). Exercise, when it produces sufficient stress on various tissues and biologic functions, results in adaptive responses from the body known as the training effect, characterized by increased cardiovascular and muscular efficiency. The possible health advantages of exercise for adults (25 to 65 years of age) include the prevention of coronary artery disease, maintenance of optimal body weight, improved psychologic status, increased bone density, and lower incidence of respiratory diseases (Haskell, 1985).

Little if anything has been written on the cost benefits of prevention or health promotion for persons with long-term disability. The efficacy of health promotion for people with long-term disability is difficult to demonstrate. In a population in which the nature of their incurable disease may be erratic, progressive, and unpredictable in terms of severity, it is impossible to know what would happen if an intervention strategy such as fitness programming was never tried. It is difficult and perhaps unethical to attach a monetary value to the quality of life.

RESEARCH

Little research exists on the effectiveness and value of aquatic programming for people with disabilities (Gehlsen et al, 1984; Weiss and Jamieson, 1987).

Research questions stimulated by this program include the following:

Can a WETSwim program help to maintain and improve strength, ROM, endurance, mobility, independence, and self-esteem?

Can weekly contact with a health-care professional help to keep participants in touch with their health status and health-care needs?

Does exposure to physically disabled individuals in a community setting improve attitudes toward the disabled?

What does participation in a health-promotion program such as WETSwim mean to participants?

What types of decisions do people make when responsibility for goal setting is transferred from health-care provider to health-care recipient?

Do participants feel that the WETSwim program has enabled them to feel more in control of their lives? Do they feel healthier and a greater sense of wellness?

SUMMARY

Recognition of the need for individuals to take responsibility for their own health—mentally and physically—is growing. Fitness centers have sprung up in every community. Stress management is recognized as a health issue in many major corporations. In addition, cost-containment efforts in the health-care industry have fostered efforts to promote and maintain health at both personal and community levels.

Health-promotion activities, such as aquatic programming, can be developed and implemented on the community level by occupational and physical therapists and can be instrumental in developing skills that enhance physical and psychosocial performance. These programs may in turn result in greater independence, social integration, and quality of life for those individuals. Health-care professionals involved in developing programs to promote health must aim to ensure access both financially and physically. By ensuring not only adequate rehabilitation but access to the community and its resources once rehabilitation is completed, we can attempt to prevent disabling conditions from becoming handicapping ones.

Because many physical activities are unavailable to this population, an aquatic program can provide a realistic alternative for maintaining physical fitness, continuing with rehabilitation goals, and participating in a leisure activity while remaining financially feasible. It can also provide opportunities for exploration and mastery of aquatic skills in an activity and environment in which physical limitations are less restrictive.

References

American Red Cross: Adapted Aquatics. Washington, DC, American Red Cross, 1977.

Gehlsen GM, Grigsby GM, Grigsby SA, and Winant DM: Effects of an aquatic fitness program on the muscular strength and endurance of patients with multiple sclerosis. Phys Ther 64(5):653–657, 1984.

Hallpike JF: Multiple Sclerosis: Pathology, Diagnosis, and Management. Baltimore, Williams & Wilkins, 1983.

Haskell WL: Physical activity and exercise to achieve health related physical fitness components. Public Health Rep 100(2):202–212, 1985.

Heckathorn J: Strokes and Strokes. Reston, VA, American Association of Health, Physical Education, Recreation and Dance, 1980.

Johnson C: Aquatic therapy for an ALS patient. Am J Occup Ther 42(2):115–120, 1988.

Johnson J: Wellness: A Context for Living. Thoroughfare, NJ, Slack, Inc, 1986.

Paffenbarger RS, Wing AL, and Hyde RT: Physical activity as an index of heart attack risk in college alumni. Am J Epidemiol 108:161–175, 1978.

President's Council on Physical Fitness and Sports: Aqua Dynamics: Physical Conditioning Through Water Exercises. Washington, DC, U.S. Government Printing Office, 1977.

Priest EL: Academic remediation in aquatics. Ther Recreation J 10(2):61–64, 1976.

Schapiro RT: Symptom Management in Multiple Sclerosis Long-Term Disability. New York, Demos, 1987.

Simons AF: Multiple Sclerosis: Psychological and Social Aspects. London, William Heinemann, 1984.

U.S. Surgeon General's Office: Healthy People: The Surgeon General's Report on Health Promotion and Disease Prevention, Vol 2. DHEW publication no. (PHS) 79–55071a. Washington, DC, U.S. Government Printing Office, 1979.

Weimer RB: Some concepts of prevention as an aspect of community health. Am J Occup Ther 26(1):1–9, 1972.

Weinstein LB: The benefits of aquatic activity. J Gerontol Nurs 12(2):6–11, 1986.

Weiss CR and Jamieson NB: Affective aspects of an age-integrated water exercise program. Gerontologist 27(4):430–433, 1987.

Bibliography

Adams R: Games, Sports, and Exercises for the Physically Handicapped. Philadelphia, Lea & Febiger, 1982.

American Red Cross: Adapted Aquatics. Garden City, NY, Doubleday, 1977.

Arthritis Foundation: Arthritis Aquatics Program—Instructors Manual. Atlanta, GA, 1983.

Bolton E and Goodwin WS: An Introduction to Pool Exercises. London, Livingston, 1967.

Cariucci J: Development of Pool Programs. Paper presented at the Physical Therapy Forum, King of Prussia, PA, November, 1985.

Champion MR: Hydrotherapy in Pediatrics. Rockville, MD, Aspen Systems, 1985.

Davis BC: A technique of re-education in the treatment pool. Physiotherapy 53(2):57–59, 1967.

Davis BC and Harrison RA: Hydrotherapy in Practice. New York, Churchill Livingstone, 1988.

Duffield MH: Exercise in Water. London, Balliere Tindall, 1976.

Dulcy F: Aquatic Programs for Disabled Children. Occupa-tional Therapy in Health Care. New York, Hayworth Press, 1983.

Finnerty GB and Corbitt T: Hydrotherapy. New York, Frederick Ungar, 1960.

Heckathorn J: Strokes and Strokes. Reston, VA, American Association of Health, Physical Education, Recreation and Dance, 1980.

Johnson CR: Aquatic therapy for an ALS patient. Am J Occup Ther 42(2):115–120, 1988.

Johnson CR: Back Strokes. Havertown, PA, Occupational Therapy Associates, 1989.

Kneipp S: My Water-Cure. Kempton, Bavaria, Germany, Jos. Koesel, 1982.

Licht S (ed): Medical Hydrology. New Haven, CT, E. Licht, 1963.

Lowman CL and Roen SG: Therapeutic Uses of Pools and Tanks. Philadelphia, 1952.

President's Council on Physical Fitness and Sports: Washington, DC, Aqua Dynamics. U.S. Government Printing Office, 1977.

Skinner AT and Thomson AM (eds): Duffield's Exercise in Water. London, Bailliere Tindall, 1983.

Skinner AT and Thomson AM: Hydrotherapy. In Wells PE, Frampton V, and Bowsher D (eds): Pain Management in Physical Therapy. Norwalk, CT, Appleton & Lange, 1988.

Special Olympics: Swimming and Diving. Washington, DC, Special Olympics, Inc, 1981.

Ther Recreation J 10(2), 1976.

APPENDIX I: EQUIPMENT AND SUPPLIERS

Aquatic Exercise Products, Inc. (underwater exercise equipment)
3070 Kerner Blvd, Unit 5
San Raphael, CA 94901
(415) 485–5323

Danmar Products, Inc. (adapted swimming equipment)
2390 Winewood
Ann Arbor, MI 48103
(313) 761–1990

E & B Discount Marine (flotation belts, $10)
201 Meadow Rd
PO Box 3138
Edison, NJ 08818–3138
(800) 533–5007

Flaghouse (paddles, kickboards, games)
18 West 18th St
New York, NY 10011
(212) 989–9700

Orthopedic Product Sales, Inc (WetVest, $105)
PO Box 14033
Columbus, OH 43214
(614) 451–2610; (800) 992–9999

Recreonics (inner tubes and "swim trainers,"
  $17)
7696 Zionsville Rd
Indianapolis, IN 46268
(800) 428–3254 (national); (800) 792–3489
  (Indiana)

Sportime (snorkels, fins, paddles, games)
2905-E Amwiler Rd
Atlanta, GA 30360

Therapeutic Systems, Inc. (flotation belts, $60)
275 S Main St, Suite 9
Doylestown, PA 18901
(215) 340–1155

18

Elissa Krasnopolsky-Levine
Lynda Olender-Russo

Nutrition in Health and Wellness: Planning for Services

The surgeon general's report on nutrition and health, released in July 1988 (U.S. Department of Health and Human Services, 1988) established dietary recommendations and national nutritional objectives for 1990 to reduce health risks, especially for chronic disease. The relationship between nutrition and health and its association with the development of certain chronic diseases have been repeatedly demonstrated. The treatment and possible prevention of these chronic diseases almost always involve some degree of dietary manipulation. In fact, diet may be the single most important factor that individuals can alter. The magnitude of this problem is realized when one notes that, among the major leading causes of death in this country, there are inherent dietary implications (U.S. Department of Health and Human Services: An Update Report on Nutrition Monitoring, 1989).

In view of the aforementioned, it is interesting to note that textbooks for the rehabilitative therapist have typically omitted or skimmed topics related to nutritional care and referral for nutrition services. Marge (1988) emphasized the inclusion of nutritional awareness as one of several necessary additives to a comprehensive rehabilitative health-promotion program. Toward that aim, nutritional health-enhancement strategies

are necessary, are needed early in the primary treatment phase, and should apply to prevention in the primary, secondary, and tertiary stages and to subsequent secondary disabilities throughout the life-cycle continuum.

Physical and occupational therapists who provide comprehensive injury rehabilitation and prevention therapies should plan to include a nutritional component as part of their therapeutic regimen. The planning of these services can be viewed from two standpoints: either (1) from a program perspective whereby a nutritional component can be included as another service within the overall rehabilitative program and the nutritionist may be a member of the existing health-care team or (2) from an outside source whereby services can be obtained via the referral of clients to an independent contractor.

To assist either in the development of a nutritional component within the rehabilitative service or to identify how to use appropriate nutritional referrals, the goals of this chapter include the following:

1. Provide the practitioner (in administration) with the theoretic framework necessary to develop or incorporate a nutrition component or program in health-promotion, disease-prevention, or injury-rehabilitation services

Figure 18–1. Development model for designing a nutrition program.

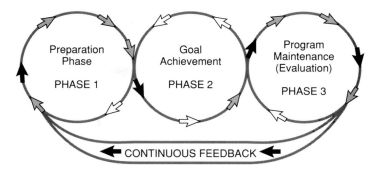

2. Define the various terms associated with the planning and intervention of nutrition programs and services
3. Increase the awareness of available nutritional treatment modalities and the types of nutrition services available either within or outside of the formal rehabilitative setting
4. Establish guidelines to determine when a dietary consultation is needed
5. Provide quality assurance measures to evaluate services provided.

Whether planning for a nutrition program within a parent rehabilitative service or establishing a mechanism for outside dietary referral services, three interrelated phases should be considered (Fig. 18–1):

Phase I: preparation phase (formulation of a theoretic perspective, an underlying philosophy, a program or service purpose, including goals and objectives)
Phase II: goal-achievement phase (actual imple-

mentation of "the what" that you have set out to do and "the how" to do it)
Phase III: program-maintenance phase (evaluates the methodology and the outcome of goal achievement, the process of staff interaction either within the existing service or with outside consultants, and the evaluation of staff and client compliance and satisfaction)

PREPARATION PHASE

As illustrated in Figure 18–2, the initial phase of program development should promote a marriage of both the parent organization's and the nutrition service's underlying philosophy, mission, goals, and objectives. In addition, the provision of any service should be mutually beneficial to those seeking the service as well as to those providing it (e.g., mutually positive outcomes should be achieved). Thus, steps to formulate program design and implementation should incorporate the combined input of the

Figure 18–2. Phase 1: Preparation phase for nutrition program planning.

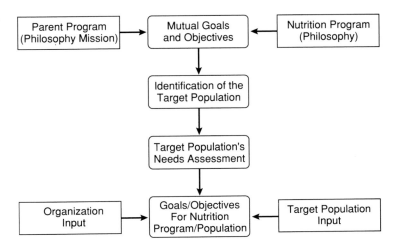

target population (once determined) and the parent organization or service. If these preliminary steps are omitted, optimal benefits may be difficult to define or impossible to achieve. For example, the occupational therapist may be helping a child to eat by improving his or her oral motor skills. The use of different food textures and consistencies may be necessary at different therapeutic stages and may require the parent or guardian to participate actively in incorporating these changes into the child's dietary regimen at home. A discussion with parents before the development of such objectives may help to prevent difficulties later. A parent may need to learn food-preparation techniques or preventive measures to deal with the fear of aspiration pneumonia during feeding or an unwillingness to perform the hands-on control during feeding. Education for the parent or support groups may be a priority for the parents or guardian of these children who may otherwise have been overlooked if their input had not been sought, and it may eventually make the difference between the program or service's success and failure as it related to improved oral motor skills.

Philosophy and Purpose

The preparation phase of a nutrition program or service either within or as an outside adjunct to a rehabilitative service should begin with a statement of the program's philosophy or beliefs that provide purpose and direction. Health-care professions have an obligation to establish an overall philosophy to serve as a guide for the parent agency, in this case, rehabilitative services. An appropriate philosophy for a nutrition service is that it operates with the following beliefs:

1. Nutrition is an important and integral component of the life cycle and contributes to an optimal level of wellness.
2. An environment for the provision of high-quality nutritional care services should be created and maintained during all aspects of a prevention or promotion program.
3. The client or consumer should be a partner in the provision of these services and throughout all three phases of the program's development.

Program-Related Goals and Objectives

Needs Assessment

A thorough needs assessment should be obtained before the development of a nutritional program or consultant service goals and objectives. This will help to identify the populations for whom the program will provide services. Potential populations may be identified by the use of demographic information such as age, sex, socioeconomic status, and the ethnicity of individuals within a given geographic area to be served. Owen (1984) described this aspect of the preparation phase of program development as a community diagnosis. Target populations are identified by their place in the life cycle (e.g., infants, children, pregnant adults, adolescents, or the elderly and community background such as geographic and cultural features). This enables the health-care provider to identify further the types of problems and thus the services most needed. Diagnoses such as iron-deficiency anemia and osteoporosis are examples of problems that afflict certain populations at various points within the life cycle and are significant enough to warrant prevention and early intervention. Chronic diseases such as cardiovascular, diabetes, and hypertension are examples of nutrition-related problems for which prevention or treatment may help to reduce the often crippling and irreversible effects. Health statistics, such as the prevalence of certain diseases and the related morbidity and mortality rates are also important and need to be considered.

A knowledge of local health statistics and social services may be especially useful in determining where and what kind of services are most needed in the community. This information may potentially be the basis for financial support and referrals to the program you are planning. What may seem to be trivial information on the population identified may be crucial to the survival of the program. For example, socioeconomic factors such as transportation needs (e.g., accessibility to and the mobility of the clients for which the program is intended) should not be overlooked because lack of funds for specialized transport (in the case of the disabled) would prevent the use of even the most desirable services. In addition to identifying adjunct services that may be needed, this example illustrates the importance of client or consumer input at the preparation stage of the program development.

The identification of the target population

within an existing service such as a hospital or school should consider groups with already identified high-risk and high-volume problems. Special education programs for children with disabilities within the public school system is one such example of a high-risk group that has already been targeted; another example is the elderly population, which is growing rapidly in this country and is a high-volume group that will certainly command the attention of the health-care community in the future.

Once the target populations have been chosen, the next step is to identify the organization's as well as the target population's needs and resources (or lack thereof) to determine the program's goals and objectives. Duplicating existing services or planning for services that cannot realistically be provided is not an effective use of resources. In the health-care setting, the improvement or prevention of disease, in the most cost-effective way, is an example of a positive outcome for both the user and the provider of the health-care service.

Budgetary Aspects

Although it may seem unethical to place a price tag on good health in today's society, budgetary constraints do exist and limit who may be able to receive what treatments. This dilemma often leads to an ethical debate among professionals having to deal with the costs placed on the quality of life. If the health-care industry is to survive and to continue providing quality care, then an adequate income must be generated to support such services.

An estimate of the costs of setting up a program or providing a service should be determined during the needs assessment (Hyman, 1984). This should include the direct costs, representing the direct expenditure of funds for items such as salaries, equipment, travel, and so on, as well as the indirect costs, defined as the overhead costs incurred by the parent agency. This includes the provision of administrative services and the maintenance and depreciation of the facility.

An adequate staff-to-client ratio should be predetermined on the basis of the level and number of nutritional services to be provided. The professional qualifications of the proposed staff should reflect the complexity and diversity of services to be rendered. If an expansion of an existing service is planned, then the qualifications of existing

personnel should be taken into consideration. Subsequent recruitment and education needs and their related costs are an important step in providing quality services.

To summarize, the outcome of the needs assessment should provide answers to questions related to the target population, the program offerings, resources currently available, and the estimated budget to provide this service.

Program Screening

Once the target population has been identified via the needs assessment, the next step is to determine who within that population is at risk. Figure 18–3 illustrates the steps to follow when planning intervention strategies within the preparation phase of program development. The first step in this process is to screen for individuals at nutritional risk. The screening process should facilitate the determination of type of service needed by the individual or population. The type and levels of care should be set by each program according to their goals and types of services to be provided. Levels of care should be assigned to individuals based on the objective data obtained during the screening process. Individuals are identified according to risk to differentiate the healthy individuals from those who are at risk (i.e., those with a diagnosed illness or problem). Within the health-care continuum, the intervention modality planned for individuals is often determined by their level of care. As outlined in Figure 18–3, levels of care may be categorized into levels of health promotion and primary, secondary, or tertiary health prevention. The subclassification of the healthy population is based on the degree of wellness and the number of risks influencing the likelihood of developing disease as follows:

1. The healthy population without any risk factors and not likely to develop disease
2. The healthy population with a minimal number of risk factors.

A comparative example of healthy individuals is a female client who has a negative family history of diabetes and cardiovascular disease and who does not smoke. In contrast is another healthy individual who is male, has a strong family history of diabetes and heart disease, and who is a smoker. Presumably, the latter individual has a much greater chance of developing

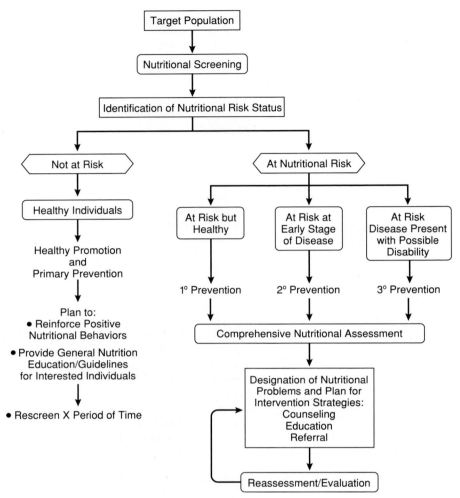

Figure 18–3. Steps to follow when planning intervention services for individuals during the preparation phase of the program.

heart disease, although both would be considered healthy individuals. The necessity for early intervention and the type of program planned for these two individuals will differ. In addition, the time frame for rescreening the healthy but potentially at-risk individual may be shorter than for the person who is healthy but not at the same level of need.

Incorporated within the screening process is the identification of abnormal biochemical parameters, stage of disease or disability, and an individual's educational and therapeutic needs. A valuable aid for identifying clients at nutritional risk is a nutritional screening and assessment tool, an example of which is illustrated in Figure 18–4. A basic nutritional screening may include the collection of the client's height, weight, usual weight, history of appetite, food-

intake changes, laboratory data, family history, and the presence of any known disease. This data must relate to the specific outcomes to be measured. For example, a program whose goal is to promote wellness via the prevention or treatment of individuals with cardiac disease must include criteria for the measurement of cardiac risk. This includes biochemical measures of total cholesterol: high-density lipoprotein (HDL) and low-density lipoprotein (LDL) cholesterol. These initial data not only reflect the type of services that will be needed but also provide a baseline value on which future measurements can be compared.

The occupational or physical therapist may already have identified nutritional risk factors present in their clients, such as weight loss, limited food choices, and so on. The rehabilita-

PART I (Nutrition Screening)

Name _M.L._

Address _Anytown, U.S.A._

Dx: _Hypercholesterolemia, osteoarthritis ℝ knee, obesity_

Meds: _Occasional aspirin_

Vitamins/Mineral Supplement: _OTC multivitamin (>100% U.S.R.D.A.)_

Diet order: _Wt. reducing, low cholesterol_

Diet Restrictions: _No self-imposed restriction_

Prior Nutrition Education: _No formal_

Factors Influencing Intake

Yes	No	
	✓	Change in appetite
	✓	Dysphagia
	✓	Sore mouth/throat
	✓	Painful swallowing
	✓	Nausea/vomiting
	✓	Diarrhea
✓		Constipation (BM q other day)
	✓	Loss of taste (or Δ)
✓		Food allergies (list)-strawberry
	✓	Food intolerances
✓		ETOH -socially 1 drink/mo
	✓	Tobacco
	✓	Other

PART II

Date ___8/17/90___

Age _38_   Sex _M_   Race _W_

Anthropometrics

Ht. _5'6½"_		Wt. _194 lb_	
UBW _180 lb._		%UBW _107%_	
IBW _147 lb_		%IBW _132%_	
Max wt. _194 lb_		Min wt. _160%_	
Hips _43"_		Waist _46"_	
TSF _16_ mm		%STD _133_	
MAC _35_ cm		%STD _107_	
MAMC _29.96_ cm		%STD _106_	
Subscapular _29_ mm		%STD _—_	

Type of Exercise: _Walking (5 ml/hr)_

Duration _20 minutes_   Frequency _2x/mo *_

Restrictions (Physical) _None_

To public transportation if lift not available

Socioeconomic Data

Location of Meals: _① Executive Dining room/Deli ⑤ Home_

Location of Shopping: _Supermarket_

Occupation: _Financial planner_

Insurance Co. _Executive's Health_

Insurance No. _00000000_

Medicare _NO_   Medicaid _No_

PART III (Nutritional Status)
Risk Status

☐ Not at risk

☑ At risk

☑ Referral for Comprehensive Nutrition Assessment

Date(s)	8/10	8/17	8/24	8/24	8/24			
B.P.	140/85	130/85						
Lab	Total chol.	—	HDL	LDL	Glu			
Value	237	—	42	160	103			

Estimated Energy Expenditure

BEE: ___1855___ kcal/day

REE (+ _20_ %) _2,226_ kcal/day

Completed by _Jane Doe_ 8/17/90

Title _Nutritionist for health U.S.A._

Figure 18–4. Sample nutritional screening and assessment tool.

Illustration continued on following page

DIET HISTORY (TYPICAL DAY RECALL)

To be completed by R.D.

TIME	FOOD ITEM	AMOUNT	
6:30	Orange juice	8 fl oz	
	Cornflakes	1½ cups	
	Milk (whole 3.3% fat)	½ cup	
9:00	Tea	10 fl oz	
	Donut (powdered)	1 whole	
12:30	Whole-wheat bread	2 slices	Sent out from deli
	Beef bologna	4 oz	Worked on report for 2:00 business
	Swiss cheese	2 oz	meeting
	Mustard	½ tsp	
	Mayonnaise	2 tsp	
	Diet soda	12 fl oz (1 can)	
6:00	Milk chocolate bar	¼ oz	Waiting for train home
7:15	Tossed salad	1 cup	
	Low calorie Italian dressing	1 T	
	Round steak (broiled)	12 oz	
	Catsup	2 T	
	Potato (boiled)	1 cup	
	Margarine	2 tsp	
	Peas and carrots	1 cup	
	Tea	8 fl oz	

TOTAL   Calories: 2,504   %CHO 33   %PRO 27   %FAT 40

FOOD FREQUENCY CHECKLIST

Food Item	Amount (per week/day)
Eggs	2-3/wk
Meat/Fish/Poultry	Beef ~10 oz 2x wk / chicken & skin 9 oz 3x/wk / Fish 6 oz/wk
Bread	4 slices/day (ww, white)
Cereal	Cornflakes or bran 1-2 c/3 x wk
Potato or Sub	1/day
Sweets	Donuts, chocolate, ice cream 4 x/wk

Food Item	Amount (per week/day)
Vegetables (grn or yellow)	5x/wk ~ 1 cup
Other	
Fruit (citrus)	orange or grapefruit jce - 8 oz/day
Non-citrus	Apples, bananas, melons q.d.
Milk or Dairy	1 cup/day (milk)
Alcohol Intake	Vodka & orange jce 1 drink q 3 wk
Other	Cashew nuts, Trail mix — handful

Suspected deficiencies: Diet is probably adequate in vitamins/minerals; however, many empty calories and high fat (particularly saturated) are in the diet. Fiber content is variable.

Figure 18–4 *Continued*

tive therapist who works closely with the client can help to verify or provide additional data to the nutritionist screening and assessing nutritional risk. Because the nutritionist or nutritional services may be available only part-time or as an outside consultative service, knowing when to refer clients is crucial. The identification of those individuals who most need these services promotes better use of limited resources and hastens the intervention time for the high-risk individual. The following guidelines are presented to help the rehabilitative therapist determine when a referral to a nutritionist or for nutrition services may be necessary.

1. A change in weight either as observed weight loss or the development of obesity (weight changes may be reported by individuals helping to lift or transfer clients or on the basis of measurements or observation by staff and family, e.g., of increasingly loose- or tight-fitting clothing and bitemporal wasting or general wasting not secondary to atrophic changes)
2. Failure to maintain adequate growth and development or to reach developmental milestones in infants and children
3. Observed functional deterioration (e.g., a decrease in handgrip strength and ambulation capacity and increasing fatigue)
4. Observed or reported limited food intake or food selections at mealtime (e.g., preference for foods with low nutritional value)
5. Observed problems in ingesting particular food items or food textures
6. Skin breakdown (i.e., the development of pressure ulcers)
7. Complaints from clients' family, guardians, or staff about changes in food habits, willingness to eat, and bowel function

Should a client meet any of these criteria, a nutritional referral is indicated. The mechanism for consult placement is determined according to the organizational plan (e.g., whether the nutritionist is part of the existing health team or is an outside contractor).

A screening program can also be used for risk prevention by identifying risk factors to determine how many individuals will require in-depth assessment and counseling before their entrance into any program. Additionally, this may in turn help administration to plan for specific additional resources. In most instances, the more complex

the problem, the longer the counselor may need to spend instructing that individual and the more appointments that will be devoted to follow-up; thus, additional resources may be needed. As noted previously, screening distinguishes individuals who require particular types of services. In the case of the individual who is healthy and not at risk, no further intervention other than rescreening at a predetermined time may be necessary. If the individual would still like to use the program, a re-enforcement of positive behaviors and education on how to continue to promote optimal wellness including prevention may be provided. For those individuals at risk, a more comprehensive assessment to determine what may be contributing to the problem is needed.

Nutritional Assessment

A nutritionist makes a comprehensive nutritional assessment of individuals within the designated target population to determine their nutritional status. Krause and Mahan (1984) defined nutritional status as the degree to which an individual's physiologic need for nutrients is met. Additionally, two other important reasons for collecting an initial assessment include (1) the early recognition of dietary habits or factors that may increase the likelihood of health risk and (2) the establishment of baseline values on which the overall effectiveness of intervention can be made. Unlike the basic screening, which provides data and allows one to identify risk factors, the comprehensive nutritional assessment should distinguish factors that contribute to a nutritional problem and to the problem itself. For example, anorexia may be a factor contributing to poor intake, or it may be a problem resulting from such factors as pain, depression, constipation, and so on.

Inherent within this assessment process is the need to identify problems known to affect the specific population being treated. For example, an evaluation of hand motor coordination and its effect on the ability to self-feed, the presence or absence of dysphagia, and the need for any special feeding instrumentation should be incorporated into the assessment of clients with physical disabilities.

Once determined, the communication of findings among disciplines (such as the occupational therapist and the dietitian) promotes a team approach. This will improve the quality and scope of the nutritional assessment and the resulting nutritional care plan.

Given the importance of a comprehensive nutritional assessment, a brief overview of the type of data obtained is warranted. The following information incorporates and expands on the data collected during screening:

1. Anthropometrics (body size and proportions, e.g., height, weight, tricep, and subscapular skin folds and frame size)
2. Biochemical data
3. Medical history, complete with physical exam
4. Economic, psychosocial, and educational needs
5. Diet history, which specifies the individual's actual or current and prior food intake (food intolerance, allergies, and diet-related behaviors or patterns should also be noted)

Many methods exist to determine dietary adequacy, including the direct observation of one's food intake (most often limited to institutional settings), dietary recalls, or a food diary or food frequency questionnaire. Each of these methods has pros and cons depending on the need for specificity and quantification. Dietary recall, diaries, and intake observation yield quantitative information. Food frequency questionnaires, although less quantitative, are generally more predictive of long-term food intake (Treiber et al, 1990). Ultimately, these methods translate one's food intake into nutrient composition. This task is easily accomplished with commercially available computerized nutrient data bases. These software programs provide a plethora of data related to macronutrient (protein, carbohydrate, and fat) and micronutrient (vitamins and minerals) consumed.

It is important to be realistic about outcome capabilities. Problems that are amenable to intervention and those that are not need to be accurately assessed. For example, the aforementioned client with hypercholesterolemia may have a number of factors contributing to his high cholesterol. One of those factors may be genetic (such as being male), which places him at higher risk for the development of heart disease. The individual cannot change his genetic makeup, but he can change his diet and exercise habits. Both factors are known to affect the level of cholesterol in his blood. If, within the nutritional assessment, it is revealed that this individual consumes a large amount of cholesterol and fat

(particularly saturated fat), then it is possible that with dietary changes the hypercholesterolemia can be eliminated. This reduces the number of risk factors and, thus, the possibility of developing heart disease. Failure to determine the factors that can and cannot be changed may result in a poor outcome. If the individual's dietary assessment revealed that he was already adhering to a heart-wise diet, then nutrition intervention would not likely help change the outcome. Perhaps referring the client for exercise or drug therapy for treatment of his hypercholesterolemia would be more effective.

This in-depth analysis (assessment), specific and individually tailored, is a necessary antecedent for planning effective nutritional care intervention.

NUTRITIONAL CARE PLANNING

Planning for nutritional care can be viewed from a broad perspective, such as program planning (based on an adequate needs assessment) to incorporate a nutrition component into a rehabilitative program, or it may refer to the planning or designing of a nutritional care plan for individuals once they have entered a program. In either case, planning should start with the formulation of goals (broader concepts of what is desired) and objectives (more narrowly focused goals that incorporate the specific outcome or behavior to be achieved as well as how this is measured).

When planning for the individual, it is necessary for the counselor or practitioner to have outlined the specific goals that he or she wishes to help the client achieve. It is also crucial to involve the client in this decision-making progress. Doing so should increase the client's compliance and help the practitioner determine the client's priorities. In a sense, this is matching the needs of the client with the goals or needs of the program just as one tries to match the needs of the community with the type of services to be provided.

To plan effectively for nutrition services, it is important to answer the following questions:

1. What are the program's goals and objectives both for the program and for the individual?
2. How can these goals and objectives be met, and what is the best way to meet them? This step is crucial and establishes the action plan

for carrying out the goals and objectives with specificity. The client's educational level and ability to follow directions are important concerns. In addition, careful consideration of the client's preferences for therapeutic options and compliance capabilities need to be considered also. The selection of tools, such as educational materials, should be made at this time. Tools selected should be user friendly and cost effective both to the participant as well as to the program. Other tools and techniques (such as individualized counseling, group classes, home visits, video or film viewing) necessary to implement the care plan should be decided on before the actual intervention process.

3. Who will be responsible for helping the client meet these goals? Staffing assignments should be specified based on the level of care needed. Other individuals helping to carry out or supervise the recommendations outside of the core facility should be identified. This will help delineate the needed resources and support systems.

4. Within what time frame should these objectives be attained? A time frame for achieving the stated goals should be established. Failure to achieve certain goals within a stated period of time may signal that some other kind of intervention or referral may be needed to help facilitate the desired outcome. For example, failure to show any improvement in the hypercholesterolemic client (as measured by a 10% to 15% decrease in the total serum cholesterol within a 3-month period or less according to the specific program's goals) may suggest that a more restrictive diet is needed or drug therapy should be considered.

A discussion of the nutritional care of individuals at all points during the life cycle is beyond the scope of this chapter. The following sections highlight some of the nutritional problems that may affect individuals at different points along this continuum and special health-care problems that may require nutrition intervention.

Nutrition in Healthy Individuals

Most individuals are considered healthy and need only consume a "balanced diet." A balanced diet supplies all of the nutrients in the proper amounts to maintain an adequate nutritional status.

Nutritionists use many methods to evaluate the nutrient intake of individuals; these methods are discussed elsewhere in this chapter. Most are ways to determine quickly whether or not the diet meets the recommended dietary allowances (RDAs). The RDAs are levels of intake judged by the Food and Nutrition Board and detail the specific level of nutrients considered necessary to meet the known nutrient needs of practically all healthy individuals (Food and Nutrition Board: Recommended Dietary Allowances, 1989). The RDA incorporates margins of safety to allow for varying needs of the population. It is not intended to serve as a guide for minimum or optimal levels of intake. Nonetheless, this standard is used frequently to guide individuals and practitioners evaluating dietary intake reports in the possible need for changes in an individual or group's dietary habits. General advice for the healthy population is moderation. An excellent resource for guiding the nutritional well-being of individuals in the United States is outlined in the surgeon general's report on nutrition and health released in 1988 (U.S. Department of Health and Human Services, 1988). Some of these recommendations include:

1. Reduction in the consumption of fat (especially saturated fat) and cholesterol
2. Maintenance or achievement of ideal body weight.
3. Decrease in the consumption of foods high in sugar (to avoid the development of dental caries, particularly in children)
4. Increase in the consumption of complex carbohydrates and fiber.

Another quick method to identify potentially inadequate or unbalanced diets involves the basic four food groups. This method may be easily applied by the rehabilitative therapist to determine the possible need for referral for nutrition services to help in planning more nutritious meals for their clients. Foods are divided into the following groups: (1) the milk group, (2) the meat or protein group, (3) the fruit and vegetable group, and (4) the grains group, which includes cereal, pasta, and bread. Another group that is not considered part of the basic four food groups but which contains fat and includes items such as salad dressings, margarine, soda, pie, and so on is called "other." Foods in this category are not recommended to be consumed in excess because they are generally low in nutrients and high in calories. Individuals who consume a variety of food items in each of the four recommended groups will likely (when consuming adequate calories) eat a balanced diet. However, if the therapist notices that any one or more of these groups are continuously omitted from an individual's intake, it may signify an inappropriate diet.

Nutrition in Childhood

After the first year of life, adequate nutrition to support growth and development continues to be just as important despite the relative growth rate decline. The nutrient needs and dietary habits of a 2-year-old are no doubt quite different from those of a 10-year-old. It is well beyond the scope of this chapter to discuss the varying nutritional needs of children; however, we would like to note briefly a few of the more controversial areas in child nutrition. Many children will experience variability in their appetite, particularly as they begin to show interest in their environment, develop relationships with their peers, and display specific food preferences. Although this often creates much anxiety for parents, these behaviors are considered to be normal for most children. It is important to note if the child fails to maintain adequate growth or development, because illness can also contribute to a diminished or a changed appetite.

The issue of hyperactivity in children and possible related dietary causes has been a concern for parents and teachers alike. Both sugar and food additives have been blamed for hyperactive behavior. However, controlled studies to determine its cause and effect have not shown that these two factors contribute to hyperkinetic behavior (Krause and Mahan, 1984). Reviews indicated that these results may be due to a placebo effect or the parents' or teacher's approach to the child's behavior. Continued research in this area is still needed to examine this relationship more closely.

Nutrition in Adolescence

Adolescence is a time of rapid growth characterized by an increase in bone and muscle mass and sexual and psychologic maturity. Adequate nutrition is necessary to support these processes. During this time, there is an increased need for calories, calcium, phosphorus, vitamin D, and iron to promote bone and muscle growth. Calcium, phosphorus, and vitamin D are also needed for bone mineralization and expansion. In girls, the increased need for iron results not only from the expansion of muscle but also from losses associated with the onset of the menses. Because of the great differences in when and to what extent the adolescent growth spurt occurs, it is necessary to evaluate nutrient needs on an individual basis. Additional demands for nutrients, such as strenuous aerobic activity, intensive physical rehabilitation, or pregnancy, may place the adolescent at nutritional risk unless his or her dietary intake is carefully planned to meet these additional needs.

An altered perception of body image in the adolescence period may lead to poor or fad diet practices. Given the importance of a balanced and adequate diet during this time, the practitioner should be aware of any dietary changes that may suggest that an inappropriate diet regimen is being practiced. Of particular concern are two eating disorders: anorexia nervosa and bulimia. According to Appenzeller (1988), an estimated 10 to 15% of adolescent girls and young women may be afflicted with these two eating disorders. Anorexia nervosa is characterized by an intense fear of being fat, with weight loss of at least 25% of original body weight (or the combined percentage) when anticipated weight gain during periods of growth is considered, which is not attributed by any physical illness. The behaviors that these individuals exhibit to promote weight loss may include the abuse of laxatives and diuretics and excessive exercise. When behaviors such as gorging, vomiting, or purging are exhibited, the individual is classified as bulimic. Bulimic individuals are often at or slightly above their ideal body weight and usually are considered to be more mature (e.g., college-age women). Both of these disorders require appropriate dietary intervention in conjunction with psychologic treatment.

Nutrition in the Athlete

One of the surgeon general's 1990 objectives included "appropriate regular physical activity." Appropriate physical exercise is defined as regular physical activity of sufficient duration (e.g., 20 minutes or longer for a minimum of 3 times weekly and intensity of approximately 60% or greater of a person's cardiorespiratory capacity; U.S. Department of Health and Human Services, 1989, 1990).

Exercise, particularly when combined with proper nutrition, has many benefits, including but not limited to the maintenance of ideal body weight, healthy bones, reduced symptoms of anxiety or mild to moderate depression, and lowered risk of developing coronary artery disease. For some diabetics, exercise has been shown to blunt the rise in blood glucose (National Institutes of Health, 1987).

The nutritional needs of athletes are not much different from those of typically healthy individuals. A balanced diet that is adequate in calories (energy) will likely supply all of the necessary nutrients to support optimal athletic performance. The particular energy requirements of athletes are, as with others, influenced by the individual's age, sex, body weight, height, and type and duration of the sport as well as one's level of fitness. The distribution of macronutrients is similar to those suggested by other national and professional organizations (surgeon general's report, American Heart Association, National Cancer Institute). These guidelines recommend that carbohydrates should supply most of the calories in the diet (e.g., 50% to 55% or more; no greater than 30% of total calories should come from fat; and the remainder of the calories, or 15% to 20% should be supplied by proteins). Although carbohydrates, fats, and proteins can all be oxidized for energy, carbohydrates are the only substrate that can be metabolized anaerobically as well as aerobically. Carbohydrates in the form of blood glucose and stored muscle glycogen are used during the first few minutes of exercise. As activity continues, usually beyond 10 minutes, aerobic metabolism, which uses carbohydrates and fat, occurs. The more fit an individual, the more likely he or she is to conserve muscle glycogen stores and thereby oxidize more fat for energy during endurance activities. This could potentially allow athletes to endure longer than others, particularly during competition (American Dietetic Association, 1988; Kris-Etherton, 1989). The type and timing of carbohydrate consumption are still areas of controversy. The consumption of concentrated carbohydrates, also known as simple sugars (such as a candy bar), before an event has, for the most part, been discouraged. This belief stems from the theory that insulin will be released and inhibit free fatty acids and fat for utilization and, therefore, could

cause a greater utilization of muscle glycogen (Hultman et al, 1988). Still others reported no adverse effects related to premature fatigue or decreased performance when this type of carbohydrate is consumed (Ernst and La Rosa, 1988). This difference in opinion may be related to newer information on how quickly specific foods may raise blood glucose levels, known as the glycemic index.

Another popular modification of carbohydrate intake in the athlete is known as carbohydrate loading. This technique depletes and then repletes muscle glycogen stores. It has been used to maximize an athlete's endurance for the reasons described previously. This method of carbohydrate deprivation is no longer recommended and may be dangerous for all individuals, especially with cardiovascular disease and diabetes and the young. The strict deprivation of carbohydrates and replenishment causes retention of water (about 3 grams for every gram of glycogen stored). A more practical approach that stresses consistently high carbohydrate intake and addresses good nutritional behaviors is now preferred. After an exercise event is completed, sufficient carbohydrates are needed to replenish muscle glycogen stores. Because glycogen synthetic rates are approximately 50% higher 2 to 4 hours after an event, this is the optimum time to replenish stores (Kris-Etherton, 1989). If possible, carbohydrate supplementation during exercise with a carbohydrate solution of no greater than 10% sugar may be helpful to spare muscle glycogen and delay fatigue. The protein needs of the athlete should remain at RDA (0.8 g/kg of body weight) or slightly above the (1 g/kg of body weight). Excess protein intake is not necessary and may contribute to hypercalciuria and dehydration. In addition, protein is not as sufficient an energy source as carbohydrates. It requires the removal of nitrogen, in a process called deamination, to first use the carbon chain it is constructed of (for energy). The use of protein supplements or their amino acid building blocks is popular among some athletes and is not warranted for the reasons discussed.

Although often forgotten, water is one of the essential nutrients for life. Its importance during exercise cannot be overemphasized because exercise may blunt one's thirst mechanism, resulting in potentially life-threatening dehydration. Water serves to regulate the body's temperature and is a component of the environment in which nutrients and waste products are transported to and from cells. During exercise, perspiration or the evaporation of sweat serves to cool the body. Electrolytes, such as sodium, potassium, chloride, and magnesium, are dissolved in this perspiration and, with vigorous exercise or in hot weather, may become depleted. When sodium or calcium becomes low, cramping may result. Under circumstances in which the risk of dehydration is high (e.g., marathon events), a solution containing carbohydrates and electrolytes may be beneficial. Many such commercial supplements are now available; however, one should choose them carefully so that a limited amount of carbohydrates (suggested previously) is supplied. According to Loosli (1990), an athlete can determine if he or she is well hydrated by simple monitoring. This includes obtaining a daily weight both before and after workouts. If more than 3% of body weight is lost, dehydration can be suspected. In addition, urine should appear clear throughout most of the day. How much fluid repletion is necessary? As recommended by Loosli (1990), 15 fluid ounces of liquid should be consumed for each pound lost.

The need for vitamins and minerals may be increased in athletes secondary to their role as cofactors in energy metabolism. Despite this increased need, there is probably no need for supplementation if the increased energy needs are supplied by a balanced diet. This would then also supply the extra vitamins and minerals needed. Given the already insufficient intake of iron and calcium for many women and the increased need in adolescents for these two minerals, supplements may be necessary. It is, therefore, important to know the type of activity and the diet of the individual. For example, ballet dancers or gymnasts who may purposely consume a hypocaloric diet for cosmetic reasons may not obtain sufficient amounts of nutrients in their diet to meet their accelerated energy needs; thus, supplementation would be warranted here as well.

Nutrition in the Elderly

Estimating the nutritional needs of the elderly (individuals 65 years and older) is difficult because of the extreme variations in the health, function, and lifestyle of this group. Chronologic age is not a good indicator of the degree of wellness. Thus, an individual assessment of the elderly's health status is necessary. Even when generally grouping cohorts, individuals' needs at 65 years of age differ from those at 80 and 90 years of age. Despite this variation, some general nutritional consequences associated with aging are evident.

As an individual ages, there are changes in his or her body composition, including a decrease in lean body mass (LBM) and an increase in the percentage of body fat (ADA, 1988). This decrease in metabolically active LBM appears to explain some of the decline in metabolic rate and strength seen with aging. Weight gain may result especially when energy needs are reduced without changes in dietary habits. Another related change is a decrease in total body water content (associated with high fat and lower LBM). Elderly men have a total body water content of approximately 52%; in women the total body water content is even lower at approximately 45% (Prendergast, 1988). This becomes a significant issue when one considers such problems as congestive heart failure and chronic renal failure that often develop as one ages. Problems requiring fluid restriction, particularly in the latter example, a malfunctioning thirst mechanism as a result of stroke, or fluid losses iatrogenically induced by diuretics may place these individuals at risk for dehydration or water intoxication. In addition to the aforementioned changes, physiologic changes occur, such as decreased sensations of taste, smell, sight, and hearing. Altered sense perception may interfere with the elderly's ability to obtain and prepare food as well as their desire to consume an adequate and balanced diet (Pritikin and Cisney, 1986). Even if good dietary habits are maintained, normal physiologic changes may suggest a need for alterations in their nutrient requirements. The RDA does not specify nutrient needs for individuals who are 65 years of age and older; rather, it categorizes all healthy individuals 51 years of age and older. This lack of further classification may be due to the lack of data and the wide variations in the nutrient needs of the elderly. Prendergast (1988) suggests that changes such as increasing calcium and vitamin D intake above the RDA level of 800 milligrams to 1500 milligrams may help prevent the development of osteoporosis. The need for an adequate calcium intake of at least the RDA remains especially true for the elderly, because a decrease in hydrochloric acid (associated with normal aging) decreases calcium's bioavailability. This decrease in the stomach's acidity can also inhibit iron absorption.

The levels of other nutrients such as vitamin B_{12} and folate have been noted to be lower in the elderly (Krause and Mahan, 1984; Prendergast, 1988). In the former, a decrease in intrinsic factor secretion may account for the decreased absorption of vitamin B_{12}. An increased need for chromium has been suggested by Solomon (RDA for the Elderly, 1987) and may explain the glucose intolerance characteristic of aging.

The effects that medication may have on ingestion metabolism and excretion can also contribute to less than optimal nutrient levels in the elderly. Because the elderly consume more prescription and over-the-counter medications than other populations, they are at greater risk for experiencing the consequences of drug–nutrient interactions (Blumberg, 1987). Medications may indirectly affect one's nutritional status by causing side effects such as anorexia, changes in taste and smell, and alterations in bowel habits, such as constipation (or exacerbating this condition, which is so prevalent in the elderly). The latter condition may in turn cause a dependency on laxatives and contribute to the subsequent malabsorption of nutrients and induce electrolyte losses. Antacids or H2 blockers, which reduce the stomach's acidity, can decrease the absorption of iron and calcium as previously noted.

In addition to diet, exercise also affects the metabolism of drugs (by increasing the blood flow and muscle organ perfusion altering the drugs' clearance). Again, sufficient data do not exist to specify how exercise affects the nutritional status of the elderly, but one should be aware that a number of factors may jointly affect the elderly's nutrient needs. According to Pelletier (1986) in his reports on centenarians, physical activity via its role in increasing energy expenditure and fat metabolism may help to offset some of the negative effects of a poor diet.

In summary, a balanced diet that is adequate but not excessive in calories and fat, combined with regular physical activity, appears to be beneficial for the elderly. Special concerns, such as the presence of heart disease, physical disabilities, and medications that are used to treat various conditions that are prevalent in the elderly, should all be considered when planning for dietary needs.

Nutrition in the Impaired and Disabled

As noted by Erickson and McPhee (1988), most diseases result in impairment, which is any loss or abnormality of psychologic, physical, or anatomic function. As stressed throughout this chapter, nutrition intervention to prevent or decrease the development of disease and disability is preferred. However, some individuals may be born with impairments, and others will develop them during their lifetime. Optimal wellness for these individuals, including adequate nutrition, should not be overlooked.

The ability to obtain and ingest as well as to metabolize and excrete food is essential to maintaining one's nutritional health. Failure to do so successfully will likely lead to malnutrition. An evaluation of the type of impairment (e.g., mental or physical) and of the modalities used to treat or maintain health is an essential part of the nutritional evaluation process. Knowledge obtained as a result of this assessment helps to minimize any existing or potentially adverse nutritional effects of the disease and its therapy. Ingestion of food depends on the desire for food as well as the physical ability to obtain and process this food. If mental impairment (e.g., injury to the hypothalamus), a central nervous defect, or a mental disability (e.g., severe depression) is present, the physical sensation or expression of hunger may be absent. This subjects an individual to both undernutrition or overnutrition. Once this risk has been identified, as noted by the development of obesity or progressive weight loss, the nutritionist can monitor intake and, if necessary, modify the nutrient composition (such as caloric content) of the individual's diet. When the ability to chew, suck, or swallow (which may manifest as spitting, dribbling, gagging, or vomiting), or the coordination of these activities, is faulty or impaired (such as might occur in individuals with central nervous system or neuromuscular conditions or gross anatomic defects), the amount of food actually ingested or digested is often reduced. In the hospital (i.e., acute-care setting), the consistency and texture of food are often reflected in varied modified menus. In contrast, a school lunch program primarily caters to the healthy school-aged child. The occupational or physical therapist should communicate with the school dietitian so that appropriate and well-balanced food selections can be planned for the children with special needs. In addition, the dietitian can be consulted on how to modify existing products to achieve the desired consistencies and textures. Products are commercially available that will change textures from a thin liquid to a thicker liquid to even a pudding-like consistency. Changes in the consistency or texture of the food, such as the use of a puree (semisolid) diet in the case of neurologic-dysphagia, may result in successful nourishment. However, if these activities are not coordinated with other bodily functions, such as breathing or when a diminished gag reflex results, these individuals may be at serious risk for aspiration. In this situation, an alternate feeding route, such as tube feeding, may need to be considered.

It is just as important not to overlook the available methodologies to foster self-feeding and oral intake when feasible. Encouraging the impaired or disabled to achieve and maintain their optimal level of function is an important aspect of the rehabilitation process. Proper positioning and techniques to improve oral function, such as jaw control, may facilitate ingestion. The use of adaptive equipment, such as cups with projecting rims, plate guards, and specialized utensils, can enhance the act of ingestion as well as self-feeding in suitable individuals and preclude the need for an alternate feeding route.

The rehabilitative health-care specialist needs to be aware of the effects of medications on appetite and nutrient and medication absorption. This is another crucial aspect to planning for the nutritional care of the individual with impairments or disabilities. A common example is the administration of phenytoin (Dilantin) with continuous tube feedings. Clinical reports, such as one noted by (Maynard et al, 1987), indicated that continuous tube feeding interferes with the absorption of this drug. Thus, changing the feeding schedule (e.g., holding the feeding for 1 hour before and after the administration of this drug) or changing to intermittent feeding may assist in the attainment of therapeutic levels.

The process of nutritional assessment not only identifies the problems or potential for problems within this population but also evaluates the nutritional status of these individuals. With this in mind, it is important to be aware of any changes in body composition that occur or that may potentially occur in this population. Muscle atrophy, secondary to disuse, or the absence of anatomic structures will necessitate allowances for differences in weight and body composition when compared with published standards for the healthy population.

Wide variations in energy needs are common, and the type and cause of impairment as well as the time that has elapsed since initial insult will affect caloric needs. When a trauma is sustained, energy needs may increase considerably during the catabolic phases and during rehabilitation. Even relative to a specific disease entity, the energy needs are variable. An example of this situation involves children with cerebral palsy. Those children who have spastic paralysis resulting in limited motion will have substantially lower energy needs than those who have athetoid palsy in which there is involuntary motor activity (Frankle, 1988; Krause and Mahan, 1984).

Ultimately, a balanced diet sufficient in energy needs is desirable. However, any impairment that prevents the selection, obtainment, ingestion, and utilization of nutrients may adversely affect an individual's nutritional well-being.

Nutrition in Musculoskeletal Disorders

Osteoporosis

Osteoporosis is a disorder in which there is a reduction in bone mass. According to researchers Mahan and Arlin (1991) and the National Dairy Council (1989), its development is multifactorial and depends on genetics, hormones, nutrition, and the amount and type of physical activity that one engages in or has engaged in during his or her lifetime. Osteoporosis is more common in women, especially in those who are postmenopausal, as a result of diminished estrogen production. Thus, athletic women who become amenorrheic (possibly resulting from low body weight and fat content, prolonged training, or dietary deficiencies) may place themselves at risk for the early development of osteoporosis. The presence of hormones and the influence of one's genetic makeup is not alterable; however, dietary factors can be changed, such as the amount of calcium and vitamin D that an individual consumes. Therefore, a lifelong regimen of adequate nutrition, particularly adequate calcium (Anderson, 1988) and vitamin D, is important in preventing skeletal loss and the crippling disease of osteoporosis.

Immobilization or lack of weight-bearing activity has also been implicated as a contributing factor in the development of osteoporosis. Studies of individuals restricted to prolonged bed rest or subject to weightlessness, such as experienced by those who are injured or astronauts, have shown resultant bone loss. According to the ADA (1988), regular weight-bearing exercise by young women may prevent this bone loss. In the elderly, exercise 3 times a week for 30 minutes has been shown to increase bone mass. In addition, regular exercise in the elderly may help to prevent falls, which often lead to fractures for those at risk. Exercise has also been postulated to promote the stimulation necessary for maintenance of calcium in bony areas and is thought to increase the dietary effectiveness of calcium utilization.

Arthritis

Arthritis can be simplistically defined as an inflammation of the joints. The two most common forms include rheumatoid arthritis and osteoarthritis (also known as degenerative arthritis). The gastrointestinal and micronutrient disorders in rheumatoid arthritis are beyond the scope of this chapter; however, the need for adequate and balanced nutrition is important in promoting recovery or improving treatment. Of potential concern in the rheumatoid group of arthritics is the ability to prepare food and self-feed especially when the hands are involved. Osteoarthritis is the most common form of arthritis and usually affects the weight-bearing joints. Prevention of obesity or weight reduction avoids or reduces the stress placed on joints. It is particularly challenging to promote weight loss in individuals with osteoarthritis, because of the inability for most to incorporate regular physical exercise into their daily routines. This inactivity may be a direct result of painful joints, although

exercise may also alleviate pain. Pain may not only limit physical activity in these individuals but, when severe, may in and of itself, or as a result of medications taken to provide relief, cause anorexia. For individuals who are already at or below their suggested weights, this may place them at even greater risk of malnutrition.

GOAL-ACHIEVEMENT PHASE

The goal-achievement phase of program development is the intervention or implementation process of executing the plan. It is the action or the setting in motion of all the hard work of assessing and planning. The types of intervention modalities that should be used will depend on both the specific objectives to be achieved as well as the resources of the program. They will also depend on the type of care needed. As shown in Figure 18–5, individual nutritional intervention modalities include varying degrees of nutritional counseling, nutrition education, and referrals that are provided over a given time period to produce a measurable outcome (Owen, 1984).

Nutrition Counseling

Nutrition counseling is the provision of advice and services to individuals or groups to meet the goals of nutrition intervention for disease man-

Figure 18–5. Phase 2: Facets of goal-achievement phase.

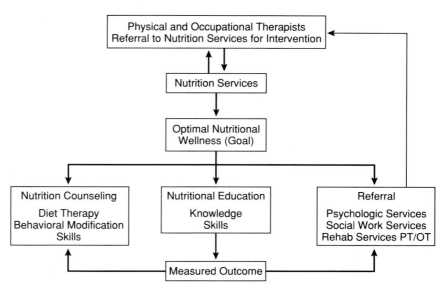

agement or prevention (ADA, 1985). Nutrition counseling often includes diet counseling, which is defined by Caliendo (1981) as nutrition advice with the specific purpose of helping individuals modify their food intake in accordance with their health-care needs. Over the last decade, behavioral modification has become an important adjunct to nutrition counseling and, therefore, should be included in this treatment category.

Nutrition Education

Nutrition education is the process by which beliefs, attitudes, environmental influences, and understanding about food lead to practices that are scientifically sound, practical, and consistent with individual needs and available food resources (Caliendo, 1981). Nutrition education is often used in conjunction with nutrition counseling to affect individuals' dietary habits that are considered to be in need of change.

Referral System

Establishing a referral system (other than for nutrition support services) is a necessary component of intervention, because individuals' needs will vary and may require the involvement of other health-care professionals or services. Referrals provide quality care by allowing the most qualified individuals to give their attention to specific problem areas. Examples of typical referrals in a nutrition program include food stamps, a meals-on-wheels program, and the Women, Infants and Children assistance program for the socioeconomically disadvantaged. Other types of referrals include individual referrals to a psychologist for further exploration or treatment of problems that may be interfering with the adaptation of favorable behaviors (which may lead to noncompliance or relapses) and referrals to a physician for further work-up, diagnostic tests, or a medical assessment of current problems, rehabilitation services, and so on. It is the counselor's and program's responsibility to coordinate such referrals and to obtain feedback from referral sources. Ultimately, this referral system, with its important feedback and communication network, should foster continuity of care as well as a team approach to the management of individuals' health-care needs.

PROGRAM-MAINTENANCE PHASE

The third phase of a comprehensive program for nutrition services is the program-maintenance phase. Figure 18–6 illustrates the three separate yet interrelated components of the program-maintenance phase of a nutritional program. The model includes:

1. An outcome-oriented program evaluation of goal and task achievements
2. A self-regulatory and self-evaluation component, which includes a process-oriented approach (e.g., group methodology and dynamics)
3. A consumer compliance and satisfaction component, which examines client adherence to and approval of program goals and objectives

Outcome-Oriented Program Evaluation

One of the most important aspects of any program is its capability to be measured or evaluated (i.e., to determine the program's outcome, its worth, and value). Through monitoring and data-collection activities, individual programs and parent agencies can effectively examine what it is that they are doing (outcome), how they are doing it (process), and whether or not it makes a difference. This process is the hallmark ingredient of quality management. It represents and involves the on-going vigilance of the provision of care, serves as a mechanism for the identification of deficiencies, and facilitates subsequent corrective or innovative actions.

Vigilant or watchful provision of care requires systematic monitoring of services and the subsequent related outcome. A program offering for the obese client requires measurement not only of individual objectives, such as percentage of individual weight loss, but also subsequent related population outcome (e.g., percentage of clients losing a certain set percentage of weight). The easiest outcome-oriented evaluation method simply answers the question, "Does the program accomplish what it set out to do and is the outcome worth the cost?" In this case, if the number of clients who lose a significant amount of weight is less than the predetermined standard, the program presently being offered is not worthwhile and thus not worth the cost outlay. The program outcome evaluation at this time would recommend that the nutritional offering be discontinued or revised.

Figure 18–6. Phase 3: Components of the maintenance phase of a nutrition program within a parent agency.

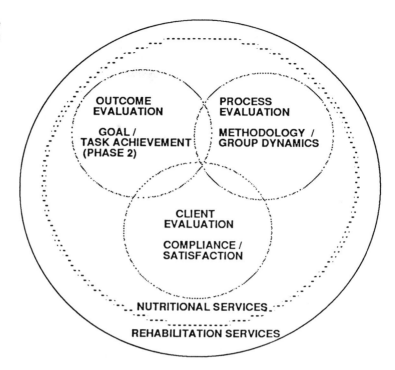

During the evaluation process, program outcomes are examined to identify deficiencies. Outcomes may be favorable or unfavorable and may provide insight into emergent needs. The favorable outcomes help to solidify aspects of the program that are successful. The unfavorable outcomes or the identification of deficiencies allow one to re-evaluate, adjust, or change population or program needs. Thus, new ideas are generated and a new needs assessment is identified. Percentage-based weight loss, behavior modification, and the lowering of a client's cholesterol level and blood pressure by a specified margin over a certain time frame are examples of positive outcomes of dietary intervention. If individualized goals or objectives such as these cannot be met (e.g., the normalization of serum cholesterol within a certain time frame), corrective and more realistic objectives may need to be formulated. Examples include the adjustment of existing time frames and the use of referrals at an earlier point in time.

Program data related to client participation (e.g., high attendance at program educational offerings or at dietary clinic services) may demonstrate favorable outcomes for the program. If an unfavorable outcome (e.g., poor attendance to program offerings) was determined, a new needs assessment might include a strong marketing component.

Self-Evaluative Component

Self-regulatory or self-maintenance issues of the health-care team and the program itself should also be included as part of the program-evaluation process. The scope of nutritional care should be delineated, and appropriately trained staff should be assigned to specific related responsibilities. What treatments and activities are performed? The threshold for staff compliance and functioning should be realistically and collaboratively set by both management and the staff involved. Did staff fulfill their responsibilities? If so, were they achieved in a timely manner? If possible, staff should self-monitor and self-evaluate their own ability to achieve what it is they set out to do. This increases staff sensitivity to program goals and objectives, outcomes, and subsequent needs. In this manner, problems or methods by which care or performance may be improved can be identified. In addition, results of the analysis of patterns or trends of care can contribute to the formulation of an action plan to continue, restructure, or cancel the current methodology as designed.

Group-interaction skills are an important part of this process. Frequent interaction between staff and management will validate the fact that each member can make a difference. The most difficult aspect of staff participation is in allocating time to group communication or process. This time-consuming activity is well worth the effort, however, because staff input significantly improves staff compliance.

Consumer-Oriented Component

The third interrelated component of the program-maintenance phase is consumer satisfaction and compliance. Programmatically useful information related to satisfaction toward the nutrition education and counseling given and the response to referral services is essential for a well-designed nutritional offering. A Likert-type scale questionnaire is one example of an instrument used to measure consumer attitude (satisfaction). Consumer concerns specific to technical and financial aspects can also be identified in this manner. An extensive waiting time for dietary counseling and a perceived costly fee-for-service program are two such examples of identifiable problems. Consumer evaluation contributes to the identification of program deficiencies, assists in the development of new needs assessment, and generates the input necessary for innovative program changes.

As previously mentioned, each aspect of a program-evaluation component must include a method of measuring the degree to which an outcome is favorable. This may be difficult to perform without a systematic approach to identify what is favorable or unfavorable to a significant degree. At what point does the favorable outcome indicate program effectiveness? How can this be accurately measured? The answer is obtained with meticulous monitoring and evaluating of the nutritional services provided. This provides a science of exactness and serves as an important link between product and effectiveness. This accurate measurement process is extremely important to the success of any quality management program and is appropriately titled quality assurance.

Quality Assurance

A quality assurance system is inherent within and the core component of an evaluation process. It is the key element to quality management. Kaufman (1980) defined quality assurance as the certification of continuous, effective, and efficient care. The goal of a quality assurance system within a nutritional care program is to improve nutritional health-care services. Whether nutrition services are being provided as a part of an existing rehabilitation service or via an outside source, a measure of its effectiveness and value to the organization is necessary. In either case, the actual documentation of the importance and value of such services to the organization will likely result in continued funding and political support for its operations.

The development of objective evaluation measures (indicators) is crucial to an effective quality assurance program. The indicator, whether at the individual level or at the organizational level, must be based on and appropriate for the program developed and the community or population to be served. Selected predetermined indicators (criteria) should be in accordance with the program's specific objectives. Criteria should be well defined, well developed, scientifically sound if possible, and based on professional standards. The basic elements important to consider when developing effective quality assurance indicators are:

1. Relevance. Indicators should be appropriate for the program goals and objectives. They should answer the question, "Is the program relevant and effective?" Because monitoring can be time consuming, indicators should be based on those aspects that are crucial to the program. Examples include nutrition screening, assessment and planning, educational offerings, counseling, and referral aspects. Community significance, such as cultural and ethnic factors and their interrelationship with socioeconomic factors, also needs to be considered.
2. Validity. Another aspect to consider is the validity of the criteria (i.e., it measures what it purports to). If one is interested in obtaining outcome of nutritional intervention, the criteria should be specific for the intervention being instituted. An example is the measurement of the reduction of cardiac risk as defined by a total cholesterol level. The ratio of HDL to LDL levels is a more valid indicator of cardiac risk.
3. Research based. Indicators must be based on predetermined elements of quality care. This

should reflect recent trends, current acceptable research in the literature, and professional standards of care.

4. Measurable. Indicators should be quantifiable. Key questions include, "Are indicators measurable? If so, in what way?" For example, should serum cholesterol levels be measured to meet normal levels by a certain time frame or should levels be lowered by X per cent? In addition, what percentage of clients have met the standard? The minimal number of clients expected to meet that standard is known as a threshold.

5. Realistic. Is the threshold set at an achievable level of compliance? A threshold percentage can assist in determining if intensive attention to a particular problem is needed. An indicator related to the lowering of serum cholesterol levels to within normal limits within 1 month's time may be set at 97%. This means that an intensive evaluation of the appropriateness of care given through the nutritional offering would be made. It may be that the threshold for lowering cholesterol levels to normal limits is unachievable in a specific population; thus, the percentage of clients who meet this criteria is much lower than previously anticipated.

6. Limitations. Limitations should include a time frame for achievement. Acceptable time limits for a desirable outcome may be measured in days, months, or, in the case of the organization or program, years. For example, a decrease of total serum cholesterol level by 10% within 3 months would not only meet the criteria but would do so within an established time frame. Another limitation to consider when establishing criteria is available resources. Staff numbers and availability as well as financial constraints diminish outcome capability.

7. Exceptions. Acceptable justifications for not meeting criteria may exist and should be identified. For example, a diagnosis of untreated hypothyroidism would interfere with weight loss and, thus, the expected standard.

Feedback

Communication of quality assurance findings, related to all three aspects of the valuative processes within the program-maintenance phase, should be made to the parent agency (such as a rehabilitative service) to identify trends or performance patterns that could assist in organiza-

tional and credentialing decisions. Outcome data can also be compared at this time both with past performance of the nutritional program as well as with other comparable nutritional programs.

Summary

The importance of nutrition in promoting health is realized to a greater extent each year. Combined with the rising costs of health care, the challenge to provide optimal health-care services to the public is difficult and the consequences of its failure are serious. Throughout this chapter, the need for adequate planning in an organized and step-like manner has been stressed to ensure comprehensive and effective programs. The establishment of goals and objectives and the formulation of a program plan that fosters mutual satisfaction have been outlined in the sections related to nutrition assessment. The integration of goals with the services to be provided and the specific types of intervention strategies available have been described. The successful implementation of any program should be heralded as such and enjoyed by all who were involved. Thus, measurement of the success of a program through an evaluation component will help to maintain desirable program function and continue to ensure its success. Given the statistics of an increasingly aging population, rehabilitation and promotion of wellness, particularly in the golden years, will continue to be a health-care concern in the United States. Providing individuals with the necessary information and skills to foster wellness will promote an optimal quality of life. It is, therefore, the duty of health-care professionals to ensure that they have sought to include services such as nutrition that will enable individuals to meet this challenge to the best of their abilities.

Case History
Part I (Sample Program). Health U.S.A. is a comprehensive medical plaza in the suburbs of a large metropolitan area. Recently, the organization revised its mission to better serve the needs of the community in which it is situated. The community is comprised primarily of individuals in the middle- and upper-middle-class socioeconimic strata. Most of the population commutes to the city where they are employed.

During the process of revising the medical plaza's mission, the local health department noted that the population had an usually high incidence of the nation's chronic diseases, in particular, coronary artery disease (CAD).

Health U.S.A. decided it would focus on health promotion and the prevention of these chronic diseases, especially CAD. As part of this overall program, an expansion in the nutrition services was recommended because nutritional factors are known to affect many chronic diseases. Of note were reports of increased revenues in other institutions incorporating nutrition services, especially those providing weight-reduction programs. The director of Health U.S.A.: Nutrition Services was asked to submit a proposal for this expansion. After discussing how to market its new services to the community with its public relations division, Health U.S.A. decided to sponsor a community health fair. For individuals who desired prevention or treatment, Health U.S.A. would provide a referral to the appropriate services.

Part II (Individual). M.L. is a 38-year-old man who is employed as a financial planner for a major corporation. Recently, M.L.'s father suffered his second heart attack, and M.L. decided to have his cholesterol level screened at a community health fair (Health U.S.A.) to determine if he should modify his current lifestyle to prevent his chances of developing heart disease. At this fair M.L. was told that his total cholesterol level was 237 mg/dl, which is borderline high. M.L. was referred to his private physician and Nutrition Services Inc. for follow-up and appropriate intervention.

At his first visit to Health U.S.A.: Nutrition Services, M.L. was screened for nutritional risk. Nutrition risk was defined by this organization as a body weight of greater than 120% or less than 90% of ideal body weight, a total cholesterol level above 200 mg/dl, or three or more negative factors influencing nutritional status as noted on the nutritional assessment form. M.L. was noted to be at nutritional risk because his weight was 132% of his ideal weight and his blood cholesterol level exceeded 200 mg/dl.

Because M.L. was placed at nutritional risk, he was referred to a credentialed nutritionist for a comprehensive nutritional assessment. The need for a comprehensive assessment was to obtain a detailed analysis of M.L.'s dietary habits to individually plan for his care. Because M.L. was already at risk, intervention and modification of undesirable eating habit, as well as encouragement of continued healthful practices would be needed. The comprehensive nutritional assessment included a more detailed interview with M.L.; a diet history (typical day recall and a food frequency questionnaire); and a review of the goals that M.L. wished to achieve from his visits. The degree of importance that he placed on each goal (i.e., a ranking of his

goals) was also obtained to consider the client's priorities when designing intervention strategies. In addition, M.L. was asked to keep a food and exercise diary for 1 week. This would assist in determining day-to-day variations in his eating habits and identify significant lifestyle behaviors that affect his dietary intake.

Following the collection of all pertinent data, an analysis or assessment is made to determine an individual's nutritional status and to formulate specific goals for desired outcomes. In this case, a nutrient intake analysis of M.L.'s diet history revealed that he consumed approximately 2,500 calories per day. This is approximately 275 calories above his estimated energy needs (2,225 calories/day) to maintain his current body weight. Given this excess in caloric intake over M.L.'s estimated energy expenditure, M.L. would be expected to continue to gain weight at a rate of approximately 1 pound every 12 days unless he makes appropriate dietary changes. In addition, M.L.'s distribution of nutrient intake is an important factor in predicting the dietary risk factors for the development of coronary heart disease. Of particular interest are the type and total percentage of fat consumed. The results of M.L.'s intake show that he consumes approximately 40% of his calories from fat, 27% from protein, and only 33% from carbohydrates. This is clearly outside of the recommendations for a healthy diet, which suggest a reduction of the total amount of fat to no more than 30%, reduction of protein to 15%, and an increase in the amount of carbohydrates to 55%. In M.L.'s analysis, 16% of his total calories are contributed by saturated fat, 18.8% from monounsaturated fat, and only 5% from polyunsaturated fat. The National Institutes of Health, in its recommendations for the treatment of high serum cholesterol, suggests that the total amount of saturated fat in one's diet not exceed 10% of total caloric intake. M.L. consumed his breakfast at home. For lunch, he would send out for a sandwich or, time permitting, eat in the executive dining room. Dinner would be consumed either at home or, occasionally, in his office.

Excess calories, a high intake of saturated fat, and little physical activity have likely contributed to M.L.'s obesity. This places him at risk for the development of heart disease as well as other chronic diseases. The clinician's recommendations for M.L. included reducing his total caloric intake. A reduction in his total cholesterol intake and fat, especially saturated fat, may be necessary at a later point in time. Reducing the total caloric intake would likely limit portion sizes and, therefore, reduce fat intake as well. In addition, encouraging M.L. to participate in mild to moderate physical activity is important to the overall diet program. The benefit of regular physical activity for M.L. was multifactorial and included increased energy expenditure, maintenance of muscle mass during caloric deprivation, its positive effect on metabolic rate, and the sense of well-being that exercise often promotes. As indicated by Apenzeller (1988), exercise has been shown to raise the HDL cholesterol level. This has a protective effect in the development of cardiovascular disease independent of the effect of weight reduction but is additive when the two are done in conjunction.

During the in-depth interview with M.L., it was revealed that he had suffered an injury to his right knee a few years ago while playing basketball. He noted occasional pain particularly when he engaged in strenuous activities. As a result, he has not actively participated in such activities. At present, M.L. denies pain or physical restrictions. M.L.'s personal physician indicated that M.L. most likely had osteoarthritis of the right knee secondary to an injury he sustained. Activity has not been restricted, and in fact weight reduction has been recommended recently to relieve the stress to his joints.

A review of M.L.'s activity log revealed a mostly sedentary lifestyle. M.L. stated that because of his long hours at work he really did not have time to exercise.

Another factor relevant to M.L.'s dietary habits was a pattern of stress-induced eating. This was not noted in the dietary recall but was seen on his diet diary. This stress eating often occurred before an important meeting or at night after a particularly stressful day.

At M.L.'s follow-up appointment, the results of his nutritional assessment were discussed. M.L.'s goals were compared with those outlined by his nutritionist. With client and nutritionist working together, a nutritional care plan outlining the specific intervention strategies and how they were to be achieved was made. In addition, a time limit was negotiated for the achievement of the various goals. M.L. was to be responsible for adhering to his dietary plan and for notifying the counselor of difficulties during this process. The counselor was responsible for providing M.L. with the knowledge and skills necessary for implementing the plan. When necessary, and with the client's approval, outside referrals would be made.

When M.L. returned for his follow-up visit, the results of his nutritional assessment and history were discussed with him. M.L.'s goals were reviewed and compared with those originally set. Goals identified by both parties as a high priority and which M.L. felt he could comfortably begin to incorporate into his lifestyle would be the focus of the first counseling and educational session.

Part III (Nutritional Care Planning). The goal-oriented nutritional care planning follows.

CLIENT-DIRECTED GOALS
1. Reduce serum cholesterol
2. Weight reduction (M.L. would like to weigh 160 lb)
3. Reduce fatigue

THERAPIST-DIRECTED GOALS
1. Promote healthful dietary habits that the client can easily incorporate into his lifestyle and maintain
2. Lower M.L.'s total serum cholesterol to less than or equal to 200 mg/dl while increasing the proportion of HDL cholesterol to LDL cholesterol
3. Promote the achievement of client's desirable (ideal) body weight
4. Promote regular physical activity and reduce fatigue

OUTCOME-ORIENTED BEHAVIORAL OBJECTIVES
1. M.L. will demonstrate an understanding of the relationship between his diet and the risk for developing heart disease by verbalizing those factors in his intake analysis that may promote hypercholesterolemia.
2. M.L. will have a 10% reduction in his total serum cholesterol within 3 months by adhering to his dietary plan.
3. M.L. will lose 4 to 8 lbs/month by adhering to his dietary plan. Adherence to dietary plan will be aided by measured weight loss as well as dietary recalls and diaries collected during this time.
4. M.L. will engage in a physical activity of his choice for a minimum of 30 minutes' duration at least 3 times per week.

INTERVENTION STRATEGIES FOR ACHIEVEMENT OF BEHAVIORAL OBJECTIVES
1. M.L. will receive nutrition education on the relationship between diet and heart disease with specific information on how total fat, cholesterol, type of fat, and other dietary factors can be modified.
2. M.L. will receive individualized diet counseling to address the specific aspects of his diet that contribute to his elevated serum cholesterol. Specific recommendations that meet with M.L.'s approval will be emphasized for trial. Behavior modification techniques and exercises will be presented to ensure compliance.
3. After behavioral modification techniques have been implemented, M.L. will sustain his weight loss.
4. M.L. will be referred to rehabilitative services for an individualized exercise plan and for evaluation of his right-knee osteoarthritis. M.L. will be instructed on how to find his target pulse during exercise.

PROCESS-ORIENTED BEHAVIORAL OBJECTIVES

1. The manner in which staff provides care will be evaluated using a set of identified, positive patterns of performance.
2. Effective group dynamics will be evaluated using a standardized group process skill check.
3. The methodology by which problems are resolved will be reviewed to determine efficiency and effectiveness.

INTERVENTION STRATEGIES FOR ACHIEVEMENT OF PROCESS-ORIENTED OBJECTIVES

1. Methods to measure the manner in which care is provided may include (1) record keeping by nutritional care staff to monitor and evaluate their own practice; (2) peer review using a survey tool that measures key areas of patient care as defined by Joint Committee on Accreditation of Health Care Organizations (JCAHO) guidelines; and (3) review of staff performance appraisals by management for areas related to professionalism and communication with clients and colleagues. A summary of findings will be reported semiannually to the parent agency.
2. Tools designed to measure the staff group processes and problem-solving abilities, such as the Phases of Integrated Problem Solving (Morris and Sashkin, 1987) and tools to assess an individual staff member's behavior in conflict situations, such as the use of the Thomas-Kilmann Conflict Mode Instrument (Thomas and Kilmann, 1974), will be used.
3. A systems analysis will be performed semiannually to evaluate methodology practices for problem resolution.

CLIENT SATISFACTION AND COMPLIANCE BEHAVIORAL OBJECTIVES

1. M.L. will show satisfaction with the nutrition services provided as exhibited by an average score of 3 or more on a Likert-type satisfaction survey.
2. M.L. will be compliant to the behavioral objectives and mutual goals established by himself and the nutritional care facility.

INTERVENTION STRATEGIES FOR ACHIEVING CLIENT SATISFACTION AND COMPLIANCE OBJECTIVES

1. A Likert-type survey will be completed at 8 weeks and again at M.L.'s exit from the program.
2. A review of outcome-oriented data will identify compliant as well as noncompliant consumers. An open-ended questionnaire will be completed 8 weeks into the program. An assessment of rationale for noncompliant clients will be made by both client and staff member to reset goals.

References

American Dietetic Association: Nutrition services payment system guidelines for interpretation. Chicago, State, American Dietetic Association, 1985.

American Dietetic Association: Sports nutrition. A guide for the professional working with active people. Chicago, American Dietetic Association, 1988.

Anderson JJB: Diet, activity, and bone status in women. Nutr M.D. 14(10):1–3, 1988.

Appenzeller O: Sports Medicine Fitness. Training. Injuries, 3rd ed. Baltimore, MD, Urban and Schwarzenberg, 1988.

Blumberg JB: Drug-induced malnutrition in the geriatric patient. Nutr M.D. 13(8):1–3, 1987.

Caliendo MA: Nutrition and Preventive Health Care. New York, Macmillan, 1981.

Erickson RP and McPhee MC: Clinical evaluation. In Delisa JA (ed): Rehabilitative Medicine. Principles and Practice. Philadelphia, JB Lippincott, 1988.

Ernst ND and La Rosa JC: Recommendations for treatment of high blood cholesterol. The national cholesterol education program adult treatment panel. Contemp Nutr 13(1):1–2, 1988.

Food and Nutrition Board: Recommended Dietary Allowances, 10th ed. Washington, DC, National Academy of Sciences, National Research Council, 1989.

Frankle DL: Nutrition. In DeLisa JA (ed): Rehabilitative Medicine. Principles and Practice. Philadelphia, JB Lippincott, 1988.

Hultman E, Thompson JA, and Harris RC: Work and exercise. In Shils and Young (eds): Modern Nutrition in Health and Disease, 7th ed. Philadelphia, Lea & Febiger, 1988.

Hyman HH: Implementing Institutional Objectives. Rockville, MD, Aspen Systems Corp, 1984.

Kaufman M: Preliminary Guide to Quality Assurance in Ambulatory Nutrition Care. Rockville, MD, Child Health Service Bureau of Community Health Services, 1980.

Kris-Etherton PM: Nutrition and athletic performance. Contemp Nutr 14(8):1–2, 1989.

Loosli AR: Athletes, food and nutrition. Food Nutr News 62(3), 1990.

Mahan LK and Arlin MT (eds): Krause's Food, Nutrition, and Diet Therapy, 8th ed. Philadelphia, WB Saunders, 1991.

Marge M: Health promotion for persons with disabilities: Moving beyond rehabilitation. Am J Health Prom 12(4):29–35, 1988.

Morris WC and Sashkin M: Phases of Integrated Problem Solving (PIPS). University Associates, Inc, 1987.

National Dairy Council: Nutrition and a physically active lifestyle. Dairy Council Digest 60(4):19–24, 1989.

National Institutes of Health: Consensus development conference on diet and exercise in non-insulin dependent diabetes mellitus. Diabetes Care 10(5):639–644, 1987.

O'Connor T: Dietary fat, colonies and cancer. Contemp Nutr 10(7):1–2, 1985.

Owen A: Planning and evaluating nutrition services to ensure quality. In Simko MD, Cowell C, and Gilbride JA (eds): Nutritional Assessment: A Comprehensive Guide for Planning Intervention. Rockville, MD, Aspen Systems Corp, 1984.

Pelletier KR: Longevity: What centenarians teach us? In Dychwald K (ed): Wellness and Health Promotion in the Elderly. MD, Aspen, 1986.

Prendergast JM: Nutritional status of the elderly. In Delafuente JC and Stewart RB (eds): Therapeutics in the Elderly (pp. 196–209). Baltimore, MD, Williams & Wilkins, 1988.

Pritikin N and Cisney N: Dietary recommendations for older Americans. *In* Dychtwald K (ed): Wellness and Health Promotion for the Elderly. Rockville, MD, Aspen, 1986.

Public Health Reports: Nutrition services in state and local public health agencies. Pub Health Rep *98*(1):7–10, 1983.

Puhl J: Iron and exercise interactions. Contemp Nutr *12*(2):1–2, 1989.

RDA for the elderly: Nutr M.D. *13*(8):3, 1987.

Ross Laboratories: Dietary Modifications in Disease: Mental and Physical Disabilities. Columbus, OH, Ross Laboratories.

Simko MD, Cowell C, and Gilbride JA: A systems approach to planning nutrition intervention programs. *In* Simko MD, Cowell C, and Gilbride JA (eds): Nutrition Assessment: A Comprehensive Guide for Planning Intervention. Rockville, MD, Aspen Systems Corp, 1984.

Stuff JE, Garza C, Smith EO, et al: A comparison of dietary methods in nutritional studies. Am J Clin Nutr *37*:300–306, 1983.

Teague ML, Cipriano RE, and McGhee VL: Health promotion as a rehabilitative service for people with disabilities. J Rehabil *56*(1):52–56, 1990.

Thomas KW and Kilmann RH: Thomas-Kilmann Conflict Mode Instrument. Tuxedo, NY, Xicom, Inc, 1974.

Trieber FA, Leonard SB, Frank G, et al: Dietary assessment instruments for pre-school children: Reliability of parental responses to the 24 hour recall and a food frequency questionnaire. J Am Diet Assoc *90*(6):814–820, 1990.

U.S. Department of Health and Human Services: Health United States 1989, DHHS Pub. No. (PHS) 90–1232. Hyattsville, MD, U.S. Department of Health and Human Services, 1990.

U.S. Department of Health and Human Services: Surgeon General's Report: Promoting Health-Preventing Disease, 1990 Objectives for the Nation. Washington, DC, U.S. Public Health Service, National Institutes of Health, 1988.

U.S. Department of Health and Human Services: An Update Report on Nutrition Monitoring, DHHS Pub. No. (PHS) 89–1255. MD, U.S. Department of Health and Human Services, 1989.

C H A P T E R

19

Susan Morrill

Holistic Stress Management

The four goals of this chapter on holistic stress management are as follows:

1. To explain the principles of holistic stress management in a meaningful and practical way for health-care practitioners
2. To teach the reader how to develop, design, and implement a holistic stress-management program
3. To encourage creativity among health-care providers who are integrating holistic stress management techniques into a particular clinical setting
4. To share some of the results and insights that clients have discovered through participating in holistic stress-management programs

It is suggested that health-care practitioners who have a desire to develop holistic stress-management programs in the clinical setting begin first by developing a stress-management program for themselves. Personal experience with a holistic stress-management program can magnify its success in the clinical setting. Clinicians could start a holistic stress-management pilot program with a small group of clients or peers before implementing a large-scale program. This idea is discussed later in the chapter. Now the terms *holism, stress management,* and *holistic stress management* are discussed.

HOLISM

Holism is a philosophy or attitude that life is viewed in terms of how each piece adds to the wholeness of a system. In the holistic model, the whole of the organism is greater than the sum of its parts. As Oberteuffer said, "the person who cannot be divided, is not divided. The fact is that a person is a whole, is one, a psychophysical organism capable of reacting in many ways to the many and various stimuli to which one is exposed in the course of a lifetime" (Oberteuffer, 1968, p. 4).

In the holistic model, health is viewed as an expression of each person functioning as an integrated whole, a totality of body, mind, and spirit (Brallier, 1982; Cmich, 1984; Dossey et al, 1989; Tubesing, 1979). Holistic health is oriented to the person rather than to the disease or symptom (Flynne, 1980). The holistic movement emphasizes individual responsibility for health maintenance and supports a team approach in working with a person who has an illness. The client and the health-care professional have dual input and together create goals so that the client can achieve the greatest degree of health or well-being possible. Holistic health includes dimensions such as self-responsibility, nutritional awareness, physical fitness, stress management, and environmental sensitivity (Ardell, 1982). One type of holistic model is discussed in detail later in this chapter.

STRESS MANAGEMENT

We hear about stress on a regular basis through television, radio, books, newspapers, and movies. Witkin (1985) maintained that "stress can be responsible for high blood pressure and low blood pressure, for overeating and loss of appetite; for fatigue and hyperactivity; for talkativeness and withdrawal; for hot and cold chills. We are advised that under stress we are more susceptible to infection, depression, accidents, viruses, colds, heart attacks, and even cancer. We are stress conscious and stress concerned. We are not, however, sufficiently stress educated (Witkin, 1985, p. 1).

From a health-care perspective, it is important to educate ourselves and our clients about stress and to teach them specific tools that will assist in the management of stress. Stress is the nonspecific response of the body to any demand placed on it (Selye, 1974). It is immaterial whether the agent we face is pleasant or unpleasant; all that counts is the intensity of the demand for readjustment or adaptation (Selye, 1974).

The body automatically goes into a fight or flight pattern when a potential stressor is perceived by the individual. This fight or flight response is appropriate in certain instances such as avoiding a car accident, defending oneself in combat, or any other survival-based incident. However, we do not need such a strong physical reaction under less stressful situations. What we do need is education in how to make behavioral changes that will alert us about our stress level so that we may prevent triggering strong stress responses or, once triggered, learn how to decrease the stress immediately. This is the basis for traditional stress management. Learning to channel the energy that is available from a stress arousal state into a creative endeavor is highly rewarding as well as health saving (Brallier, 1982). When people do not manage stress effectively or have chronic stress behavior, the effects

are numerous. Some of the physical effects include elevated blood and urine catecholamines and corticosteroids; increased blood glucose, heart rate, and blood pressure; shallow breathing; numbness; tingling and coldness in the extremities; queasy stomach; tight muscles; back head pain; dry mouth; and sweating (Jaffe and Scott, 1984). Other effects of stress range from severe depression and anxiety to job burnout and substance addiction (Brallier, 1982; Cmich, 1984; Cooper, 1989; Flynne, 1980; Jaffe and Scott, 1984). It is therefore essential for health-care practitioners to become educated in stress management to facilitate health in their clients.

HOLISTIC STRESS MANAGEMENT

Holistic stress management incorporates the principles of holism as its foundation. In this section we examine the physical, mental, emotional, and spiritual levels as the keystones to the holistic model. The model used in this chapter is an adaptation of a holistic model developed by Drs. Ron and Mary Hulnick, President and Vice president, respectively, of the University of Santa Monica, California. It was chosen as an exemplary holistic stress-management model that is easily adapted into a clinical setting.

The first level of this model is the *physical level*. This level includes the physical body as well as the physical environment. Issues to study in this level include health habits, relationships, living environment, work environment, and leisure activity (Table 19–1).

The second level of this holistic model is the *mental level*. This level involves all of the thoughts, judgments, beliefs, and attitudes about ourself and others. The mental level includes

Table 19–1. Components of the Physical Level of the Holistic Stress-Management Model

Component	Description
Physical health and health habits	Overall physical health, nutrition, exercise, sexuality, habits or addictions (smoking, drinking, drugs, food and exercise addictions, and so on), sleeping patterns, health-awareness issues (routine physicals, obstetric-gynecologic visits, dental visits), energy level for activities of daily living
Relationships	Includes all relationships with family, friends, neighbors, co-workers, health-care providers, teachers, and so on
Living environment	Includes the location of the home, type of home, inner home environment (space factors, cleanliness, toxic factors [radon, water quality]) and outer environment (pollution, noise, crowdedness)
Work environment	Includes type of employment, hours of employment, work satisfaction
Leisure activity	Includes all leisure activities (e.g., relaxation, entertainment, laughter and spontaneous play, hobbies)

such concepts as imagination, creativity, decision making, mental awareness and clarity, and internal dialogue.

The third level is the *emotional level*. This involves the feeling state of an individual at a particular time. It also relates to a person's ability to express his or her feelings openly with self and with others. The emotional range is unlimited and spans from the most comfortable emotions (love, joy, peace) to the most uncomfortable ones (despair, isolation, rage). This level includes a person's ability to accept emotions as part of life. It also includes appropriately sharing feelings with others, listening to and understanding others' feelings, trusting one's feelings, and following natural intuition in difficult situations.

The fourth level of this model is the *spiritual level*. This level involves the concept of a person's connection with the world. This connection can be expressed, for example, as a connection with nature, life, or God. It is a highly individual choice. To some this level "involves the development of the Higher Self—the transpersonal self. The experience of transcendence is described as a feeling of oneness, inner peace, harmony and wholeness and connection with the universe" (Dossey et al, 1989, p. 15). This level includes concepts such as living life with a sense of direction and meaning, sharing a sense of connection by service to others, and feeling protected by a source greater than oneself.

By understanding the dynamics of this holistic model, we can begin to identify areas in the four levels that may be out of balance. This can assist us as health-care providers in developing individual programs for clients who are suffering from stress at any level. According to the Hulnick model, we can view health as a continuum, with a balance point B representing the line of homeostasis of the person (Fig. 19–1). The line pulls us in two directions: toward a positive polarity of optimal health or in a negative polarity away from balance and optimal health. *Positive* and *negative* refer only to direction. We can then chart where we are on the health continuum on each level of the holistic model. Figure 19–1 gives examples of negative and positive polarity under the physical, mental, emotional, and spiritual realms. It is important to note that this is a dynamic model. The points are not fixed and can change in either direction based on the choices we choose for our own health and well-being.

We can use this model to identify which direction clients are moving, either toward or away from health in any of the four levels of the holistic model. We then can begin to educate clients in health-promoting strategies that will support them in gaining greater health in these areas.

The key is that movement in any area toward balance will shift the line of homeostasis in the individual toward a more positive polarity. As clients effect changes on one or many levels of the holistic model, there is a greater propensity toward achieving balance. The keys to developing a holistic stress-management design that supports clients in achieving their goals of optimal health include adequate client education, tracking of results, feedback, and follow-up.

DEVELOPING INDIVIDUAL DESIGNS FOR YOUR CLIENTS

The principles in developing a stress-management design are similar to developing any physical or occupational therapy treatment plan. They include evaluation of the client, which provides information such as:

1. Definition of the problem
2. Data base
3. Subjective and objective findings
4. Assessment
5. Short- and long-term goals
6. Treatment plan (including holistic stress-management education, tracking, feedback, and follow-up)

Stress could be documented under many of these headings, integrated with the rest of the empiric data collected. Only the stress-management components are discussed here. The following is an example of how holistic stress management was incorporated into a regular evaluation and treatment plan.

CASE HISTORY

R.M., a 35-year-old woman, sustained an acute onset of lower extremity, trunk, and cervical spine weakness. She was referred for home physical therapy by her physician. An active person, R.M. had no previous significant medical problems before onset. She worked as a nurse 5 days a week. As part of her subjective history, she mentioned stress and anxiety as a main problem in her life, which she believed could be a contributing factor in her illness. Her mother

Negative Polarity	**Positive Polarity**

<———————————————————— B ————————————————————>
< . . . . .Direction Away From Optimal Health   Direction Toward Optimal Health . . . .>

PHYSICAL LEVEL

Negative
- Chronic illness, low endurance, poor body image
- Poor eating habits, excesses of fat, sugar and red meat products, poor food preparation
- Smoking, drinking, drug abuse
- Either excessive or insufficient sleep
- Fatigue, low energy for ADL
- Dysfunctional relationships
- Home and work environment reflect unclean, unsafe conditions
- Unemployed or unsatisfactory job
- Life lacks fun and entertainment

Positive
- Strong healthy body, positive self-image
- Healthy food choices, balance of vegetables, fruits, meat and dairy products
- Moderation of recreational substances
- Normal sleeping pattern
- Sufficient energy level for day-to-day activity
- Satisfying relationships
- Home and work reflect good health habits and good living
- Positive work life
- Balance of play and fun

MENTAL LEVEL

Negative
- Obsession with negative thoughts and negative consequences
- Loss of creative and imaginative ideas and thoughts
- Unclear in decision making
- Foggy mental state

Positive
- Moderation of positive and negative thinking
- Focuses on beneficial outcome
- Thinks with creativity and imagination
- Able to make decisions
- Clearly expresses ideas

EMOTIONAL LEVEL

Negative
- Inhibited in expressing emotion, a situation
- Fearful of one's feelings
- Fighting, yelling, screaming at inappropriate times or exaggerated emotions in a situation
- Not regarding the feelings of others
- Not trusting one's own feelings

Positive
- Expressing genuine feelings in the moment
- Trusting one's feelings and accepting the whole range of emotions as part of life
- Concerned with others' feelings

SPIRITUAL LEVEL

Negative
- Feeling abandoned by God
- Experiencing a sense of isolation from friends and family
- Experiencing extreme sarcasm toward human existence
- Sense of "I don't matter"
- Experiencing a sense of no meaning or purpose in life
- Suicidal thoughts

Positive
- Feeling connected to the world at all levels
- Searching for acceptance and love in one's own life
- Contributing in life
- Enjoying nature and all its beauty
- Connecting to a spiritual source (from within or from the outside)

Figure 19–1. Health can be viewed as a continuum, with a balance point *(B)* representing the line of homeostasis. We are pulled in one of two directions: toward a positive polarity of optimal health or toward a negative polarity, away from balance and optimal health.

had just died 1 month before this illness developed. She mentioned that she had been having problems sleeping and that she had developed tension headaches since her illness as well as depression and decreased enthusiasm for any activities of daily living (ADL.)

Objectively this client had deficits in all gait, posture, transfers, bed mobility, muscle strength, active range of motion (ROM), sensation, and proprioception. She also developed a higher pulse rate, higher blood pressure, and higher respiratory rate since the onset of her illness, which her doctor indicated secondary to stress. Normal goals, objectives, and treatment plans were developed for her ADL, strength, ROM, posture, and gait. In addition, R.M. and her therapist developed strategies to deal with her stress, which were incorporated into her physical therapy program.

The therapist's first step in working with R.M. in the area of stress was education. The therapist discussed what stress is, and how it can affect the body and answered R.M.'s questions about stress. The therapist then introduced the holistic health model to the client, reproducing the holistic model just described in this chapter. The next step in this process was having R.M. identify and prioritize the areas of stress in her life that she wanted to work on.

She outlined the areas as follows (in order of importance):

1. Inability to relax and the onset of higher blood pressure, pulse, and respiratory rate
2. Tension headaches
3. Decrease in energy and decreased enthusiasm for living

The next step was to develop short-term and long-term goals. As a team, the therapist and the client developed the following goals:

1. *Short-term goal*: Decrease in anxiety and tension as evidenced by a drop in heart rate, blood pressure, and respiratory rate by 20% within 3 weeks. *Long-term goal*: Normalized blood pressure, heart rate, and respiratory rate.
2. *Short-term goal*: Decrease in the frequency of tension headaches by 50% and in the pain associated with the tension headaches by 50% over a 3 week period. *Long-term goal*: Elimination of tension headaches by 100%
3. *Short-term goal*: Energy level increased by 30%

over a 3-week period. *Long-term goal*: Sufficient energy for all ADL.
4. *Short-term goal*: Increased enthusiasm for living evidenced by increased laughter, interaction with others, and a feeling of purpose in life developing over a 3-week period. *Long-term goal*: Establishing a normal balance of enthusiasm.

The third step is important in developing a personalized holistic stress-management program for clients. This is the strategy development part of the process. Together therapists and clients decide on a holistic plan that will enable clients to meet their goals. Later in this chapter, strategies are discussed under each level of the holistic model. R.M. and her therapist discussed potential strategies under each level of the holistic model, and ultimately R.M. decided on the following strategies she wanted to use initially in her program:

Physical Level

1. *Relaxation education*: to assist in both anxiety and tension headaches. The methods R.M. chose were breathing-exercise education and the relaxation response as developed by Benson (1975).
2. *Drawing*: R.M. enjoys art and decided to draw when she was feeling anxious.
3. *Energy conservation*: to assist R.M. in learning how to use her energy effectively for all ADL.

Emotional and Spiritual

R.M. classified her decreased enthusiasm under both categories. She chose the following to assist her in reaching her goal of increasing enthusiasm:

1. **Comedy:** R.M. would watch comedy on television (she subscribed to cable television and Home Box Office) a minimum of once per week.
2. **Hugs:** R.M. would reach out physically to others on a regular basis and ask for physical support (hugs, back rubs) when she needed it.
3. **Grief Counseling:** R.M. would contact and make an appointment with a grief counselor.

The next step was to implement a tracking system so that R.M. could accurately track her progress in each area. R.M. used the tracking sheet shown in Figure 19–2.

At the end of each week, R.M. and her therapist went over the tracking sheet. The therapist gave R.M. feedback on her performance and reviewed any parts of the educational component that needed reinforcing. R.M. also provided feedback on how she was doing in all areas of her program, and together R.M. and her therapist course-corrected where necessary. R.M. discovered that initially she took too many strategies on in the first week and decided to renegotiate the frequency of the items the following week.

All physical therapy goals were re-evaluated at this time as well. By spending 10 to 15 minutes once a week to review each week's accomplishments and struggles, maximum compliance was achieved. By following this program, R.M. was able to meet all of the goals she initially developed with the therapist, including all physical therapy goals and stress-management goals.

R.M. was discharged after 6 weeks of therapy. She had recovered full motor function and total ADL independence and had learned to manage her own stress effectively. The final component of a well-designed holistic stress-management plan was then implemented by the therapist: follow-up. R.M. decided to send the therapist her strategy sheets every 2 weeks for the first month after discharge and once a month for the next 2 months. The therapist would comment where appropriate and return the sheets to R.M. At the end of 3 months, R.M. was maintaining good health habits and was well on her way in establishing those habits in her life. She no longer needed supervision in her program at that time.

When asked about the most significant part of the program, R.M. said, ''Definitely the most important parts were that, number one, I was included in developing my own program and gave and received feedback, and, number two, I could use my creativity to get well.''

This holistic stress-management model can be used by any health-care professional in virtually any setting. The key is to design a program that includes education, tracking, feedback, and follow-up.

CREATING A PERSONAL HOLISTIC STRESS-MANAGEMENT PROGRAM

Often health-care professionals will ask **how** to develop strategies for personal programs and where to get information on teaching strategies to clients. It is recommended that health-care members try strategies on themselves before implementing them with clients to gain a better understanding of the strategy. Literature, videotapes, and audio equipment can assist as teaching tools, especially in the area of relaxation and imagery. Table 19–2 provides a brief listing of strategies that can be used in holistic stress management. This is only a beginning list of strategies. The Bibliography and Appendix I provide a resource list for more information on these and other strategies.

IDEAS FOR IMPLEMENTATION OF HOLISTIC STRESS MANAGEMENT IN THE CLINICAL SETTING

Now that we have a beginning list of holistic health strategies and an understanding of how to design a program for clients, the next step is to actually experiment with the concepts at your own facility. There are various ways to implement any part of a holistic program at your particular setting. Here are just a few ideas to consider:

1. *Develop* a holistic stress-management support group among staff members and run a pilot stress-management program among yourselves. Create your own individual design, choose certain strategies you want to try, and have weekly or biweekly feedback from the group or a group member. Group members could research certain strategies and develop educational in-services on various topics of interest.
2. *Implement* one stress-management strategy with clients who complain of stress in their life. Begin small. Try developing one strategy between you and each client. Educate, implement, track, give feedback to, and receive feedback from each client. Follow up on progress.
3. *Develop* audio tapes or visual aids to assist in holistic stress management at your own setting. Develop relaxation tapes that your clients can listen to while waiting for their treatment, in treatment booths, or waiting for transportation. Holistic stress management does not have to take away from your priority treatment time; it can be an adjunct to it. Have literature available in waiting rooms on stress management.

I AM making a commitment to myself for the following week that I AM:

PHYSICAL: M T W TH F S S SUMMARY

1. Practicing relaxation for _____   X   X   _2 times_
_____5 minutes 2x a week_ _____
2. Drawing when I feel anxious _____   X   X   X   _3 times_
3. Performing cleaning and washing _____   X X X X   X _5 times_
4. Exercise daily _____   X X X X X X X _7 times_

MENTAL:

_____

_____

_____

_____

_____

EMOTIONAL:

_____

1. Watch comedy on H.B.O |x   X   X _2 times_

2. Receive hugs _____ X X   X   X _4 times_

3. Make an appointment _____ X _____ _1 time_

_____with a grief counselor_ _____

SPIRITUAL:

_____

_____

_____

_____

_____

Copyright 1986 by Ron and Mary Hulnick

Figure 19–2. R.M.'s tracking sheet for her first week in her personalized stress-management program. (Form adapted from Drs. Ron and Mary Hulnick.)

Table 19–2. Strategies for Holistic Stress Management

Physical Strategies
1. Relaxation techniques
   a. Goals: decrease the state of anxiety of a client; assist client in releasing muscle tension, assist client with sleeping; assist client with pain management.
   b. Techniques used (examples): breathing exercises; Jacobson's relaxation or progressive muscle relaxation; therapeutic massage and also therapeutic touch and Trager psychophysical integration; meditation; biofeedback; autogenic training; self-hypnosis; t'ai chi ch'uan or yoga.
2. Imagery
   a. Goals: Decrease fear and anxiety; develop more healthy images about oneself; increase the sense of connection with all the levels of the holistic model.
   b. Techniques used (examples): guided imagery; memory imagery; imagination imagery; drawing.
3. Environment
   a. Goals: Create the optimal safe environment both at home and work; become more sensitive to the environment and learn how to conserve energy and resources.
   b. Techniques used (examples): recycling all paper, cans, and plastics; evaluate noise level, space, lighting, air, and water at the workplace and at home (includes evaluating computer and telephone habits and adding adaptive equipment when necessary, e.g., telephone shoulder rests, lumbar rolls, computer screen shields, adjusting computer for maximum hand and wrist safety, and so on); conserve water, paper products, and electricity at home and work; create an environment that reflects the individual via color schemes, plants, paintings, pictures, and so on; asking questions such as "Do I really need this?" when shopping for new clothes, appliances, and so on.
4. Exercise and movement
   a. Goals: For rehabilitation, to restore strength, range, and freedom in the musculoskeletal system, and to normalize normal movement patterns including posture, gait, and all functional movements associated with activities of daily living; for prevention as it relates to increasing longevity and delaying or preventing the onset of diseases such as heart disease, respiratory illnesses, and obesity; for enhancing one's self-image and increasing a sense of well-being; for competition in sport.
   b. Techniques used (examples): traditional therapies (occupational therapy, physical therapy, speech pathology, exercise physiology, dance and movement therapy); all sports and gym activities; other methods (martial arts, yoga, t'ai chi ch'uan, Alexander technique, Feldenkrais, dancing [folk, ballroom, ballet, jazz, tap, improvisational, square dancing]).
5. Nutrition
   a. Goals: With the help of a nutritionist or another skilled health-care professional to create a diet that is healthy and meets the needs of the individual, taking into consideration all medical and social aspects.
   b. Techniques used (examples): reducing sugar, fat, salt, caffeine, and alcohol gradually from a diet plan; reducing red meat consumption and replacing it with other protein sources; choosing foods that are free of chemicals, preservatives, and toxins; increasing the amount of fresh fruits and vegetables and whole grains into one's diet plan; ensure proper vitamin and mineral intake by eating foods that are high in vitamin and mineral content; reading literature from the American Heart Association and nutritional guidelines developed from other health associations.

Mental Strategies
   a. Goals: The goals of strategies that work with the mental level are to create realistic and appropriate beliefs about ourselves as well as to enhance our skills in imagination, decision making, and cognitive awareness.
   b. Techniques used (examples): creative visualization; affirmations; thought journals; psychologist referrals in many areas including Rogerian, gestalt, psychosynthesis, rational emotive therapy, art therapy, addiction counseling; dream journals; human resource trainings, which include education in creative decision making, decision-making styles, and other cognitive education.

Emotional Strategies
   a. Goals: The goals of strategies in the emotional realm are to support an individual in appropriately expressing feelings with self and others as well as to incorporate feelings into day-to-day decisions and activities.
   b. Techniques used (examples): maintaining journal; practicing communication techniques such as exploring feelings, reflecting feelings, giving and receiving effective feedback, and positive reinforcement; psychodrama; art therapy; free-style drawing; counseling, social work, or psychology interventions; sharing true feelings with those close to the individual; writing letters to others expressing true feelings.

Spiritual Strategies
   a. Goal: To support the individual in establishing or re-establishing a sense of connection with the world and to support a person in areas such as serving others and feeling a sense of purpose in life.
   b. Techniques used (examples): Prayer; meditation; pastoral counseling; attending church or synagogue; nature walks; horticulture therapy; spending time with loved ones; service to others (i.e., volunteering in a hospital, assisting the homeless, joining a service organization, and so on); buying or spending time with pets or animals; spending time with infants or children.

4. *Develop* questionnaires for clients relating to issues such as home safety and environmental concerns. Inform your clients as to how to increase the safety of their home and work environment.

5. *Talk* to various counselors, social workers, psychologists, and psychiatrists at your setting to determine how they view stress management. Perhaps they use strategies that your clients could benefit from. Do not be afraid to make referrals if you and your clients feel extra support would be helpful.

6. *Learn* a holistic stress-management strategy that you have always wanted to try. For example, try different movement classes such as yoga, t'ai chi/ch'uan, or dance. Explore if it adds more creativity to your treatments with clients.

7. *In-service* other members of your facility with whom you may not deal on a regular basis about holistic stress-management strategies (e.g., administration, ancillary help, security).

8. *Develop* stress-management strategies as a family! Volunteer to be a feedback person for friends who are undergoing much stress and assist them in developing strategies that will help them decrease their own stress.

The key is to start small and proceed at your own pace when integrating holistic stress-management concepts into your own life. Evaluate the effectiveness of strategies you use. Determine which strategies are appropriate for you to use in your professional environment. Allow yourself to make mistakes when beginning any stress-management program. No one is perfect. Renegotiate strategies, change your design, and experiment with feedback methods. Remain open-minded for learning that may occur within yourself and within your client. The following quotes are from patients who have worked on or are still actively working on a holistic stress-management program:

The first area I worked on was the physical level. I began to gain control through proper diet and exercise. I was then ready to move on to the mental level. I began [a journal for] my thoughts every day and wrote eight affirmations, which I read each morning. Slowly I began moving toward the emotional level. I found that internal strength for me meant listening to my heart and trusting myself. That fact has changed my life. I have not had an anxiety attack for over a year. I am slowly developing my spirituality. I am just beginning this process. I am grateful I have come this far.

I am a person who never could stick to anything, a diet, exercise program, you name it, I couldn't stick to it. When Susan suggested to choose one small thing to commit to each week, I decided I would try it. I chose to, in the beginning, breathe five times deeply when I was feeling anxiety. I only committed to one time a week to try this. I was successful the first week and each week thereafter. Receiving encouragement allowed me to look deeper into the causes of my stress, and slowly I have developed strategies to overcome the negative impact of stress. It has taken time to learn, I have made mistakes, but I am not perfect.

The physical healing I have received is incredible. I had been in a car accident in September 1989 and injured my neck and back. By utilizing various strategies in the holistic model my entire body has changed. By focusing on lightness and freedom in my joints, my posture has changed dramatically. My commitment to myself has increased each week. I learned how to manage my own pain and how to conserve my own energy.

My headaches disappeared. It took time to learn biofeedback, but it worked. I continue to write a strategy sheet each week and so does my family. We are all closer now.

After I had my stroke, I was depressed for months. At 29 years of age, I decided that my life was now meaningless. Fortunately, I was referred for physical and occupational therapy at home. Both therapists worked with me on stress-management strategies. I saw them both a total of 4 times a week. The constant reinforcement and feedback on my progress made a big difference. I began listening to relaxation tapes, and I began painting with my left hand. Not only was I making gains physically, I was making gains emotionally. I regained my self-esteem.

I never thought my environment was the cause of so much of my tension. It was. I discovered that the ventilation in my office was below standard, the lighting was inadequate, and my computer was placed too low for my height. Just by making small changes in my environment my tension has decreased.

At first I was offended when my therapist suggested I seek counseling. I swallowed my pride because I knew inside I needed to work on some things in my life. I sought professional assistance and now am coping with my own stress in a healthy way.

Do you have any idea how good it feels to be listened to?

In summary, a holistic stress-management program can be used in a variety of ways. The model described in this chapter is easily adaptable to any setting. The keys in developing a holistic stress-management design that supports optimal wellness are client education, goal setting, strategy development, tracking of results, feedback, and follow-up. The strategies listed in this chapter and Bibliography are meant to serve as guides for the health-care practitioner who is interested in beginning a holistic stress-management program or for the practitioner who is ready to add more depth to an existing program.

References

Ardell D: 14 Days to a Wellness Lifestyle. Mill Valley, CA, Whatever Publishing Inc, 1982.

Benson H: The Relaxation Response. New York, William Morrow, 1975.

Brallier L: Successfully Managing Stress. Los Altos, CA, National Nursing Review, 1982.

Cmich D: Theoretical perspectives of holistic health. J Sch Health 1:30–32, 1984.

Cooper R: Health and Fitness Excellence: The Scientific Action Plan. Boston; Houghton Mifflin, 1989.

Dossey B, Keegan L, Kolkmeir L, et al: Holistic Health Promotion: A Guide for Practice. Rockville, MD, Aspen Publications, 1989.

Flynne P: Holistic Health: The Art of Science and Care. Bowie, MD, Prentice-Hall, 1980.

Hulnick R and Hulnick M: University of Santa Monica, California.

Jaffe D and Scott C: From Burnout to Balance: A Workbook for Peak Performance and Self-Renewal. New York, McGraw-Hill, 1984.

Oberteuffer D: A Holistic Point of View for Physical Education. Paper presented at the annual meeting of the Australian Association for Health, Education, and Recreation, Melbourne, January 18, 1968.

Selye H: Stress Without Distress. Philadelphia, JB Lippincott, 1974.

Tubesing D: Holistic Health. New York, Human Sciences Press, 1979.

Witkin G: The Female Stress Syndrome. New York, Berkley Press, 1985.

Bibliography

MEDITATION AND RELAXATION
Benson H: The Relaxation Response. New York, William Morrow, 1975.

Jacobson E: You Must Relax. New York, McGraw-Hill, 1987.

Lamott K: Escape from Stress. New York, GP Putnam, 1975.

LeShan L: How to Meditate. New York, Bantam Books, 1972.

Naranjo C and Ornstein R: On the Psychology of Meditation. New York, Viking Press, 1971.

Selye H: The Stress of Life. New York, McGraw-Hill, 1951.

Stroebel C: QR: The Quieting Reflex. New York, Berkley Books, 1982.

BIOFEEDBACK AND IMAGERY
Achterberg J: Imagery in Healing. Boston, Shambhala Publications, 1985.

Assagioli R: Psychosynthesis: A Manual of Principles and Techniques. New York, Hobbs, Doorman, 1965.

Fuller G: Biofeedback: Methods and Procedures in Clinical Practice. San Francisco, The Biofeedback Institute, 1977.

Gawain S: Creative Visualization. San Rafael, CA, New World Library, 1978.

Green A and Green E: Beyond Biofeedback. New York, Delacorte, 1977.

Samuels M and Samuels N: Seeing with the Mind's Eye. New York, Random House, 1975.

MENTAL STRATEGIES
Colligan D and Locke S: The Healer Within. New York, Dutton, 1986.

Flanagan O: The Science of Mind. Cambridge, MA, MIT Press, 1984.

Gazzaniga M: Mind Matters: How the Mind and the Brain Interact to Create Our Conscious Lives. Boston, Houghton Mifflin, 1988.

Hay L: You Can Heal Your Life. Santa Monica, CA, Hay House, 1984.

McWilliams P and Roger J: You Can't Afford the Luxury of a Negative Thought. Los Angeles, Prelude Press, 1988.

Pelletier K: Mind as Healer Mind as Slayer. New York, Delta Books, 1977.

Rossi E: The Psychobiology of Mind/Body Healing. New York, Norton, 1987.

NUTRITION, EXERCISE, AND ENVIRONMENT
Calliet R and Gross L: The Rejuvenation Strategy. New York, Doubleday, 1987.

Cooper KH: Running Without Fear: The Comprehensive New Guide to Safe Aerobic Exercise—Running, Swimming, Cycling, Skiing and More. New York, Bantam Books, 1985.

Earthworks Group. 50 Simple Things You Can Do to Save the Earth. Berkeley, CA, Earthworks Group, 1989.

Feldenkrais M: Awareness Through Movement. New York, Harper & Row, 1977.

Halpern S and Savary L: Sound Health. San Francisco, Harper & Row, 1985.

Jacobson M and Brewster L: The Changing American Diet. Washington, DC, Center for Science in the Public Interest, 1984.

Lange R: The Nature of Dance. London, MacDonald and Evans Ltd, 1975.

HOLISM AND HEALING MODALITIES
Cousins N: The Anatomy of an Illness as Perceived by the Patient. New York, Norton, 1979.

Creighton C, Simonton O, and Simonton S: Getting Well Again. New York, Bantam Books, 1978.

Dass R and Gorman P: How Can I Help? New York, Knopf, 1988.

Flynne P: The Healing Continuum: Journeys in the Philosophy of Holistic Health. Bowie, MD, Robert J. Brady, 1980.

Krieger D: The Therapeutic Touch: How to Use Your Hands to Help or Heal. Englewood Cliffs, NJ, Prentice-Hall, 1979.

Matson F and Montagu A: The Human Connection. New York, McGraw-Hill, 1979.

APPENDIX I

University of Santa Monica, 2107 Wilshire Blvd. Santa Monica, CA 90403. (213) 829-7402

Relaxation, Imagery, and Music Tapes

Halpern Sounds, 1775 Old Country Rd., 9, Belmont, CA 94002

Music Rx, P.O. Box 173, Port Towsend, WA 98368

Sources Cassette, Dept. 99, P.O. Box W, Stanford, CA 94305

Windham Hill Records, P.O. Box 9388, Stanford, CA 94305

National Association for Music Therapy, 1133 15th St NW, Washington, DC 20005

General Health

American Journal of Health Promotion, 746 Purdy St., Birmingham, MI 48009

Harvard Medical School Health Letter, P.O. Box 10945, Des Moines, IA 50340

Hippocrates: Magazine of Health and Medicine, P.O. Box 52431, Boulder, CO 80321.

Prevention, Emmaus, PA 18099

University of California, Berkeley Wellness Letter, P.O. Box 10922, Des Moines, IA 50340

Nutrition

Environmental Nutrition. 52 Riverside Dr., New York, NY 10024.

Nutrition Action Healthletter. Center for Science in the Public Interest, 1501 16th St NW, Washington, DC 20036

Tufts University Diet and Nutrition Letter, 475 Park Ave S, New York, NY 10016

Environmental

Mother Earth News, P.O. Box 3122, Harlan, IA 51593

Sierra. Sierra Club, 530 Bush St., San Francisco, CA 94108

Whole Earth Review. P.O. Box 428, Sausalito, CA 94965

Workplace and Environment

PART

III

Workplace and
Environment

CHAPTER

20

Ruth E. Levine
Laura N. Gitlin

Use of the Environment for Promoting Optimal Function in the Chronically Disabled*

The focus of this chapter is the environment: the human and nonhuman factors that surround and influence clients and their caregivers. Individual activities occur in settings that promote, neutralize, or hinder behavior, and this offers the therapist opportunities to promote functional performance by using environmental factors in treatment. This is because physical, social, and cultural influences shape human behavior and provide external stimuli to which individuals react and modify their responses to fit personal needs.

In rehabilitation, individuals are viewed as the primary focal point for prevention of disease; but we rarely look beyond clients and consider their setting as the context for treatment decisions. The environment can be described as a hidden treatment modality that can be adjusted to promote treatment goals, wellness behaviors, and adaptation and accommodation to disabilities (Kiernat, 1982).

In this chapter, we describe the importance of

the environment as a component of health-care delivery. First, we begin with a case study, an overview of environmental theories, and key concepts and definitions. Second, effects of environmental stimuli on client care are described, including ideas for goal setting, treatment planning, and evaluation. Finally, we explore how therapists might use the environment to improve treatment and ameliorate barriers that hinder functional performance.

CASE HISTORY 1

We begin with a case history to demonstrate the extent of environmental influence, especially the social and physical dimensions that impact client compliance with a prescribed medical regime.

Mr. S. is a 38-year-old pipefitter who owns his own mechanical construction business, designing solutions to heating and air-conditioning installation problems and supervising field and office staff. His leisure activities include attending large-equipment auctions, gardening, and hunting deer using a bow and arrow.

After 10 years of back problems. Mr. S. experienced sciatic pain, which was so severe that he walked in a bent-over position. Still undaunted, he continued field supervision, which included demonstration of how to level quick-drying ce-

*This Chapter is based on research funded in part by grants from the American Occupational Therapy Foundation (AOTF) and the National Institute on Disability and Rehabilitation Research (NIDRR), Department of Education, Grant No. H133G00160. Opinions expressed in this chapter are those of the authors and should not be construed to represent opinions or policies of AOTF or NIDRR.

ment with a rake. He experienced acute pain and remained in bed for several days, noting numbness in his left lower extremity. As the pain increased, he realized that he had no sensation in his foot. No longer able to walk, he agreed to seek emergency treatment and was admitted and recommended for L5 surgery to remove the protruding disk.

Before surgery, the orthopedist questioned Mr. S. about his work and assumed from the response that Mr. S. was a manager who did not lift heavy loads. Thus, the doctor reasoned that there was no need to fuse the spinal column and, therefore, recommended a laminectomy. Six weeks after surgery, Mr. S. resumed work and leisure activities such as climbing trees to make a stand for hunting. The advice of the physician regarding rest was interpreted by Mr. S. to include resumption of hands-on supervision in the mornings but work from a prone position on a drawing table in the office in the afternoons. Mr. S. also classified tree climbing and hunting activities as leisure pursuits and resumed these activities one weekend but quickly experienced increased pain. He returned to the surgeon, who advised more rest. Mr. S. reasoned that he was resting and questioned the advice. This chain of events occurred again, and Mr. S. decided that the doctor could not help him. Six months later, Mr. S. still had pain, could only walk for short distances early in the day, could not lift effectively, or participate fully in leisure activities.

Mr. S.'s behavior was motivated by his need to earn a living and control his own recovery, although he had little knowledge of the consequences of his choices. He interpreted the doctor's words as friendly advice rather than a home program that should be followed to avoid further complications. The doctor, alternatively, did not understand Mr. S.'s interpretation of his orders. He assumed that he and Mr. S. were communicating and shared the same meaning of words such as "rest," "lifting," "pain," and "work." An understanding of Mr. S. as an individual with distinct needs, values, and goals would have prompted the development of a more effective follow-up and prevention program.

Additionally, Mr. S. would have greatly benefited from an assessment of his work and home environments to identify strategies that were safe, yet allowed for Mr. S.'s need for independence and control. Additionally, in view of Mr. S.'s mechanical skill and knowledge, a technical description of the surgical procedure of the back repair should have been offered with anatomic photographs depicting the consequences of stress after surgery. This might have increased compliance. A detailed description of the chances for future complications and further injury could help Mr. S. make an informed decision about the amount of lifting and bending he chose to do.

Mr. S.'s situation was ultimately resolved by a physical therapist who listened to Mr. S.'s description of his symptoms and took the time to explain the mechanics of the spine using an anatomic model. The therapist also offered options for lifting, ideas for increasing endurance, and exercises for strengthening weakened muscles. Finally, the therapist described the types of degenerative changes that Mr. S. would experience as he aged. Now Mr. S. had the information he needed to make informed decisions regarding his activity level, positioning for lifting, and choice of leisure pursuits.

Although environment has been discussed in occupational therapy literature since the turn of the century, it continues to be an underemphasized facet of treatment in both occupational therapy and physical therapy practice. In particular, environmental assessments and alterations that effect behavioral changes are not included routinely in treatment. The following overview of environment theories and definitions will promote an understanding of the relationship between environment and treatment success. Throughout the chapter, the client's interests are intertwined with his or her environment, and neither can be understood without comprehending the other. Thus, Mr. S. could have benefited from treatment that included the human and nonhuman aspects of his environment.

CONCEPTUAL OVERVIEW

Psychology has taken the lead in research on the impact of the environment on behavior. However, theory development is described as prescientific or descriptive (Lawton, 1982, p. 35). At this point, theories of the environment can be classified into three categories: (1) *internal system theories* or those that maintain that individuals can overcome environmental forces through **internal resources** (e.g., medical model, rehabilitation model); (2) theories that view environment as a determinant of human behavior (e.g., Goffman, Mead); and (3) theories that conceive environment as composed of potential resources and limitations in view of an individual with explicit competencies (e.g., ecology of aging theories, environmental congruence models, occupational therapy environmental theories). Each theory group is reviewed here (Table 20–1) although the last category offers the most potential for therapists in designing and complementing effective prevention and rehabilitation programs.

Table 20–1. Environmental Theories

Label	Theory Base	Perspective of Individual	Example
Internal system theories	Medical model, rehabilitation model	Internal resources needed to overcome press	Injured person will "want" to be independent in self-care
Environment as determinant	Sociologic models	Environment shapes behavior; person conforms	Authoritarian institutions make patients feel dependent and passive
Person–environment transaction	Psychology, gerontology, occupational therapy models	Person interacts in multidimensional ways with environment	Teaching clients to climb stairs in own home to reinforce training

Internal System Theories

Medical and rehabilitation models address environment factors indirectly. Both consider environment as a backdrop for intervention because the primary therapeutic focus is on affecting change in the individual.

The success of the medical model is based on identification and eradication of pathogens. Once labeled, the pathogen can be attacked and the illness cured. Thus, practitioners concentrate on pathology and disease using technical tools to comprehend body systems. The clients' account of their illness and pain is not valued as much as objective data. The physical, social, and cultural context in which individuals function is often overlooked, and this represents a critical limitation of the medical model (Borysenko, 1987; Capra, 1983; Cousins, 1979; Ferguson, 1980; Illich, 1976).

Rehabilitation, an outgrowth of the medical model, is based on the assumption that individuals want to be self-sufficient. Although a cure is sought for the disabling condition, clients are expected to adapt to their disability within a statistically derived average time frame. Accommodation to losses is expected as normal, and few practitioners understand or take the time to recognize the psychosocial process of recovery and grieving for lost function (Kaufman, 1988). These ideas are presented in greater depth in Chapter 25 in which Rubenstein describes the need to understand one's own personal values in view of those displayed by clients.

Medical training promotes categorizing individuals by diagnosis; thus, a commonly held assumption is that individuals can be treated the same. A vague understanding of individual differences based on education level, ethnic background, interests, and activities creates a belief that clients share the same values and beliefs

about illness and wellness. However, we do not all process stimuli the same way nor do we view events from a shared perspective. For example, a 50-year-old man who never assisted in meal preparation and household chores before his disability may not value these instrumental activities after his rehabilitation training. His assumptions about independence may not be congruent with those of his rehabilitation team. He may reason that it is his wife's "duty" to care for him. Alternatively, as one client commented as she was being shown a dressing technique, "I raised 10 children in my time so the ten of them can get together and take care of one—me."

Environment as a Determinant of Behavior

The next category is derived from a social systems perspective. Instead of focusing on the individual, sociologists consider the environment as an overpowering, all-encompassing influence on human behavior. Goffman (1961) posited that the environment was so pervasive that individuals behaved in a similar manner when exposed to the same stimulation. Thus, he described similar reactions of novices who entered convents, prisoners, and patients in asylums as they tried to live in authoritarian social systems that ignored individuality. These theorists posit that environment is pervasive and shapes human behavior patterns.

Hall, a theorist who described how cultures and people affect individual behavior, examined how individuals deal with space and the meaning it has for them. Hall (1977 and 1969) and others demonstrated how physical distance between individuals influenced communication patterns. For example, studies indicate that Arabs tend to stand close to each other when talking, whereas Western Europeans require more distance between each communicator. Hall offered an example of an Arab trying to be polite to an American by moving closer as he talks and the American, trained to keep "safe" distances, demonstrates annoyance by backing away (p. 156). These theorists and cross-cultural studies contributed to therapists' understanding of the critical impact of social systems on client behavior. However, from this theoretic perspective, the domination of environment precludes human initiative to change, modify, or impact behavior.

Person–Environment Transactional Theories

Theories developed by gerontologists, psychologists, and occupational therapists have considered environment in interaction with individuals who possess distinct competencies. This perspective tends to view the interaction and transaction of person and environment as jointly influencing and shaping human behavior. Theorists can use these theories to view the environment as a complex, multidimensional concept that explains some ties between external stimuli and individual reactions, perceptions, and behavior. This group of theories holds the most potential for use by therapists in developing prevention and rehabilitation programming.

Building on Lewin (1948) and Murray's (1938) work, Lawton, an environmental psychologist, suggested that the way individuals experience any given environment is largely determined by functional performance and level of competence. He defined competence as the "theoretical upper limit of capacity of the individual to function in the areas of biological health, sensation, perception, motoric behavior and cognition" (Lawton, 1975, p. 21). Competence is "a diverse collection of abilities residing within the individual which may be influenced by environmental factors and change from setting to setting" (Lawton and Nahemow, 1973, p. 659). In an earlier work, Lawton and Simon (1968) suggested that highly competent people will rise above their environments and those with reduced competence or ability to function in an environment will be more vulnerable to the external world (p. 108). That is, as "competence of the individual decreases, the proportion of behavior attributable to environmental, as contrasted with personal, characteristics increases" (p. 114). Individuals with decreased functional abilities become more

vulnerable to the effect of the world around them because they do not possess as many skills to adapt and change their behavior. This is called *environmental docility*. The stimulation of the outside world is referred to as *press*, a physical, interpersonal, or social need that activates or arouses a person to behave in a given environment. Press can be modified or altered as competence declines (Murray, 1938). Lawton and Nahemow (1973) established a predictive model in which individual competence is compared with environmental press in a formula with optimal zones of performance. For example, consider how therapists adjust the environmental demands or press placed on clients by using different size weights, by adjusting heights of equipment, and by building up or reducing handles of activities of daily living (ADL) equipment. Press is not a new idea in occupational and physical therapy practice.

On the basis of Lawton's work, Kahana (1975) developed a *congruence model*, which emphasizes goodness of fit between environmental characteristics and individual needs. This fit, she hypothesized, strengthens psychologic well-being. Lawton described psychologic well-being as an optimal fit between person and environment, whereas Kahana implied an interactive, multiplicative relationship between humans and environment in which the level of congruence becomes a predisposition to satisfaction or well-being. Other theorists sharing this perspective examined the importance of control over stressful environmental events such as a relocation and found that an individual's participation in this process enhances well-being (Pastalan, 1982 Schooler, 1982;). In a later study, Kahana and colleagues (1980) described the complexity of the variables that create a fit between elderly persons and their environment and urged researchers to consider multiple dimensions that create well-being (p. 594).

More recently, Lawton (1989) expanded the concept of environmental docility to include *proactivity* or an individual's conscious manipulation and control over environmental forces. In this extension of his work, individual control and purposeful activation are viewed as offsetting environmental press and contributing to psychologic well-being (Lawton, 1989). In other words, decreased competence may not necessarily lead to susceptibility to environmental forces. Rather, an individual's ability to compensate within a given environmental and competence framework is also of critical importance to the well-being of that individual.

COMPONENTS OF THE ENVIRONMENT

Environment, defined broadly as "all that originates outside the skin of the person" (Lawton, 1989, p. 6), consists of the world around the clients and the circumstances or conditions that affect functional performance. The environment has human and nonhuman components. The human components include family, friends, colleagues, social groups, and culture, whereas nonhuman aspects include animals, material possessions, objects, and places that surround people. Theorists view environment as consisting of distinct and varying dimensions.

For example, Lawton and Nahemow (1973) explained environment as consisting of physical, interpersonal, and social forces and characterized by potential constraints and resources for an individual with specific needs, competencies, and personal goals and values. Adaptation or the ability to act competently requires a match between environmental demands and the person's abilities. In this ecologic model, human development requires "continual adaptations in which both the organism and the environment change over time in a nonrandom manner" (Lawton and Nahemow, 1973, p. 621).

Dunning (1972) classified environment as consisting of space, people, and tasks. The task environment includes environmental expectations or press, which relates to the person's performance level. Barris expanded these ideas (1982 and 1987; Barris et al, 1985) and developed a model of the environment as consisting of four concentric and interrelated layers: objects, tasks, social groups and organizations, and culture. Objects are tangible, stable, visible things used by clients. Tasks are a set of activities with a common purpose. Social groups and organizations are individuals who form collective opportunities for interaction. Culture is the collective way of living and performing activities that is taught during childhood and creates an enduring belief system shared by group members. Each one of these layers is further characterized by distinct attributes that can then be manipulated or modified to achieve a behavioral goal as demonstrated in a study of clients with Alzheimer's disease (Corcoran and Gitlin, 1991).

Neurophysiologic researchers view environ-ment as consisting of sensory stimulation. Some theorists concentrate on how the input is interpreted by the person and how a change in stimuli might change the person's performance. Many therapists rely on their knowledge of the sensory and motor systems to improve the individual's functional performance. Hearing aids, walkers, braces, wheelchairs, reachers, splints, and larger signs are all examples of environmental adaptations that promote performance.

KEY CONCEPTS FOR PRACTICE

Arousal and press are two critical concepts linking person–environment and behavioral outcomes. *Arousal* refers to an internal state of an organism, with physiologic and subjective manifestations influencing choice of behavior (Barris et al, 1985). It is the degree to which an individual is stimulated by the environment: an internal state in which both physical and emotional experiences are processed. Stimulation comes from the external world, and each person interprets these cues according to their own internal system, which includes the nervous system, emotional needs, and cultural factors. People naturally and continually seek a satisfying match or balance between external stimulation and internal needs. Effective therapy can use this principle to evoke curiosity and motivation rather than resistance and anxiety.

Choices about behavior are also based on the press of environment or the expectations for certain behavior that emerge from the setting (Lawton, 1989; Lawton and Nahemow, 1973). As described earlier, press, initially identified by Murray (1938), refers to stimuli possessing some motivating quality that activates an individual need. The demand can be objective or individualistic. Press is the "force that together with an individual need evoke a response" (Lawton and Nahemow, 1973, p. 659). Therapists manipulate press to promote optimal learning among clients.

Successful performance requires a match between person and press of the environment. Adjustments in the arousal and press can promote or retard individual performance. Too much stimulation may create feelings of being overwhelmed, whereas too little stimulation may lead to boredom. Therapists work to create a "just-right" challenge balancing the person's ability with demands of the environment (Burke, 1977). Manipulation of environment to achieve this fit may include modification of the physical, task, or social layers.

For example, a woman with a high-risk pregnancy who is confined to bed may find her world boring and difficult because she is separated from the stimulation of her daily life (Johnson et al, 1991). In contrast, an older adult with dementia may experience his or her environment as overwhelming and too stimulating. Therapists would challenge the bedridden woman with an activity that increased concentration such as volunteer solicitation for a favorite charity or the introduction of a "control center" where household or work tasks could be directed. These are two solutions that might enhance environmental stimuli and increase feelings of well-being. The opposite would hold true for the older adult for whom environmental modifications would include assurance of a clutter-free work surface, use of two- or three-step instructions, and repetition of cues.

ENVIRONMENT AND CLIENT CARE

The inclusion of environment in prevention and rehabilitation programs leads to a consideration of the individual from a more holistic vantage point. Therapists should consider three factors: the nonhuman environment, the human environment, and culture. Prevention thus becomes contextual and nonmedical in orientation and, we argue, more cost effective and efficient. In the medical model paradigm, a practitioner concentrates on pathology and defines rehabilitation and prevention needs based on diagnosis and disability. In an environmental perspective, the practitioner discerns need based on assessment of individual functioning within a specific environmental context, such as home, work, or school.

How do therapists assess the client's level of arousal and press and determine the correct match that stimulates interest without overwhelming clients? Therapists analyze behavior and use cues or feedback. These signs and symbols, especially nonhuman ones, can be interpreted to increase understanding of the culture, values, and lifestyle of clients. Nonhuman environment refers to everything that is not human, such as clothing, jewelry, photographs, plants, toys, tools, animals, and furniture (Searles, 1960).

Therapists intuitively rely on cues to establish rapport; however, this analysis can be continued

during treatment and can include manipulation of the nonhuman environment to increase or limit press and to promote functional performance. Modifying the level of difficulty of an activity so that it is either more (increased press) or less challenging so to prevent injury and reduce anxiety can promote feelings of accomplishment and self-worth. For example, therapists commonly teach stair climbing on a five-step model stairway. Clients do not feel skilled when they return to their homes that have 15 steps and only one-side rails. In another example, clients are taught to dress in the ideal conditions of their hospital room. No provision is made for their lower bed, bureau placed across the room, or bathroom with no safety rails. In short, many clients initially feel overwhelmed by the consequences of illness or disability. In this case, graduation of environmental stress may be an effective treatment strategy.

Culture is the blueprint or map for human behavior, influencing thoughts and actions (Leininger, 1978, p. 80) and hence how treatment is understood. This multifaceted influence is learned by direct and indirect daily experiences based on what people do (cultural behavior), say (speech messages), make, and use (cultural artifacts). In short, a child learns a life pattern of beliefs and values that shape the way he or she believes, thinks, perceives, feels, and behaves (Spradley and McCurdy, 1980, p. 2). Culture imposes a conditioning variable that is internalized in the human psyche and not easily forgotten (Lifroeber, cited in Laudin, 1973, p. 4).

The pervasive influence of culture affects how treatment is perceived, how the client will pursue treatment goals, how the illness or disability is viewed, and how future goals are formulated and acted on. Illness is not the same to all individuals. Members of subgroups decide when to seek professional health care, how and when to care for ill members, how to organize and use caregiver networks, how and when medication is used, how daily regimes are interrupted by illness, how pain is interpreted and endured, and how family members are organized to cope with a chronically disabled member.

The labeling of illness, reaction to it, and definition of acceptable behavior as a result of the illness are determined by culture. Thus, therapists need to consider how clients perceive therapy. If clients feel that they should be cured by someone else, they may find a therapeutic regime difficult to tolerate. If, however, clients want to do things themselves, they may find the supervision of a therapist annoying. The meaning that the client derives from therapy should be understood and discussed to promote alignment among therapist, client, and caregiver goals for behavioral change. Clients judge their programs through a cultural filter, which is based in part on past learning and emotions, and three levels of belief: (1) perception of illness, (2) perception of therapy, and (3) belief in the meaning of his or her own life and activities (Levine, 1987, p. 9).

Consider the myriad reactions to a simple illness such as a cold. Some individuals ignore it until they are too sick to work, others continue to work even if they have fever, some take to bed as soon as they feel ill, others use home remedies, some consult a physician, and others prescribe their own over-the-counter medication. Levels of participation in normal life activities vary with the individual's definition of their cold. If the person feels "sick," events may be postponed or canceled. If the cold is considered inconvenient but not serious, events may be continued but shortened. If the person refuses to admit that he or she is ill, events and obligations may be continued as if nothing were wrong. Prevention and health promotion are not merely a commonsense set of behaviors. There are no standard health or lifestyle practices that bridge all family cultures. Thus, instruction that is culturally relevant and meaningful to an individual becomes a more effective approach for treatment.

CASE HISTORY 2

Another case story illustrates the use of the principles discussed in this chapter.

Mrs. M., 70 years old, had a cerebrovascular accident. She was hospitalized for 1 week and sent to a rehabilitation center for 2 weeks. During that time she received occupational and physical therapy including ADLS, upper and lower extremity exercises, a kitchen and bathroom checkout, and stair ambulation. Her performance required supervision with cuing and minimal supervision in ADL. The team members explained their program to a caregiver: the oldest daughter, Gloria, who frequently came to visit her mother. However, once Mrs. M. arrived home, she remained in bed and was completely dependent in all aspects of her care, denied having any training, and wanted her daughter to take care of her until she got "better."

Mrs. M. was followed by a home visiting team; therapists confirmed her dependence. At this point, neighbors were caring for Mrs. M. in shifts and Gloria visited only on weekends when she was not working. The home visiting team reported that Mrs. M. was fearful of descending stairs and denied her training in stair climbing, ambulation, transfers, kitchen, and ADL.

Although Mrs. M. received rehabilitation, she was unable to adapt the institutional program to her home needs. In her mind, the training had little resemblance to her own familiar schemes. She assumed that she was sick and would be taken care of until she was well again. Gloria did not live near her mother and could visit only on weekends because she worked full time and had four children. During rehabilitation, no one had asked about Mrs. M.'s home layout or questioned Gloria about her availability. The structure of rehabilitation services pre-empted a home visit. Thus, the rehabilitation team was unable to understand Mrs. M.'s human and nonhuman environment.

This case illustrates how the home environment becomes the client's context for retaining newly acquired skills. The usual practice of assigning adaptive equipment in a medical setting and training in transfer and other self-care techniques may not provide older clients with the necessary knowledge and skill to integrate these tools into daily routines in familiar environments. This may be particularly true for the elderly with a first-time disability who may need additional teaching support and time to substitute a compensatory technique or piece of equipment for a once-familiar life task. Research of adult learners further highlights the importance of providing repeated practice opportunities in the environment in which the behavior is to occur (Brown, 1975, p. 7).

As we see in the case of Mrs. M., inadequate training experiences and personal fears increased her vulnerability to the physical and social press of her environment, which in turn led to maladaptive behavioral outcomes. The home occupational and physical therapists used cues from Mrs. M.'s world to reinforce her previous knowledge of stair climbing, ambulation, kitchen, and ADL training. Mrs. M. was soon independent in her own home.

BARRIERS TO USING ENVIRONMENT

Although we have advocated the use of environment as a treatment modality, several limitations or barriers exist. First, within the present reimbursement structure, therapists have limited time to spend with their clients and their care-givers. Although using an environmental per-spective may in the long term be cost effective and an efficient form of therapy, it may involve greater contact with an individual in their envi-ronment whether it be at work, home, school, or play. Second, the use of environment in treat-ment planning and implementation hinges on the therapist's ability to be sensitive to client and care-giver goals, interests, and values. This has implications for how both occupational and phys-ical therapists are educated and trained. Tradi-tional educational experiences focus on individ-ual pathology rather than the more contextual approach that includes the person's environ-ment. Third, reimbursement and financial con-siderations restrict the extent to which modifica-tion of the physical environment is possible. Therapists must often select adaptive equipment for their clients without adequate time to explore the person's level of performance or demon-strated need over time. However, introduction of low-technologic and low-cost modifications, drawn from the client's home, can be effective in promoting increased activity level and pre-vention of injury for individuals with a wide range of chronic conditions (Levine and Gitlin, 1990).

Finally, we lack appropriate assessment instru-ments to reliably measure how environment im-pacts individual competence and functional per-formance. Valid and reliable instrumentation is critical for sound treatment planning and imple-mentation, especially with the multidisciplinary team of specialists who participate in rehabilita-tion.

References

Barris R: Activity: The interface between person and environ-ment. Phys Occup Ther Geriatr 5:39–49, 1987.

Barris R: Environmental interactions: An extension of the model of human occupation. Am J Occup Ther 36:637–644, 1982.

Barris R, Kielhofner G, Levine RE, et al: Occupation as interaction with the environment. In Kielhofner G (ed): A Model of Human Occupation: Theory and Application. Baltimore, MD, Williams & Wilkins, 1985.

Borysenko J: Minding the Body: Mending the Mind. Reading, MA, Addison-Wesley, 1987.

Brown GI: The Live Classroom: Innovation Through Con-fluent Education. New York, Viking Press, 1975.

Burke JP: A clinical perspective on motivation: Pawn vs. origin. Am J Occup Ther 31:254–258, 1977.

Capra F: The Turning Point: Science, Society, and the Rising Culture. New York, Bantam Books, 1983.

Corcoran M and Gitlin LN: Environmental Influences on the Elderly with Dementia: Principles for Intervention. Occup Ther Phys Ther Geriatr Care 9 (No. 3 and 4) Fall/Winter 1991.

Cousins N: Anatomy of an Illness. New York, Norton, 1979.

Dunning H: Environmental occupational therapy. Am J Oc-cup Ther 26:292–298, 1972.

Ferguson M: The Aquarian Conspiracy: Personal and Social Transformation in the 1980's. Los Angeles, JP Tarcher, 1980.

Gitlin LN and Corcoran M: Training occupational therapists in the care of the elderly with dementia and their care-givers: focus on collaboration. Educ Gerontol 17 (5) Sept./Oct., 1991.

Goffman E: Asylums. Garden City, NY, Anchor Books, 1961.

Hall ET: Beyond Culture. Garden City, NY, Anchor Books, 1977.

Hall ET: The Hidden Dimension. Garden City, NY, Anchor Books, 1969.

Illich I: Medical Nemesis. New York, Bantam Books, 1976.

Johnson C, Kolodner EL, and Gitlin LN: Health Promotion Strategies for Women with High Risk Pregnancies. OT Practice (in press)

Kahana E: A congruence model of person-environmental interaction. In Windley PG, Byerts TO, and Ernst FG (eds): Theory Development in Environment and Aging. Wash-ington, DC, Gerontological Society, 1975.

Kahana E, Liang J, and Felton BJ: Alternative models of person-environment fit: Prediction of morale in three homes for the aged. J Gerontol 35(4):584–595, 1980.

Kaufman SR: Stroke rehabilitation and the negotiation of identity. In Reinhartz S and Rowles G (eds): Qualitative Gerontology. New York, Springer, 1988.

Kiernat JM: Environment: The hidden modality. J Phys Occup Ther Geriatr 2(1):3–12, 1982.

Laudin H: Victims of Culture. Columbus, OH, Charles E. Merrill, 1973.

Lawton MP: Competence, environmental press and the ad-aptation of older people. In Windley PG, Byerts TO, and Ernst FG (eds): Theory Development in Environment and Aging. Washington, DC, Gerontological Society, 1975.

Lawton MP: Competence, environmental press and the ad-aptation of older people. In Lawton MP, Windley PG, and Byerts To (eds): Aging and the Environment: Theoretical Approaches. New York, Springer, 1982, pp 33–59.

Lawton MP: Ecology and aging. In Pastalan LA and Carson DH (eds): Spatial Behavior of Older People. Ann Arbor, MI, Institute of Gerontology, University of Michigan, 1970.

Lawton MP: Environment and other determinants of well-being in older people. Gerontologist 23:349–357, 1983.

Lawton MP: Environmental proactivity in older people. In Bengtson V and Schaie KW (eds): The Course of Later Life: Research and Reflections. New York, Springer, 1989.

Lawton MP and Nahemow L: Ecology and the aging process. In Eisdorfer C and Lawton MP (eds): The Psychology of Adult Development and Aging. Washington, DC, Ameri-can Psychological Association, 1973.

Lawton MP and Simon BB: The ecology of social relation-ships in housing for the elderly. Gerontologist 8:108–115, 1968.

Leininger M: Transculturat Nursing: Concepts, Theories and Practices. New York, Wiley, 1978.

Levine RE: Culture: A factor influencing the outcomes of occupational therapy. Occup Ther Health Care 4(1):3–15, 1987.

Levine RE and Gitlin LN: Home adaptations for persons with chronic disabilities: An educational model. Am J Occup Ther 44:923–929, 1990.

Lewin K: Resolving Social Conflicts. New York, Harper, 1948.

Murray HA: Explorations in Personality. New York, Oxford University Press, 1938.

Pastalan LA: Research in environment and aging: An alternative to theory. In Lawton MP, Windley PG, and Byerts TO (eds): Aging and the Environment: Theoretical Approaches. New York, Springer, 1982.

Schooler KK: Response of the elderly to environment: A stress-theoretical perspective. In Lawton MP, Windley PG, and Byerts TO (eds): Aging and the Environment: Theoretical Approaches. New York, Springer, 1982.

Searles HF: The Non-Human Environment. New York, International Universities Press, 1960.

Spradley JP and McCurdy DW: Conformity and Conflict. Boston, Little, Brown, 1980.

CHAPTER

21

Susan J. Isernhagen

Corporate Fitness and Prevention of Industrial Injuries

PROMOTING HEALTH: THE CORPORATE FITNESS ROLE

Corporate Strategies

In the mid-1900s, a corporation would have been considered unusual to take a proactive role in its workers' general health. As health awareness progressed through the 1960s and 1970s, however, corporations became more interested in the effect of health and wellness. Why? The rising costs of health care and work injuries were becoming unmanageable for many companies. This trend has continued.

With the necessity for cost containment in health matters for both on-the-job and off-the-job illness and the growing awareness that the fitness fad had some positive attributes, industry and business began to examine incorporating health and fitness into their own corporate culture (Isernhagen, 1988).

Although costs were one of the early reasons for corporations' interest in fitness, many other reasons have surfaced. With productivity an issue, with labor relations a factor, and with teamwork of growing importance, the theme of health and fitness fits into the total scheme of a better-equipped work force.

Wellness Programs

Each corporation or business has its own reasons for sponsoring a wellness program. Some of the motives behind the corporate plan are now discussed.

Improved General Health of the Workers

This can be translated specifically into dollars when there is less absenteeism from work, fewer cases of illness requiring medical attention, and less decrease in productivity as a result of poor health. This is reflected in the costs of health insurance. If a company purchases health insurance, its rates will depend on the medical costs of its particular work force. The healthier the work force, the lower will be the rates. Thus, because health insurance is usually a fringe benefit, there is less expense to the employer. In cases in which the business is self-insured, the monetary savings can be seen more directly. The amount paid out is related directly to the amount of medical attention sought by the work force. Therefore, a healthy work force results in cost savings to the employer.

Some insurance companies offer a business

356

discounts on their policy (Kyes, 1990). The amount and type of discount vary depending on the type of risk-reduction or injury-prevention program offered by the business. This can be interpreted as a proactive approach taken by the firm in reducing costs, preventing injury, and promoting employee well-being.

Increased Productivity

A healthier work force is likely to be better prepared for its work. Fewer physical problems will interfere with physical activity. Strength, coordination, and endurance should be at higher levels for the physical work. In addition, a healthy body is likely better able to ward off the effects of stress and production changes and better able to adapt to production schedules. Therefore, increased productivity may well be a factor in a healthier group of employees.

Increased Efficiency

Current employees are best at performing their own work. If ill employees need to be replaced, productivity often declines because the replacement worker is not as efficient as the original worker. In addition to the double cost to the employer (health-care costs for the ill worker plus replacement costs of the new worker), there most likely will be a general decline in the output or quality of the services provided. In the service industry, a person unfamiliar with the clients or structure will not be nearly as efficient as one who has already learned the nature of the business or the industry's clients. Loss of workers can also produce loss of morale in entire departments. Therefore, the protection of on-the-job status is important for efficiency and morale.

Fewer Work Injuries

Work injuries are usually reduced with a healthier work force. Other chapters in this book (by Brayley, Williams, Rothman, O'Callaghan, and Barbis) reflect on prevention programs that espouse increased knowledge of the employee coupled with ergonomic principles. In addition to this, a fit worker will be less susceptible to sprains, strains, overuse problems, and errors resulting from a lack of endurance. The feeling of health that comes with fitness and exercise also may lend itself to coping with physical problems rather than giving in to them.

Attitude and feeling of well-being are extremely important in the worker's compensation system. An ill worker who feels unimportant and not valued by the employer is much more likely to produce worker's compensation claims than one who feels strong, valued, and like an important part of the work force.

Camaraderie

Camaraderie, when it exists, is one of the most powerful facets of work. In addition to spurring productivity and reducing the likelihood of wanting to be off work, camaraderie can make for a healthful atmosphere. A happy worker will do his or her job better. A healthy and fit worker is more likely to be a happy worker. Part of this reason is the camaraderie that can be generated by working together on fitness projects. The old adage, "Those who play together stay together," can also be true of a work force. By having valuable goals such as fitness and health outside of work, the feeling of loyalty, teamwork, and friendly competition can come into the workplace. Therefore, the fitness and health programs can bring people together for common purposes outside of the general work ethic.

Valuable Older Employees

The long-time worker is a highly valued team member. Often the older workers have strong work ethics and are positive examples for younger workers. Older workers also know how to perform the job efficiently and well, because of their years of practice and experience. Health and fitness programs can add years to productive lives, thus enabling older workers to stay on the job longer. In addition, many corporate fitness programs continue beyond termination of work as a result of retirement. Older workers who have formerly worked with a company are sometimes eligible for health and fitness benefits.

In addition to making the older worker more fit and less vulnerable to the effects of aging, a strong feeling of continuity can be facilitated. There is strength in a "family" of older, middle, and younger workers. Work forces in which there is constant turnover and distress only promote more distress. Therefore, the fitness of older workers is helpful not only to protect them from the effects of aging but also to foster the feeling of loyalty throughout the lifetime of all workers.

Summary

Corporations may have many initial reasons for promoting worker fitness and health. Despite the initial reasons, however, the varied positive effects of such a program are a product of the fitness program regardless of the initial intent of the corporation. The totality of fronts on which the health changes can be seen is amazing. In these days of corporate raiding, massive layoffs, international competition, and economic uncertainty, the physical health and wellness of employees are great combatants to the stress caused by other outside sources.

Currently, many types of programs can be offered and implemented by a corporation. Typically, they take on the flavor of a wellness or fitness program. The delineating factor is that wellness programs tend to focus on behavioral aspects such as nutrition, weight control, and smoking cessation, whereas fitness tends to address the physical well-being of the individual (Gebhardt and Crump, 1990). However, to ensure success with a health and fitness program, a corporation should include components of both wellness and fitness programs. As a result, a multitude of factors can be addressed to make the corporate program applicable to all employees.

Types of Programs Made Available for Corporate Health and Fitness

Blood Pressure Moderation

The first step in reducing the risk of high blood pressure in a work force is to assist the work force in understanding the basics and specifics of their own blood pressure. If general questions about blood pressure were aimed at a group of laypeople, few would know their exact blood pressure. Only those identified as having a problem would readily know. At that, those individuals are often at the mercy of their clinic where they can receive blood pressure information only once a month or at scheduled visits. Therefore, education on blood pressure is more meaningful if employees understand their own situation. The first step is education in their individual needs.

The factors that cause high blood pressure also need to be discussed: diet, stress, heredity, activity, and general fitness. In addition, discussions should include the effects of aging, medications, interaction with other medications, and the cyclic nature of blood pressure.

Once all the factors regarding blood pressure are known, healthful actions can be taken. One of the most powerful factors is the fitness level. Aerobic fitness increases cardiovascular and cardiopulmonary abilities. Blood pressure can be decreased merely by becoming more aerobically fit. The informed consumer of exercise programs will moderate his or her blood pressure as it relates to his or her activity level.

The Centers for Disease Control pointed out the link between coronary heart disease and risk factors of physical inactivity, smoking, high serum cholesterol, and high systolic blood pressure (Gebhardt and Crump, 1990). Because a regularly attended fitness program has been shown to decrease resting heart rate and lower the systolic blood pressure (Gebhardt and Crump, 1990), employees can see for themselves the benefits of such a program. They will know that they are improving their overall health.

Heart Rate

In connection with blood pressure, heart rate is a factor in the fitness level of the individual. Although certain individual differences in heart rate exist and the heart rate does change with aging, workers can bring about a very positive effect on lowering the heart rate through a fitness program. Again, aerobic exercise 3 to 4 times weekly for 20 to 30 minutes can have a long-term effect of reducing the heart rate. Most important, however, it will also increase the ability to tolerate changes of activity without a skyrocketing heart rate. Unconditioned individuals may find that their heart rate increases rapidly with activity and takes a long time to come down. This precludes heavy work or home activity. Alternatively, fit individuals will be able to take on additional stress while maintaining a relatively low heart rate. Therefore, their tolerance for heart rate demands is greater. In addition, fit individuals will see a decrease in time for recovery after the stressful activity.

Those who have lower and more stable heart rates can feel the difference at work and in their everyday activities. The ability to tolerate activity, such as carrying, lifting, walking up hills or stairs, and so on will be markedly felt. This produces not only a healthier person but also one who has a greater feeling of well-being.

Healthy Heart and Hunger

All workers need to eat according to the level of their daily needs. A manual materials handler requires a different nutritional and caloric base than an office worker. Therefore, one of the main prerequisites in studying eating habits of workers is to discuss their work caloric demands. In addition, specific needs for fluids, proteins, and carbohydrates affect alertness, muscle building, and replenishment of nutrients and body fluids. A nutrition base is important for the worker.

In addition, the types of food eaten will have a great impact on the cardiovascular system. A thorough education in cholesterol levels must again begin with the workers' own understanding of their particular situation. Cholesterol tests are very important. As a result, information on the relationship between cholesterol and the changes of heart disease becomes more pertinent.

Wise workers are wise eaters. Both for nutritional competence and to avoid the ill effects of fatty or high-cholesterol diets, workers must be wise about their food intake.

To Smoke or Not To Smoke

Smoking has been strongly linked to some very powerful health hazards, including an increased risk of heart disease, cancer, and lung problems and a degeneration of the fitness level. Smoking has, since the 1960s, been shown to be very detrimental to health.

In addition to the effects of smoking on oneself, smoke in the workplace can lead to problems with employee morale, health of other employees, and general air quality, which can affect the work. As a result, many workplaces now either are entirely smoke-free or have large areas that are smoke-free. This is commendable and actually necessary for the health of the workers who inhale passive smoke.

The direct approach for reducing smoking problems in a work force is not only to discontinue smoking in the workplace but to encourage all workers to eliminate smoking as a habit. Therefore, even corporations and businesses that do not have large employee-fitness programs often pay for or encourage the use of smoking-cessation programs for their employees. This is generally of low cost and does not necessitate in-house staff to manage.

Barriers to smoking, however, can become an emotional issue for many workers. People who have smoked for years feel it is their right and privilege and are often angered by anti-smoking campaigns. Therefore, the issue of smoking cessation must be handled diplomatically to discourage smoking in the workplace and to encourage total health, of which smoking cessation is only one part. The smoker who is cornered into feeling rebellious to protect the habit will not be a happy worker. Alternatively, if total corporate fitness is promoted to the level at which the smoker can see the health benefit of not smoking, this will become an internal decision.

Smoking-cessation programs can be performed in several different ways. The key aspect, again, must be the employees' overall well-being. As a result, a simple stop-smoking campaign or "going cold turkey" may not achieve the desired outcome. Because smoking is an addiction, the cessation program would do well to offer a support group or buddy system. Another way to improve its success rate would be to offer competition or incentives (Maheu et al, 1990). Maheu and colleagues (1990) demonstrated results of a 50% cessation rate for people who participated in competitive or cooperative programs after 52 weeks compared with a cessation rate of only 25% in a noncompetitive program.

Alcohol or Chemical Abuse

Many corporations do not directly address alcohol or chemical abuse. Instead, self-questionnaires point out high-risk behaviors that cause health problems. Questionnaires and general awareness may encourage people to seek help. For example, if one drinks more than 15 to 25 alcoholic beverages per week, he or she may see a "red flag" after filling out a health survey. Chemical abuse also involves other drugs in addition to alcohol. Although drug screening is still a very controversial issue in industry, it is important that the corporation encourage workers to analyze their own situation. It may shock some workers to find that they are in a "danger" category. The workers ultimately make their own decision, but the awareness has been raised by the workplace.

For those with chemical or alcohol abuse, many employers will fund counseling to handle the problem further. This is often provided by employee-assistance programs. Confidentiality and support make these programs successful.

Cancer Alert

Because cancer is a killer with preceding illness, awareness of predisposing cancer factors is important. The American Cancer Society is instrumental in providing education on cancer prevention and early detection.

Some of the factors important in a wellness program associated with reducing risk of cancer are yearly or routine checkups by physicians, monthly breast self-examinations, awareness of the warning signals of cancer, and, again, the individual awareness that some types of cancer may run in families. Although companies do not usually pay for cancer checkups over and above that covered by health insurance, merely increasing workers' awareness of cancer factors and encouraging early detection can contribute greatly to a healthy work force.

In addition to understanding the risks of cancer, it is extremely important for a company to deal with such problems once they are discovered in the work force. For example, people with cancer often work for years while undergoing treatment. Many of them live without recurrence, and many of them who die eventually have intervening productive years. The attitude of maintaining wellness and health for people with cancer is extremely important. Therefore, cancer—one of the most dreaded diseases—must be treated with an enlightened attitude in the workplace.

Other Safety Programs

In addition to the specific health- and wellness-promoting factors discussed previously, a company may choose to jump on the bandwagon for other known causes. One of the most prevalent of these is the *"buckle up" campaign*, which has been embraced by many businesses and industries. In addition to the national campaign, there can be significant support from workplaces for seat belt use. Although encouraging seat belt use in all situations is important, policies *mandating* seat belt use at work are extremely effective in changing habits.

Policies not only can enforce the principle of safety at work but, it is hoped, will make changes in the workers' own lives and in their families' lives. Graphic displays such as in filmstrips or demonstrations may be effective. In addition to seat belt use, other safety programs may involve driving speed, vision checks, and knowledge of traffic laws.

Corporate programs are benefited greatly by an education center where filmstrips, pamphlets, books, and counseling are available on the afore-

mentioned subjects. Paycheck stuffers, use of safety signs, "thought-for-the-month" slogans, and other reminders that health is important can be obtained or can be developed by management. By creating a positive relationship with employees, management can foster a total teamwork concept of wanting the best for each employee. These techniques are most beneficial, however, when management is seen taking the same necessary steps for health and wellness as they desire their employees to take.

Specific Fitness Programs

Exercise fitness can be generated within the entire work force by the provision of a health facility for exercise. This can be provided on-site with a gymnasium, staffed personnel, and programs to be designed and undertaken by all levels of employees. It may also be accomplished when industry pays all or a portion of membership at a fitness center. Whatever the choice, some of the following concepts are important for the exercise program.

First, the program itself should be developed by a professional skilled in evaluation of fitness levels and prescription of exercise programs. This might include a physical therapist or an exercise physiologist. A physician should also be involved when the person has risk factors, such as age, heart disease, a smoking habit, and so on. The physician will give approval for the person to undertake a program to certain levels.

Second, the professional involved in the evaluation must perform individual testing on each worker. This is important because the individual heart rate, projected exercise heart rate, musculoskeletal attributes, and any physical precautions must be taken into consideration when assigning exercise programs. This affects duration, intensity, and speed of the workouts.

Third, not all pieces of exercise equipment should be used by each person. A degenerative back condition, an old joint injury, or a deconditioned athlete may be reason enough to restrict an employee's use of a certain piece of equipment. Not only should all pieces of equipment be tried out by the evaluator and the employee but there should also be specific directions for use of that piece of equipment. This is particularly important if the method of use of the equipment is different from standard protocols.

Fourth, it should be important to the individuals that the circuit training comprises aerobic, strengthening, endurance, and stretching activities (Smith, 1990). In this way circuit training will have the greatest effect.

Fifth, exercise equipment should be purchased or prescribed for its safety of motion, adaptability of weight level, and use of safe body positioning. Aerobic equipment that allows the heart rate to be monitored during exercise is an important safety factor. If heart-rate monitoring is not possible with equipment, then the individuals must be instructed in proper monitoring. Therefore, flexibility in equipment, professional evaluation and supervision, and adaptable schedules are very important in beginning and maintaining fitness and exercise profiles.

Who Exercises?

Interestingly, in many corporate cultures, the first groups chosen for exercise programs were the executive-level groups. There was an underlying impression that high stress, high blood pressure, long work hours, and lack of physical activity were detrimental to the mental and physical well-being of those who managed the companies. Therefore, executive fitness programs are popular and in some companies are the only programs offered.

Another method opens up programs to all workers. There is a perception that blue-collar workers participate in health and fitness programs less often than white-collar workers, but the evidence is not clear. Those blue-collar workers who do not avail themselves of fitness programs may have the perception that their physical work is "keeping them in shape." This may or may not be true. Nygard and colleagues (1987), in their work in Finland, showed that the laborers who performed heavier manual work often were less fit by their later years than those who performed lighter work. This may have been due to the overall trauma received over the years from heavy work. It definitely showed, however, that heavy work in itself is not a conditioning factor for health or fitness.

If teamwork is to be fostered throughout the company, it is very helpful if the exercise facility is open to all levels of workers at the same time. It is less productive for morale to have executives exercise at one time or in one place and blue-collar workers in another. This does nothing for positive teamwork and camaraderie, which is important in fitness building. It is important, rather, that all people in the fitness program be seen as individuals working toward the same goals: health and fitness on the job and in their personal lives.

Each corporation must determine the level of involvement to be subsidized. If total insurance costs and worker's compensation costs are to be considered, *all* workers should have equal opportunities for fitness. Having "coaches" at all levels of management and among workers is very helpful for indoctrinating new employees into the fitness program.

Whether white or blue collar, all workers need health and fitness promotion. In the individual motivational aspect, there may be a difference in values, but the more people who participate and are positive about the program, the more who will be subtly influenced to improve their own health and fitness with such a workout program.

Funding the Fitness Programs

The major source of funds for fitness programs is the business itself. The costs are carefully weighed against the projected benefits. The corporation must trust that their investment in the health and fitness of its workers will provide benefits to all.

General Mills' Experience

A study completed by General Mills was reported in 1989 by Wood and associates. Wood and co-workers reported that the fitness program instituted in 1985 and continued through 1986 showed marked results not only in health awareness but in reduced absenteeism. Wood and associates reported:

> Twelve hundred field sales employees were initially targeted to participate in this program, which focused on improving participants' physical, mental and social well-being. Participants were asked to fill out a computerized lifestyle appraisal form before they started the program. The rates of absenteeism were monitored for each individual in the participant and non-participant groups. . . . Observations show that after two years in the Tri-Healthalon Program, there was an increase in healthy lifestyle behaviors in the participant group with a 5% decrease in the number of smokers, a 37% increase in the number of people who use their seat belts, and

a 23% increase in the number of people who exercise three times a week. There was no significant difference in absenteeism between the groups in 1984 before the program began. [However,] absenteeism was significantly . . . less in the participant group during 1985 and 1986 after initiation of the program. (p. 130)

This prospective study is helpful in examining specific changes that can be made in a large organization. Wood and co-workers (1989) took the concepts from the World Health Organization, which defined health as a balance of physical, mental, and social well-being. By dividing it into these categories, Wood and colleagues were able to study a 2-year plan for accomplishing goals in each category.

1. Physical well-being included: fitness, nutrition and weight control, safety, and cancer prevention.
2. Mental well-being included: stress management, recreation, relaxation and entertainment, positive thinking, and goal setting.
3. Social well-being included: smoking, chemical usage, interpersonal relations, and safety.

In addition to having corporate sponsorship and employees who were directly overseeing this project, General Mills also added incentives for individuals participating in the program. These incentives ranged from gift certificates to jogging suits. In addition, competition was established among sales regions for the largest percentage of successful participation. Therefore, General Mills not only set up the program, sponsored and encouraged it but also interacted with competitiveness and individual reward goals, which go over and above many health and fitness programs.

Of additional note in this study are the lifestyle changes from 1984 through 1986. Seat belt users increased from 44 to 81%. Those who exercise three times a week increased from 48 to 71%. Other significant changes were reflected in lowering of cholesterol—the percentage of people with high cholesterol dropped from 37 to 32%—and lowering of high blood pressure from 14.5 to 10%. These risks are significant and especially interesting because the participants were also aging during the time when they were having "younger" medical analyses. In addition, even though nutrition and weight control were part of the program, the percentage of people who were more than 10% overweight decreased only

from 45 to 43%. This coincides with current thinking that it is not the weight of the individual that is important but rather the overall health. This may be of interest to future planners of health promotion.

One of the most helpful features of this study was the authors' dedication to demonstrating its cost effectiveness. They studied the decrease in lost time days (absenteeism) and put this into dollar terms. They then compared the dollars saved as a result of decreased absenteeism over the 2 years with the amount of money spent on the program for the 2 years. The Tri-Healthalon produced paybacks of $3.10 the first year and $3.90 in 1985 and 1986 for every dollar spent on the program. Therefore, those corporations undergoing health promotion from a cost-containment standpoint may be well advised that in decreasing absenteeism alone they may be able to receive significant payback for the time and effort.

Contracting

A second method of increasing health promotion and fitness is for the company to contract with an outside organization to promote these programs. The cost is borne primarily by the employers. In some cases, the basic program will be purchased by the employers with optional packages to be paid for by the employees. This allows a company to develop a basic plan of health promotion but also offer components that can be obtained on an individual basis. Another format for increasing health and fitness is the use of outside exercise or health facilities. In this way, the company may pay part or all of the monthly membership fee, with another part and participation donated by employees. Therefore, funding of the actual programs is primarily by the employer but in some aspects can be a combination of employer and employee responsibility.

Insurance Company Involvement

Another situation that is having a larger impact on health and fitness programs is the relationship between insurance companies and employers. Both the health insurance and the worker's compensation insurance companies will benefit by promoting lower cost of claims. Therefore, insurance companies are finding that staffing with specialists to aid companies in promoting safety and wellness will also produce a payback for them.

Joe Manion, a risk manager of a large national insurance company, found that the company can interface with industry (personal communication, April 1990):

> The rising costs of work-related injuries have reached a crisis level for businesses nationwide. The 1988 National Safety Council statistics reveal that 84 million Americans are covered by compensation laws in the United States. According to the Social Security Administration, $22,470 million was paid out under Worker's Compensation in 1985. This is an increase of 14 percent from 1984. Of this total $15,089 million was income benefits—and $7,381 million was for medical costs.
>
> To impact the anticipated future increases in Worker's Compensation payments, insurance companies are establishing or improving upon programs through their respective claims or loss control departments that directly involve their insureds—such programs as:

Improving upon job design to reduce the potential for musculoskeletal injuries such as strains and sprains of the upper extremities, low back and lower extremities

Providing educational materials to inform workers of proper lifting or posture while performing their work tasks

Providing consultative type services to provide companies with current and appropriate information on pre-employment physicals, pre-employment strength testing, job safety analysis, accident investigation and reporting

Providing ergonomically based recommendations for administrative or engineering controls

Assisting companies with establishing injury management programs that are designed to minimize lost work days, reduce unnecessary medical treatment and rehabilitate workers who have suffered work-related injuries

> Insurance companies will continue to provide and improve upon programs that will assist businesses with controlling the medical and income benefits resulting from a work-related injury.

Additional Industry Examples

Johnson and Johnson strategized their program, "Live for Life." It was developed in conjunction with consultants from the National Institutes of Health and Stanford and Harvard Universities. It provides comprehensive health menus for employees. Its purpose is to enhance lifestyles, and it involves fitness, exercise, smoking cessation, weight control, nutrition, stress management, and blood pressure intervention. It is free of charge to employees.

A study on this program in 1986 showed that the mean annual inpatient cost increases for insurance had been reduced substantially. The cost increases were $43 for the group that participated in the fitness programs versus $76 for the nonprogram group. In addition, absenteeism dropped 18% by the third year of the program (Bly and Jones, 1986). This mirrors the General Mills experience.

In 1988 Texas Instruments, a company dedicated to worker health and fitness, designed and built a building—a 2,800 square-foot AT&T Texins activity center—specifically for recreation for its workers. Its health and fitness director, Kelley Shaw, stated that many workers changed their lifestyles and made lifetime commitments to fitness improvement.

In the Texas Instruments program, there is an initial screening and use of weight equipment, a pool, and a track. One of the aspects that Kelley Shaw found most helpful is the dedication to providing the worker with an adaptable format. The center stays open until 2 A.M. 2 days a week so that the late-shift personnel can work out. This, in addition to tournaments and proactive classes, has made a very positive change in the health and fitness of the work force at Texas Instruments (Taylor-Thomas, 1989/1990).

The U.S. Surgeon General set a goal of having 60% of adults regularly engaged in vigorous activity by 1990. An article in *Executive Fitness* (Corporate America, 1989) reported that corporate America will likely meet that objective, but the public at large will fall short. Statistically in 1985 one third of worksites with 250 to 749 employees and over one half of those with 750 or more employees offered fitness programs. "Company sponsorship of health programs within business and industry is a response to the awareness that healthy people are also healthy productive employees" (Isernhagen, 1988a, p. 30). "Having reviewed the literature for several years, we are surprised to find that the amount of uncertainty [on worker fitness and risk evaluation] that we initially encountered has not diminished; in many instances, we have become even less confident about medical judgments and predictions of fitness or risk" (Himmelstein and Pransky, 1988, p. 168).

> The scope of ergonomics is broad and its practice embraces several major topics. For example, it is concerned with the particular characteristics of the person, both physical (including body size, physical ability, working posture) and psychological (e.g., learning ability, reacting to directions and decision-making). Ergonomics relates to a person's relationship to the workplace and his [or her] effectiveness while working within it, his reaction to work load and stress, his level of endurance and the rate at which he becomes fatigued. Safety factors and the likely incidence of accidents are also points of concern. Man-machine-task relationships are an important consideration within ergonomics and encompass reference to physical use of controls or equipment within work arrangement or visibility and interpretation of displays. Since all activity takes place within an environment, ergonomics is concerned also with the environmental conditions including lighting, noise, temperature control and ventilation. (Bullock, 1990, p. 3)

SPECIFIC INJURY PREVENTION

Although injury prevention is primarily covered in other chapters, it is important to integrate injury prevention with health promotion. Once a worker is imbued with the idea of maintaining a positive health and fitness profile, this will extend to the work and worksite as well. It would be counterproductive for an employer to promote health and fitness outside of work and yet have the worker be at a dangerous or inefficient worksite for most of the workweek.

Although stronger, more fit workers are less likely to get injured, repetitive motions, sudden trips or falls, or improper movement technique can cause injury even in the fit worker.

Therefore, to be consistent with the principles of health and fitness, the employer should ensure that employees not only have a safe place in which to work but also understand safety principles as they relate to injury prevention and productivity.

Back Schools

Since 1980, back schools have been quite prevalent throughout the United States. Arthur White was quoted in context of the effectiveness of back schools: "There is definitely an awareness in

forward movement of these types of industrial programs. Ten years ago there were only one or two well-known industrial programs in the world; now there are thousands. It requires a corporate commitment. When we were dealing with middle management without the support of dollars from the top, we were working with our hands tied. Now that most large industries are self insured, they can better see their losses and the benefits of these programs" (Isernhagen, 1988a, p. 30).

Without corporate commitment to health, fitness, and safety as well, workers will not long stay safe in the workplace. Back schools have been implemented to teach the workers proper back position, proper body mechanics, and awareness of safe principles of movement. They are only effective, however, when supervisors and management encourage the use of safe procedures and write policies that enforce them.

What often happens, however, is that back schools are presented, and then the workers are left to "get the work done the best way I can." If, in fact, workers find themselves struggling with a heavier load than recommended, often pressures will be created when workers use procedures that injure the back. This can be prevented only when proper assistance or mechanical devices are given to the workers so that time pressure in itself does not mean that the workers must injure themselves to get the job done. Supervisors must constantly ensure that all workers are using safe procedures. In addition, workers should be commended and rewarded for working without injury or for using proper body mechanics. Any accident involving back injury, whether cumulative or sudden, should also be investigated to find the source of the problem.

The investigation can uncover trends. Depending on the firm, some common reasons for injury could range from "did not have safety belt anchored appropriately" to "was in a hurry to complete job assignment/task so did not wait for assistance." From this information, then, management can take steps to remedy the situation to prevent similar injuries in the future. Some steps could include changing the rules and regular training sessions on equipment use (Eisma, 1990).

Another important aspect to address regarding injury prevention and safety promotion is the employees' behavior. Krause and colleagues (1990) pointed out that behaviors are measurable and can lead to changes in attitudes. By focusing on behavior (a measurable objective), the firm is taking on a more proactive approach. It also rewards safe behavior instead of assuming a punitive approach to safety. After all, negativity could foster ill feelings about safety, whereas positive feedback is more effective in changing behavior for the best (Krause et al, 1990).

Cumulative Trauma Prevention

Recently cumulative trauma and overuse syndrome have also been found to be major culprits in injuries in industry. In 1990 the Occupational Safety and Health Administration (OSHA) published recommendations regarding repetitive strain injuries in a meat packing plant as well as the previously documented policy on manual materials handling.

Therefore, workers must be educated in preventing not only sudden injury but cumulative trauma of any part of the body. Cumulative trauma can be a factor in hand and wrist injuries, shoulder problems, neck and upper back discomfort, low back strain or sprain, and lower extremity injuries. The factors involved with repetitive strain such as repetition, force, static position, and angle of repetitive movement must be identified ergonomically and education provided to the worker. In this case, education is a component of providing an ergonomically safe workplace (Isernhagen and Schmitz, 1989).

One issue involved in any injury-prevention program is how to ensure participation by the employee. The following are educational principles that should enhance the instructor's ability to reach the worker with injury-prevention education.

1. The injury-prevention program must be attended first or simultaneously by management and supervisors to gain an appreciation of the concepts taught to the workers.
2. The supervisors and management must agree to allow safe procedures in the workplace and also to be sympathetic to workers when they bring problems to management.
3. It is helpful if supervisors or management personnel take the course with the workers in a group process.
4. The educational materials should be directed at the level of the workers. They should not be filled with medical jargon, large words, and information that is not relevant to the daily work.

5. The workers must become involved with the material. In other words, a point of interest is needed at which workers can internalize some of the content. One way is through the case example, which allows workers to deal with the problems of another human being and to learn solutions.
6. Opportunities for group problem solving by the workers and the instructor should be provided. The instructor who reads rules is not teaching effectively. The workers and the instructor who jointly discuss problems and find solutions, however, are ensuring learning. This also gives ownership of solutions to both the supervisors and the workers.
7. There should be some direct problem solving of workers on their own work load after the presentation of the material. This might be in the form of group discussion or questions and answers. There must be no negative feedback from supervisors or the instructor as to problems brought out during this discussion period.
8. There should be some related postprogram of problem solving so that the teaching of injury-prevention principles and safety in the workplace can be continued.

Another important aspect in a cumulative trauma (or any trauma) prevention program is ergonomics. An ergonomic team should have members from all levels in the corporation including management and employer, supervisory personnel, line workers, a union representative (if applicable), and an outside occupational medicine consultant. To maintain equity, all corporation members should be represented equally. The outside occupational medicine specialist should be trained in ergonomics and should understand the effects of prolonged activity and positioning. Typically, the specialist is a registered physical or occupational therapist.

In order for the ergonomic team to meet its goal, it must abide by points 6 and 7 just listed. Team participation and communication is of utmost importance. Employers and management may be out of touch with what occurs on the production floor. Line workers may be unaware of other management considerations (e.g., budgets). As a result, some conflict may arise. By becoming involved in problem-solving situations, each person will get a feel for what the other must do, thus increasing their ownership of the problem and solution.

PREVENTION OF REINJURY: REHABILITATION PRINCIPLES

Industries cannot completely prevent injury. In the spirit of health and wellness, employers must recognize that some work-related injury is inevitable. The severity and quantity of injury, however, are definitely subject to intervention and ergonomic principles. In addition, as mentioned, the healthy work force may be less susceptible to injury. When injury occurs, the healthy and fit work force is likely to recover more quickly. Thus, the health and fitness in industrial programs will manifest in lesser problems when work injury does occur.

Employer Attitude

Companies can avoid alienation of their workers in the event of injury by preparing them for that contigency. Workers should be educated in their rights and the procedure in which to report work injuries when they do occur. Employees then understand that, although the employer does not wish for an injury to occur, if it does happen they will receive good care. This is the first line of defense against a negative attitude from employees who have been injured. By knowing that the employer stands ready to help at any moment and that the employer will be proactive in following through with the employees' rights, the employees will then have a more positive attitude when injury occurs.

Swanbum pointed out in detail the informed employer's approach to dealing with immediate care of work injury (Swanbum, 1988).

From her point of view, a critical component of immediate care after injury is the employer's caring attitude. A representative of the employer should be present when injured employees initially consult the physician, maintain contact with support, and constantly assure employees that they are welcome back to work when they are physically ready. When employees are ready to return to work after an injury, the employer representative can facilitate a smooth transition.

Early Intervention

Early medical intervention is also critically important (Barnett-Queen and Bermann, 1990; Isernhagen, 1988). The corporation that has a health and fitness program most likely has also sought to have, within its own facility or within close proximity, close medical care for immediate diagnosis and treatment of injury. The corporation no doubt will work closely with physicians so that physicians understand what kind of light duty or immediate return to work is possible for workers who are not severely injured. If the physician deems that returning to work can be immediate, this is better for all concerned psychologically and physically. Of course, injured employees must be protected from further injury, so the physician must decide whether rest at home or return to work is most conducive to healing.

In the case of thorough, early medical intervention, communication must exist between the industry and the medical field. This communication must be constant so that both the employer and the employee never feel out of touch with the progress of the injured workers and the prognosis for return to work as soon and safely as possible. Immediate health-care delivery systems are on the increase throughout the United States (Isernhagen, 1988d). Physicians, physical therapists, occupational health nurses, and other allied health personnel combine their expertise to reduce the impact of injury as soon as possible. Bed rest and loss of work time are not necessarily seen as beneficial. In fact, the reverse might be true; they may increase the physical and psychologic debilities of the workers.

Return-to-Work Process

After early intervention, a decision must be made as to when the worker can return to work. This decision can be made by the treating medical professional, who may be a physician or a physical therapist. If healing time is appropriate, then a fitness program for the parts of the body that are not involved in active healing can be started. Exercise and fitness programs for the injured area can also be started as soon as possible. Rehabilitation and prevention of deconditioning can be simultaneous with healing of an injured part.

With attention to the functioning and healing of the individual, the physician can release the person to return to work as soon as it is safe. Functioning of the rest of the body can be preserved, and protection of the part that has been injured is necessary as long as there is dysfunction or potential for reinjury.

Return to full duty is dependent on an evaluation of the recovery and of the critical demands of the job. When the functioning matches the critical demands, injured employees can return to full duty. If healing has been somewhat prolonged or the injury affects the work directly, then a functional capacity evaluation is extremely helpful (Isernhagen, 1988c). This is performed by a physical therapist or an occupational therapist based on a list of work activities such as lifting, carrying, bending, stooping, standing, sitting, climbing, reaching, crawling, and so on. An analysis of the individual's abilities can then be matched with the functional critical demands of the job. When there is a match, the client can return to work. If the functional capacity evaluation shows a discrepancy between the abilities of the worker and the demands of the work, then a rehabilitation program such as work conditioning or work hardening can be appropriate.

Work conditioning and work hardening are short-term but intensive interventions in which the worker reaches a higher physical ability level through the use of exercise, work simulation, aerobic training, and education.

Professional Roles in Health Promotion

The concepts of health promotion, injury prevention, and immediate care have been discussed. The health-promotion aspect has been detailed without the use of specific professionals who are to direct these programs. Corporate health and fitness in general have myriad professionals involved.

Small businesses may have their entire health and fitness program under the auspices of one professional who can contract out for services that he or she is not able to provide. In other cases, large corporations may have specialists who can provide each aspect of health and fitness promotion.

In general, those professionals whose work encompasses exercise, aerobic work, immediate care, and injury prevention may fall under the category of a medical professional such as a physical therapist, exercise physiologist, or occupational therapist. Other certified professionals with musculoskeletal or cardiovascular background may also be appropriate.

There are professionals who specialize in chemical dependency, nutrition counseling, cholesterol level, smoking cessation, and stress man-agement. It is more effective for a nutritionist to oversee the weight-control section and a psychologist to supervise the stress-management portion than for an unqualified individual to tackle these professional subjects. If the respective professional is not available to lead the sessions, then information must be obtained and responsibly incorporated into a program. If there is not a professional in charge of the sessions, there can be a reference list. Referral to the appropriate professional should be made if any problems arise.

Through teamwork, workers will feel in a healthful atmosphere. Health and fitness should be promoted at every level and by every professional presenting concepts. Workers should be left with a well-rounded sense of fitness and appropriate resources if illness, lack of fitness, or injury occurs.

CHALLENGES FOR THE FUTURE*

Future trends in health promotion will be directly influenced by the quality and results of current research on the monetary effectiveness of such programs. As stated early in this chapter, cost effectiveness in industry has led corporations to provide health and fitness benefits for their workers. Although it is important from a human perspective to know that workers are safe and healthy, the dollar continues to drive the American economy. The good news is that studies do show that promoting health both on the job and off the job is effective. Health-insurance costs and worker's compensation costs are continuing to be a major problem for business and industry. Avenues that can promote a reduction or maintenance of these costs will continue to be important.

Countries are competing to be world leaders in industrial production. The productivity of workers is essential. The demise of edges in businesses such as the automobile industry and steel manufacturing shows that countries are vulnerable when decreased productivity and increased costs occur. Although it is important not to blame any one factor, it is critical to realize that all portions of industry need to be responsible for solutions. In this, corporations can take a proactive stand by involving supervisors, work-

---

*E. Andrew Wood, Manager of Health Promotion and Fitness, General Mills, Minneapolis, contributed to this section.

ers, and medical and other professionals to increase not only the health and wellness of their workers but also productivity at work and loyalty to the employer.

Health and wellness will be here to stay as long as the financial pressures on corporations remain and as long as the programs continue to show evidence of cost effectiveness.

In addition, the following trends may be observed in the 1990s and into the next century:

1. As fitness continues to be emphasized as a lifestyle, Americans will continue to be more open to the suggestions of employers that health and fitness are important.
2. Business and industry simultaneously will become more involved in health and fitness programs not only from within their own corporation but also resulting from the general health trends.
3. As more information on health and fitness becomes available to the general public, it will be easier for corporations to promote health and fitness in the workplace. Exercise equipment and educational sessions will be better used and attended because the workers will have a broader background than they did previously.
4. Because fewer corporations will be able to afford large programs, there may be an increase in the number of programs that are "purchased" for integration into the corporation. Health and fitness programs may be contracted to industry rather than every industry's developing its own program.
5. Corporations will see that fitness and health is not a stand-alone program. It will be seen as part of a total program for incorporation of increased health and decreased injury and illness in the workplace.
6. To ensure a healthier worker, companies will be emphasizing prework screening. Although it is not yet established what factors relate to health risk at work, there will be continued research into what health risks are acceptable in workers and better matching of workers to work.
7. There will be a greater use of ergonomics to make the workplace safer and easier. This, in addition to a healthier work force, should reduce overall illness and injury at work.
8. Early intervention after injury will be available.
9. Chronic injury situations will be reduced with

more effective treatment, early modified return to work, functional capacity evaluation programs, and work-hardening programs.

SUMMARY

Corporate health and fitness benefits all. Corporations are rewarded by having a healthier, happier, more productive work force. Workers feel better about themselves because they are now more in control of elements of their lives. Health and wellness do just that: They place the individual in control. Lifestyle changes cannot be mandated; they must be individually selected.

Medical and insurance costs should be reduced by decreased injury and illness. Incidence may not decrease as much as expected, however, because increased health and wellness generally means increased early intervention. With increased awareness of health, people seek medical care sooner and fewer injuries and illnesses progress to serious stages.

The goals of health and wellness for the entire work force will result in better industrial relations. Management that is willing to sponsor programs that benefit workers and workers who are prepared to spend time and energy becoming healthier should bring labor and management closer together. This produces a major step forward in productivity and corporate management for the future.

The future holds promise of a healthier, more productive work force. Words such as proactive, empowerment, communication, and health are powerful indicators of what a thoroughly integrated corporate fitness and health program can accomplish.

References

Barnett-Queen T and Bermann L: Response to traumatic event crucial in preventing lasting consequences. Occup Health Saf 59(7):53–55, 1990.
Bly J and Jones R: Impact of worksite health promotion on health care costs and utilization. JAMA 256:3240–3253, 1986.
Bullock M: Introduction. In Bullock M (ed): Ergonomics. London, Churchill Livingstone, 1990.
Corporate America Meets 1990 Fitness Objectives. Executive Fitness, p. 3, November 1989.
Eisma T: Rule changes, worker training help simplify fall prevention. Occup Health Saf 59(3):52–55, 1990.
Gebhardt D and Crump C: Employee fitness and wellness programs in the workplace. Am Psychol 45(2):262–272, 1990.

Himmelstein J and Pransky G: Preface. *In* Worker Fitness and Risk Evaluation. Philadelphia, Hanley and Belfus, 1988.

Isernhagen S: Back schools. *In* Isernhagen S (ed): Work Injury: Management and Prevention. Rockville, MD, Aspen, 1988a.

Isernhagen S: Fitness and health promotion programs. *In* Isernhagen S (ed): Work Injury: Management and Prevention. Rockville, MD, Aspen, 1988b.

Isernhagen S: Functional capacity evaluation. *In* Isernhagen S (ed): Work Injury: Management and Prevention. Rockville, MD, Aspen, 1988c.

Isernhagen S: Immediate care delivery systems. *In* Isernhagen S (ed): Work Injury: Management and Prevention. Rockville, MD, Aspen, 1988d.

Isernhagen S and Schmitz M: Cumulative Trauma Prevention Manual. Duluth, MN, Isernhagen & Associates, 1989.

Krause T, Hidley J, and Hedson S: Broad-based changes in behavior key to improving safety culture. Occup Health Saf 3:31–36, 1990.

Kyes K: Reducing liability costs. Rehab Management 3:27–29, 1990.

Maheu M, Gevirtz R, Sallis J, et al: Competition/cooperation in worksite smoking cessation using nicotine gum. Prev Med *18*:867–876, 1990.

Nygard C-H, Suurnikki T, Landau K, et al: Musculoskeletal load of municipal employees aged 44-58 years in physical, mental, and mixed work. Eur J Appl Physiol *56*:555–561, 1987.

Schwartz G, Watson S, Galvin D, et al: The Disability Management Sourcebook. Washington, DC, Washington Business Group on Health/Institute for Rehabilitation and Disability Management, 1989.

Smith RB: Workplace stretching programs reduce costly accidents/injuries. Occup Health Saf *59*:24–25, 1990.

Swanbum N: The employer point of view. *In* Isernhagen S (ed): Work Injury Management and Prevention. Rockville, MD, Aspen, 1988.

Taylor-Thomas M: Corporate fitness: For good reasons, it's here to stay. *Cybex Times*, pp. 2–5, Winter 1989/1990.

Tharrett S and Sey A: Corporate fitness. Rehab Management 3:14–17, 1990.

Wood EA, Olmstead G, and Craig J: An evaluation of lifestyle risk factors and absenteeism after two years in a worksite health promotion program. Am J Health Prom *58*(11):128–133, 1989.

CHAPTER
22

JANE O'CALLAGHAN

Primary Prevention and Ergonomics: The Role of Rehabilitation Specialists in Preventing Occupational Injury

Technology changes, but people remain an essential element in every industry. The ideal relationship between people and their work is one that minimizes occupational injury or illness while ensuring productivity and personal fulfillment. Primary prevention through ergonomics is not only an attack on disease but also a vehicle for promoting organizational and individual well-being. Health in the individual equals health in the organization and vice versa.

The goal of this chapter is to introduce rehabilitation therapists to primary intervention and ergonomics.

Rehabilitation professionals are increasingly committed to ergonomic prevention and health promotion in their own working areas. The sequence of prevention and promotion can be seen in the simplest of rehabilitation problems. For example, a rehabilitation specialist who sees a worker with back strain for the second time begins to think about ergonomics and prevention. The therapist then visits the workplace and recommends changes in job design and worker

back education as preventive measures. This not only reduces the likelihood of further back strain for the worker but prevents similar injuries to other workers.

In this case the rehabilitation specialist has introduced ergonomic prevention into the workplace. It is sometimes termed secondary prevention because the worker's primary injury was overcome, but it is also primary prevention because the worker was assisted in achieving a higher level of health than would otherwise be possible. Rehabilitation experts, who are knowledgeable about the normal and traumatized musculoskeletal system, disability, anatomy, physics, biomechanics, and behavioral sciences, are particularly well equipped to recommend ergonomic changes in the workplace.

Ergonomic prevention of occupational injury and health promotion form a valuable dyad that presents a challenge to health professionals, offers hope to recipients, and promises relief to those whose increasingly difficult responsibility is to fund health services (Warrick, 1990).

DEFINITIONS

Ergonomics

The word *ergonomics* is derived from the Greek words *ergon* (work) and *nomos* (natural law). Ergonomics is the science that addresses human performance and well-being in relation to the job, equipment, tools, and the environment. The goal is to improve the health and efficiency of both the individual and the organization. Ergonomics began as a specialty in industrial engineering that examined the efficiency of the human–machine interface. Recently, the field has expanded to consider the impact of machine and workstation design on the worker.

Ergonomics assumes that objects for human use can be designed to suit human characteristics, capabilities, and limitations. A fundamental principle is that all work activities cause some level of physical and mental stress, and the intensity of this stress can produce musculoskeletal symptoms. Overuse of a segment of the musculoskeletal system is often due to the poor match between the worker's capabilities and the demands of the job.

Primary Prevention

Primary prevention aims at reducing the occurrence of injury. It includes generalized health promotion as well as specific protection against disease, precedes disease or dysfunction, and is applied to a population generally considered to be both physically and emotionally healthy.

Some examples of ergonomics as primary prevention are:

Evaluating tasks and workstations to determine biomechanical stresses
Redesigning high-risk tasks to ensure that stresses on joints and muscles do not lead to injury
Changing workstation layouts to reduce postural stresses
Assessing awkward postures to eliminate fatigue and cumulative trauma
Assessing highly repetitive manual assembly operations to identify the risk of disorders such as tendinitis, epicondylitis, and carpal tunnel syndrome
Educating workers and managers to increase their awareness of ergonomic prevention

MAGNITUDE OF OCCUPATIONALLY RELATED DISORDERS

Occupationally caused or aggravated musculoskeletal disorders are one of the serious health problems affecting workers according to the National Institute of Occupational Safety and Health (NIOSH, 1985). Musculoskeletal disorders can occur in all parts of the body, but the back and the upper extremities are most commonly affected.

Injuries to the musculoskeletal system are the result of many different factors, several of which may relate to the ergonomics of the workplace. NIOSH (1986) rated the musculoskeletal system second only to the cardiovascular system in work-related disability. Twenty-seven million workdays per year are lost at a cost of at least $15 billion (Frymoyer and Mooney, 1986). It is remarkable that between 1971 and 1981 the population disabled by low back pain increased at a rate 14 times that of the growth of the U.S. population. This rate of increase was far greater than that of any other disease (National Center for Health Statistics, 1985).

Low back pain is a major cause of industrial disability. Pope and colleagues (1986) concluded that low back pain will affect up to 70% of the population at some time during their working lives. Manning and associates (1984) reported that 25% of all time lost as a result of industrial injuries is attributable to low back pain. To reduce the enormous costs of low back pain to industry and the community, primary prevention is essential.

SETTING THE STAGE

Given the magnitude of the problem, rehabilitation specialists must become more actively involved in primary prevention and ergonomics. This section describes what the rehabilitation therapist must do to establish the "need" of the organization for an ergonomic program.

Planning for ergonomic prevention begins with establishing contact with the health and safety departments of a company to gather information for a proposal. There are four ways to gather information for planning ergonomic services: injury and compensation analysis, ergonomic survey, worker interviews, and related ergonomic research.

Injury and Compensation Analysis

For this analysis, you need to review the company's injury statistics and the jobs with high rates of turnover and absenteeism and evaluate the medical claims that are related to occupational diseases and injuries. Caution is advised when using accident and injury data bases because they have weaknesses such as biases in reported information, under-reporting (selective nonreporting of events), and insufficient data for valid analysis. Moreover, the detailed information required for a meaningful diagnosis is often not in the data base; you need to get out of the office and onto the floor.

Ergonomic Survey

This activity involves conducting a survey of the workplace. If you want to establish a prevention program, begin by telling the company what they are already doing right. Take photographs on the site of both low-risk and high-risk areas. Walk through with managers and supervisors.

To measure stresses imposed on workers, the following tools are necessary:

A strain gauge to measure forces
A scale to measure weights
A measuring tape to obtain work space, equipment, and product dimensions
Camera and video recorder

In addition, a computerized version of the NIOSH (1981) formulas is useful in determining the acceptable and maximum permissible weights for each manual materials-handling activity.

For effective primary intervention, the ergonomic survey should be done in response to a building plan, job description of a new position, or prepurchase equipment specification rather than an injury or accident report. Look for high-risk factors. The musculoskeletal risk factors associated with work have been amply summarized by Armstrong (1986) as being predominantly force, posture, and time (repetition) as well as cold, vibration, and unsuitable gloves.

Worker Interviews

Workers are your best teachers and major source of information about the hazards. Rehabilitation therapists need to regard workers as members of the occupational health team. Worker participation in primary prevention does not mean a loss of management control of the workplace; rather, it increases personal responsibility for health and safety.

After talking with the workers, videotape the jobs. View the film and make your own list of problems. Then call a meeting with the workers, the union representative, the supervisor, management, and the health and safety committee. Show the video, and ask the group to identify their concerns and possible solutions. Schedule a strategy meeting several weeks after this session so that all the participants have time to investigate their solutions.

Ergonomic Research

Related ergonomic research is another source of information. This section describes some of the ergonomic research related to low back pain.

Occupational low back pain has become a focus for prevention because it costs so much in lost productivity (Frymoyer et al, 1983) and compensation payments (Snook, 1982). The prevention measures used by industry have included education, pre-employment screening, and modifications to the workplace. Training provides benefits to both workers and employers. Lepore and associates (1984) reported significant reductions in the average annual cost of expenditures for back injuries (67.5%), average annual cost per claim (76%), and severity of injuries as measured by absenteeism (71%).

Hall and Iceton (1983) found that low back schools reduced both the frequency and cost of lower back injuries. Andersson (1984) found that pre-employment radiographic screening is ineffective in identifying employees at risk for future back pain. Chaffin and associates (1984, pp. 274–291) found that workplace modifications are effective in reducing mechanical stressors.

SELLING THE PROGRAM

When you have all the information, put it together and present it to the decision makers. Find out who is ultimately responsible for integrating change in the company. Do not make the presentation unless the company president commits to attending! If the president and upper management are not committed to a participative prevention and health-promotion program, the program will not succeed.

First, present an overview of injuries and absenteeism. Demonstrate the seriousness of the problem using statistics and costs. Talk about lost production time, insurance costs, medical costs, and lost wages. Illustrate why problems are not usually caused by a single injury but develop gradually through repeated trauma. You can also use this meeting to suggest the formation of an ergonomic task force, with management and union representatives, that would work with the joint safety committee.

CREATING AN ERGONOMIC TASK FORCE

An ergonomic task force can play a significant role in establishing ergonomic policies in an organization by helping to ensure that primary ergonomic prevention is incorporated into the company's strategic business plan. This task force needs to establish clear principles and direction before recommending any changes. It needs to have cross-sectional representation from the organization, including management, union representatives, employees with different types of jobs, and ergonomic specialists (physiotherapists and occupational therapists) and others with expertise or interest in championing the process.

The task force needs to establish a framework for implementing ergonomic change within the organization, which should include the following elements:

Principles: philosophy, beliefs, values
Purpose: vision, mission, goals
Plans and practices: strategic and tactic

Developing Guiding Principles for the Ergonomic Task Force

The task force needs to develop guiding principles both for itself and for the ergonomic program. Developing the team principles gives the group an opportunity to review their past working relationships and to reach an agreement as to how they want to work together in this forum. It helps the group to clarify what the members can expect from each other regarding decision

making, communication, trust, responsibility, leadership, and so on. This is an important step because management, unions, and employees have traditionally been in adversarial positions; they have often not worked well together or communicated effectively. This process of jointly deciding how to work together helps to unify the group and enhances the commitment of all parties to live with the decisions they make.

Next, the task force needs to develop program principles to clarify what they jointly believe about an ergonomic approach in the organization. It is useful for the ergonomic task force to meet and discuss how they are going to work with the rest of the organization. This exercise allows the task force the opportunity to discuss their various beliefs about ergonomics, customer service, quality versus cost, training, involvement, integrity, long-term versus short-term investment, and so on. These principles are the foundation for the work of the task force. Some examples of program principles are:

The long-term health of the employees has first priority.
Employees are important members of the ergonomic team.
Employees have a right to a safe workplace.

These principles can then be translated into plans, strategies, policies, and procedures. They are the foundation for all the decisions that will be made around the issue of ergonomics.

Developing a Mission and Goals for the Ergonomic Program

The truth is that the task force cannot do everything; it must focus its resources wisely to ensure that it accomplishes as much as possible. The task force needs to help the organization identify what it actually wants to accomplish through an ergonomic program. It needs to identify how the organization will focus its time, money, and energies in the area of ergonomics to meet these goals.

To gain broad support and commitment for this mission, the task force may want to involve not only management but a large number of employees to help identify the overall goals of the program. "When people plan the battle, they don't battle the plan." This principle encourages high-level participation from all the major stake-holder groups.

An example of a mission for the ergonomic task force is to create a working environment that encourages efficient productivity by the safe design of the workplace and the promotion of health and wellness. The task force must also define short-term and long-term goals to ensure that the overall mission is achieved.

Integrating Plans into Practices

Plans are wonderful, but they may never get put into practice unless there is a watchful eye. It is one thing to talk about the task force philosophy and purpose and another to put it into action. Plans are just descriptions of how we are going to accomplish our goals. Everyone needs to know what is going to happen, why it is going to happen, and how it will happen.

The task force also needs to test what is currently happening against what they say they want to have happening. They may ask questions like, "To achieve our proposed 50% reduction in back injuries, are the employees on the loading dock using the techniques that they learned in the educational program?"

The task force needs constantly to review how their philosophy, purpose, and plans are being put into practice by monitoring the process of implementation on many fronts. Some of the questions to ask are:

Are we working with each other in the way in which we agreed? (How are we making decisions? How are we communicating?) Where do we need help? Do we need training, new systems, methods, and so on?

Are we putting our program principles into practice? Are we putting our money where our mouth is? Are we "walking what we talk?"

If we only do what we have planned to do, will we accomplish our mission? Are our plans clear and well understood and supported by the management as well as staff?

A Personal Opinion

The preceding points suggest a need for an organizational development approach in bringing about ergonomic changes. My experience supports that premise. It is not essential that the rehabilitation specialist play that role; however, he or she needs to be a part of the process. Every task force will not go through all of these steps formally. However, experience has shown that each step is a contributing factor to the success of ergonomic change.

METHODS: ERGONOMICS TASK ANALYSIS

The preceding two sections addressed ways to sell the concept of ergonomics and establishing an environment for successful, ongoing ergonomic change. However, before a job can be effectively redesigned, it must be appropriately and thoroughly evaluated. Experimental ergonomic changes waste time and money and lead to a lack of confidence and trust. Planning for the ergonomic analysis is as important as the analysis itself. The survey and information-gathering step enables you to focus on more detailed analysis and measurement.

Several approaches to ergonomic analysis are possible for the occupational and physical therapist. A description of some of these approaches follows.

Job-Demands Analysis

In the past, job analysis was used by many companies as a means of designing jobs for maximum production. However, job analysis can also be used to evaluate and reduce the load on the worker's musculoskeletal system and reduce the risk of injury or illness.

When you are assessing jobs with differing physical requirements, use a checklist of physical tasks to document the general physical requirements and to highlight those demands that may lead to worker injury or illness. An example of such a checklist is shown in Figure 22–1; it is based on one developed by the Canadian Ministry of Labour. A physical or occupational therapist observes the job and fills out the form, noting the average frequency of occurrence and the weight handled during the performance of the physical tasks.

This information can also be used to return injured workers to appropriate jobs by comparing these job-demands data with a clinical assessment of a worker's specific mobility and strength.

Name:
Department:
Job:
Date:

PHYSICAL DEMAND	NOT AT ALL	OCCASIONALLY (less than 1 hr)	FREQUENTLY (1–3 hr)	MAJOR DEMAND (more than 3 hr)	COMMENTS
Lifting					max wt usual wt
Carrying					max wt usual wt
Pushing					max wt usual wt
Pulling					max wt usual wt
Fine finger work					max wt usual wt
Handling					max wt usual wt
Gripping					max wt usual wt
Reach above shoulder below shoulder					max wt usual wt
Neck motion					
Throwing					
Sitting					
Standing					
Walking					
Running/jumping					
Climbing					
Bending/stoop					
Crouching					
Kneeling					
Crawling					
Twisting					
Balancing					
Hearing					
Vision: Far Near Color Depth					
Perception					
Feeling					
Reading					
Writing					
Speech					
Inside work					
Outside work					
Hot/cold					
Humid					
Dust					
Vapor fumes					
Noise					
Proximity to moving objects					
Hazardous machinery					
Electrical					
Radiant energy					
Slippery					
Congestion					
Chemicals					
Vibration					
Travelling					
Work alone					
Interact					
Operate machinery					
Irregular hours					

Figure 22–1. Job-demands checklist. (Adapted from the Centre For Disability and Work, Ontario Ministry of Labor, Toronto, Canada, 1984.)

Job-demands analysis is important in identifying jobs that could be potentially hazardous to a worker's musculoskeletal system. It is particularly useful with jobs composed of many tasks rather than those that are highly repetitive. Such job-demands analysis is helpful in motivating ergonomic changes when combined with your injury data analysis.

Discomfort and Comfort Scale

The presence of discomfort over long periods may be evidence of an unhealthy work environment. Figure 22–2 shows a possible method of screening workers for occupational discomfort. This scale is filled out before work starts, before the first break, before the meal break, after the meal break, before the next break, and at the end of work.

This type of scale can be used with job-demands analysis or postural evaluations to document potentially high-risk tasks.

Evaluation of Upper Extremity Activities

Armstrong and colleagues (1986) found many of the necessary upper extremity postures to observe and evaluate for the prevention of injury and illness. Cumulative trauma to the wrist area may be caused by the following factors:

Checklist for the Identification of Upper Extremity Injuries	
Disorder	**Risk Factors**
Carpal tunnel syndrome	Repetitive hand work; repeated extreme flexion or extension with strong pinching; repeated forces on the base of the palm or wrist
Tenosynovitis and peritendinitis of the abductor and extensor pollicis tendons of the radial styloid (De Quervain's disease)	>2,000 manipulations/hour; unaccustomed work; repeated radial deviation with strong thumb exertions; repeated ulnar deviation with strong thumb exertion
Tenosynovitis of the finger flexor tendons	Exertions with a flexed wrist
Tenosynovitis of the finger extensor tendons	Ulnar deviation of the wrist with outward rotation
Epicondylitis	Radial deviation of the wrist with inward wrist deviation

Figure 22–3 shows a general checklist for the identification of upper extremity injuries. As the number of "no" answers increases, so does the likelihood of injury.

Postural Evaluation Methods

Awkward postures can be caused by poor workstation layout, incorrect methods, or the body size of the individual worker. Non-neutral postures may contribute to injuries. Another approach to recording potentially stressful tasks is the postural evaluation methods. Resources for analyzing postures are plentiful (Corlett et al, 1976; Karhu et al, 1981; Keyserling, 1986).

Corlett and co-workers (1979) developed a method called *postural targeting*. The physical or occupational therapist observes the worker at random times during the workday and records the angular configurations of various body segments with the aid of the body diagram.

Another postural observation system was developed in Finland. The Ovaco working posture analysis system is a practical method for identifying and assessing unsuitable working postures (Karhu et al, 1977 and 1981).

Evaluation of Seated Work Postures

Because of the prevalence of bench work in industry, some general comments on seated work are appropriate. In general, the posture of a seated person depends not only on the design of the chair but also on individual sitting habits and the task to be performed.

Many seated work tasks lead to high frequencies of musculoskeletal problems. Examples of such tasks are office work, small-parts assembly, inspection, automobile operation, and sewing-machine operation. Some tasks involve high muscle load, repetitive loadings, or cramped postures.

Sitting should be seen as a dynamic activity. People need to be able to move around in their seats, lean in different directions, and get up and down easily. For detailed information on chair evaluation, consult Grandjean (1980).

Job-Design Solutions

The Canadian Standards Association (1989) published a book entitled *A Guideline on Office Ergo-*

DISCOMFORT SCALE

Name: _____   Job: _____

Date: _____   Time of Day: _____

Please use the scale below to rate your present sense of well being.

1   2   3   4   5   6   7

Feeling   Feeling   Feeling   Feeling
very well   alright   not well   terrible

Please rate your feelings of discomfort in the listed different parts of your body.

Use the scale below to rate any discomfort that you are feeling and enter a number representing that discomfort for each body part in the spaces provided.

If you have no discomfort (1) in a body part please fill that in.

1   2   3   4   5   6   7   8   9   10

Just   Some   Clearly   Very   Intolerable
uncomfortable   discomfort   uncomfortable   uncomfortable

A. Eyes _____
B. Neck _____
C. Upper back _____
D. Mid back _____
E. Low back _____

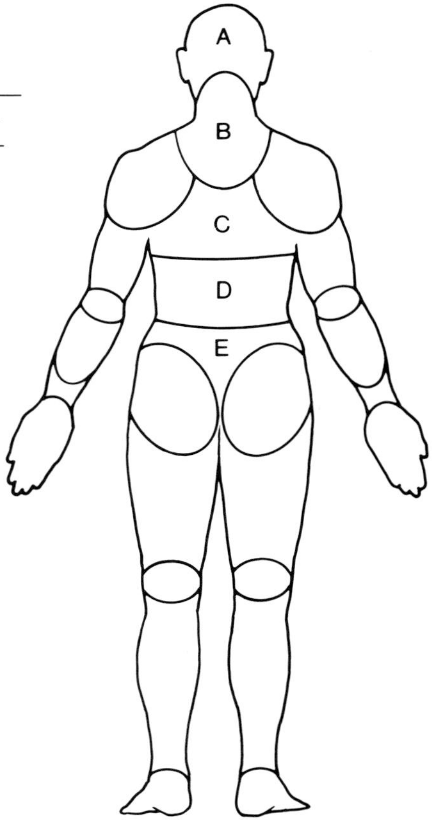

L. Shoulder _____   R. Shoulder _____

L. Upper arm _____   R. Upper arm _____

L. Elbow _____   R. Elbow _____

L. Forearm _____   R. Forearm _____

L. Wrist _____   R. Wrist _____

L. Hand _____   R. Hand _____

L. Buttock _____   R. Buttock _____

L. Thigh _____   R. Thigh _____

L. Knee _____   R. Knee _____

L. Leg _____   R. Leg _____

L. Foot and ankle _____   R. Foot and ankle _____

Figure 22–2. Discomfort Questionnaire (Modified from Corlett EN and Bishop RP: VA technique for assessing postural discomfort. Ergonomics *19*:175–182, 1976.).

1. Can the task be done without the fingers or wrist touching sharp edges?
2. Is the tool operating without vibration?
3. Are the worker's hands exposed to moderate temperature?
4. Can the task be done without using gloves?
5. Can the task be done without using finger pinch grips?
6. Can the task be done without bending (flexion or extension) of the wrist?
7. Can the tool be used without flexion or extension of the wrist?
8. Can the task be done without deviating the wrist from side to side (ulnar or radial deviation)?
9. Can the tool be used without ulnar or radial deviation of the wrist?
10. Can the worker be seated while performing the task?
11. Can the task be done without "clothes wringing" motion?
12. Can the orientation of the work surface be adjusted?
13. Can the height of the work surface be adjusted?
14. Can the location of the tool be adjusted?
15. Is the cycle time above 30 seconds?
16. Can the thumb and finger slightly overlap around a closed grip?
17. Is the span of the tool's handle between 5 and 8 cm?
18. Is the handle of the tool made from material other than metal?
19. Is the weight of the tool below ten (10) lb?
20. Is the tool suspended?

Figure 22-3. Upper extremity evaluation (Modified from Lifschitz Y and Armstrong TJ: A Design Checklist for Control and Prediction of Cumulative Trauma Disorder in Intensive Manual Jobs. Proceedings of the Human Factors Society, 30th Annual Meeting, 1986, pp 837–884. Copyright 1986 by The Human Factors Society, Inc. All rights reserved.)

nomics. This book helps people choose and configure equipment, assess environmental conditions, and optimize job design. Its recommendations are practical. For example, the optimum work level/surface height is level with, or slightly below, the elbow. The shoulders should be supported through the elbows when writing. An adjustable work height from 630 to 760 mm will accommodate 90% of the population. A reasonable compromise for a fixed height surface would be 710 to 720 mm, with adjustable seat height and footrest (Canadian Standards Association, 1989).

MANUAL MATERIALS-HANDLING ACTIVITIES

Because lifting is so prevalent and is often the cause of serious musculoskeletal disability, a specific evaluation of lifting tasks is often warranted.

In evaluating manual materials-handling activities, the amount of force transmitted to the back is a function of the object weight and the horizontal distance between the center of the mass of the object and the center of the worker's body (NIOSH, 1981). This is called a *moment of force* or *torque* and is a fundamental principle of ergonomics. Increasing the horizontal distance increases the forces transmitted to the spine (primarily L4/L5 and L5/S1). As this distance increases, the muscular forces generated in the back to oppose the weight of the object increase to keep the body in an upright position. These opposing forces produce compression of the discs. Prolonged repetitive or forceful compression leads to degenerative changes in the disc and ultimately permanent damage of the lumbar spine.

NIOSH Guidelines

Guidelines exist that provide a simple equation for estimating safe lifting limits (NIOSH, 1981). According to NIOSH, object weight and horizontal distance combine with factors such as the height of the object at the start of the lift, the vertical travel distance of the object, the frequency of lifting, and the duration of the lifting activity. To determine the recommended weight limits for any given task, all of these factors must be considered. Under ideal conditions, NIOSH recommends a maximum weight of 40 kg as suitable for 99% of all men and 75% of all women for infrequent lifting. When one of the lifting parameters changes from the ideal, only lower weights can be tolerated.

To determine the acceptability of the manual handling activities, lifts can be evaluated by using the NIOSH modeling program. Two limit values can be derived for each activity: the action limit (AL), which provides an acceptable weight that can be lifted, given the observed lifting parameters, with risk of injury to 99% of men and 75% of women; and the maximum permissible limit (MPL), which indicates that the frequency and severity of injuries increase significantly when work exceeds the MPL.

In algebraic form:

AL (kg) = 40 (15/H) (1 − (0.004[V − 75]))
(0.7 + 7.5/D)
1 − (F/F$_{max}$) and
MPL (kg) = 3 (AL)

H is the horizontal distance (in centimeters) from the center of mass of the object to the midpoint between the ankles of the body with a minimum value of 15 cm (body interference) and a maximum of 80 cm (reach distance for most people). V is the vertical distance (in centimeters) from the load's center of mass at the start of the vertical lift measured from the floor, with no minimum value and a maximum of 175 cm (upward reach for most people). D is the vertical travel distance (in centimeters) of the object assuming a minimum value of 25 cm and a maximum of 200 cm minus the vertical origin height (V). If the distance moved is small (D less than 25 cm), the effect is nominal, so D is set equal to 25 cm. F is the average frequency of lifts (per minute) with a minimum value for occasional lifts of 0.2 (once every 5 minutes) and a maximum value defined by both the period of lifting (less than 1 hour or for 8 hours) and whether the lifting involves only arm work or significant body stabilization or movement. F$_{max}$ is the maximum frequency that can be sustained (from NIOSH tables). Values for F$_{max}$ vary from 12 to 18 lifts per minute.

Manual Handling Solutions

In general, lifting tasks above the MPL require engineering controls to reduce the risk. Tasks between the MPL and the AL may require a combination of administrative controls (through job rotation, team lifting, and so on) and engineering controls. Tasks below the AL are considered acceptable.

Engineering and workplace design considerations to minimize musculoskeletal stress might include (Chaffin and Andersson, 1984):

Roller conveyors that allow objects to be pulled in toward the body before lifting
Slides that work by gravity and present items to the worker at standing knuckle height (75 cm)
Machines that have work parts close to operator
Tilting fixtures or racks of large stock bins to present parts closer to the worker
Enough room for workers to walk around the

bin or pallets to avoid having to reach and lean forward to remove parts from the opposite side
Carts for pushing and pulling that require hand forces not exceeding 23 kg on the handle
Carts with vertical handles that can be grasped at different heights and that have large rubber tires with good bearings and two wheels that pivot easily (inclination should be no greater than 4 degrees)
Clean, dry floors to avoid slipping or high-traction shoes (coefficient of friction [ratio of foot shear divided by normal force] should exceed 1.0)

Example

Imagine that a female worker is moving electronic boxes from a pallet on the floor to a shelf 1.5 m (150 cm) above the floor at a rate of 5 lifts/min for 1 hour. The horizontal distance from the midpoint between her ankles to her hands on the box was measured to be 45 cm. The vertical starting position of her hands on the box above the floor was 25 cm. The boxes were all the same weight.

Is this woman at risk of back injury? What changes in the workplace would make the largest differences in reducing the risk?

Information

H = 45 cm
V = 25 cm
D = 125 cm (shelf height − V)
F = 5 lifts/min

F$_{max}$ = 15 lifts/min (from F$_{max}$ table for 1-hour stoops)

Factor Values

Hfac = 15/H = 15/45 = 0.33
Vfac = 1− 0.004 V − 75 =
1 − 0.004 25 − 75 = 0.80
Dfac = 0.7 + 7.5/D = 0.7 + 0.06 = 0.76
Ffac = 1 − F/F$_{max}$ = 1 − 5/15 = 0.67
AL = 40 (Hfac) (Vfac) (Dfac) (Ffac)
AL = 40 (0.33) (0.80) (0.76) (0.67)
AL = 5.4 kg
MPL = 3 × AL = 16.2 kg

Interpretation

The weight of the boxes was 15 kg. The NIOSH AL, given the conditions of the lift, is 5.4 kg. Thus, these lifts far exceed the AL. However, the MPL is calculated to be 16.2 kg. These lifts are slightly below the MPL.

NIOSH guidelines suggest that this worker has a moderate risk of musculoskeletal injury. Either the job should be changed or a stronger worker should be assigned to this job and instructed on safe techniques.

The values of the factors point to the most profitable workplace changes. A value of 1 is the largest any factor can be. The farther from 1, the greater the room for improvement. Therefore, the Hfac and the Ffac should be considered first. Getting the worker closer to the load and reducing the frequency would raise the AL. (This example was adapted from a course given by Robert Norman entitled "Measurement of Low Back Injury Risk," University of Waterloo, Ontario, Canada, 1989.)

Snook Tables

Snook (1978) stated that two thirds of low back injuries linked to heavy handling tasks could be prevented if the tasks were designed to fit at least 75% of the population. Snook based this assertion on 191 compensable back-injury cases that were investigated by measuring the load-weight demands of the injured workers' jobs.

The threshold limit value is the weight, push, or pull force that 75% of the population felt that they could handle. Weights higher than this make a worker three times more susceptible to back injury.

Snook presented these data for men and women performing lifts, lowers, pushes, pulls, and carries over different vertical distances, different distances of the load from the body, and different rates of work. These data are available in Snook (1978).

OTHER ERGONOMIC APPROACHES

Organizational and Administration Factors

Job Rotation

Job rotation has been used to compensate for stressful repetitive work. Slightly different tasks may lead to changes in loading and to decreased fatigue rates (Hagberg, 1986). Jonsson and colleagues (1988) noted that reducing static loading and increasing the variety of jobs can lead to improvements in worker health. Note that the jobs should have different musculoskeletal stresses in order for job rotation to be effective.

Quotas

The use of a quota or piecework system may contribute to musculoskeletal problems. High individual productivity has been found to be a relatively strong predictor of deteriorating health in electronic assembly line workers (Jonsson et al, 1988).

Appropriate Packaging

In terms of size, large objects that extend the arms impede the worker's vision. Packaging needs to be small enough and symmetrical in shape to handle efficiently. Objects should have easy-to-grasp handles or handholds. The total weight of the object should be clearly marked on the outside.

Job Placement (Selection)

Although previous injury is a factor, it is not causally related to deteriorating health. However, Nathan and associates (1988) found age, irrespective of previous employment, to be the best predictor of developing carpal tunnel syndrome.

Pre-employment Screening

Chaffin and associates (1978) noted that pre-employment strength testing did reduce the frequency of injuries causing low back pain. Cady and colleagues (1985) reported that those who are least physically fit are more likely to have an acute lower back injury. However, the more physically fit employees may have the most expensive injuries.

Andersson (1984) found that pre-employment radiographic screening is ineffective in identifying employees at risk for future back pain.

Although these findings suggest that stronger individuals are more likely to withstand job-related musculoskeletal stresses, this has not been shown to be true for upper limb tasks. Jonsson and colleagues (1988) found that stronger workers placed greater loads on their shoulders and had a higher deterioration of symptoms. They recommended against using static strength pre-employment testing.

The authorities on pre-employment screening are not in agreement, so the jury is still out on pre-employment screening related to strength and fitness.

Education

Education of the Workers

An essential factor in effective health and safety programs is education. Therefore, give careful consideration to the methods used to present information to workers. Training should be developed jointly, given jointly, and received jointly. Adult education guidelines for learner-centered programs include the following:

Develop the program in the employees' first or technical language. Employees must be familiar with the language used to educate; if the employee's first language is Portuguese, then the program must be in Portuguese.
Clearly define the goals of the program.
Begin the session with a concise overview, and summarize the most critical points.
Design an evaluation that is applicable to each program.
Use participatory teaching methods. Adults learn more effectively by doing rather than by listening passively. Incorporate the learners' experiences into the course material. Participation by workers and employees is vital to building successful primary intervention into the work process.

(These points were adapted from Quinn, 1983.)

Safe Lifting

Lifting is the most common event associated with the onset of low back pain (Bigos et al, 1986). Thus, training workers to lift safely has been a major focus of prevention programs. Unfortunately, the experts in lifting have not reached a consensus about the elements of a safe lift. Many lifting programs apply a single set of rules for handling, which in the real workplace may not be effective or safe.

However, authorities do agree on some prin-

ciples that help to protect the disc and other structures, such as the following:

The object being lifted should be kept as close to the trunk as possible. Increasing the horizontal distance of the center of gravity of the load from the trunk causes unnecessary flexion and increases the load on the disc.
The speed of the lift is important. The object should be lifted as quickly as possible once the position is set. This avoids sustained flexion, which puts undue elongation and decreased tautness on the annulus and ligament. The force is removed before maximal displacement occurs.

In addition to these axioms, some authorities emphasized the bending of the knees, whereas others emphasized a straight back. NIOSH recommended that training in safe lifting include the following elements (NIOSH, 1981):

Risks to body of unskilled lifting
Physics of lifting
Awareness of body's strengths and weaknesses
Avoidance of unexpected physical factors that might contribute to low back pain
Development of handling skills
Use of handling aids

Strength and Fitness Training

Strength and fitness training requires the voluntary participation of the employees. Often the workers who would benefit most do not attend these programs.

Cady and associates (1985) reported that fire fighters with higher fitness levels are at lower risk of sustaining injury, specifically back injury. Fitness was gauged by endurance, strength, flexibility, and exercise blood pressure and heart rate. However, the more recent study by Battie and associates (1989) on aircraft workers did not reveal a similar relationship.

However, other health benefits associated with physical fitness exist. Bowne and associates (1984) reported sustained decreases in absenteeism and medical costs after introducing a fitness program. Also, it has been demonstrated that exercise can reduce depression and anxiety.

Training Managers

Training and education of management are as important as that of the workers. Without the understanding, feedback, and support of management, the training of workers will have little effect. In the literature, Wood (1987) found that compliance with safety rules and supervisor involvement was necessary for their manual handling program to be successful. The following discussion is adapted from Snook and associates (1988).

Early Care and Response to Pain

Be sure to emphasize the importance of employer and management support, because their attitude will have a marked influence on the extent of the changes implemented. Fitzler and Berger (1983) reported on a management-training program at American Biltrite. Management was educated in the importance of the positive acceptance of and early intervention in low back pain. Instead of taking an adversarial stance, immediate in-house treatment was provided along with an appropriate modified job that was consistent with the worker's condition. Low back claims were reduced from $200,000 per year to $20,000 per year over a 3-year period.

Early Return to Work

Management should be cognizant of the physical demands of the jobs in order to appropriately place new and injured workers. Lindstrom and associates (1989) reported that job-placement techniques can reduce injury and work-loss days.

Often management is unwilling to accept a worker unless he or she is completely recovered, an assurance that even a rehabilitation expert would be uneasy making. The decisions to be made are: When should one return to work and to what job should one return? To make an intelligent decision, consider the specific nature of the worker's injury and the type of demands placed on the different body tissues by the available tasks. Some designated light jobs may be stressful if they load previously injured tissue. Job analysis is essential for identifying the stresses placed on the body.

EVALUATION

The benefits of an ergonomic program are difficult to express concretely. Attention to ergonomics demonstrates that a company cares about its workers. Productivity and job satisfaction in-

crease. Reduction in lost-time injuries means less need for relief workers and lower work force costs. Reduced worker's compensation claims lower administrative costs and may result in a more favorable assessment. Clearly, ergonomics saves money; exactly how much is difficult to measure because of other factors.

The ergonomics program at Ethicon (Lutz and Hansford, 1987) is based on a multidisciplinary approach created through an ergonomic task force. Some of the functions of this task force are:

Identifying problems
Analyzing jobs to determine possible design problems
Appropriating funds
Planning orientation and education sessions

The effectiveness of this program has led to a reduction in the rates of injury, a related reduction in medical costs, and a significant improvement in worker attitude.

Workers at Goodyear's automotive plant in Logan, Ohio, are reported to have experienced significant ergonomic improvements between 1986 and 1988 (Moretz, 1989). For example, employees work at stations that are adjustable for their height and muscular structure, and designers were informed about how workers actually do their jobs. The number of lost-time cases dropped from 559 in 1986 to 8 in 1988. In the same period, the injury rate dropped from 5.2 to 1.0%, and each year their worker's compensation costs decreased 10%.

CONCLUSIONS

No chapter on primary intervention is complete without some comments on the change process.

Do not make any assumptions about the workers' psychologic or physical responses to work. Always ask.

Obtain permission from the management to enter a workplace. It is always preferable to have the blessing of the trade union as well. You are a guest.

Talk to the managers, the supervisors, the workers, and the health and safety professionals to obtain all points of view.

Do your homework. Know the nature of the industry or ask for a detailed briefing first.

Do not attempt too much too soon. Be realistic. Start with simple things.

Understand that change is threatening to people. Introduce change gently. Do not expect too much too soon. Change strategies are more successful if they originate with the workers.

Discuss what you intend to suggest first. Present a draft to check possible misinterpretations or errors.

This chapter describes a rehabilitation therapist's role in primary prevention and ergonomics. Its major thesis is that workplace trauma can be decreased by introducing an ergonomic program as primary prevention and that ergonomics and primary prevention is an emerging field of practice for rehabilitation therapists. Although some guidance for primary prevention and ergonomics is offered, further information is needed in many ergonomic texts for prevention programs to be fully effective.

References

Andersson MH: Pre-employment screening. *In* Pope MH, Frymoyer JW, and Andersson G (eds): Occupational Low Back Pain. New York, Praeger, 1984.

Armstrong TJ: Upper extremity posture: Definition, measurement and control. *In* Corlett N, Wilson J, and Manenica I (eds): The Ergonomics of Working Postures. London, Taylor & Francis, 1986.

Battie MC, Bigos SJ, Fisher LD, et al: A prospective study of the role of cardio-vascular risk factors and fitness in industrial back pain complaints. Spine *14*:141, 1989.

Bigos SJ, Spengler DM, Martin N, et al: Back injuries in industry: A retrospective study: II. Injury factors. Spine *11*:246, 1986.

Bowne DW, Russell ML, Optenberg SA, et al: Reduced disability and health care costs in an industrial fitness program. J Occup Med *26*:809, 1984.

Cady LD Jr, Thomas PC, and Karwasky RJ: Program for increasing health and physical fitness of fire fighters. J Occup Med *27*:110–114, 1985.

Canadian Standards Association: A Guideline on Office Ergonomics. Toronto, Ontario, Canadian Standards Association, 1989.

Chaffin DB and Andersson GBJ: Occupational Biomechanics. New York, Wiley, 1984.

Chaffin DB, Herrin GD, and Keyserling WM: Pre-employment strength testing: An updated position. J Occup Med *20*:403–408, 1978.

Chaffin DB, Pope MH, and Andersson GBJ: Workplace design. *In* Pope MH, Frymoyer JW, and Andersson G (eds): Occupational Low Back Pain. New York, Praeger, 1984.

Corlett EN and Bishop RP: A technique for assessing postural discomfort. Ergonomics *19*:175–182, 1976.

Corlett EN, Madeley SJ, and Manenica I: Postural targeting: A technique for recording work postures. Ergonomics *22*:357–366, 1979.

Fitzler SL and Berger RA: Attitudinal change: The Chelsea back program. Occup Health and Safety Feb, pp. 24–26, 1983.

Frymoyer JW and Mooney V: Occupational orthopedics. J Bone Joint Surg *68A*:469, 1986.

Frymoyer JW, Pope MH, Clements JH, et al: Risk factors in low-back pain: An epidemiological survey. J Bone Joint Surg *65A*:213–218, 1983.

Grandjean E: Fitting the Task to the Man. London, Taylor & Francis, 1980.

Hagberg M: Optimizing occupational muscular stress of the neck and shoulder. *In* Corlett N, Wilson J, and Manenica I (eds): The Ergonomics of Working Postures. London, Taylor & Francis, 1986.

Hall H and Iceton JA: Back school: An overview with specific reference to the Canadian Back Education Units. Clin Orthop *179*:10–17, 1983.

Jonsson BG, Persson J, and Kilbom A: Disorders of the cervicobrachial region among female workers in the electronics industry— a two year followup. Int J Industrial Ergonomics *3*:1–12, 1988.

Karhu O, Harkanen R, Sorvali P, et al: Observing work postures in industry. Appl Ergonomics *12*:13–17, 1981.

Karhu O, Kansi P, and Kuorinka I: Correcting working postures in industry. Appl Ergonomics *18*:199–201, 1977.

Keyserling W: Postural analysis of the trunk and shoulders in simulated real time. Ergonomics *29*:569–583, 1986.

Lepore BA, Olson CN, and Tomer GM: The dollars and sense of occupational back injury prevention training. Clin Management *4*:38–42, 1984.

Lindstrom I, Ohlund C, Eek C, et al: Work return and low back pain disability: The results of a prospective randomized study in an industrial population. Abstract presented at the annual meeting of ISSIS, Kyoto, Japan, May 15–19, 1989.

Lutz G and Hansford T: Cumulative trauma disorder controls: The ergonomics program at Ethicon, Inc. J Hand Surg *12A*(5):863–866, 1987.

Manning DP, Mitchell RG, and Blanchfield LP: Body movements and events contributing to accidental and nonaccidental back injuries. Spine *9*:734–739, 1984.

Moretz S: Ergonomics power plant's safety upsurge. Occup Hazards March, 1989, pp 27–29.

Nathan PA, Meadows KD, and Doyle LS: Occupation as a risk factor for impaired sensory conduction of the median nerve at the carpal tunnel. J Hand Surg *13B*:167–170, 1988.

National Center for Health Statistics: Prevalence of Selected Impairment, Series No. 10, U.S.-1977 DHHS Publication No. (PHS) 134. Hyattsville, MD, U.S. Department of Health and Human Services, 1985.

National Institute for Occupational Safety and Health: Prevention of leading work related diseases and injuries— United States. MMWR (Suppl):XXX–XXX, 1986.

National Institute for Occupational Safety and Health: Prevention of Musculoskeletal Injuries: A Proposed Synoptic Strategy. Cincinnati, OH, National Institute for Occupational Safety and Health, 1985.

National Institute for Occupational Safety and Health: Work Practices Guide for Manual Lifting. Technical Report No. 81-122. Cincinnati, OH, U.S. Department of Health and Human Services, 1981.

Pope MH, Andersson GBJ, Browman H, et al: Electromyographic studies of the lumbar trunk musculature during the development of axial torques. J Ortho Res *4*(3):288–297, 1986.

Quinn MM: The preventing occupational disease. *In* Levy BS

and Wegman DH (eds): Occupational Health. Boston, Little, Brown, 1983.

Snook SH: The design of manual handling tasks. Ergonomics 21:963–985, 1978.

Snook SH: Low back pain in industry. *In* White AA and Gordon SL (eds): American Academy of Orthopaedic Surgeons Symposium on Idiopathic Low Back Pain. St. Louis, CV Mosby, 1982.

Snook SH, Campanelli S, and Hart H: A study of three preventive approaches to low back injury. J Occup Med 20:478–481, 1978.

Snook SH, Fine LJ, and Silverstein BA: *In* Levy BS and Wegman DH (eds): Musculoskeletal Disorders in Occupational Health: Recognizing and Preventing Work-Related Disease, 2nd ed. Boston, Little, Brown, 1988.

Warrick J: Health promotion: A life-long spectrum for health care facilities. Health Care Manage Forum Spring, 1990.

Wood DJ: Design and evaluation of a back injury prevention program within a geriatric hospital. Spine *12*:77, 1987.

CHAPTER

23

Pascale Carayon
Roger O. Smith

Physical and Mental Strain in Computerized Workplaces: Causes and Remedies

COMPUTERS IN OFFICES

Historically, rehabilitation professionals applied their interventions primarily in health and education-related settings, such as hospitals and public schools. In the past decade this has been changing. More and more rehabilitation professionals are targeting interventions for workers in the workplace to help prevent work-related injuries and to accommodate work-related disabilities. An indication of this phenomenon can be seen with any quick review of the classified advertisements in rehabilitation trade newspapers. For example, in occupational therapy, a substantial portion of recruitment advertisements are searching for personnel who have knowledge and expertise in work-related interventions. About 20% cite work-rehabilitation components of jobs. This suggests that information such as that in this text is vital for rehabilitation professionals to move their practices into this new arena of work disabilities.

A second phenomenon in the past decade impacts the issues discussed in this text and is the focus of this chapter. Early this century, industrialization transformed the United States from a trade/farming-oriented work force to a manufacturing work force. Recently, the work force has shifted again, this time from manufacturing to service-oriented jobs. Moreover there is a substantially increased proportion of jobs in offices and specifically computer workstations.

This increase in computer-oriented jobs has begun to require new skills of rehabilitation professionals. Although providing therapy to people with disabilities or intervening to prevent disabilities is not new, the focus on computers and how technology may cause disability has invited increased attention to specific disorders such as repetitive motion injuries like carpal tunnel syndrome; pain disorders of the neck, shoulders, and arms; and visual strain problems. Rehabilitation professionals discovered that their backgrounds in anatomy, physiology, psychosocial pathology, and activity analysis can significantly contribute to optimizing worker productivity. This is especially true for workers who may have a historic sensitivity or a predisposition to strains encountered on the job.

The rehabilitation field, however, has not yet adequately researched this area, and its scholarly relationship to providing interventions for workers in office and computer jobs is not clear. Practitioners are not waiting for a research directive because the need for intervention is obviously present. It is, therefore, all the more

WORKPLACE AND ENVIRONMENT

critical to examine the work already being performed in this area by related disciplines.

One field of study that has devoted intensive research to the issues of computerized workplaces and their impact on workers is human factors engineering. This chapter reviews pertinent information from human factors and its related disciplines. Approaches that can serve as interventions to promote health in computerized workplaces are then summarized. These interventions address workstation design, task design, and the sociotechnical environment.

The use of computers in offices is pervasive. The Office of Technology Assessment (1985) estimated that about 15 million office workers use computers. This number was expected to rise to over one half of the work force by the year 2000. Over the last 10 to 15 years, public interest in the influence of office work on employee health has increased dramatically. This interest has been spurred by worker outcries about the adverse health effects of office computerization. Complaints of visual dysfunction, muscular aches and pains, and psychologic disturbances have been the primary areas identified.

Solutions to these problems depend on a good understanding of the physical and mental strain experienced by office workers. One useful framework to identify the causes of physical and men-

tal strain in computerized workplaces is the balance theory of job design for stress reduction proposed by Smith and Sainfort (1989). This model states that working conditions produce a stress load on the person. That load can have both physical and mental strain consequences such as back pain or adverse mood state. The stress load is influenced by individual perceptions. For example, an individual might perceive a 50-hour work week as enjoyable. Another person alternatively, might perceive working 30 hours per week as taxing and stressful. The stress load is also influenced by its objective properties independent of the perception of those properties. For example, a nonergonomically sound chair can create back discomfort or pain because it does not provide adequate support for the entire back. When the load becomes too great, the person displays stress responses, which are emotions, behaviors, and biologic reactions that are maladaptive. When these reactions occur frequently over a prolonged time period, they lead to health disorders.

Figure 23–1 illustrates a model for conceptualizing the various elements of a work system, that is the loads that working conditions can exert on workers. At the center of this model is the *individual* with his or her physical characteristics, perceptions, personality, and behavior. The in-

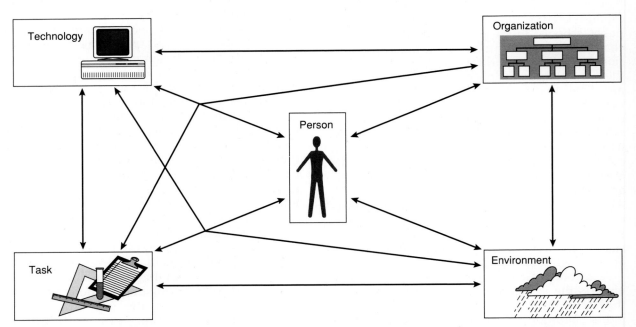

Figure 23–1. Model of the work system. (From Smith MJ and Sainfort PC: A balance theory of job design for stress reduction. Int J Industrial Ergonomics 4:67–79, 1989.)

dividual has *technologies* available to perform specific job *tasks*. The capabilities of the technologies affect performance and also the worker skills and knowledge needed for its effective use. The task requirements also affect the skills and knowledge needed. Both the tasks and technologies affect the content of the job and the physical demands. The tasks with their technologies are performed in a work setting that comprises the physical and the social *environment*. There is also an *organizational* structure that defines the nature and level of individual involvement, interaction, and control.

The various elements of this model interact to determine the way in which work is done and the effectiveness of the work in achieving individual and organizational needs and goals. This is a systems concept in that any one element will influence any other elements. Demands are placed on the individual by the other four elements, which create loads that can be healthy or harmful. Harmful loads lead to physical and mental strain that can produce adverse health effects.

The relevance of the balance theory to computer technology jobs is that, according to the balance theory, jobs are (or can be) affected by many elements of the work system. The causes of physical and mental strain in computerized workplaces are tied to this interactive set of elements. One of the major premises of this theory is that it does not accuse any one factor. Rather, it examines the design of jobs from a holistic perspective to emphasize the potential positive elements in a job that can be used to compensate for other adverse aspects.

RESEARCH ON PHYSICAL AND MENTAL STRAIN

Visual Problems

The causative link of video display terminals (VDTs) on visual stress-related problems remains a bit ambiguous. Even though some researchers concluded that they have observed problems, others have not. Furthermore, even if VDTs cause some visual strain, it remains unknown whether it is a health hazard.

Field studies of VDT users repeatedly demonstrate the effects of visual strain, such as visual discomfort, dysfunction, and visual fatigue. In some studies more than three quarters of the VDT users report visual problems (Sauter et al, 1983; Smith et al, 1981). In many of these studies, there are more complaints from VDT users than nonusers, but this is not true of all studies (Starr et al, 1982). Whether or not VDT use is worse than non-VDT use, however, is not the concern. What is of concern is that over one half of the VDT work force is reporting visual complaints and symptoms. It is clear that future research needs to identify whether these complaints indicate a serious threat to health or whether they are simply a discomfort issue.

In the area of the impact of VDTs on visual function, both field and laboratory studies (Gunnarsson and Ostberg, 1977; Gunnarsson and Solderberg, 1980; Haider et al, 1975 and 1980; Ostberg, 1975 and 1986; Wu et al, 1986; Yamamoto et al, 1986) demonstrated changes in various visual functions ranging from accommodation to convergence to dark focus when working at a VDT. In all cases, these changes have been quite small and have returned to normal after a short period of rest. Other studies (Dainoff et al, 1984; Gould and Grischkowsky, 1984; Stark, 1984; Taylor and Rupp, 1986; Voss et al, 1986; Zwahlen et al, 1984) failed to show any changes in visual functioning, including accommodation, convergence, pupillary response, eye movements, and saccade pattern and under simulated laboratory conditions of high visual load VDT work. Because the most demanding VDT conditions demonstrate only very small changes in visual functioning, it is questionable whether normal daily use of a VDT has visual health significance.

Although most research today has been cross-sectional field studies and intensive laboratory investigations, there have been a few limited longitudinal studies and medical evaluations that have assessed vision function changes and pathology in VDT users. In Montreal (Association of Ophthalmologists of Quebec, 1982), a group of ophthalmologists studied a population of VDT users over a 5-year period and recorded standard optometric measures such as visual acuity, phorias, muscle balance, and convergence. The findings indicated no changes in functional visual capabilities over the 5-year period between VDT users and nonusers. However, the VDT users did show greater levels of eye irritation than the nonusers.

Studies examining visual pathology using detailed ophthalmologic evaluations (Grignolo et al, 1986; Smith et al, 1982) failed to show any relationship between VDT use and vision disease. However, Smith and colleagues (1984) showed relationships between inadequate ergonomic conditions and VDT operator eye complaints.

The research evidence seems to indicate that VDT use does not produce pathologic changes in vision. In fact, the potential to cause pathologic changes is quite small (National Academy of Sciences, 1983). In addition, it seems there is mixed evidence of functional vision changes as a result of VDT use and, even when observed, such changes have been of little practical significance and return to normal with rest. What is clear is that VDT use is highly visually demanding and produces visual discomfort and fatigue. These conditions do not appear to be a serious health concern but can contribute to diminished worker performance, reduced satisfaction, and increased worker worry and stress.

The search for causes of visual discomfort and fatigue has identified many contributors. They include overuse of the eyes, poor screen images that affect focusing, fluctuating screen luminance, screen glare, improper illumination, and high-contrast sources in the work environment (Dainoff, 1982; Grandjean, 1979; Smith et al, 1984). These causes of visual discomfort and fatigue fall in the "environment" and "technology" elements of the work system. Other causes are due to interactions among several elements of the work system. For instance, high levels of illumination can cause visual discomfort because of reflections or glare on the computer screen. In this example, the interaction of the environment (illumination level) and the technology (computer screen) is the source of visual discomfort.

Musculoskeletal Problems

Although vision complaints were the first to emerge with VDTs, musculoskeletal problems were not far behind and have become the foremost health concern associated with VDT use. Early studies of VDT operators showed large percentages reporting musculoskeletal disturbances (Cakir et al, 1979; Coe et al, 1980; Gunnarsson and Ostberg, 1977; Hunting et al, 1980). Although fewer VDT operators reported muscular problems as opposed to visual problems, the extent of the effects were less transient and more pronounced. More recent studies confirmed that

VDT users have more musculoskeletal complaints than do nonusers (Sauter et al, 1983; Smith et al, 1981). The influence of a VDT does not seem to be directly affecting the musculoskeletal system but rather affects the physical behavior of the user. It induces poor posture if placed at an unergonomically designed workstation, causes workers to spend more time in static seated postures, and frequently demands ongoing repetitive motions. These conditions have been shown to produce back discomfort, neck and shoulder aches and pains, and wrist disorders.

Early research dealt with health complaints and discomfort. Current studies have become more focused, keying in on repetitive strain injuries, chronic trauma, and specific diseases and syndromes such as carpal tunnel and cervical-brachial syndromes. These latter studies have been successful in defining specific impairments as a result of VDT work and have economic implications such as worker's compensation payments for disability.

Smith (1986) suggested that the most immediate health risk in VDT work was chronic trauma. He identified back disorders and wrist disorders as two emerging problem areas. Arndt (1983) proposed that improper wrist bending and repetitive keying could produce tenosynovitis and carpal tunnel syndrome. Arndt's colleagues (Sauter et al, 1986) provided support in later research. In a clinical evaluation, Sauter and associates (1986) conducted mechanical examinations of VDT operators reporting trouble using wrist rests during keying. In one subject, inflammation and tenderness at the ulnar border of the right hand in an area surrounding the pisiform bone was found. The pisiform was found to be enlarged, suggesting the development of a small ganglion cyst or calcific mass. This result was caused by the hand rubbing the keyboard or the wrist rest during keying. Although this is just one case, it demonstrates the application of clinical methods in defining musculoskeletal problems associated with VDT use as well as potential health effects of such use.

There is an abundance of anecdotal evidence that VDT use can lead to serious wrist problems such as carpal tunnel syndrome given high keying demands (AFL-CIO, 1984). However, there is a lack of evidence to support this contention. Findings from Australia (Bammer, 1986; McPhee, 1986) indicate that disability from wrist pain and tenosynovitis is prevalent among VDT users with high keying requirements. These disorders are the precursors of more serious wrist disorders that take more time to develop.

One of the most significant musculoskeletal problems associated with VDT keying and postural demands is the cervical-brachial syndrome. Neck problems have been a major complaint of VDT operators. Cakir and associates (1979) found that 70% of VDT copy typists reported neck aches, whereas only 39% of the editors and 22% of the programmers reported such problems. As with other VDT health concerns, neck problems also vary by the extent of VDT use and by job task demands.

Kemmlert and co-workers (1986) used a questionnaire designed to reveal neck and shoulder problems in a group of 550 male and female office employees. Approximately 50% of the group reported neck and shoulder trouble at some time; these problems were more prevalent among women than men and increased with age. However, a greater proportion of women (43%) spent time typing and working with office machines than did men (7%); the different results between genders could be due to job demands and task requirements. This is likely because a significant correlation was found among typing, use of office machines, and neck and shoulder problems. There was no difference in the percentage of VDT users and office machine users who had neck and shoulder problems, but this could be due to the predominance of the VDT group in the office machine category. Overall, about 30% of the office machine workers reported a neck and shoulder problem. These results are subject to question, however. There was little correspondence between the questionnaire responses and clinical observations.

The most often reported musculoskeletal problem is back pain (Bergqvist, 1984; Cakir et al, 1979; Smith et al, 1981; Sauter et al, 1983); upward of one third to one half of VDT users report symptoms. In highly demanding jobs, over three quarters of the VDT operators reported back pain (Sauter et al, 1983; Smith, 1986). The primary factor associated with back pain is seated posture that places undue loading on the spine and back muscles because of improper positioning or static posture causing isometric muscular contraction. Hagberg and colleagues (1986) examined the muscular load on the trapezius muscle of secretaries when working at a word-processing task. Electromyographic activity from the right and left descending points of the trapezius was recorded

with surface electrodes in six secretaries during two work sessions of 3 to 6 hours. The static load on the trapezius muscle exceeded recommended acceptable load level of 2% of the maximal voluntary contraction for long-term work, with a mean maximal voluntary contraction of approximately 4% (Jonsson, 1982). These results confirmed complaints of cervical-brachial pain by secretaries using VDTs.

Grandjean and associates (Grandjean, 1984; Grandjean et al, 1983; Hunting et al, 1980; Nakaseko et al, 1982) at the Swiss Federal Institute examined the relationship between seated posture of VDT operators and potential musculoskeletal problems. In a field study of 162 VDT worksites and 100 worksites not using VDTs, it was shown that constraining postures of VDT work were associated with musculoskeletal physical health impairments in the hands, arms, shoulder, and neck. This was also true for typists not using VDTs. Ergonomic design considerations such as the keyboard thickness, height of the keyboard from the floor, inability to rest hands on the desk, keyboard, or wrist rest, lateral deviation of the hands while keying, and inclination or turning of the head were associated with the reported physical impairments. These findings were confirmed by Nakaseko and colleagues (1982).

Grandjean and associates (1982 and 1983) evaluated the preferred seating characteristics of VDT users in both laboratory and field experimental studies. In the field study, they established model workstations that allowed for VDT operator adjustments to preferred settings and rotated workers into these workstations where they performed their normal work activities. The findings correlated with those of the laboratory study in demonstrating that most of the VDT operators did not prefer an upright posture; rather, they preferred a slight backward inclination (97 to 121 degrees). This posture required that keyboard heights needed to be higher than with an upright posture, and other critical elements of the workstation dimensions such as viewing distance and leg room were also changed. As Grandjean (1984) pointed out, these preferred dimensions are not in agreement with many recommendations, guidelines, and standards even though they may be more healthful.

Finally, sedentary seated work that does not provide for muscular activity may play a role in circulatory dysfunction of the legs. Thompson and colleagues (1986), in a series of animal and human blood-flow studies, demonstrated that static postures may impede venosomatic reflexes that are crucial to neuromuscular excitability, which is important in controlling blood pooling. Thus, excessive blood pooling may occur in the lower legs and feet because of static postures. Winkel (1986) showed that lower limb discomfort and vascular strain may increase during leg inactivity as well as high leg activity. In fact, sitting with no leg movements appears to be the most susceptible condition for foot and lower leg swelling, which decreases with moderate activity such as alternate sitting and walking.

In conclusion, the research evidence for disabling health problems of the musculoskeletal system associated with VDT work is mounting. Field studies demonstrated many VDT users reporting a variety of muscular complaints, most notably of the back, neck and shoulders, and hand and wrists. In a small percentage of VDT operators, clinical studies showed serious disorders such as carpal tunnel syndrome and cervical-brachial disorders, with related minor disorders such as tenosynovitis. More research is still on-going, and evidence is also accumulating that static seated postures that contribute to cervical-brachial disorders additionally contribute to lower back pain and disorders of the spine. Given that the majority of VDT users experience back pain, this issue is a critical public health concern and is the most significant worker's compensation issue emerging from VDT work. Finally, static seated postures are also being tied to circulation problems of the lower legs and feet. Ergonomic research is underway in scientific agencies, in universities, and by furniture manufacturers to deal with the causes of these problems. Proper workstation design, VDT keyboard design, and tasks with movement requirements are central directions of this research. However, more needs to be done to define the specific causal mechanisms for many of these musculoskeletal disorders before designs are developed that may shift the problem from one muscular location to another.

Stress Problems

Interest in the influences of psychosocial job demands and VDT operator health has been apparent as early as the late 1970s (Cakir et al, 1979; Gunnarsson and Ostberg, 1977). That these job demands may also be stressful has been investigated (Sauter et al, 1983; Smith et al, 1980). Recent reviews of the health issues surrounding the use of VDTs (Bergqvist, 1984; Office of Technology Assessment, 1985; Smith, 1986) implicate psychosocial and stress considerations as important issues in the overall impact of VDT technology on worker physical symptoms and complaints. Although the literature on VDT stress concerns is quite small and is limited in terms of methodologies used, consistent findings provide some insight about the stressful nature of VDT work. The reactions of employees to their displeasure is reflected many times in high levels of job stress, stress that can be tied to the way in which the computer technology is used. This computer technology changes job tasks and may produce job conditions that are stressful. Thus, it is not the computer technology *per se* that is the basic consideration in job stress but rather how it has changed the nature of work through productive improvements in its applications (Smith, 1986).

Office workers in general, especially clerical office workers, are at high risk for stress-related disease (Cohen, 1982). Haynes and Feinleib (1980) described a markedly higher incidence of coronary heart disease for clerically employed women who have children than for homemakers and women in other occupations. Smith and colleagues (1978), in an epidemiologic examination of stress diseases in 130 occupations, found that secretaries ranked second in the incidence of stress-related diseases. Although these studies suggest a significant health risk in clerical occupations, they do not define the job factors that account for this risk. It is fair to say that environmental and chemical hazards are not primary concerns here, so the most likely contributors are working conditions and job features that produce physical or psychologic stress. These issues have yet to be thoroughly assessed for clerical workers. Smith and colleagues (1981) compared psychologic disturbances and job stressors in professional VDT users, clerical VDT operators, and, as a control group, clerical workers not using VDTs. They found the highest levels of anxiety, depression, anger, confusion, and mental fatigue in the clerical VDT operators. The clerical operators also reported higher levels of irritability than did members of the control group (80% versus 63%) as well as nervousness (50% versus 31%), fatigue (74% versus 57%), fainting (36% versus 17%), stomach pains (51% versus 35%), and pain down the arms (37% versus 20%). The professional VDT users also reported more irritability than members of the control group (76% versus 63%) but less fainting (8% versus 17%) and pain down the arms (11% versus 20%). In this study, participants identified aspects of their jobs that could be problematic. Clerical VDT operators reported more problems with the following job features than either the professional VDT users or the clerical control group members: peer cohesion, job autonomy, work pressure, work load, supervisory control, and career goals. The clerical VDT operators also reported less work-load satisfaction, more boredom, and lower self-esteem than other study participants, thus demonstrating general dissatisfaction with their jobs.

Sauter and co-workers (1983) confirmed some of these findings. Clerical VDT users in this study experienced more work pressure, less job autonomy, and more management control than clerks not using VDTs. However, they found levels of reported depression, anger, and confusion lower in VDT operators. This suggests that factors beyond VDT use and reported levels of stress might influence psychologic disturbances.

These studies indicate that certain classes of VDT operators report high levels of psychologic disturbances and job stress. The effects are selective in that certain types of VDT jobs produce more problems than others. Examination of specific stressors indicates that different levels of perceived problems are linked to job task requirements. The stress factors that differ among occupations are work content (meaningfulness, repetitiousness), work load, and career concerns. Clerical VDT operators reported that their jobs were boring and subject to a great deal of structure and control. They felt that work loads were heavy and constant and thus produced work pressure.

In conclusion, VDT work is associated with job dissatisfaction, stress, mood disturbances, and psychosomatic symptoms in select VDT jobs in which the nature of the work increases job demands, reduces worker control and job content, and increases close supervision. In other jobs in which the VDT acts as a tool to enhance the work tasks, there is not an increased risk of stress because of the use of a VDT. However, the precise nature of how VDT technology influences worker stress is not clear, and there is a critical need for continued research into the mechanisms of organizational and job-design influences of computer technology.

REMEDIES FOR REDUCING PHYSICAL AND MENTAL STRAIN

Ergonomic Design

Ergonomics is the study and practice of fitting the environment and activities to the capabilities, dimensions, and needs of people. Ergonomic knowledge and principles are applied to adapt working conditions to the physical, psychologic, and social nature of the person. The goal of ergonomics is to improve performance while enhancing comfort, health, and safety. Basically, VDT-related health and safety problems can be solved by applying ergonomic principles. Although no set of rules can specify all the conditions necessary for healthful and productive computerized work, the use of the proper principles can help in making the right choices.

A major feature of the ergonomics approach is that the job task characteristics will define the ergonomic interventions and the priorities that should exist for workplace design requirements. A discussion of five critical areas—the VDT, visual and auditory environment, heating, ventilating and air conditions, and workstation design—highlights the major factors that one should be aware of to minimize VDT operator health complaints and to enhance the potential for improved productivity. Recommendations and specifications may have to be modified to account for personal, situational, or organizational needs as well as improved knowledge about strain concerns in computerized workplaces.

The Visual Environment

Much of the visual discomfort reported by VDT users can be decreased by providing an appropriately designed visual environment. Lighting is an important aspect of the visual environment, which influences readability and glare on the VDT screen and in the environment.

The intensity of illumination or the illuminance being measured is the amount of light falling on a surface. The illumination required for a particular task is determined by the visual requirements of the task and the visual ability of the employees concerned. The illuminance in VDT workplaces should not be too high. An illuminance in the range of 300 to 700 lux measured on the horizontal working surface (not the VDT screen) is normally acceptable. The lighting level should be set according to the visual demands of the tasks performed. Conflicts may arise when different tasks are performed (e.g., hard copy and VDTs are used by the same employee or different employees who have differing requirements and who work in the same office). As a compromise, room lighting can be set at the lower level (300 lux) or intermediate level (500 lux), and additional task lighting provided for the hard copy as needed.

Luminance is a measure of the brightness of a surface. High-luminance intensity sources (such as windows) in the peripheral field of view should be avoided. In addition, there should not be a large difference in the luminance of objects that can be viewed.

Large differences in luminance or high-luminance lighting source can cause glare. Direct glare is caused by light sources in the field of view of the VDT operator, whereas reflected glare is caused by reflections from polished or glossy surfaces.

Direct and reflected glare can be limited through one or more of the following techniques:

Controlling the light from windows. This can be accomplished by closed drapes, shades, and blinds over windows or awnings on the outside, especially during sunlight conditions.

Controlling the view of luminaires: (1) by proper positioning of VDTs with regard to windows and overhead lighting to reduce direct or reflected glare and images; (2) using screen hoods to block luminaires from view.

Controlling the screen surface by (1) adding antiglare filters on the VDT screen; (2) proper adjustment up or down and left or right of the screen.

Controlling the lighting sources using (1) appropriate glare shields or covers on the lamps; (2) properly installed indirect lighting systems.

The Auditory Environment

One advantage of the VDT is that it is less noisy than other technologies. However, it is not unusual for VDT operators to complain of bothersome noise. Office employees expect quiet work areas. Their tasks often require concentration and a noise-free environment. Annoying noise can disrupt their ability to function properly and may produce stress.

Actually, there may be many sources of noise in VDT offices. Fans and airflow controls in VDTs

are noisy as are the click of keys or the high-pitched squeal of the VDT. These types of noise may be distracting and even irritating in an office environment. The peripheral equipment associated with VDTs, such as printers, can also be a source of annoying noise. Adequate printer covers and location can reduce the noise level.

Problems of noise may be exacerbated in open-plan offices in which noise spreads more easily than in individual offices. Attention to sound control is a critical factor in the open-plan automated environment. Acoustical control can rely on ceiling, floor, and wall materials as well as furniture and equipment finishes. The most common means of blocking a sound path is to build a wall between the source and the receiver. Walls not only are sound barriers but are also a place to mount sound-absorbent materials. In open-plan offices, free-standing acoustical panels can be used to reduce the ambient noise level and also to separate an individual from the noise source.

Acoustical control can also be achieved by proper space planning. For instance, workstations that are positioned too closely do not provide suitable speech privacy and can be a source of disturbing conversational noise. As a general rule, a minimum of 8 to 10 feet between employees, separated by acoustical panels or partitions, will provide normal speech privacy.

Heating, Ventilating, and Air Conditioning

Temperature, humidity, airflow, and air exchanges are important parameters for employees' performance and comfort. Thermal comfort is an important consideration in employee satisfaction that can influence performance. Research has shown that VDT employees and other office employees are not satisfied with their thermal comfort. As a general rule, it is recommended that the temperature be maintained between 20 to 24°C (68 to 75°F) in the winter and between 23 to 27°C (73 to 81°F) in the summer. To minimize foot discomfort, the surface temperature of the floor should be between 18°C (65°F) and 29°C (84°F).

The temperature regulation in a VDT workplace may be more difficult because of the heat generated by VDTs, particularly if many VDTs are installed in the same area. Office ventilation can be set up to exhaust the VDT-generated heat and to provide additional cooling to the areas affected by the VDTs. It is important that ventilation not produce currents of air that blow directly on employees. This is best handled by proper placement of the workstation and air ducts.

Some types of visual discomfort (e.g., eye dryness) have been partly attributed to the effects of air movements. Visual and respiratory discomfort is also caused by air that is not humid enough. Relative humidity is an important component of office climate and strongly influences employees' comfort and well-being. Air that is too dry leads to a drying out of the mucous membranes of the eyes, nose, and throat. Individuals who wear contact lenses may be made especially uncomfortable by dry air. In cases in which intense, continuous near-vision work at the VDT is required, very dry air has been shown to irritate the eyes. As a general rule, it is recommended that the relative humidity in VDT environments be at least 50% and less than 60%. Air that is too wet enhances the growth of unhealthy organisms that can cause disease.

The Computer

Poor screen images, fluctuating and flickering screen luminances, and screen glare cause visual discomfort and fatigue. In terms of the screen, a range of issues concern readability and screen reflections. One issue of concern is the adequacy of contrast between the characters and screen background. To give the best readability for each operator, it is important to provide computers with adjustments for character contrast and brightness. These adjustments should have controls that are obvious and easily accessible from the normal working position (e.g., located at the front of the screen).

Good character design can help improve image quality. Image quality is a major factor for reducing eye strain and visual fatigue. The proper size of a character is dependent on the task and the display parameters (e.g., brightness, contrast, glare treatment) and the viewing distance. Character size that is too small can make reading difficult and causes the visual focusing mechanism to overwork. This produces eye strain and fatigue.

Experts traditionally recommended a viewing distance between the screen and the operator's eye of 45 to 50 cm but no more than 70 cm. However, experience in field studies showed that, given proper ergonomic design of the workstation, operators may adopt a viewing distance greater than 70 cm and still not develop visual problems. Thus, viewing distance should be determined in context with other considerations. It varies depending on the task requirements, VDT screen characteristics, and individual characteristics. For instance, with poor screen or hardcopy quality, it may be necessary to reduce viewing distances for easier reading. Typically, viewing distance should be 50 cm or less because of the size of characters on the VDT screen.

Adjustable monitor stands and adjustable height tables can help set up the monitor in the proper location. Furthermore, adjustable systems allow flexibility for multiuser workstations.

The keyboard should be detachable and movable, thus providing flexibility for independently positioning the keyboard and screen. The keyboard should be able to be fixed to ensure that it does not slide on the tabletop. To guarantee a favorable arm-height position, the keyboard should be as thin as possible. It is recommended that the thickness of the keyboard (i.e., the distance from the desk to the home row keys) should not exceed 30 to 50 mm. The slope or angle of the keyboard should be between 0 and 15 degrees measured horizontally. Adjustability of keyboard angle is useful when several employees use the same VDT.

When using the keyboard, a wrist rest can also help to minimize extension of the hand. A separate wrist rest influences the workstation design because the table has to be deeper than a conventional typing table. A good wrist rest should have a fairly broad surface (approximately 5 cm) with a rounded front edge to prevent cutting pressures on the wrist and hands. Padding further minimizes compression and irritation. Height adjustability is important so that the wrist rest can be set to a preferred level in concert with the keyboard height and slope. A variety of wrist-support systems are available today. Some provide stationary support. Others float on a horizontal plane to allow movement but with antigravity support.

Related to the keyboard is the repetitive striking of keys, which can aggravate hand or wrist problems for persons who are predisposed to joint or tendon pain syndromes. Software that provides keyboard acceleration can be implemented to reduce the number of keystrokes a typist must use. Keyboard acceleration programs work as computer shorthand. For example, a person has to key in only their initials in order to type their entire name. Other common or lengthy words can be abbreviated to increase keyboard efficiency. A variety of acceleration programs are available, many of which run in the background with standard computer software.

The Workstation

Workstation design is a major element in ergonomic strategies for improving office working conditions and particularly for reducing musculoskeletal problems. The relative importance of the screen, keyboard, and hard copy (i.e., source documents) depends primarily on the task, and this defines the ergonomic interventions necessary to improve operator comfort and health. Data-entry positions, for example, are typically hard-copy oriented. The operator spends little time looking at the screen, and the job is characterized by high rates of keying. For this type of task it is logical to position the keyboard and the hard copy in front of the operator because these are the primary tools used in the task, and the screen off to the side. Alternatively, data-acquisition operators spend most of their time looking at the screen and seldom use hard copy. For this type of task, the screen and the keyboard should be placed directly in front of the operator and the hard copy (if any) off to the side. Interactive VDT operators have a wide variety of job tasks. In some cases, the keyboard is not important and this may be placed off to the side with the source documents placed directly in front of the VDT operator. The task requirements determine critical layout characteristics of the workstation.

The size of the work surface is dependent on the task, the documents, and the VDT. The primary working surface (e.g., those supporting the keyboard, the display, and the documents) should be sufficient to (1) permit the screen to be moved forward or backward, (2) allow a detachable keyboard to be placed in several locations, and (3) permit source documents to be laid out. Additional working surfaces (i.e., secondary working surfaces) may be required to store, lay out, read, and write on documents or materials. Sometimes VDT workstations require that multiple pieces of equipment and source materials be equally accessible to the user. In this case, additional working surfaces may be necessary to support these additional tools.

The tabletop should be as thin as possible to provide clearance for the operator's thighs and knees. Moreover, it is important to provide unobstructed room under the working surface for the feet and legs so that operators can easily shift their posture. Knee-space height and width and leg depth are the three key factors for the design of clearance space under the working surfaces. It has to be stressed that, under the table, space is not just an issue of foot, leg, and thigh clearance but, more important, requires adequate clearance to allow operators free postural movement. Thus, good workstation design accounts for individual body sizes and often exceeds minimum clearances to allow for free postural movement.

Tables that are too high cause the keyboard to be too high for many operators. This puts undue pressure on their hands, wrists, arms, shoulders, and neck. Table height has to be coordinated with VDT operator height so that shorter operators have lower table heights.

It is desirable for table heights to vary with the height of the operator. This may mean that it is necessary to have adjustable height tables. Key factors in determining the suitability for adjustable working surfaces are (1) the number of individuals using the workstation, (2) the variety of tasks performed at the station, and (3) the type of VDT used. Adjustable multisurface VDT tables enable good posture by allowing the keyboard and display to be independently adjusted to appropriate keying and viewing heights. Tables that cannot be adjusted by the user or that are not adjusted easily without assistance or special tools are not appropriate when used by several individuals of differing sizes. If adjustable tables are used, ease of adjustment is essential. The more difficult it is to adjust the workstation, the less likely it is that employees will take the time to make the adjustments.

Not only should adjustments be easy to make but operators should be informed that they should adjust the workstation to be comfortable, and they should be taught how to make the adjustments. Workstation adjustability and ease of adjustment are crucial factors when the same workstation is used by several individuals or when jobs of a single VDT operator produce long periods of sitting, necessitating frequent posture shifts to reduce musculoskeletal problems.

The keyboard height is a critical factor in hand, wrist, and arm strain. The working surface height should primarily be adjusted to accommodate the recommended keyboard height. Once this is achieved, the display height should be adjusted so that the viewing or gaze angle is in the range of 10 to 40 degrees. The display height adjustment can be made using an independently adjustable display surface when using multisurface tables or by placing something under the screen to raise it on single-surface tables.

Poorly designed chairs can contribute to office employees' discomfort. Chair adjustability in terms of height, seat angle, and lumbar support reduces the pressures and loading on the musculoskeleture of the back, leg, shoulders, and neck. In addition, the action of the chair helps maintain proper seated posture and encourages good movement patterns. A chair that provides swivel action improves movements, and backward tilting increases the number of postures that can be assumed. The chair height should be adjustable so that the feet can rest firmly on the floor with minimal pressure beneath the thighs. To enable very small women to sit with their feet on the floor without compressing their thighs, it may be necessary to add a footrest.

The seat "pan" is where the person sits on the chair. It is the part that directly supports weight. The seat pan should be wide enough to permit operators to make slight shifts in posture from side to side. This not only helps to avoid static postures but also accommodates a large range of individual sizes.

The tension and tilt angle of the backrest should be adjustable. Inclination of chair backrest is important for operators to lean back in a comfortable manner while maintaining a correct relationship between the seat pan angle and the backrest inclination. A back to seat inclination of about 110 degrees is considered the best position by most experts.

High backrest chairs are preferred because they provide both lumbar and shoulder support for employees seated in an upright position. This allows employees to lean backward or forward, adopting a relaxed posture and resting the back muscles. A full backrest with a height of approximately 45 to 51 cm is recommended. To prevent back strain, it is also recommended that chairs have lumbar support. The lumbar region is one of the most highly strained parts of the spine, and the provision of an appropriate backrest helps to minimize static muscular strains.

For some VDT workstations, chairs with rolling castors are desirable. They are easy to move and facilitate postural adjustment, particularly when the operator has to reach for equipment or ma-terials that are on the secondary working surfaces. Many experts proposed that chairs have five supporting legs rather than four because they are more stable.

Another important chair feature is armrests. Pros and cons to the use of armrests at VDT workstations have been advanced. On one hand, some chair armrests can present problems of restricted arm movement, interference with keyboard operation, pinching of fingers between the armrest and table, restriction of chair movement such as under the worktable, irritation of the arm or elbows, and adoption of awkward postures (e.g., if the space between the armrests is too wide, the operator may lean awkwardly to one side to rest his or her arms on them). On the other hand, well-designed short armrests or elbow rests can be a place to rest arms to prevent or reduce fatigue. Properly designed armrests can overcome the problems mentioned previously. Removable armrests are advantageous because they provide greater flexibility for individual operator preference. For specific tasks such as using a numeric keypad, a full armrest can be a beneficial place to support the arms.

Job Design

Computerization can potentially provide significant improvements in the quality of jobs but also can bring about job changes that reduce employee satisfaction and increase stress. Designing jobs that meet both the aims of the organization and the needs of employees can be difficult. It requires attention to important aspects of work that contribute to employee self-esteem, satisfaction, motivation, health, and safety. These job-design aspects include work load, the physical environment, job content, employee feedback, rewarding excellence in performance, and social interaction.

Job Demands

A major complaint of office employees who have undergone computerization is that their work load has increased substantially. This is most true for clerical employees who typically have an increased number of transactions to process when computers are introduced into the work routine. This increase in transactions means more keystrokes and more time at the workstation. These can lead to greater physical effort than before and possibly more visual and muscular discomfort. This discomfort reinforces the feeling of increased work load and adds to employee dissatisfaction with the work load.

Quite often the work load of users of computers is established by the data-processing department in concert with other staff departments such as human resources and line managers. An important consideration is the cost of the computer equipment and related upkeep such as software and maintenance. The processing capability of the computers is a second critical element in establishing the total capacity that can be achieved. The technology cost, the capability to process work, and the desired time frame to pay for the technology are factored together to establish a staffing pattern and the required work load for each employee. This approach is based on the capacity of the computers coupled with investment recovery needs and does not necessarily meet the objective of good human resource utilization.

Work load should not be based solely on technologic capabilities or investment recovery needs but must include important considerations of human capabilities and needs. Established methods for work load assessment and determination based on technologic capabilities have long been used by industrial engineers and organizational psychologists. These methods define appropriate performance for the average employee, which can serve as a yardstick for estimating economic benefits of technology, necessary staffing needs, and investment payoff timing. These methods can also define acceptable performance standards that can be used to evaluate employees and to determine when remedial action is necessary.

Factors such as attentional requirements, fatigue, and stress should be taken into account in establishing the work load. Work load problems are not concerned solely with the immediate level of effort necessary but also deal with the issue of work pressure. This is defined as an unrelenting backlog of work or work load that will never be completed. This situation is much more stressful than a temporary increase in work load to meet a specific crisis. It produces the feeling that things will never get better and only worsen. Supervisors have an important role in dealing with work pressure by acting as a buffer between the demands of the employer and the daily activities of the employees. Work pressure is a perceptual problem. If the supervisor deals with daily work load in an orderly way and does not pressure the employee about a pileup of work, the employee's perception of pressure will be reduced, and the employee will not suffer from work-pressure stress.

Work pressure is also related to the rate of work or work pace. A very fast work pace that requires all of the employee's resources and skills to keep up will produce work pressure and stress. Stress is exacerbated when this condition occurs often. An important job-design consideration is to allow the employee to control the pace of the work rather than having this controlled automatically by the computer. This provides a pressure valve to deal with perceived work pressure.

A scientific basis must be used for establishing work load to achieve the most effective gains from the technology. A work load that is too great will cause fatigue and stress, which can diminish work quality without achieving desired quantity. A work load that is too low will produce boredom and stress and also reduce quality and economic benefits of computerization.

Job Content

The amount of esteem and satisfaction an employee achieves from work is tied directly to the content of the job. For many jobs, computerization brings about fragmentation and simplification, which act to reduce the content of the job. Jobs need to provide an opportunity for skill use, mental stimulation, and adequate physical activity to keep muscles in tone. In addition, work has to be meaningful for the individual. It has to provide for an identification with the product and the company. This provides the basis for pride in the job that is accomplished.

Computerization can provide an opportunity for employees to individualize their work. This lets them use their unique skills and abilities to achieve the required standards of output. It provides cognitive stimulation because employees can develop a strategy to meet their goals. This requires that software be flexible enough to accept different types and ordering of input. Then it is the job of the software to transform the diverse input into the desired product. Usually computer programmers will resist such an approach because it is easier for them to program using standardized input strategies. However, such strategies build repetition and inflexibility into jobs, which reduces job content and meaning.

Being able to perform a complete work activity that has an identifiable end product is an important way to add meaningfulness to a job. When employees understand the fruits of their labor, an element of identification and of pride in achievement is provided. This is in contrast to simplifying jobs into elemental tasks that are repeated over and over again. Such simplification removes meaning and job content and creates boredom, job stress, and product-quality problems. New computer systems should emphasize software that allows employees to use existing skills and knowledge to start out. These then can serve as the base for acquiring new skills and knowledge.

Training can serve to enhance employee performance and to add to new skills. Such growth in skills and knowledge are important aspects of good job design. No one can remain satisfied with the same job activities over a period of years. Training is a way to assist employees in using new technology to its fullest extent and to reduce the boredom of the same job tasks. New technology by its nature will require changes in jobs, and training is an important approach for not only keeping employees current but also in building meaning and content into their jobs.

Job activities should exercise employee mental skills and should also require a sufficient level of physical activity to keep the employee alert and in good muscle tone.

Some job-design consultants are beginning to focus on the advantage of taking breaks, how to make the most out of break periods, and training workers. For example, Mayfield and Voge (1990) wrote and illustrated a document entitled "Computer Comfort: A Guide to Working at Your Computer with Less Strain on Your Neck, Back, Hands and Eyes." It highlights exercises that can be performed to break potentially damaging repetitive motions, and accompanying software helps to demonstrate the effects of poor workstation design on posture. These types of educational media can increase the workers' awareness to help avoid strain and assist in developing healthy habits and skills. However, they are usually limited in scope and do not discuss important task, organizational, and environmental factors that can affect physical health.

Decision Making and Control

Employees are a good source of information about productive ways to work. Their daily con-

tact with the job gives them insight into methods, procedures, bottlenecks, and problems. Many times they modify their individual work methods or behavior to improve their products and rate of output. Often these are unique to the individual job or employee and cannot be adopted as a standardized approach or method.

If work systems are set up in a rigid way, then this compensatory behavior cannot occur. Thus, it is in the interest of the employer to allow employees to exercise at least a nominal level of control and decision making over their own task activity. Here again, the computer hardware and software have to be flexible so that individual approaches and input can be accommodated as long as set standards of productivity are met.

One approach for providing employee control is through employee involvement and participation in making decisions about work (e.g., helping management select ergonomic furniture through comparative testing of various products and providing preference data; being involved in the determination of minimum work load requirements for a new job; or voicing opinions about ways to improve the efficiency of their work unit). Participation is a strong motivator to action and a good way to gain employee commitment to a work standard or a new technology. However, participation will be effective only as long as employees see tangible evidence that their input is being considered and used in a way that benefits them.

Feedback

If employees are to be able to exert control over their jobs, they need to receive feedback to help them make decisions and to guide their behavior. This feedback should occur on many levels. The first level concerns the job activity and should be about individual performance. Computers can provide minute-by-minute information about individual output (usually only quantity information is available on a minute-by-minute basis). Such information can help employees improve their performance and can act as a motivator. However, minute-by-minute feedback provides a much too narrow time frame for assessing overall performance and contributions to the company. Such frequent feedback could produce feelings of work pressure. To reduce this pressure, it is reasonable to give feedback on employee performance directly to that employee on an hourly basis. This is frequent enough to provide the employee with trends in his or her performance that are meaningful and to allow for necessary behavior changes to meet production goals.

Because the hourly feedback is only about the quantity of work, it would also be useful to provide employees with some information about the quality of their work. This might best be obtained directly by the employee through a personal audit of a small sample of his or her own outputs. This could be done once daily toward the end of the day. Such self-checks remove the fear of errors being used as a punishment and make the quality checking a positive process of self-improvement. The quantity and quality feedback is solely for the individual employee.

Supervisors should be given aggregated performance data only for the work unit. This encourages supervisors to be helpful, not monitors, and also provides valuable performance information for managing the work unit.

Feedback on how the employer perceives the employees' performance is also necessary. This is one element in an employee performance appraisal system that can be used for justifying salary modifications and merit awards. This feedback differs from the previous types of feedback discussed in that it has a value judgment attached that can influence pay and career advancement. This type of feedback should be given infrequently (e.g., a quarterly basis) using objective indicators of the employees' contributions to the company. This frequency of feedback allows for improved behavior before serious problems get out of hand and also provides frequent reward opportunities that are more motivating than annual reviews. This approach also supports the concept of not using feedback as a means of harassing employees for greater efforts through nagging supervisors. Rather, it provides objective evidence of how the employee has managed his or her own behavior in meeting production goals and standards.

Rewards

Employees who make positive contributions to the success of the organization should be rewarded for their efforts. Rewards can be administrative or social. Examples of administrative rewards are additional rest breaks, extended lunch periods, or special parking spaces. They

identify the person as someone special and deserving. Social rewards provide special status to the individual. This is best exemplified by the receipt of praise from the supervisor for a job well done. This enhances personal self-esteem. If the praise is given in a group setting, it can enhance peer-group esteem toward the individual. Monetary rewards can also be used, but these can be a two-edged sword because they may have to be removed during low-profit periods, and this can lead to employee resentment, thus negating the entire purpose of the reward system.

Integration

The purpose of job design is to make work more effective and efficient so that employees can be productive, satisfied, and healthy. Good job design improves the motivation of employees to work toward the betterment of the employer. The considerations of job content, work load, and other features of a good job that have been discussed in this chapter have to be recognized as an integrated whole. That is, keying in on just one or two features will not bring about the desired improvements in worker performance or improved health (reduced stress). Rather, small improvements made incrementally in the whole job will provide the necessary integration of features and the desired results. This also allows the employer the ability to fine-tune the job-design process for specific groups of workers such that when the desired level of performance and safety are achieved additional modifications and resource expenditures are unnecessary. This allows valuable resources to be saved or applied to other endeavors.

Organizational Design

The introduction of new technology produces changes in the way work is accomplished by introducing new tasks, requiring new employee skills, and changing relationships among employees. This requires that organizations rethink their basic approaches in dealing with employees. The previous section on stress problems illustrated a number of potential stress-producing situations in VDT work, many of which are related to organizational considerations. The way in which an employer introduces new technology, the maintenance of fair and equitable work standards and pay, the nature of supervision of employees, skills upgrading of employees for effective use of the new technology, and establishing career paths have all been identified as critical organizational considerations for reducing employee stress and obtaining the most production from the new technology.

Introduction of New Technology

Any kind of change in the workplace produces fears in employees. New technology brings with it changes in staff and the way work is done. The fear of the unknown, which in this case means the new technology, can be a potent stressor. A good strategy to introduce new technology is to keep employees well informed of expected changes and how they will affect the workplace. Informational memorandums and bulletins should be provided to employees at various stages of the process of decision making about the selection of technology and during its implementation. These informational outputs have to be made frequently (at least monthly) and need to be straightforward about the technology and its expected effects. A popular approach proposed by many organizational design experts is to involve employees in the selection and implementation of the new technology. The benefit of this participation is that employees are kept abreast of current information, employees may have some good ideas that can be beneficial to the process, and participation in the process builds employee commitment to the use of the technology.

Work Standards

A major mistake that some employers make in applying new technology is to establish new work standards without using scientific methods. Employees perceive such attempts to capitalize on technology as unfair, and they respond negatively. This can have a particularly serious effect on product quality and customer relations. There are established methods from industrial engineering and industrial psychology for work-load allowances and rest breaks. These must be the basis for developing work standards, not the unscientific needs of management to meet pro-

duction levels based on a technology payoff timetable. A primary reason for acquiring new technology is to increase individual employee productivity and to provide a competitive edge. Getting more work out of employees means that fewer are needed to do the same amount of work. Often employees feel that this increased output means they are working harder even though the technology may actually make their work easier. Using scientific methods helps establish the "fairness" of new work standards.

Employee Evaluation

Once work standards have been established, they can serve as one element in an employee performance-evaluation scheme. An advantage of computer technology is the accessibility to instantaneous information on individual employee performance in terms of the rate of output. This serves as one objective measure of how hard employees are working. However, managers have to understand that this is just one element of employee performance, and emphasis on quantity can have an adverse effect on the quality of work. Therefore, a balanced performance-evaluation system will include quality considerations as well. These are not as easy to obtain and are not as readily available as are quantity measures. However, managers must resist the temptation to emphasize quantity measures. A key consideration in any employee-evaluation program is the issue of fairness just as it is an important consideration in work-load determination. This leads into the concept of equitable employee compensation.

Compensation

Computer technology can bring about changes in jobs that make them simpler and more repetitive, thus requiring fewer skills and less knowledge. Many employers feel that this entitles them to reduce employee pay. However, such a policy is contrary to the concept of fairness. Because employees are producing more as a result of the technology, they feel they deserve a share of the improved profits that are attainable because of the technological advantage. Even if the jobs are easier in terms of functions, they are harder because of increased work load. Employees feel that if their jobs are jeopardized by technology and if they have to work harder, they should realize some benefit from the increased productivity. Employers must be careful in how they share the benefits and profits from the new technology if they expect to continue to obtain high-quality and high-quantity output from employees. Therefore, even if jobs become simpler and easier, employees need some benefits from the new technology in keeping with the concept of fairness. If they perceive the system as unfair, then quality will suffer and stress will increase.

Career Development

A significant employee fear and potent stressor is concern over job loss as a result of improved efficiency produced by new technology. Many research studies demonstrated that the anticipation of job loss and not whether one's job is secure is much more stressful and more detrimental to employee health than knowing right away about future job loss. Telling those employees who will lose their job early provides them with an opportunity to search for a new job while they are still employed. This gives them a better chance to get a new job and more bargaining power regarding salary and other issues. Some employers do not want to let employees know too soon for fear of losing them at an inopportune time. This is not fair, and by not being honest to employees who are laid off, employers can adversely influence the attitudes and behavior of those employees who remain.

For those employees who are retained, there is the concern that the new technology will de-skill their jobs and provide less opportunity to be promoted to a better job. Often the technology flattens the organizational structure, producing similar jobs with equivalent levels of skill use. Thus, there is little chance to be promoted except into a limited number of supervisory positions, which will be less plentiful with new technology. If this scenario comes true, then employees will suffer from the blue-collar blues that have been prevalent in factory jobs. This impacts negatively on performance and stress.

Career Opportunities

Averting the negativity associated with no career path requires a commitment from the employer for enhancing job design that builds skill use into jobs as well as the development of career paths so that employees have something to look forward to besides 30 years at the same job. Career opportunities have to be tailored to the needs of the organization to meet production requirements. Personnel specialists, production managers, and employees have to work together to design work systems that give advancement opportunity while using technology effectively and meeting production goals. One effective technique is to develop a number of specialist jobs that require unique skills and training. Workers in these jobs can be paid a premium wage reflecting their unique skills and training. Employees can be promoted from general jobs into specialty jobs. Those already in specialty jobs can be promoted to other more difficult specialty jobs. Finally, those with enough specialty experience can be promoted into troubleshooting jobs that allow them to rotate among specialties as needed to help make the work process operate smoothly and more productively.

Supervision

Computerization has been shown to have an important impact on how supervisors interact with their employees. It is natural that, when supervisors are suddenly provided with instantaneous, detailed information about individual employee performance, they feel a commitment, in fact an obligation, to use this information to improve the performance of the employees. This use of hard facts in interacting with employees often changes the style of supervision. It puts inordinate emphasis on hourly performance and creates a coercive interaction. This is a critical mistake in a high-technology environment in which employee cooperation is essential.

Supervision has to be helpful and supportive if employee motivation is to be maintained and stress is to be avoided. This means that first-line supervisors should not use individual performance data as a basis for interaction. The supervisor should be knowledgeable about the technology and serve as a resource when employees are having problems. If management wants employees to ask for help, then the relationship with the supervisor has to be positive (not coercive) so that employees feel confident enough to ask for help. If employees are constantly criticized, they will shun the supervisor, and problem situations that can harm productivity will go unheeded.

Performance Monitoring

Monitoring employee performance is a vital concern of labor unions and employees. Computers provide greatly enhanced capability to track employee performance, and this will follow from such close monitoring. As we noted previously, this fear is not unfounded and is almost inherent in the use of computer systems unless conscious efforts are taken to promote helpful supervision.

Monitoring of employee performance is an important process for management. It helps to know how productive your work force is and where bottlenecks are occurring. It is vital management information that can be used by top management to realign resources and to make important management decisions. However, it is not a good practice to provide individual employee performance information to first-line supervisors because it can lead to a coercive supervision style. To enhance individual performance, it is helpful to give periodic feedback directly to employees about their own performance. This can be done in a noncoercive way directly by the computer on a daily basis. This will help employees judge their performance and also assist in establishing a supervisory climate that is conducive to satisfied and productive employees.

Disability Accommodation

Beyond the generic improvement of computer-oriented jobs, special considerations must sometimes be made for persons with existing disabilities and impairments. The Americans with Disabilities Act of 1990 federally mandates that institutions and employers provide reasonable effort to accommodate workers with disabilities. Many people with physical disabilities and who use wheelchairs are attracted to jobs that are more sedentary. This emphasizes the need to consider ergonomic access and accommodation in computer-oriented occupations such as programming, telephone operation, telemarketing, mail-order processing, and so on.

Enabling a match between computer workstations and people with disabilities cannot be ad-equately covered in this chapter nor is it the mission of this text, but obviously it is important for rehabilitation professionals to recognize this need and to obtain more resources in this area as accommodation situations present. Basically, however, there are three approaches; the third is preferred because it is a combination of the first two.

First, the computer workstation can be initially set up to accommodate many types of disabilities with little extra expense or effort. Allowing for maximal adjustability in the positioning of computer components permits access by people who have wheelchairs, hand and arm movement limitations, and visual impairments. Many decisions, however, need to be made when equipment is purchased, not after. Some computers and workstations are more accessible than others. More and more computer companies are aware of this. In 1986, section 508 of the Rehabilitation Act of 1973 as amended by P.L. 99-506 was passed, which required all computer manufacturers who sold equipment to the federal government to incorporate reasonable features to improve their accessibility for use by people with disabilities.

Second, hundreds of special products are available to adapt computers and workstations to accommodate persons with disabilities. These are cataloged in a national data base, and this information is available to the public (Berliss et al, 1991; HyperABLEDATA, 1990). This data base includes items such as screen readers for people who are blind, large-print displays for people with visual impairments, adapted keyboards for people with motor disorders, head pointing access systems for people who cannot use their hands, and so on. Several resources that have additional information on accommodation of computers and their workstations to people with disabilities are listed in Appendix I.

Third, in many situations that involve people with some disabilities, true access to the computer workstation relies on having generally accessible computer stations as well as some special hardware and software. Performing this match usually requires an interdisciplinary team computer-access evaluation. Some accommodation problems can be adequately solved with simple measures. Others, however, depend on the most current knowledge of computer-access technologies available. Today computer-access experts tend to be based in regional evaluation centers, although computer accommodation is increasingly becoming understood by more and more rehabilitation professionals.

Systemic Approach: Using the Balance Theory

Each of the remedies described previously focuses on a small part of the work system (see Fig. 23–1). Ergonomic design emphasizes the physical environment, the technology, and workstation elements of the work system. It is mainly concerned with the physical aspects of the work system. Job design and organizational design table the problems related to the task and work-organization elements of the work system. Each remedy will be limited as to its effect on physical and mental strain. Because any one element of the work system influences the other elements, any one remedy will affect the entire system. It is important to understand the interrelationships among the elements of the work system. Remedies that focus on only one element of the work system are not likely to suppress all physical and mental strain problems. This approach requires careful examination and diagnosis of the causes of physical and mental strain in computerized workplaces. In this way, effective remedies can be generated. The previous sections provide a long list of remedies that can be used to reduce physical and mental strain problems.

CONCLUSION

Workers in computerized jobs encounter problems, actual and potential, that were not recognized years ago. This has been due in part to the shift to a service-oriented work force and the significant rise in the proportion of jobs that depend on computers.

This evolution in job characteristics has changed not only the way we work but the way in which our health may be threatened. This chapter reviewed the literature on computerized jobs and discussed the known impact of these jobs on the health of the workers who deal with computers as part of their occupational role. Fortunately, much of the research leads us to some rational methods for intervening in health-taxing situations. The balance theory gives us a systemic perspective, and specific therapeutic interventions have been described that can be implemented to improve specific components of the computerized workstation, its tasks, and its physical and sociotechnical environments.

Although countless areas of research have yet to clearly define the impact of computerized jobs on our lives, we have the tools to begin to improve how we as human beings interact with computers. As is always the case, tools can be used for our benefit or for our own destruction. It is up to us to design and apply computers in our best short- and long-term interest.

References

AFL-CIO: Conference on Office Automation. New York, AFL-CIO, Industrial Union Department, 1984.

Arndt R: Working posture and musculoskeletal problems of videodisplay terminal operators: Review and appraisal. Am Industrial Hygiene Assoc 44:437–446, 1983.

Association of Ophthalmologists of Quebec: Cathode Ray Tube Display Terminals and Their Effects on Ocular Health. Quebec, University of Laval, 1982.

Bammer G: VDUs and musculo-skeletal problems at the Australian National University, unpublished document, 1986.

Bergqvist UO: Video display terminals and health: A technical and medical appraisal of the state of the art. Scand Work Environ Health 10:1–87, 1984.

Berliss J, Borden P, Ford K, and Vanderheiden G: Trace Resource Book: Assistive Technologies for Communication, Control and Computer Access. Madison, WI, Trace Research and Development Center, 1991.

Cakir A, Hart DJ, and Stewart TFM: The VDT Manual. Darmstadt, Germany, InceFry Research Association, 1979.

Cohen BGF: Proceedings of a Conference on Occupational Health Issues Affecting Clerical/Secretarial Personnel. Cincinnati, OH, National Institute for Occupational Safety and Health, 1982.

Dainoff MJ: Occupational stress factors in visual display terminal operation: A review of empirical research. Behaviour Information Technol 1:141–176, 1982.

Dainoff MJ, Frazier L, and Taylor B: Workstation and environmental design factors in best and worst case conditions and their effects on VDT operator health and performance. Cincinnati, OH, National Institute for Occupational Safety and Health, 1984.

Gould JD and Grischkowsky N: Doing the same work with hardcopy and with cathode ray tube (CRT) computer terminal. Hum Factors 26:323–337, 1984.

Grandjean E: Ergonomical and Medical Aspects of Cathode Ray Tube Displays. Zurich, Switzerland, Federal Institute of Technology, 1979.

Grandjean E: Postural problems at office machine workstations. *In* Grandjean E (ed): Ergonomics and Health in Modern Offices. London, Taylor & Francis, 1984.

Grandjean E, Hunting W, and Piderman M: VDT workstation design: Preferred settings and their effects. Hum Factors 25:161–175, 1983.

Grandjean E, Nishiyama K, Hunting W, et al: A laboratory study on preferred and imposed settings of a VDT workstation. Behaviour Information Technol 1:289–304, 1982.

Grignolo FM, DiBari A, Brogliatti B, et al: Ocular tonometry in VDT operators. *In* Proceedings of International Scientific

Conference: Work with Display Units. Stockholm, Sweden, National Board of Occupational Safety and Health, 1986.

Gunnarsson E and Ostberg O: The physical and psychological working environment in a terminal-based computer storage and retrieval system. Report 35. Stockholm, Sweden, National Board of Occupational Safety and Health, 1977.

Gunnarsson E and Soderberg I: Eye-strain resulting from VDT work at the Swedish Telecommunications Administration. Stockholm, Sweden, National Board of Occupational Safety and Health, 1980.

Haider M, Idollar J, Kundi M, et al: Stress and strain on the eyes produced by work with display screens: Report on the work-physiological study performed for the union of employees in the private sector. Vienna, Austria, Austrian Trade Union Association, 1975.

Haider M, Kundi M, and Weissebock M: Worker strain related to VDUs with differently coloured characters. In Ergonomic Aspects of Visual Displays Terminals. London, Taylor & Francis, 1980.

Haynes SG and Feinleib M: Women, work and coronary heart disease: prospective findings from the Framingham Heart Study. Am Public Health 70:133–141, 1980.

HyperABLEDATA: Co-Net: Cooperative Database Distribution Network for Assistive Technology, 2nd ed. Madison, WI, Trace and Development Center, 1990.

Mayfield M and Voge L: Computer Comfort: A Guide to Working at Your Computer with Less Strain on Your Neck, Back, Hands, and Eyes. Menlo Park, CA, Computer Comfort, 1990.

McPhee B: Occupational cervicobranchial disorders. In Proceedings of International Scientific Conference: Work with Display Units. Stockholm, Sweden, National Board of Occupational Safety and Health, 1986.

Nakaseko M, Hunting W, Laubli T, et al: Constrained posture and some erogonomic problems of VDT operators. Labour 58:203–212, 1982.

National Academy of Science: Video Displays, Work and Vision. Washington, DC, National Academy Press, 1983.

Office of Technology Assessment: Automation of America's Offices. Washington, DC, U.S. Congress, 1985.

Ostberg O: CRTs pose health problems for operators Int Occup Health & Safety XX:24–26, 46, 50, 52, 1975.

Ostberg O: Visual accommodation before and after VDU work with split screen versus traditional screen paper mode of operation. In proceedings of International Scientific Conference: Work with Display Units. Stockholm, Sweden, National Board of Occupational Safety and Health, 1986.

Sauter SL, Chapman LJ, Knutson SJ, et al: Wrist trauma in VDT keyboard use: Evidence, mechanisms and implications for keyboard and wrist rest design. In Proceedings of International Scientific Conference: Work with Display Units. Stockholm, Sweden, National Board of Occupational Safety and Health, 1986.

Sauter SL, Gottlieb MS, Rohrer KM, et al: The well-being of video display terminal users. Madison, WI, Department of Preventive Medicine, University of Wisconsin–Madison, 1983.

Smith AB, Tanaka S, and Halperin W: Correlates of ocular and somatic symptoms among video display terminal users. Human Factors 26:143–156, 1984.

Smith AB, Tanaka S, Halperin W, et al: Cross-sectional survey of VDT users at the Baltimore Sun. Cincinnati, OH, National Institute for Occupational Safety and Health, 1982.

Smith MJ: Job stress and VDUs: Is the technology a problem? In Proceedings of International Scientific Conference: Work with Display Units. Stockholm, Sweden, National Board of Occupational Safety and Health, 1986.

Smith MJ, Cohen BFG, Stammerjohn LW, et al: An investigation of health complaints and job stress in video display operations. Human Factors 23:389–400, 1981.

Smith MJ, Colligan MJ, and Hurrell JJ Jr: A review of NIOSH Psychological stress research 1977. In Occupational Stress. Report No. 78-156. Cincinnati, OH, National Institute for Occupational Safety and Health, 1978.

Smith MJ and Sainfort PC: A balance theory of job design for stress reduction. Int J Industrial Ergonomics 4:67–79, 1989.

Smith MJ, Stammerjohn L, Cohen BGF, et al: Video display operator stress. In Grandjean E and Vigliani E (eds): Ergonomic Aspects of Visual Display Terminals. London, Taylor & Francis, 1980.

Stark L: Visual fatigue and the VDT workplace. In Bennette J (ed): Visual Display Terminals, Usability Issues and Health Concerns. Englewood Cliffs, NJ, Prentice-Hall, 1984.

Taylor SE and Rupp BA: Display image characteristics and visual response. In Proceedings of International Scientific Conference: Work with Display Units. Stockholm, Sweden, National Board of Occupational Safety and health, 1986.

Thompson FJ, Yates BJ, and Franzen DG: Blood pooling in leg skeletal muscles prevented by a "New" venopressor reflex mechanism. In Proceedings of International Scientific Conference: Work with Display Units. Stockholm, Sweden, National Board of Occupational Safety and Health, 1986.

Voss M, Nyuman KG, and Bergqvist U: VDT work and changes in binocular vision: Some results. In Proceedings of International Scientific Conference: Work with Display Units. Stockholm, Sweden, National Board of Occupational Safety and Health, 1986.

Winkel J: Macro- and micro-circulatory changes during prolonged sedentary work and the need for lower limit values for leg activity: A review. In Proceedings of International Scientific Conference: Work with Display Units. Stockholm, Sweden, National Board of Occupational Safety and Health, 1986.

Wu SS, Stark L, Veretto F, et al: Blink rate as a measure of effort in visual task performance. In Proceedings of International Scientific Conference: Work with Display Units. Stockholm, Sweden, National Board of Occupational Safety and Health, 1986.

Yamamoto S, Noro K, Kurimoto S, et al: VDT operators' variation of the accommodation of the eyes during VDT work. In Proceedings of International Scientific Conference: Work with Display Units. Stockholm, Sweden, National Board of Occupational Safety and Health, 1986.

Zwahlen HT: Pupillary responses when viewing designated locations in a VDT workstation. In Grandjean E (ed): Ergonomics and Health in Modern Offices. London, Taylor & Francis, 1984.

APPENDIX I: LIST OF RESOURCES ON DISABILITY ACCOMMODATION

RESNA: An Interdisciplinary Association for the Advancement of Rehabilitation and Assistive Technologies
1101 Connecticut Ave NW
Suite 700
Washington, DC 20036
(202) 857-1199

Trace R & D Center
Rehabilitation Engineering Center on Accessibility of Computers and Electronic Equipment
S-151 Waisman Center
1500 Highland Avenue
Madison, WI 53705
(608) 262-6966

Cerebral Palsy Research Foundation
Rehabilitation Engineering Center on Modification to Worksites and Education Settings
2021 North Old Manor
Box 8217
Wichita, KS 67208
(316) 688-1886

Stout Vocational Rehabilitation Institute
Rehabilitation Research and Training Center on New Directions for Rehabilitation Facilities
School of Education and Human Services
Menomonie, WI 54751
(715) 232-1389

CHAPTER
24

Karen A. Williams

Consultative Work Programs for Cumulative Trauma Disorders

Throughout the United States and other parts of the world, cumulative trauma disorders (CTDs) of the upper extremities are becoming increasingly more prevalent. As our society moves from heavy industry into a more service-oriented society, which requires more desk work and small assembly or hand machine manipulation, it is becoming increasingly more difficult for workers to maintain the required high levels of productivity.

CTDs are synonymous with the following terms: repetitive motion disease, repetitious strain injury, upper limb syndrome, overuse syndrome, occupational overuse syndrome, and variations using different combinations of the aforementioned terms.

Although it may appear that CTDs of the upper extremity are a relatively new phenomenon, Ramazzini, the father of occupational medicine, was the first to identify these types of disorders. In 1713, Ramazzini recorded a "disease of clerks and scribes" (Isernhagen, 1988). In 1882, the *British Medical Journal* noted the existence of telegrapher's cramp (Isernhagen, 1988). Similar occupational injuries have been discussed in medical journals from America, Australia, Great Britain, Japan, and Scandinavia. These journals discuss sewing cramp, scissors cramp, writer's cramp, typist's cramp (in 1920), and rope making hazards (in 1951) (Isernhagen, 1988). Most recently, CTDs have been associated with the use of keyboards.

CTDs develop in soft tissue, most frequently in the tendons, muscles, and nerves. Also the vascular system may be involved in response to repeated overexertion and excessive movements.

CTDs can be defined as those disorders that are caused, precipitated, or aggravated by repeated exertions or movements of the body. The following five diagnoses represent common, specific types of CTDs of the upper extremities:

1. Carpal tunnel syndrome is a condition in which the structures in the carpal tunnel of the wrist are compressed mechanically or by swelling. Frequently, workers involved in repetitious handwork that requires repeated wrist flexion, forceful ulnar or radial deviation, localized pressure at the base of the palm of the hand, and forceful pinching experience symptoms related to carpal tunnel syndrome.
2. De Quervain's syndrome is characterized by tenderness and pain over the upper portion of the wrist on the thumb side. De Quervain's syndrome is caused by inflammation of the tendons of the thumb and radial wrist exten-

sors, which is aggravated by high numbers of repetitions during thumb manipulations, repeated ulnar deviation of the wrist, or sustained forceful posturing of the thumb.

3. Ganglion cysts are hard, small areas of fluid in the tendons of the wrist or digits. They may be caused by sudden or strong use of a tendon. They also may be associated with repeated manipulations with extended or deviated wrists and forceful grip.

4. Epicondylitis (tennis elbow, golfer's elbow) is generally related to inflammation and pain in the elbow region. Epicondylitis can be caused by continued stressful use of the wrist and digit extensors and by ulnar deviation and is often combined with forearm pronation and supination.

5. Tendinitis is an inflammation of a tendon. Quite often, this inflammation can extend into its sheath. When this occurs, it is called tenosynovitis. Causative factors are as follows: (1) direct blows to the tendon; (2) repetitive motion causing strain and fatigue; (3) infection from arthritis, tuberculosis, or venereal disease (Peterson, 1979).

The symptoms of CTDs tend to appear weeks, months, or even years after continuous performance of the offending activity. Traumatic injuries at work are usually clear cut and of an accidental nature. The documentation with regard to cause and effect of traumatic injuries is more well defined and the prevention definable by removing dangerous work-site conditions or educating against accidents.

The conditions of CTDs are much more difficult to document and to pinpoint in terms of onset. Aches, pains, and stiffness can be noted far in advance of the injury actually being reported.

Documented controversy exists among investigators regarding the cause of CTDs of the upper extremity. One of the greatest controversies pertains to the relative contribution of occupational versus nonoccupational factors.

Occupational factors may include the following:

1. Repetitive exertions
2. Forceful exertions
3. Stressful postures, either end-ranges or awkward sustained postures (e.g., extreme wrist flexion with carpal tunnel syndrome)
4. Low temperatures causing stiffness and decreased circulation and sensation
5. Vibration, which decreases circulation and may cause microtrauma in the soft tissue
6. Poorly designed workstations that do not take into account anthropomorphic differences in workers
7. Production rates and incentive programs
8. Poorly fitted gloves that require the worker to exert excessive force to perform the task, resulting in early fatigue
9. Poorly maintained equipment (e.g., dull knives) that increases worker fatigue

Nonoccupational factors may include:

1. Congenital defects
2. Chronic diseases
3. Age
4. Gender
5. Recreational activities and avocational interests
6. History of previous upper extremity injury

When an individual experiences an upper extremity CTD, activities of daily living (ADL) are significantly impaired. It is not uncommon to remove what was thought to be the antagonist mechanism (e.g., work demands) only to have the individual continue to be symptomatic. Returning the upper extremity CTD worker back to work after a medical absence presents another challenging problem. Does the worker return to his or her previous job, which may exacerbate the condition? The success rates over the years for both conservative and surgical intervention have been, at best, fair. When symptoms produced from CTDs cannot be decreased or alleviated, the ability of clients to return safely and effectively to their previous vocational and avocational tasks has been hindered.

Prevention of upper extremity CTDs is the key. Education of individuals at the workplace is imperative. Education programs must be oriented differently for managers and workers. Early recognition of workers' complaints and symptoms, specialized ergonomic assessments, and upper extremity screenings will aid in the prevention of upper extremity CTDs.

PREVENTION AND EDUCATION PROGRAMS

The need for well-planned programs of education for all concerned with hand-intensive work has been realized, and increased emphasis has been placed on the aspect of prevention within the overall ergonomic approach (Isernhagen, 1988).

The Handle with Care program was effective in reducing the cost and incidence of industrial hand injuries in Oklahoma. The Handle with Care program originated in 1983 as an hour-long pilot program that was presented to supervisors of a company in Oklahoma. From that point on, Handle with Care grew into an 8-hour training seminar, which enabled participants to present, recognize, and correct hand hazards in their places of business (Smith, 1987).

Ethicon, Inc., developed a successful on-site prevention program to decrease the incidence of upper extremity CTDs in 1978. Today CTDs are managed by an ergonomic task force, which creates a working environment that enhances productivity by the safe design of the workplace and the promotion of wellness. The Ethicon, Inc., program uses early recognition of upper extremity CTDs by encouraging workers to seek medical attention as early as possible. In 1982, a physical therapy clinic was established on-site. Workstations are evaluated for the following: repetitive motion requirements, mechanical force concentrations, and static muscle tension situations. Exercises also are used intermittently throughout the day (Lutz and Hansford, 1987).

On-site prevention programs are becoming increasingly prevalent, particularly in hand-intensive industries. Prevention programs provide an innovative way to reduce workers' injuries while promoting a safe and healthy work environment.

At Michigan Hand Rehabilitation Center, Inc., an industrial consultative program is available to assist industry with the identification of problem areas and to provide recommendations for remediation of those problems. The industrial consultative program consists of the following services:

Prevention/education programs
Upper extremity screenings
Specialized work assessments

The prevention/education programs ideally are effective in changing attitudes and work practices. Program objectives differ depending on who is receiving the information. Possible overall objectives for managers include sensitization of the need for ergonomic programs, overview of relevant legislation and standards, ensuring an understanding of the manager's responsibility for

the safety and well-being of employees, general education of the ergonomic principles of prevention, provision of guidelines for stress reduction, and the increase of overall plant safety and wellness.

General educational objectives for supervisors might include providing a reasonable depth of understanding of body mechanics and mechanisms of injury, designing principles and work techniques, introducing efficient methods of data collection for incidence of injury, and emphasizing the responsibility of the supervisor regarding the safety and wellness of employees.

Possible general educational objectives for prevention programs for workers include the introduction of the concept of ergonomics, provision of an understanding of the mechanism of injury, encouragement of new approaches to movement or new techniques for performing tasks that are ergonomically more sound, and demonstration of the need for physical fitness and overall wellness.

The prevention programs at Michigan Hand Rehabilitation Center, Inc., for industry target three separate, different audiences: managers, workers, and high-risk workers.

The management training program is a 4-hour program designed for administrators, supervisors, superintendents, group leaders, and medical personnel. The goals of the manager's program are as follows:

1. Increase the manager's knowledge of the causes of CTDs
2. Improve the manager's knowledge of upper extremity anatomy
3. Assist the manager in basic ergonomic modifications
4. Improve the manager's knowledge of the use of splints and gloves

The management training program is limited to 10 participants per group. By keeping this group small, it promotes participation from group members. The room should be set up with the tables in a U shape with the chairs on the outside. The speaker, as well as any visual aids, should be visible to all group members.

The management training begins with an introduction of the speaker and then an introduction of all group members using both names and titles. The group members introduce themselves and also rate their level of understanding of CTDs of the upper extremity. This assists the speaker with customizing his or her discussion with the group.

The participants are then provided with a descriptive lecture on the upper extremity through the use of an anatomic limb and a slide presentation. The anatomic review is pathology-specific relating to common upper extremity CTDs. The participants are encouraged to ask questions. The group leader then defines the causes of upper extremity CTDs and provides the managers with methods of early detection of specific pathologies via "red flag signals." A review of controls that can be used to decrease the incidence of upper extremity CTDs and specific examples of ergonomic modifications are given. Proper pacing, posturing, and positioning are stressed via verbal, written, and demonstrative techniques, including videotaping. Specific splints and gloves are presented to demonstrate the proper fit.

The participants learn in an environment in which exchange of ideas, comments, and questions is encouraged. Each participant is provided with a folder that includes information on carpal tunnel syndrome, copies of articles relevant to CTDs of the upper extremity, and an extensive outline of course content on which to take notes. A sample of the flexibility exercises, which the employees receive in their training program, is included (Fig. 24–1). A course-evaluation sheet is also included to allow for feedback regarding course content and presentation.

The employee training program is designed for workers. This training program is based on a maximum of 25 participants per group and is 1 hour in length. During the employee training program, the terms carpal tunnel syndrome, tendinitis, and any other upper extremity CTD are not mentioned. This training program is strictly about employee health and wellness.

The goals of the employee training program are to make employees aware of:

1. Upper extremity structures that can be injured
2. The causes of upper extremity disorders and how they can decrease their occurrence
3. The proper use and fit of splints and gloves

The overall goal of the employee training program is to educate the worker to work smarter, not harder!

The training area may be anywhere in the plant. It is set up in a classroom style with clear view of the speaker and visual aids. The speaker introduces him or herself and then proceeds to the course content. The anatomy of the upper extremity is briefly reviewed in lay terms with the anatomic limb. The five postures to avoid while working or at home and during leisure time (extreme wrist flexion, ulnar deviation, supination, pressure over the base of the palm, and wearing constricting bands at the wrist) are reviewed (Fig. 24–2). Employees are then instructed in proper pacing and flexibility exercises to perform intermittently while at work and at home. Employees are provided with a pocket-sized handout that clearly shows all flexibility exercises. Employees with specific questions are asked to talk with the speaker after the training session. An optional 30- to 60-minute long plant tour to address specific employee questions and comments is available.

High-risk workers have already been identified as having an upper extremity CTD. These individuals will benefit from specific education provided in an individualized employee education program. This 1-hour program is designed to educate the employees about their specific condition and what they can do to prevent further problems with regard to work demands and ADL. This training is performed on a one-to-one basis with an occupational therapist specializing in upper extremity disorders.

The individual employee education program may be performed at the plant or at a rehabilitation facility. It is preferable to perform the education program on-site where specific work demands are more readily discussed.

The goals of the individual employee education program are as follows:

1. Assess each worker's lifestyle and work style in respect to influences on CTDs
2. Provide workers with an understanding of the basic upper extremity anatomic structures affected by CTDs
3. Inform and provide workers with the postures and positions that should be avoided to decrease the symptoms with their CTD
4. Educate workers in basic pain-management techniques
5. Provide workers with splints, gloves, and other protective supports needed to assist in decreasing symptoms

The workers are asked to complete a lifestyle assessment sheet developed at Michigan Hand Rehabilitation Center, Inc., and are questioned regarding any identified problem work areas.

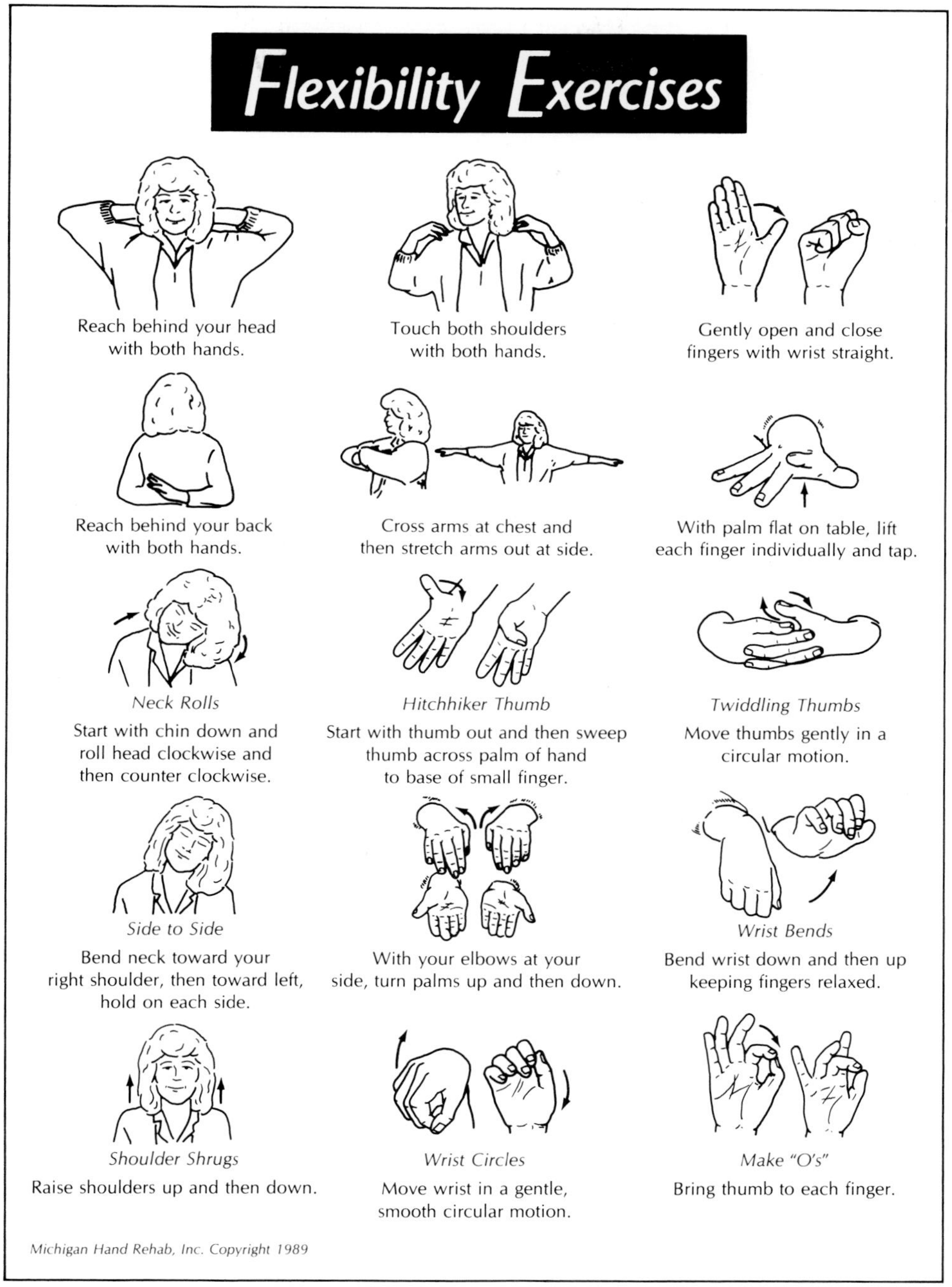

Figure 24–1. *Flexibility Exercise Poster published and used at Michigan Hand Rehabilitation Center, Inc.* This poster is ideal for placement in the work site to remind employees to utilize warm-up and cool-down exercises prior to, during, and after each work session.

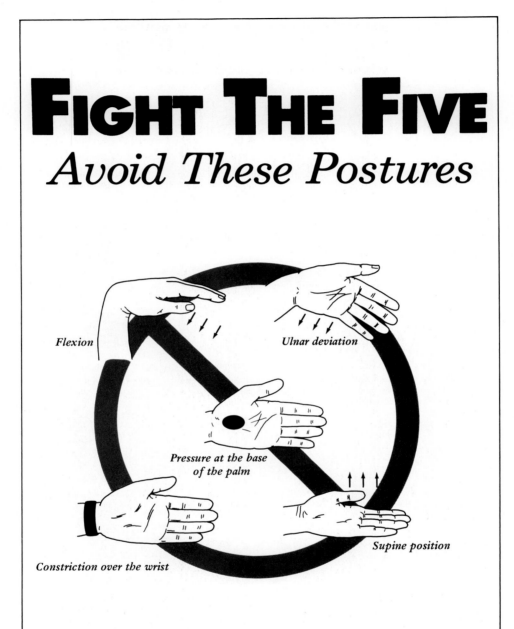

Figure 24–2. *"Fight the Five" Poster published and used at Michigan Hand Rehabilitation Center, Inc.* This poster is used to remind workers of the hand positions to avoid while performing their job tasks.

The therapist makes specific recommendations regarding work performance and proper use of upper extremities during avocational activities and ADL. Proper pacing, positioning, and posturing are reviewed with the workers. All techniques are specifically applied to these individuals and their work and leisure activities. Techniques for pain management specific to these workers' types of pain are provided. The workers are fitted with splints, gloves, elbow cuffs, and protective supports as deemed necessary. The workers then view the clinic videotape on techniques for hand protection. If necessary, specific ergonomic recommendations are made to the employer regarding workstation design. The employees are instructed to notify the proper medical personnel if symptoms continue.

These three prevention and education programs—the management training program, employee training program, and individual employee education program—are most beneficial when administered within a relatively close time frame. It is most effective to begin with the management training and then, within 1 week, employee training sessions followed by individual employee education. A specialized ergonomic assessment (which is discussed later in this chapter) is very useful for all three prevention and education programs.

SCREENINGS FOR UPPER EXTREMITY CTDs

Upper extremity screenings can aid in the early detection of carpal tunnel syndrome and various other CTDs. When these disorders are recognized early, it allows the employer the opportunity to assess promptly the worker's job and institute protection and prevention procedures for him or her. Early medical attention can prevent costly problems for everyone involved. Many times, simply educating the worker in proper pacing, positioning, and posturing will eliminate the painful symptoms of many CTDs.

An annual upper extremity screening program assesses workers' potential for developing a CTD, identifies problem areas within the plant in respect to CTDs, determines if ergonomic modifications will be beneficial, and facilitates early detection and subsequent early intervention with treatment and management of CTDs.

The annual upper extremity screening takes approximately 15 minutes per employee. Costs are nominal for each screening. The workers are asked to fill out a data sheet, which examines demographic information, previous job and medical history, and leisure time activities. The data sheets are then reviewed by the therapist with each worker. An examination is then performed by a registered occupational therapist.

The evaluation includes an assessment of the physical appearance of the extremities; specifically, the presence of atrophy, hypertrophy, scars, enlarged joints, erythema, and edema are noted. The therapist then evaluates active range of motion of both upper extremities for finger flexion and extension, thumb opposition, forearm pronation and supination, wrist flexion and extension, elbow flexion and extension, and shoulder abduction and adduction. Any deviations from normal are recorded. Distal strength is then assessed via a dynamometer in the second or third handle positions (depending on hand size), and the recording is compared with normative data.

The following diagnostic tests are then performed: Phalen's test, Tinel's sign, abduction test, Finklestein's test, Mill's test, and resistive extension (Fig. 24–3). The worker scores either positive or negative on each test. Pain, if present, is then discussed.

Once all screenings have been completed, overall recommendations are made to the contact person at the plant. Recommendations may be, but are not limited to, the following:

1. Worker would benefit from an evaluation by a physician specializing in the upper extremity.
2. Worker would benefit from an individual employee education program.
3. Tool, machine, or workstation ergonomic modifications are necessary.
4. Worker would benefit from wearing a splint or glove.
5. Worker would benefit from working in an alternative job at the plant.

ERGONOMIC CONSIDERATIONS

Specialized work assessments (SWAs) evaluate the worker's ability to perform specific job demands. The assessment is performed with respect to safety and the promotion of wellness in the workplace.

During an SWA, the physical demands of the

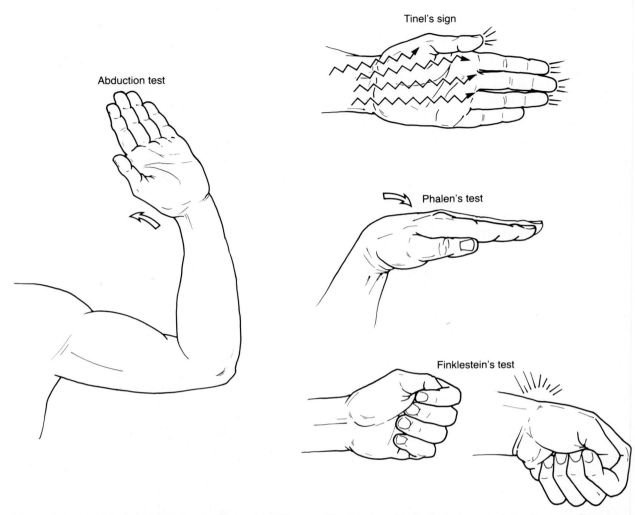

Figure 24–3. *Finklestein's test for de Quervain's disease, Tinel's sign, Phalen's test, and abduction test.* These are some of the various diagnostic tests used at Michigan Hand Rehabilitation Center, Inc., to identify cumulative trauma disorders.

job are evaluated with the following goals in mind:

1. Determine if the worker is suited for specific job stressors with respect to CTDs.
2. Determine if specific job responsibilities could contribute to the development of upper extremity CTDs.
3. Determine if or what ergonomic changes are required to assist in the reduction of CTDs of the upper extremity.
4. Determine if splints or gloves are necessary to assist in the prevention of upper extremity CTDs.

Information for the SWA is obtained via the recording of objective information either from a video camera, 35-mm camera, Polaroid camera, sketching of the workstation, and documentation of specific assessments. Some of the specific assessment areas may include force and repetition considerations (Table 24–1).

The specifics of proper tool fit and use cannot be understated. Incorrect hand tool designs can cause a variety of CTDs (Meagher, 1987). Elements important in tool design from the human factor aspect include size, shape, texture, purpose, ease of operation, shock absorption, and weight.

Table 24–1. Some Evaluation Considerations During a Specialized Work Assessment*

Repetitiveness	Mechanical assists; process changes; product changes; work enlargements; worker rotations; rest allowances
Forcefulness	Decrease weight of objects held in hand; increase friction of objects held in hand; balance tools; use air shutoff or external torque bars to control tool torque; use mechanical assists for holding tools and lifting parts; slide, do not lift, parts; use roller or powered conveyors to move parts; maintain quality control on part fit; replace or service dull and worn tools; avoid gloves that are excessively bulky

*From Armstrong T, Fine L, et al: Ergonomics considerations in hand and wrist tendinitis. J Hand Surg *12A-5-2:*830–837, 1987.

When evaluating tool size, it is important to consider that one size does not fit all. When the handle diameter is too wide, increased energy expenditure is required for tool retention, and thus the hand is susceptible to intrinsic muscle strain.

Ideally, the tool handle should allow the small joints of the hand to flex gently (mid range of flexion). This posturing provides good tool retention while allowing the muscle to be partially stretched. Gawitzke and Milner (1989) showed that a partially stretched muscle contracts more forcefully than when it is relaxed at the time of activation.

The shape of the tool should fit in the curve of the transverse palmar arch to permit an even application of force. Improperly contoured and ill-fitting handles are used forcefully over long periods of time and can thus cause finger problems. Intrinsic muscle strain may also occur.

The texture of the tool can influence energy expenditure. A slippery finish requires added energy expenditure for tool retention.

Weight of the tool is extremely important when considering excess energy expenditure and muscle fatigue. Heavy tools, by virtue of their weight alone, can cause intrinsic muscle spasms, myositis, tendinitis, epicondylitis, and other upper extremity disorders when used repetitively.

Grip-strength differences between male and female workers provide a basis for using female grip strength as a standard for tool design (Meagher, 1987).

When performing an SWA (sometimes referred to as a job analysis, work assessment, and so on), it is advantageous to have the following equipment on hand:

1. Force gauge (Fig. 24–4)
2. 120-foot measuring tape
3. Scale
4. Polaroid camera or 35-mm camera
5. Video camera
6. Dictaphone

The documentation of the SWA should represent all information obtained during the data-collection phase of the on-site SWA. Information should be presented in a concise manner in a language familiar to all individuals reviewing the report (medical and nonmedical individuals). The SWA report should include a summary and recommendations section, which provides alternative plans for remediation of identified problem areas. Assistance with the implementation of the outlined recommendations should also be offered.

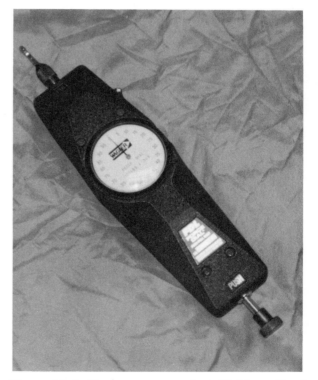

Figure 24–4. *Force gauge used at Michigan Hand Rehabilitation Center, Inc.* The force gauge is utilized to determine exactly how much force a client may be exerting while pushing or pulling objects or performing everyday tasks (e.g., opening a door, lifting a purse).

The SWA report should be mailed within 1 week to all individuals involved, and follow-up discussions regarding the contents of the SWA report should be encouraged by the therapist performing the SWA.

A variety of customized programs may evolve from either the prevention and education programs or the SWAs. Although each of these programs could warrant lengthy discussions themselves, it is not feasible in this chapter to devote much discussion to them other than to list them as possible outcomes of the aforementioned programs:

1. New employee orientation
2. Safety programs
3. Specialized ergonomic assessment libraries
4. Ergonomic committees
5. Functional capacity evaluations
6. Transitional work programs
7. Restricted work

PAYMENT

The costs of implementing a prevention and education program or an SWA will be significantly less than the costs incurred with one worker with carpal tunnel syndrome who has surgery and is unable to return to work. Although wellness programs and SWAs for specific workers may be reimbursed under many worker's compensation insurance programs, Michigan Hand Rehabilitation Center, Inc., has found that industries are allocating a certain portion of their budget toward the prevention and management of upper extremity CTDs. Companies are generally invoiced for services rendered within 1 week of those services being performed. Payment is expected within 30 days. The average costs of the prevention and education programs are listed in Table 24–2.

MARKETING

Many people equate marketing with selling; however, marketing is much more than selling (Wolters, 1989). Marketing encompasses many areas of business, such as determining customer needs and wants, developing services to address these demands, and the promotion of services.

In marketing industrial consultative services such as prevention programs, SWAs, and upper

Table 24–2. Evaluation Costs*

Program Description	Cost
Management program: Half-day session based on a maximum of 10 participants per group	$500.00
Employee program One-hour program based on a maximum of 25 participants per group	$250.00
Individual employee program	$100.00
Upper extremity screening	$ 15.00†
Specialized work assessment	$ 90.00‡

*Figures are based on averages gathered at Michigan Hand Rehabilitation Center, Inc. Travel expenses and materials charges are extra.
†Per employee.
‡Per hour.

extremity screenings, it is imperative to identify the population of potential users. Hand-intensive industries (such as the plastic industries, poultry and meat industries, electronic small assembly, data-entry positions, and so on) will most certainly be interested in information regarding effective ways to decrease their injury incidence and increase their profit margin.

In developing a marketing strategy, it is beneficial to conduct a thorough analysis in the following four areas:

1. Customer needs and wants
2. Your facility's strengths and weaknesses
3. Your competition
4. The general business environment

Meet with potential customers in person. Listen carefully to their requests and ask questions to determine preferences in various services. Satisfying the customer must be your priority.

Do some soul searching of your facility's strengths and weaknesses. Be honest! Capitalize on your strengths and strive to improve areas that may limit your growth.

Know the competitor! What are its strengths and weaknesses? Never criticize a competitor's services as a strategy to make your facility look better.

Finally, analyze the general business environment. Keep abreast of health-care and business trends via professional organizations, journals, newspapers, and networking.

Once you have completed your analysis, develop a marketing plan. Outline goals and objectives and use as many different activities to achieve your goals and objectives. The following

Table 24–3. Average Costs To Treat One Worker's Compensation Case*

Client No.	Approximate Physician Charge	Approximate Therapy Charge	Approximate Surgery Charge	Total Cost of Treatment
	Ford Motor Company			
Client 1	$3,675.00	$5,340.00	$4,000.00	$13,015.00
Client 2	$2,900.00	$5,990.00	$4,000.00	$12,890.00
	Kroger Company (Grocery)			
Client 1	$2,100.00	$1,300.00	$4,000.00	$ 7,400.00
Client 2	$3,200.00	$9,990.00	$4,000.00	$17,190.00

*Figures were obtained from a review of the costs for treating employees of each company who were seen at Michigan Hand Rehabilitation Center, Inc.

are some examples of ways to solicit your services:

1. Advertise
2. Develop high-quality promotional materials that have a consistent theme
3. Develop and publish a newsletter
4. Sponsor seminars for potential customers
5. Contact local newspapers regarding innovative programs and success stories
6. Network with other professionals in both the medical and business environment
7. Obtain letters of recommendation from satisfied customers
8. Make "cold calls" on potential customers; qualify them on the telephone and then set up an appointment to meet with them

A well-developed marketing plan will provide your facility with the competitive edge necessary to succeed in the business.

STAFF

Undoubtedly, the most important component in determining the success of your program will be your personnel. The occupational or physical therapist who engages in industrial consultative services must possess a high degree of proficiency in the prevention and management of upper extremity CTDs and must be able to communicate this information effectively to others. A high degree of flexibility, reliability, and credibility must be apparent to those individuals with whom he or she is working. Good organizational skills are mandatory because this therapist will most likely assume the role of coordinator or manager of services rendered. The therapist becomes a liaison between the medical profession and the industrial environment. The ability to

present information to others in a clear, concise verbal or written, and demonstrative manner is imperative, as well as the ability to take the initiative when circumstances dictate.

Work hours may be random. When providing prevention and education programs or SWAs to companies that operate on three shifts, the therapist may find himself or herself working at different hours of the day and night. Excellent time-management skills are also beneficial.

SUMMARY

Therapists can have a positive impact on reducing the incidence of upper extremity CTDs through prevention and education programs, upper extremity screenings, and SWAs.

The greatest benefit to the worker is that education programs increase the level of injury awareness. Workers assume an active role in the prevention of their own injuries.

Benefits to the employers of prevention and education programs and SWAs include not only a reduction in injury incidence rates but also a cost savings (Table 24–3).

References

Armstrong T, Fine L, et al: Ergonomics considerations in hand and wrist tendinitis. Hand Surg *12A* (No. 5, Part 2):830–837, 1987.

Gawitzke and Milner: Current topics in occupational safety: prevention of upper limb injuries. Paper presented at the meeting of Engineering Summer Conferences, University of Michigan College of Engineering, Ann Arbor, MI, August 1989.

Isernhagen S: Work Injury Management and Prevention. Rockville, MD, Aspen Publications, 1988.

Lutz G and Hansford T: Cumulative trauma disorder controls: The ergonomics program at Ethicon, Inc. Hand Surg *12A-5-2*:863–866, 1987.

Meagher S: Tool design for prevention of hand and wrist injuries. Hand Surg *12A* (No. 5, Part 2):855–857, 1987.

Peterson RR: Prevention! A new approach to tendinitis. Occup Health Nurs, May:19–23, 1979.

Smith BL: An inside look — hand injury prevention program. Hand Surg *12A* (No. 5, Part 2):940–943, 1987.

Wolters S: Marketing your contract agency. Occup Ther Forum, May 8, 1989, pp 8–11.

Bibliography

Adamo D: Upper extremity injury prevention programs. Industrial Rehabil Q 2 (1), 1989.

Armstrong T, Radwin R, et al: Repetitive trauma disorders: Job evaluation and design. Hum Factors 28 (3):235–336, 1986.

Arndt R: Work pace, stress and cumulative trauma disorders. J Hand Surg *12A* (No. 5, Part 2):866–869, 1987.

Blair SJ and Bear-Lehman J: Editorial comment: Prevention of upper extremity occupational disorders. J Hand Surgery *12A* (No. 5, Part 2):821–822, 1987.

Bleecker M: Medical surveillance for cumulative trauma disorders in workers. J Hand Surg *12A* (No. 5, Part 2):845–848, 1987.

Buckle P: Musculoskeletal disorders of the upper extremity: The use of epidemiologic approaches in industrial settings. Hand Surg *12A* (No. 5, Part 2):885–889, 1987.

Feldman R, Travers P, et al: Risk assessment in electronic assembly workers: Carpal tunnel syndrome. J Hand Surg *12A* (No. 5, Part 2):849–855, 1987.

Hadler N: Illness in the workplace: The challenge of musculoskeletal symptoms. J Hand Surg *10A* (No. 5, Part 4):451–456, 1985.

Hansford BH, Ken B, and Lutz G: Blood flow changes at the wrist in manual workers following preventative interventions. J Hand Surg *12* (No. 5, Part 2):503–508, 1986.

Louis D: Cumulative trauma disorders. J Hand Surg *12A* (No. 5, Part 2):823–825, 1987.

Mattila M: Job load and hazard analysis: A method for the analysis of workplace conditions for occupational health care. Br J Industrial Med *42*:656–666, 1985.

Muffly-Elsey D and Flenn-Wagner S: Proposed screening tool for the detection of cumulative trauma disorders of the upper extremity. J Hand Surg *12A* (No. 5, Part 2):931–935, 1987.

Rudolph M: Therapist applies expertise to occupations. Occupational Therapy Weekly, May 12:16–17, 1988.

PART

IV

Issues for the Therapist and Educator

CHAPTER
25
Robert L. Rubinstein

How to Find Meaning in Client Interaction

The purpose of this chapter is to focus on the human dimension of client interaction. That a special effort should be made to do so suggests that this obvious element is somehow missing in many client-practitioner interactions and further suggests that its absence should be of concern. The chapter's title indicates that the health-care practitioner—the occupational or physical therapist in this case—should be concerned with the issue of meaning: not only, of course, how she or he might find meaning in client interaction but also what a sense of meaning consists of for a client. This latter concern is the subject matter of this chapter.

Basic to our concern is the idea that meaning in client interaction is not and should not be considered anything but integral to the healing process. Some may consider what we discuss here above and beyond the mere sympathetic application of technical knowledge to aid recovery and rehabilitation. The reality is that personal factors that shape meaning are basic to the amelioration of suffering, the positive valuation of human life, and the ability of the health-care facilitator to tailor appropriate and realistic plans of recovery and improvement. Thus, a concern with meaning should not be considered extra or somehow above and beyond what the practitioner does professionally; rather, it is basic in producing effective therapy.

THE CHANGING FACE OF HEALTH CARE

The present concern with meaning comes as a reaction to the increased tendency in medicine—which mirrors that in society at large—toward increased specialization, commercialization, dehumanization, and distancing. Medicine and the allied health specialties have undergone radical transformation in the last 2 decades, which has dramatically altered the way health care is conducted, the image of health specialists, the function of health care in communities, and the relationship between health-care professional and client (Raffel, 1989; Smith and Kaluzny, 1986; Starr, 1982). Events in health care highlight and in an exaggerated way represent changes in society: increasing and almost unbelievable technologic advances combined with increasing social distance, separateness, anomie, rudeness, incivility, and a commercial mentality. To an observer, it appears as if every function and every combination of body segments are the subject of a medical or health-care specialty. Furthermore, the health domain is suffering in part from the commercialization of care. That this is occurring should be of extreme concern to frontline health-care professionals. Moreover, health promotion and disease prevention, certainly enviable goals, have in part served to expand the domain of

419

health far beyond the more narrow profile of health care that was formerly observed.

Although these events have many ramifications, they are perhaps most completely typified in one aspect of client interaction: the lack of time that the health-care professional may have to spend with clients. Rules and regulations about reimbursements and procedures, the constant pressures of client loads, and the circumscription of the professional-client relationship through specialization, status inequality, and miscommunication are culprits here (Fisher and Todd, 1983; Illich, 1976; Mischler, 1984). Yet, increasingly, studies showed that what might be termed the social effects of specialist-client interaction, or the ability to listen and to act interested in what the client has to say, have direct benefits on recovery and well-being. For example, the role of storytelling as therapeutic, beneficial, or necessary in the relationship between the client and the health-care professional has recently been rediscovered (Brody, 1987; Churchill and Churchill, 1982; Kleinman, 1988). The lack of time with clients, too, relates directly to the change in the structure of health care. Practitioners rarely have roots in the communities in which they practice or have firsthand or systematic information or knowledge about the people they see. They have no appreciation for *the whole life* of the client and see him or her only in segments or thin slices, after times of crises or trauma, without much meaningful appreciation of who that person was or is. By and large, the community and situated context of healing is gone, but many consider that these qualities are necessary for the proper conduct of health practice.

Given these circumstances and the need to focus on client interaction meaningfully, we can address in a preliminary way the question that forms the title of this essay. Briefly, then, the answer to the question, "How does one find meaning in client interaction?" is through listening carefully to and taking an interest in the client as a whole person not just as a representative of a disease state.

Not everybody intuitively knows how to do this. The goal of this chapter is to facilitate these aims for health-care practitioners by presenting some guidance in understanding what types of topics and frameworks might be important in approaching the client meaningfully. These derive from insights gained in the social and behavioral sciences that enable us to see the whole person and develop some sense of what might be meaningful for each client. Thus, in this chapter, we examine five key ideas that influence and shape the worlds of clients and practitioners: (1) culture, (2) society, (3) the person, (4) the life course, and (5) the environment.

Culture

Definitions of culture derive from two traditions, both of which are important here. On the one hand, culture may be thought of as the historically derived set of lifeways that are passed down from one generation to another. On the other hand, following anthropologist Geertz (1973), culture may be thought of as the web of meaning that people themselves have spun. Thus, culture may be thought of as meaning that is generally shared.

Cultures exist on many levels. The anthropologist Linton (cited in Kluckhohn, 1985) wrote that each person shared something with all others, with some others, and with no others. Thus, for example, all Americans share certain aspects of lifeways, values, and meanings, although much is not shared. Similarly, groups of Americans share values and meanings that are distinctive to them. For example, historically derived ethnic groups may share patterns of living, lifeways, worldviews, values, and meanings that derive from their unique experiences and that are more or less shared among the group's members. Individuals, too, have their own cultures; that is, their own habitual ways of doing, being, and understanding (see later discussion).

Professions of all sorts have their own cultures as well (Fisher and Todd, 1983; Martin, 1987). This is certainly true for various allied health and other medical professions. Professional training includes not only the learning of technical knowledge and abilities that enable practitioners to work in their fields but also socialization to a set of values and a way of relating. Thus, occupational therapists learn to act like occupational therapists, physical therapists like physical therapists, psychiatrists like psychiatrists, and so on.

Each of these professions borrows from the dominant culture to a greater or lesser extent, and this sense of values often operates both consciously and unconsciously in attempts by health-care professionals to get a client up and about, remotivated or back into life, after a trauma.

In an important paper, medical anthropologist Kaufman (1988) described how individuals' ideas about identity—their overall sense of who they as individuals are in the world—need to be negotiated, adjusted, tested, revised, reviewed, and selectively picked over after the occurrence of stroke, a traumatic medical crisis affecting primarily older people. Stroke profoundly disrupts life; after a stroke the sufferer may not reacquire full functioning. In analyzing the issues that shape the poststroke formation of personal identity, Kaufman differentiated between two processes that are based on two very different cultural notions of what should be done after a traumatic event and what recovery consists of. Thus, she contrasted the rehabilitation process with recovery. The rehabilitation process—the medical model or the notion of what is to be done from the perspective of medical culture—is undertaken by health-care professionals, in her case occupational therapists, and focuses on "observation and measurement of discrete, physical tasks or behaviors on the part of the patient" (1988, p. 83). Thus, clients in her study by and large performed the tasks that were requested of them in therapy. In contrast, the clients themselves operated from the perspective of what Kaufman called recovery, a process she defined as "a nonspecific, diffuse goal . . . which implies notions of normality, continuity and identity" (1988, p. 83). Recovery includes aspects of being a person that are not usually included in the medical—the rehabilitation—model such as who these individuals feel they are, what has gone on in their lives. Thus, people often have their own ideas about what the key issues are in their recovery that are at odds with those of health professionals but that are fundamental in the overall recovery process. We return to Kaufman's example later.

In a complex society such as in the United States, another important aspect of culture is ethnic identity. Although ethnic identity (or ethnicity) has been the result of the historic circumstances and interactions following the immigration of large groups of diverse people with distinctive cultural traditions, ethnicity has also been shown to affect not only overt behavior and values but also unconscious behavioral patterns. Indeed, concerning the domain of mental and physical health, ethnicity has been shown to account for discernible differences in the experi-

ence and expression of pain (Mechanic, 1969; Zborowski, 1969); knowledge of illness (Suchman, 1964); family configurations, support, and the nature of presenting symptoms (Cacciola, 1982; Cohler and Grunebaum, 1981; McGoldrick et al, 1982; Winch et al, 1967; Wylan and Mintz, 1976); in medical symptoms (Breen, 1968; Clough and Garland, 1979; Croog, 1961; Lerner and Noy, 1968; Snyder, 1981; Zola, 1966 and 1979; McGoldrick et al, 1982); the context of life crisis and ritual (Myerhoff, 1978; Parthun, 1976); beliefs about death (Kalish and Reynolds, 1976); death anxiety (Myers et al, 1980); health practices (Chrisman and Kleinman, 1980; Kleinman et al, 1978; Moriwaki, 1976); institutionalization (Markson, 1979); alcohol consumption (Greeley, 1979; Stivers, 1978); preference for formal support services (Johnsen, 1988); and mental health and mental illness (Al-Issa, 1982; Favazza and Oman, 1977; Giordano, 1976a, 1976b, and 1976c; Leighton and Murphy, 1965; Lerion, 1976; Olukayode, 1981; Spiegel, 1976).

Zborowski's classic study, *People in Pain* (1969), illustrates some of these dimensions. Zborowski (1969) studied clients at a Veterans Administration Hospital in New York in an attempt to understand "cultural components in response to pain." Interviews were conducted with 146 subjects of Jewish, Irish, Italian, and Old American (White Anglo-Saxon Protestant) backgrounds. Subjects included both a group with a constant diagnosis (a herniated disc) and a group with variable diagnoses. Significantly, Zborowski found that there were systematic and profound differences among ethnic groups in how subjects responded to and experienced pain. The Old Americans were "nonexpressive. The patient tends to appear unemotional and calm and is not vocal about his pain" (1969, p. 49). Members of this group in the study sample denied manifestations of pain, attempted to hide it, and tried to be rational and in control of behavior. Jewish subjects used "a dramatic vocabulary to convey their discomfort and anxieties to the fullest extent," a procedure that emphasizes their concern "that the doctor may not fully grasp the impact of the situation" (1969, p. 99). Italian-Americans were found to be similar to the Jewish subjects in open expressivity. Zborowski noted that "on the whole, the behavior of the Italian patients is seen as nonconforming to the standards of the hospital, which emphasizes restraint and self-control" (1969, p. 136). The Irish-American subjects were similar in many respects to the Old

Americans: "Their reactions to pain tend to be nonexpressive, nonvocal and noncomplaining" (1969, p. 188) and even more reserved in speaking about pain than the Old Americans.

Although these are brief vignettes, Zborowski exhaustively documented how the experience of pain, which in part is the experience of a psychophysical phenomenon, is shaped by cultural expectations and patterns for expression and affect. Differences, he found, run even deeper; there are distinctions among groups even in the extent to which pain is perceived as a symptom of disease or as an independent agent.

Society

Society is an abstraction, representing the aggregate totality of people who live in some bounded domain such as a nation. The term *society* represents a group of people, and society is said to be the locus of such things as norms and standards for behavior. Society at large shares some aspects of culture. Particular social segments such as communities, families, ethnic groups, occupational specializations, and the like share more particular aspects of culture.

Although society as an abstraction has little importance to specific clients, discrete components of society such as a family or a social support network obviously have great importance. It has long been noted that each person in society has a social network, defined variously as an aggregate of all those persons who an individual knows or considers important. A social network can include close family members, kin, friends, acquaintances, and neighbors. Clearly, when a person is ill, vulnerable, old, or alone, this social network may be extremely important (Cohen and Syme, 1985). Thus, it is significant to distinguish between the social network, defined as *all* the people one knows or who are important in some way, from one defined as people on whom one can count for various sorts of help when one is in need. Interestingly, the inner capital of the social network is based on long-term mutuality of transactions; that is, that people in one's network both give and receive. In contrast, social support may be more one-sided. People who need help may "cash in" on the help that they have earned: Elderly parents receive help from children for whom they have cared, or dependent children receive care that is inherent in their child and vulnerable status.

Social support has been implicated in a number of health outcomes (Berkman, 1985). Most important here is what has been called the *buffering* hypothesis. This states that having adequate social support buffers one from the deleterious effects of illness, radical change, and negative life events such as loss. More simply, having people to rely on helps keep one relatively more healthy.

Social support becomes more important in situational and health difficulties. For example, Stack (1974) described the role of social networks in the "strategies for survival" used by urban African-Americans. In such a materially poor but humanly rich social milieu, phenomena such as exchange and swapping, personal kindreds, child keeping, and domestic social networks are central for individual and group survival. As with other groups, such mutuality contributes to well-being and may be applied in special times of need.

The Person

Personhood (or selfhood) is a cultural construct. By this I mean that what it is to be a person, what components a person is said to have, vary among cultures and among places (Marsella et al, 1985). Personhood extends to include both the body, the physical self, and the psychologic self. Thus, cultures differ with regard to what constitutes acceptable or normative body types as well as modalities of psychologic patterns.

In American culture, there is a very strong sense of what is an acceptable body type and personality organization. Healthy, active, and young bodies are preferred; older bodies and those that show evidence of deformity or nonstandard range of form are less valued. An independent and self-motivated person is similarly valued; those who are said to be dependent or mentally ill are not valued. Valued types are said to be normative or preferred; unvalued types are said to be marginal or deviant.

Unfortunately, society marks those who are not standard, who do not measure up to the preferred or normative markers in body or psyche through the use of stigma. A *stigma* (Goffman, 1963) is a kind of social embarrassment, that is, shame, on the part of normative members of society when faced with someone who is not "normal"; someone with a stigmatized body identity, such as an obvious physical disability, wrinkling, deformity, and the like; one who uses a wheelchair or walker; one with a stigmatized social identity such as chronic mental illness; (Estroff, 1981;) or one who is different in any number of ways. Society polices itself through the use of stereotyping and stigma, suggesting that certain people are "worse than" others even to the point of being embarrassed over their presence or existence. Often persons with stigmatized identities are relegated to society's margins such as special health-care settings or districts of cities. They are often negatively labeled or blamed for their own misfortune (Cohen and Sokolovsky, 1989).

Those who represent the center of society often do not understand that, despite disabilities and social stigma, those who are marginalized or stigmatized often develop rich cultural lives of their own as members of communities or as individuals (Becker, 1980; Zola, 1982). In considering the lives of marginal or stigmatized persons, a number of factors are important. An important question is the origin of the standards that such people use to evaluate themselves. Standards that are developed for the normative context may not only be inappropriate for such individuals but they may also be developed in a milieu that actually devalues or even hates such persons. Thus, it may be more difficult for a person with a stigmatized social identity to exist as an individual without reference to standards and values developed by community members for their own lives. This is a question of empowerment and self-determination. People may gain self-esteem through resisting the standards of a society that devalues them, through ignoring such standards, or through developing some of their own. The anthropologist Frank described (1984) the life story of a "congenital amputee" called Diane DeVries. This informant's life story makes ample use of normative life-course markers such as "the normal cultural and developmental expectations of her age, gender and social background" (1984, p. 641). It also includes a number of references to the various institutional supports that have occurred in her life. Frank noted of her research that "an important finding is that this individual's own account of her life downplays her extensive medical history and that her encounters with stigma are reported in a way that highlights the positive image she holds of her body and its capabilities" (1984, p. 640).

The conflict between medical culture and assessment and personal culture and assessment is important. This, too, is taken up by Kaufman (1988). She contrasted the medical goal of implementing functional independence of a stroke victim with the world of personal goals. She noted, "To be sure, physicians' and therapists' goals are usually relevant and important to the patient, especially in the first few months following a stroke. However, as time passes, patients are ultimately engaged in a personal struggle for recovery. This goal is subjectively perceived and is not within the scope of physicians' or other providers' interventions or, indeed, frameworks of understanding" (1988, p. 85).

Kaufman described the case of a stroke victim, Mrs. Jones, who only succeeded partially toward the medical goal of functional independence. This goal, Kaufman noted, represents a medical ideology that is akin to the dominant American cultural ideology of autonomy, action, and the mastery of disease. It was clear that Mrs. Jones enjoyed the social aspects of the visits of physical and occupational therapists; however, she failed to comply with many of their behavioral requests. For much of her life, Mrs. Jones had in fact never subscribed to such an ideology. Mrs. Jones was labeled as "difficult" because she failed to demonstrate or share these values.

The Life Course

The aforementioned example suggests that behavioral patterns and key values often have an extensive history before a medical incident that turns a person into a client. Alternatively, in the case of those with chronic, long-term illnesses, values and behaviors have coevolved with such conditions.

It is important to note that social and cultural ideas on normative and proper behavior have a very strong influence on the nature of the values people hold, but it is not a simple equation. Such norms represent ideas on what people properly *should* do in life, that is, an idealized and often diffusely shared vision of the life course and the events that should happen therein. People who for whatever reason cannot or choose not to subscribe to these shared values nevertheless must deal with them either by turning their back on them or by creating individually or in a community adequate replacement values. They thus situationally interpret what is right for them.

Nevertheless, those who can be said to subscribe, in whatever sense, to normative social values also engage in an act of interpretation by creating personalized versions of normative ideas about the life course. Thus, for example, what is important to people is not only the normative image of marriage but also the particulars of their own marriage.

In one sense the most difficult problem for people is that of maintaining a sense of coherence or continuity over the life course in the face of normative life-course transitions, such as retirement or widowhood, as well as non-normative ones, such as sudden or chronic illness or disability. This problem is especially acute in American culture with its conflict between a focus on youth, autonomy, and an active orientation and the reality of limitations that occur through functional declines of illness or aging.

Two sorts of issues about stability and change in the life course are discussed here. They concern the mechanisms of coherence through the life course and aspects of reactivity to transition and change.

It appears that people build a sense of coherence through the establishment and management of a sense of identity. Often this sense of identity is constructed thematically; that is, through the use of certain key statements or ideas that summarize to oneself and to others who a person thinks he or she is (Kaufman, 1981 and 1988). We may hear such summarizations when, for example, people, often in an off-the-cuff manner, say such things as, "I'm the kind of person who . . . " These are public, self-conscious, narrative, reflexive statements that summarize what a person deems significant in presenting himself or herself to others.

In understanding reactivity to radical change in the life course, we encounter terms such as depression, control, normalcy, adjustment, and empowerment.

Depression represents a normal reaction to dramatic and deleterious changes in life. Although, of course, some people never seem to get depressed in reaction to such changes, most are challenged to build a new sense of self. This is a daunting task. Increasingly, evidence demonstrates that depression and other types of negative emotional reactions are not only indicators of incipient negative change in health status but also are indexes of commitment to a process of recovery and act as potential predictors of mortality. Mossey and colleagues, in their 12-month study of 196 older women who suffered a hip fracture, found that subjects who persistently reported few symptoms of depression were significantly more likely than those with high depression scores to walk again and to return to the level of prefracture abilities in many areas of physical functioning. They noted (1990, p. M163) that "these findings emphasize the importance of persistently elevated depressive symptoms for recovery."

The person's sense of control is implicated in radical change. For most people the ability to control one's own body has been unquestioned and unconscious before illness or injury. To oversimplify a complex area, psychologists suggested that by and large people exhibit an internal sense of control (i.e., they believe life is in their own hands) or an external sense of control (i.e., their fate is controlled by powerful others or by chance). In American culture, the internal sense of control is highly valued; we want to be masters of our own fate. The threat to self through the loss of control is profound. Those who have had control taken from them may eventually look for one small area over which they still have control to represent all that they had control over in the past, to be a marker of self-esteem and performance. These small areas are important to know and to honor. Adjustment to change and the relationship of such adjustment to control has received a great deal of attention (Kerson and Kerson, 1985; Moos, 1977; Pitzele, 1986; Register, 1987; Roth and Conrad, 1987; Strauss, 1984).

After radical change, over time eventually a new pattern of normalcy is attained. Such a pattern may be characterized as a lifestyle that revolves around regular features, exhibits set routines, and has a characteristic daily and weekly schedule and rhythm. Most important, such normalcy achieves a degree of comfort so that it seems natural; one does not think much about it, and time generally passes without too much stress.

Such a pattern of normalcy is established by the person at the nexus between his or her physical and mental capacities and the demands of the overall environment, both physical and social. In a model that primarily concerns the aged but that may certainly be extended to all people, Lawton (1980) noted that the interface between weak and strong environmental press, or demand, and low and high personal competence, or capacities and abilities, creates a number of possible performance zones. Thus, those who experience high competence and weak press or low competence and strong environmental press exhibit maladaptive behavior. In contrast, there is a zone of maximum comfort in which competence is matched with press. Slightly beyond this adaptational level is a zone of maximum performance potential in which the demands of the environment slightly exceed capacities at a given moment and in a way that requires slightly greater efforts toward competence on the part of the person.

Given a wide definition of environment as all that is external to the person, such a model provides a theoretic underpinning for rehabilitation of the person in that it graphically represents the gradual increase in competence accomplished through selective manipulation of the physical or social environment.

The degree that society, or any situation, is in charge or that clients are permitted to feel in charge of their life may be significant in recovery and in a sense of well-being. The term *empowerment* refers to the degree a person is permitted to take charge of and be a major determining factor in his or her own life in contrast to the extent that these are controlled by society or by a specific situation. For example, American society is now only emerging from a period in which persons with disabilities were not socially empowered, and such a posture eventuated in a variety of situational nonempowerments. This has had profound and subtle effects. Even a street curb that has not been made accessible for wheelchairs or a curb that has been transformed for a wheelchair but has been done so poorly and without concern for quality of work represents situational nonempowerment that is directly related to a climate of social nonempowerment. Similarly, feelings of being "less than" or "not sufficiently" internalized by some disabled are eventuated from the overall attitude of society. To a certain extent, however, individuals can provide their own sense of empowerment to overcome this.

The Environment

The last component of meaning making discussed here is the environment (see also Chapter 20). The environment may be thought of as the domain that surrounds the person, both physically and socially. Although the environment is itself external to the person and subject to the rules and ideation of collective culture, it also may be a fertile medium for the expression of individual identity. This is particularly so as the environmental aspect becomes closer to or a more intimate representation of the person. Thus, environmental domains such as the home or key objects within the home may take on meanings that represent key aspects of identity or in fact function to maintain key aspects of identity.

In a significant article, Rochberg-Halton (1984) described how cherished personal possessions act as signs or representations of the self over the life course. Such signs of the self may not only represent the self but may also act to express being, relationships, self-concepts, growth, change, and identity. Rubinstein (1987), in interviews of 88 senior adults about objects that were special to them, found the meaning of objects to be assigned to categories that represented relations with other people; the dialectic of giving and getting; objects that refer to the self; those that served as defenses against negative change and events; objects of care or generativity; objects that represent the past; and those that were prized for their affective or qualitative natures. It is interesting to note that the role of adaptive devices such as canes, walkers, or wheelchairs is now beginning to be studied in such a manner (Luborsky, in press), and it is likely that such objects should, like others, have significant personal meaning attached to them in some cases.

Meaning in the home environment has received greater study. This is very important to consider for health professionals who make home visits. There may be a great deal to learn about individuals from the way meaning seems to be projected into the home environment. At the very least, decoration such as photographs, memorabilia, and bric-a-brac offer an opportunity as points of entry into discussion of what is important to the client; at a more central level, such objects may deeply represent what the person feels about himself or herself or who the person considers himself or herself to be.

Although a number of processes that bind the person to place in the home environment have been described, two are especially important to health-care workers who deal with clients in home settings and are concerned with meaning. First, all people personalize their environments to a greater or lesser extent; however, some, who through diminished functioning or who are brought low in spirit, turn to the home environment as a most profound representation of self. This process of deep attachment to the home environment has been called *embodiment*, a process in which there is a degree of merging between the person and the environmental object such as the home. The home, as it were, becomes the person; the person feels incomplete without the home; the home affords a great deal of comfort and significance. Second, *environmental centralization* refers to the process of centralizing space in reaction to diminution of physical or cognitive functioning. With loss of abilities, people may now be able only to maintain less space or maintain themselves at a higher quality in a smaller space. Areas of the home may be shut off, or there may be trade-off in function, such as giving up certain aspects of cleaning the home or certain chores or activities, to muster more energy and time for tasks that are subjectively deemed more essential to being (Rubinstein, 1989).

In working at home with a client, the health-care practitioner can become aware of the personal meaning that is assigned to the objective environment. Such cues may be "read." If there is a disjunction between a person's sense of who he or she was and who he or she is now after injury or accident, these too may be accessed through the medium of environmental objects and feelings. A sense of reunification or renewed coherence between disjointed portions of a life course may also be represented through environmental objects.

CONCLUSION

In this chapter, I briefly reviewed five conceptual areas that provide frameworks for the affordance of personal or social meaning by clients. Although I have separated these for ease of description, in fact, these are inseparable and are mutually interdigitated. What underlies these conceptual areas are three deeper concerns that act to unify them. The first is the realm of personal meaning; that is, each person's "slant" on the world, what he or she sees as important, and how he or she interprets the world. The second is the life course; that is, what has gone on in the person's life before the present time and how previous key events may contribute to a present-day sense of well-being and self-worth.

The third concern is the world immediately around the person, both social and environmental. On whom can the client rely for help in living? What aspects of the environment offer affordances for well-being or act as barriers to it?

This chapter has provided some conceptual and technical contexts for evaluating these questions. Although looking, listening, and asking questions are good ways of coming to understand others, the provision of conceptual contexts may aid health-care professionals in organizing their thoughts and honing skills in this way.

In facing and addressing these concerns, health-care workers require access to the inside or experiential world of the client. This knowledge may be an important part of the treatment process, for how can one know which treatments or procedures are and will be efficacious unless one understands the specific contexts in which they will be experienced and used?

References

Al-Issa I: Culture and Psychopathology. Baltimore, MD, University Park Press, 1982.

Becker G: Growing Old in Silence. Berkeley, CA, University of California Press, 1980.

Berkman L: The relationship of social networks and social support to morbidity and mortality. *In* Cohen S and Syme S (eds): Social Support and Health. New York, Academic Press, 1985.

Breen M: Culture and schizophrenia: A study of Negro and Jewish schizophrenics. Int J Soc Psychiatry 14:282–289, 1968.

Brody H: Stories of Sickness. New Haven, CT, Yale University Press, 1987.

Cacciola E: Some aspects of working with Italian elderly. J Geriatr Psychiatry 15:197–208, 1982.

Chrisman N and Kleinman A: Health beliefs and practices among American ethnic groups. *In* Thernstrom S (ed): The Harvard Encyclopedia of American Ethnic Groups. Cambridge, MA, Harvard University Press, 1980.

Churchill C and Churchill S: Storytelling in medical arenas: The art of self-determination. Literature Med 1:73–79, 1982.

Clough L and Garland T: Ethnicity and Health: A Bibliography. Monticello, IL, Vance, 1979.

Cohen C and Sokolovsky J: Old Men of the Bowery: Strategies for Survival Among the Homeless. New York, Guilford, 1989.

Cohen S and Syme S: Social Support and Health. New York, Academic Press, 1985.

Cohler B and Grunebaum H: Mothers, Grandmothers and Daughters: Personality and Child Care in 3-Generation Families. New York, Wiley, 1981.

Croog S: Ethnic origins, educational level, and responses to a health questionnaire. Hum Organization 20:65–69, 1961.

Estroff S: Making It Crazy: An Ethnography of Psychiatric Clients in an American Community. Berkeley, CA, University of California Press, 1981.

Favazza A and Oman M: Anthropological and Cross-Cultural Themes in Mental Health: An Annotated Bibliography. Columbia, MO, University of Missouri Press, 1977.

Fisher S and Todd AD: The Social Organization of Doctor-Patient Communication. Washington, DC, Center for Applied Linguistics, 1983.

Frank G: Life history model of adaptation to disability: the case of a 'congenital amputee'. Soc Sci Med 19:639–645, 1984.

Geertz C: The Interpretation of Culture. New York, Basic Books, 1973.

Giordano J: Community mental health in a pluralistic society. Int J Ment Health 5:5–15, 1976a.

Giordano J: Group identity and mental health. Int J Ment Health 5:3–4, 1976b.

Giordano J: Introduction. Int J Ment Health 5:1–2, 1976c.

Goffman E: Stigma: Notes on the Management of Spoiled Identity. New York, Simon and Schuster, 1963.

Greeley A: Ethnic Drinking Subcultures. Brooklyn, NY, Bergin, 1979.

Illich I: Medical Nemesis: The Expropriation of Health. New York, Pantheon, 1976.

Johnsen P: Women as caregivers to the elderly: The filial imperative in anthropological perspective. Unpublished doctoral dissertation, Department of Anthropology, Bryn Mawr College, 1988.

Kalish R and Reynolds D: Death and Ethnicity: A Psychosocial Study. Los Angeles, Andrus Gerontology Center, University of Southern California, 1976.

Kaufman S: The cultural components of identity in old age: A case example. Ethos 9:51–87, 1981.

Kaufman S: Stroke rehabilitation and the negotiation of identity. In Reinharz S and Rowles, GD (eds): Qualitative Gerontology. New York, Springer, 1988.

Kerson T and Kerson L: Understanding Chronic Illness: The Medical and Psychosocial Dimensions of Nine Diseases. New York, The Free Press, 1985.

Kleinman A: The Illness Narratives: Suffering, Healing and the Human Condition. New York, Basic Books, 1988.

Kleinman A, Eisenberg L, and Good B: Culture, illness and care: Clinical lessons from anthropologic and cross-cultural research. Ann Intern Med 88:251–258, 1978.

Kluckhohn C: Mirror for Man; The Relationship of Anthropology to Modern Life. Tuscon, AZ, University of Arizona, 1985.

Lawton MP: Environment and Aging. Monterey, CA, Brooks/Cole, 1980.

Leighton A and Murphy J: Cross-cultural psychiatry. In Murphy J and Leighton A (eds): Approaches to Cross-Cultural Psychiatry. Ithaca, NY, Cornell University Press, 1965.

Lerion R: Ethnicity and mental health: An empirical obstacle course. Int J Ment Health 5:16–25, 1976.

Lerner J and Noy P: Somatic complaints in psychiatric disorders: Social and cultural factors. Int J Soc Psychiatry 14:145–150, 1968.

Luborsky M: Adaptive device appraisals by lifelong users facing new losses: Cultural, identity and life history factors. In Hey S and Kiger G (eds): New Perspectives in Disability Studies. Salem, OR, Willamette University, in press.

Markson E: Ethnicity as a factor in the institutionalization of the ethnic elderly. In Gelfand D and Kutzik A (eds): Ethnicity and Aging: Theory, Research and Policy. New York, Springer, 1979.

Marsella A, DeVos G, and Hsu FLK: Culture and Self: Asian and Western Perspectives. New York, Tavistock, 1985.

Martin E: The Woman in the Body. Boston, Beacon Press, 1987.

McGoldrick M, Pearce J, and Giordano J: Ethnicity and Family Therapy. New York, Guilford, 1982.

Mechanic D: Illness and cure. In Kosa J, Antonovsky A, and Zola I (eds): Poverty and Health: A Sociologic Analysis. Cambridge, MA, Harvard University Press, 1969.

Mischler E: The Discourse of Medicine: Dialectics of Medical Interviews. Norwood, NJ, Ablex, 1984.

Moos R: Coping with Physical Illness. New York, Plenum Press, 1977.

Moriwaki S: Ethnicity and aging. In Burnside I (ed): Nursing and Aging. New York, McGraw-Hill, 1976.

Mossey J, Knott K, and Craik R: The effects of persistent depressive symptoms on hip fracture recovery. J Gerontol: Med Sci 45:M163–M168, 1990.

Myerhoff B: Number Our Days. New York, Dutton, 1978.

Myers J, Wass H, and Murphy M: Ethnic differences in death anxiety among the elderly. Death Education 4:237–244, 1980.

Olukayode J: A study of the role of socio-cultural factors in the treatment of mental illness in Nigeria. Soc Sci Med 15A:49–54, 1981.

Parthun M: The incidence of mental illness among Italians in an English-Canadian city. In Grollig F and Haley H (eds): Medical Anthropology. The Hague, The Netherlands, Mouton, 1976.

Pitzele S: We Are Not Alone: Learning to Live with Chronic Illness. New York, Workman, 1986.

Raffel M: The U. S. Health Care System: Origins and Functions. New York, Wiley, 1989.

Register C: Living with Chronic Illness: Days of Patience and Passion. New York, The Free Press, 1987.

Rochberg-Halton E: Object relations, role models, and cultivation of the self. Environ Behav 16:335–368, 1984.

Roth J and Conrad P: The Experience and Management of Chronic Illness. Greenwich, CT, JAI Press, 1987.

Rubinstein R: The significance of personal objects to older people. J Aging Studies 1:225–238, 1987.

Rubinstein R: The home environments of older people: A description of the psychosocial processes linking person to place. J Gerontol: Soc Sci 44:S45–S53, 1989.

Smith D and Kaluzny A: The White Labyrinth: A Guide to the Health Care System. Ann Arbor, MI, Health Administration Press, 1986.

Snyder P: Ethnicity and folk healing in Honolulu, Hawaii. Soc Sci Med 15B:125–132, 1981.

Spiegel J: Some cultural aspects of transference and countertransference revisited. J Am Acad Psychoanal 4:447–467, 1976.

Stack C: All Our Kin: Strategies for Survival in a Black Community. New York, Harper & Row, 1974.

Starr P: The Social Transformation of American Medicine. New York, Basic Books, 1982.

Stivers R: Irish ethnicity and alcohol use. Med Anthropol 2:121–135, 1978.

Strauss A: Chronic Illness and the Quality of Life. St. Louis, C V Mosby, 1984.

Suchman E: Sociomedical variation among ethnic groups. Am J Sociol 70:328–329, 1964.

Winch R, Greer S, and Blumberg R: Ethnicity and extended

familism in an upper-middle class suburb. Am Sociological Rev 32:265–272, 1967.

Wylan L and Mintz N: Ethnic differences in family attitudes toward psychotic manifestations with implications for treatment programs. Int J Soc Psychiatry 22:86–95, 1976.

Zborowski M: People in Pain. San Francisco, Jossey Bass, 1969.

Zola I: Culture and symptoms: An analysis of patients' presenting complaints. Am Sociological Rev 31:615–630, 1966.

Zola I: Oh where, oh where has ethnicity gone? In Gelfand D and Kutzik A (eds): Ethnicity and Aging: Theory, Research and Policy. New York, Springer, 1979.

Zola I: Missing Pieces: A Chronicle of Living with a Disability. Philadelphia, Temple University Press, 1982.

CHAPTER
26

Katherine LeGuin White

Ethical Considerations in the Prevention and Rehabilitation of Injuries

Since the middle of the 19th century, Americans have professed and practiced concern for bodily fitness and participation in sports. Religious and patriotic ethics have structured many of the individual and team sports and games that American citizens have played during the past 150 years. Grover (1989), in her book *Fitness in American Culture: Images of Health, Sport and the Body, 1830–1940*, chronicled the growing popularity of sports for individuals and health professionals alike.

It is not mere pursuit of pleasure that motivates us to participate in sports. Indeed, athletes, whether professional or amateur, and health professionals who specialize in sports medicine may all be said to help create and advance a better society. Sanctions abound throughout popular culture and professional health care for achieving and maintaining health through active participation in sports and fitness programs.

Scientific medicine, technologic sophistication, increased leisure time, and commercial exploitation of the health promotion–illness prevention philosophy contributed significantly to the demand for allied health professionals to learn to work as effectively with amateur and professional athletes as they do with sick clients.

This chapter explores some ethical considera-tions that are important for allied health professionals who serve injured athletes and workers as well as those health professionals who help individuals pursue activities that promote health and prevent injury. First, a framework for raising ethical questions is discussed. That framework is then applied to the structure of therapeutic and collegial relationships as the forum for balance and interaction between scientific and humanistic issues in health care.

ETHICS

Most allied health professionals who work with rehabilitation and prevention of injury rarely confront life-threatening situations. Most of us usually deal with situations that can be described as happy or pleasant and not dangerous. However, behind the image of the rugged athlete or laborer, the beautiful young student, and the healthy octogenarian alike lurks the threat of annihilation or a sudden heart attack. This real but invisible human frailty often structures ethical issues and forces the questions we had rather leave unasked. Some ethical issues, on the other hand, beset us every day whether we are working with sick, injured, or healthy individuals or

429

pursuing our own health lifestyle: confidentiality, informed consent, and compliance for example.

All of us who profess to be experts in health care have a responsibility to frequently confront ourselves, our families, and our colleagues with questions that help us explore and refine our own and each other's frameworks for ethical living and practice. Here are some questions we can ask as we pursue that goal.

The first question is often not asked because we assume everyone knows the answer: "What is ethics?" Some people distinguish ethics from morals; some equate ethics with values or humanities. According to Veatch, a leading medical ethicist, "Ethics is the enterprise of disciplined reflection on the moral intuitions and moral choices that people make. Medical ethics is the analysis of choices in medicine" (Veatch, 1989, p. 2). Medical ethics, Veatch stated, is a matter of choices by physicians and other health professionals as well as clients, public officials, and family members; hence, the earlier admonition that we health professionals have the responsibility to articulate ethical questions and choices when talking with ourselves, our families, and our colleagues.

Framework for Exploring Ethical Questions

Another essential question for exploring ethical issues is, "What are my own thoughts, beliefs, and values about ethics in general and about a particular situation under exploration?" That question implies that we reflect on our feelings and relationships as well as on our thoughts. Sometimes we realize only in discussion with colleagues or with clients that we hold positive or negative views regarding a particular issue or question. It is also possible through discussion to realize that we harbor neutral feelings, have no beliefs about the question at hand, or attach no value to a specific choice. It is furthermore not infrequent that we consciously express strong beliefs and values without knowing what, if any, ethical tradition, code, or theory we may be embracing.

The following discussion is intended as an intellectual framework within which we can examine our own, our colleagues', and our family's articulated ethical choices. It is also a framework that can help us arrive at choices and articulate them. Although not an exhaustive framework, it

is a synthesis of the most commonly expressed and applied ethical theories used by participants in dilemmas that demand reflection on ethical issues in health care. All the theories can easily be applied to specific situations arising in the prevention and rehabilitation of injuries. These same theories can be applied equally well to the more commonly known, dramatic issues such as human experimentation, organ transplantation, or withdrawal of life support.

Existentialists tell us that humans always have a choice; they also say that choice structures freedom. Postmodernists tell us that we live in an age characterized by differences and diversity. Pursuit of ethical questions exemplifies both existential and postmodern qualities: We explore choices when we examine ethical questions; through those choices we are confronted quickly with the facts that there are many different ways to look at the questions and that our own point of view may differ from that of our colleagues, clients, and families.

The most commonly applied theories of ethical analysis express normative principles such as justice, goodness, fairness, duties, or obligations. Two theoretic constructs traditionally invoked in the structure of medical ethics questions are utilitarian, or consideration of the good to be achieved by an action, and deontologic, or study of the obligations expressed by rules and actions. These latter theories are usually more precisely called rule-deontology or act-deontology theories. More recently, some ethicists began to advocate virtue theories as the basis for raising and answering questions of medical ethics. Virtue theories examine qualities such as compassion and honesty of the person who is making a moral decision. The following discussion defines these commonly applied ethical theories using examples from situations in the prevention and rehabilitation of injuries.

Deontologic Theories

A discussion of deontologic theories is a good way to elucidate the assertion by postmodernists that our contemporary world is characterized by differences and diversity. Daily newspapers as well as daily clinical practice with injury prevention and rehabilitation provide us with numerous examples of the vastness of diversity expressed in our present world. Proponents of deontologic theories also differ among themselves about what constitutes the theory and which choices are properly articulated by so-called deontologic analyses of issues and dilemmas. Any discussion of ethics in health care, therefore, must be prefaced by an admonition to avoid oversimplification and creation of the impression that all ethicists who espouse a particular theory share a common philosophic framework or emphasis.

Indeed, Frankena (1973) instructed us in deontologic theory within the context of diversity, difference, and even conflict among moral philosophers who profess to be deontologists. In his book *Ethics*, Frankena distinguished act deontologists from rule deontologists. Act deontologists, he stated, assert that we should look at the situation itself, free from any appeal to or application of rules such as "We should always keep our promises." Rule deontologists, alternatively, insist that there are rules, independent of situations, that serve as standards for moral choices and judgments (Frankena, 1973, pp. 16–17).

Act-Deontologic Theories

As this title states, many theories may be called deontologic, even among the group of people who call themselves deontologists. While spelling out the points on which there is disagreement among philosophers who espouse the same general theoretic framework, Frankena (1973) was careful to show us how those very differences can enhance our reasoning about ethical issues. The diversity of premises, conclusions, questions, and answers generated by ethical issues and theoretic frameworks requires us to reflect often and seriously on our own responses when we deliberate over ethical choices. That same vastness of difference requires us to tolerate and respect views and values of our clients and colleagues whose ethical premises or choices may be antithetical to ours. In so doing, we may all grope together toward the truth or goodness that eludes us when we work alone.

If we can honestly generalize from Frankena's discussion of act-deontologic theories, we may say the following about those theories as an ethical framework. The term *situation ethics* that we heard so frequently in the 1960s and 1970s is one way of describing act-deontologic theories. Situations themselves, not rules or religious imperatives, supply answers to the questions raised by ethical dilemmas or situations that confront us.

Decisions are generated out of deliberations over the complexity of situations. It is possible that general rules may be built up over time as we examine many specific situations that raise the same issues. Those general rules, however, never supersede the situation itself. In other words, for act deontologists, the supreme, universal ground for decision making is the situation and its obligations. The reasoning and judgment derived from critical examination of a particular situation's obligations establish the rationale for one's ethical behavior.

The most commonly used method for examination of ethical issues in health care is casuistry, or the study of specific cases. We use the same approach to teach our students technical and professional problem solving. We also use the case-study approach when we determine a client's fitness or rehabilitation program. We may venture to say therefore that allied health professionals implicitly give credence and high value to act deontology as a theoretical framework for clinical decision making.

Allied health professionals often assert that we honor and serve our clients' individuality and uniqueness. Because act-deontologic theories also afford primacy to the uniqueness of the obligations of an individual situation, it is little wonder that we seem to favor this ethical stance for most of our educational and clinical problem solving. Because it accepts and glorifies the differences among situations, act deontology may be the ethical theory of choice for allied health professionals in the postmodern culture.

Yesterday's choices may be forgotten or irrelevant when we face the dilemmas of today. The conclusions we reached in one case or situation may not be reached in a similar case simply because of the finite differences in the situations. To those who are not act deontologists, such lack of sameness could be judged inconsistent, perhaps even indecisive or unreliable. The tension thus generated by this difference of viewpoint could create conflict that is difficult to resolve. Awareness that we and our colleagues may be acting on incompatible implicit ethical theoretic frameworks should help us tolerate and work to resolve those kinds of conflict. That same awareness can also help us structure questions and communicative encounters that result in resolution of apparent conflict.

Rule-Deontologic Theories

Rule-deontologic theories are more comforting and have more utility for those among us who prefer to stand on principles and standards when participating in ethical decision making. As their name implies, rule deontologists generally derive their choices from rules rather than from situations; in this regard, they are a contrast to their colleagues who espouse act-deontologic theories.

Frankena (1973) stated that rule-deontologic theories are built on principles that are valid regardless of whether they promote good. He also indicated that those principles show us how to act in all situations that are the same or similar. Rules such as "We should always tell the truth," "We should always do what the occupational therapist tells us to do," or "The doctor knows best" are the kinds of principles by which rule-deontology theorists make their ethical choices in clinical situations (Frankena, 1973, p. 25).

However, Frankena also pointed out some things we all know: There may be exceptions to any rule and there may be times when a heretofore unapplied rule supersedes a previously honored rule. For example, there may be a good reason not to tell the truth, to refuse to follow the doctor's advice, or to fail to do what the occupational therapist tells us to do. In abandoning any of those principles, however, the rule deontologist will replace it with a rule thought to be more pertinent for the situation under discussion.

In summary, the two kinds of deontologic theories are distinguished by whether the situation or the law is given primacy. Act deontology gives precedence to the situation and focuses its decision making on examination of the specific facts and obligations of the situation. In rule deontology, a principle that exists a priori is applied to a situation to achieve an ethical decision.

Virtue Theories

For those of us who dislike rules and lean toward the existentialists, virtue theories give us a way to explore ourselves as moral agents. The emphasis here is on being rather than on doing. That is, virtue theories focus on the virtue of the persons involved in the decision making. Virtue theorists do not examine deeds, rules, situations, outcomes, or consequences; instead, they examine the integrity, compassion, and honesty of the moral agent, the person making the decision (Veatch, 1989, p. 44). As with the utilitarians and the deontologists, the ethicists who are propo-

nents of virtue theory by no means speak with one voice; they also differ among themselves.

Virtue theorists emphasize two major premises according to Veatch in his book *Medical Ethics*. Some insist that "a virtuous professional can *discern* the right course of action in the situation without reliance on principles and rules." Others assert "that a virtuous person will *desire* to do what is right and avoid what is wrong" (Veatch, 1989, p. 44).

What, then, are virtues, and how are they expressed or lived by the virtuous health professional? The American Heritage Dictionary (1985) defined virtue as goodness or righteousness. Aristotle defined virtue as excellence and told us that virtue is that "state of character which makes a man good and which makes him do his own work well" (Aristotle, in McKeon, 1947, p. 338). Examples of virtues are service, courage, charity or benevolence, integrity, truthfulness, and sympathy.

Brody (1989), in his discussion of virtue theories, indicated that there are no clear answers to the questions such as "What would a virtuous health professional do?" or "What kind of character should a virtuous health professional have?" There are also the matters of an individual's motivation to do what is right and the need for principles as well as virtues to validate ethical decisions and inform effective therapeutic relationships (Veatch, 1989, p. 77).

Further questions are raised when we ponder virtue as a theoretic basis for ethical decision making. The cultivation and reward of virtue in a world dominated by scientific methods and beliefs are difficult at best. Competition among virtues for the guiding force in problem solving can also make it difficult for us to serve one or another chosen virtue. Furthermore, if virtue is an expression of goodness or righteousness, we must surely be concerned with the lifetime of an individual health professional or client instead of his or her reasoning and behavior in a specific situation. Finally, the complexity of virtue-theory reasoning is enhanced when that moral stance is juxtaposed with utilitarian or deontologic viewpoints during attempts to resolve moral dilemmas or make ethical decisions about client care.

There is nothing clear-cut or easy about raising and answering ethical questions. None of the theoretic positions alone is sufficient in most cases for good and equitable decision making. Great tolerance and forbearance are called for in each of us whenever we participate in ethical dilemmas or discuss ethical situations. Furthermore, our own lack of clarity—either cognitive or affective—about which viewpoint we favor heightens the complexity of trying to resolve ethical issues.

All this is not to dissuade us from facing, exploring, and deciding the questions as they present themselves to us in our practice of allied health professions. Rather, it is intended to elucidate the complexity and magnitude of the task. Understanding this one point alone could help us become more responsible and mature and more responsive to ethical issues we face daily in our work with sick and well individuals, institutional managers and policies, and the sociopolitical world we inhabit.

APPLICATION OF ETHICAL THEORIES: AN INJURY-REHABILITATION SITUATION

Mr. Ecks is a 50-year-old skilled laborer employed in a processing factory. Three months ago he sustained injuries on the job that required extensive, comprehensive rehabilitation. He responded well to short-term inpatient rehabilitation and is now receiving outpatient rehabilitation 3 times a week. The rehabilitation team estimates that Mr. Ecks will need at least 1 more month of comprehensive rehabilitation services before he is able to work again. The cost of those services is estimated at $2,000. Without completion of the course of rehabilitation, Mr. Ecks will suffer permanent loss of mobility, independence in activities of daily living, and the ability to engage in remunerative work.

Two weeks ago, the processing plant where Mr. Ecks was employed was destroyed by fire. He received notice today that the plant will not be rebuilt and that all his health-care benefits will be terminated 2 weeks from today. Mr. Ecks kept his appointment today for outpatient therapy; he asks your help in finding a way he can continue his outpatient rehabilitation and prepare for work similar to what he was doing at the time of his injury.

DISCUSSION

Utilitarians would approach the discussion of Mr. Ecks' situation by asking the question, "What is the greatest good to be accomplished?" The

search for answers would lead a utilitarian to identify carefully what good could be achieved by following two or more courses of action. To whom and for whom the good would be accomplished also have to be specified and balanced. Cost-benefit ratios need to be posited; and some consideration has to be given to the negative side of that ratio. That is, the consequences of both the most costly and least beneficial courses of action also require deliberation.

For the purpose of discussion, one could take the stand that the questions that need to be asked are more important than the answers. As we stated earlier, individuals who participate in ethical decision making need to clarify early for themselves what their dominant ethical stance is going to be in any specific situation. That is, one needs first to decide whether the applied theoretic approach is going to be utilitarian, deontologic, virtue, or some combination. Beyond that individual choice, every participant must be mindful of the range of theoretic approaches available to help decide the course of action to be taken. Finally, each person involved in the decision making needs to be tolerant of the diversity of theories applied, the ethical choice that prevails, and the conclusions reached.

It can be instructive, as an alternative to the stance that struggles with asking the right questions, to assume the role of iconoclastic utilitarian. In that position, we rigorously apply the test of what constitutes the greater good in this situation. Lacking the luxury that face-to-face communication allows, I arbitrarily pursue the latter alternative in the interest of elucidating the utilitarian point of view.

First, consider the context: the injured individual, his family, the processing plant within the community, the hospital where the client's rehabilitation has been in progress, and you, the therapist who is a member of the team working to rehabilitate Mr. Ecks. A determination of the greatest good in this situation therefore means deciding on and comparing the benefits to the community from continuing Mr. Ecks' rehabilitation even though the cost may not be reimbursed or he may have to pay for it directly himself against the benefits to the client, the community, and the hospital arising from the termination of services to Mr. Ecks before he has reached the desired state of rehabilitation.

Questions such as who pays for Mr. Ecks' care or whether he can find other employment are of secondary concern to the iconoclast. The ethical decision in this case is made by concentrating on answering only this question: Is the greatest good to be accomplished by terminating Mr. Ecks' rehabilitation when his health-care benefits terminate?

Clearly, the greatest good would be accomplished if Mr. Ecks completed his rehabilitation, thus rendering him once again a productive member of society, a self-sufficient and independent man. Not continuing his rehabilitation, while saving the hospital from possible financial loss because of nonpayment or delayed payment, would mean that Mr. Ecks could not work for a living and therefore he would have to be supported by family or community resources for a probable 30 to 40 years.

Because the utilitarian point of view fails to consider situational complexities and exigencies, its value may be minimal and easily dismissed as being impractical. Critics could say that utilitarians ignore important considerations such as how is Mr. Ecks' care going to be paid for, can Mr. Ecks be retrained for a new job in another industry, and would he need to relocate to find work.

Therapists who treat injured workers would want to explore alternatives to their 3 days a week outpatient rehabilitation program. Can Mr. Ecks achieve the same goals through a home program with minimal outpatient sessions? Has he made sufficient progress so far to reasonably expect that he will be employable after 1 more month of therapy? Can the care be provided without concern for payment or for payment after Mr. Ecks has returned to work? Are the therapists willing to work with Mr. Ecks, his physician, and the hospital administrator to develop alternative treatment and payment options? How much flexibility do the hospital and local health-care system allow for structuring treatment options for Mr. Ecks? Assuming that there are other treatment facilities where Mr. Ecks can receive his outpatient therapy, are those facilities accessible to him?

Although the question of the accomplishment of the greatest good is both valid and important, it seems simplistic to ask only that one question when trying to reach ethical decisions in situations of injury rehabilitation such as that faced by Mr. Ecks. Deontologic theories seem to offer us more help and a more pragmatic and less abstract rationale for ethical decision making in Mr. Ecks' situation.

Application of rule- and act-deontologic theo-

ries open up many of the questions that the utilitarians fail to consider. Some of those questions are now discussed and answers that deontologists might formulate explored.

To begin with, rule deontologists determine what ethical principle would appropriately be applied to Mr. Ecks' situation. One possibly pertinent principle is that we should do unto others as we would have them do unto us. Another applicable principle is that we should provide the necessary care regardless of its cost or who pays for it. In other words, health care is a right. A third possible yardstick is the principle of autonomy (i.e., the client's right to make his own decisions, live his life as he sees fit). Finally, the rules of justice or informed consent may be invoked in deciding what to do in Mr. Ecks' case.

All persons who participate in rule-deontologic decision making about continuing Mr. Ecks' rehabilitation need to clarify the grounds on which they select an applicable principle. That alone can be difficult, controversial, and ridden with conflict. As stated, at least five moral principles may be pertinent for Mr. Ecks' situation: the "golden rule," the right to health care, autonomy, justice, and informed consent. Assume that it is clear to you that justice is the principle with the most pertinence for Mr. Ecks. All other participants, including Mr. Ecks himself, may feel equally committed to different principles. Resolving this conflict could be the most important contribution you could make toward helping Mr. Ecks.

To participate in ethical conflict resolution, one would need to be informed about the range of ethical theories, to be tolerant of all views being expressed, and to be skilled in achieving compromise and agreement essential for development of a concrete action plan. It could be especially difficult to participate constructively in ethical conflict resolution if one harbored negative feelings about Mr. Ecks, the processing plant where he used to work, the hospital administration, or a colleague involved in the decision making.

To proceed with the application of rule-deontology theory in assessing Mr. Ecks' situation, we need next to follow through the rule that we have judged to be most pertinent for his situation. Let us start with the principle of justice. What, then, does justice require us to question, to choose, to do?

Justice would be done for Mr. Ecks when he

is restored to his preinjury or normal state of health and occupational productivity. In other words, when Mr. Ecks is fully rehabilitated, justice will be served. For that to happen, his employer needs to fulfill his obligation to provide health care sufficient to return Mr. Ecks to his usual independent and productive self. In this case the possibility of justice is severely compromised because the processing plant has been destroyed by fire and will not be rebuilt; therefore, Mr. Ecks could not return to his preinjury employment even if he were rehabilitated. Furthermore, the threatened termination of payment for rehabilitation services before his completion of the projected necessary course of treatments also renders justice an unlikely outcome in Mr. Ecks' situation.

If we are committed to the principle of justice, we are then required to advocate for Mr. Ecks' continued rehabilitation through dialogue with his employer, the employer's insurance carrier, and Mr. Ecks. Legal counsel and services may also be required to bring about justice for Mr. Ecks.

Whereas rule deontologists turn to principles that may establish the rightness or wrongness of choice of action, act deontologists examine the acts themselves when elucidating ethical choices. In the case of Mr. Ecks, act deontologists would want to know what is the right thing to do: Should his care be continued as it is presently structured in order to be judged as the right action, or could the right choice be either to terminate his rehabilitation in 2 weeks or structure an alternative plan of rehabilitation?

From the point of view of the therapists, the right thing to do probably is to persist in the rehabilitation plan agreed on at the time Mr. Ecks began his therapy. That is probably also the choice that Mr. Ecks himself would select as being the right one for him. Representatives of the hospital, processing plant, and insurance carrier, on the other hand, are likely to have very different views of what constitutes the right action.

Representatives of the processing plant, faced with rehabilitating an injured worker on the one hand and closing a business that was accidentally destroyed on the other hand, bring a dimension to the dilemma that neither the therapist nor Mr. Ecks could be expected to share. That dimension is the corporate entity. Consequently, conflict is brewing. Two persons in the situation—the therapist and Mr. Ecks—have individual perspec-

tives; the processing plant representative has the business as his or her perspective. Without the input of any other persons, such as physicians, family members of Mr. Ecks, or health insurance staff, there are two potentially opposing values that are being applied to determine the rightness or wrongness of a choice.

Because the processing plant spokesperson is concerned primarily with closing out a business, the right thing for him or her at this time may be determined more by loyalty to the corporation than by compassion for an injured employee.

The hospital administrator, in a similar manner to the processing plant representative, must balance organizational and individual imperatives when deciding what he or she thinks is the right thing to do in this situation. Like the hospital administrator and the processing plant spokesperson, therapists who own private practices are in the position of having to balance organizational and individual values and concerns when they struggle with trying to determine the right thing to do in a case such as Mr. Ecks'. There are no clear-cut answers for any of these corporate representatives.

Finally, there is the insurance carrier, which is also a participant in this ethical dilemma. What constitutes rightness of an act or choice for the carrier? Chances are that legalistic and monetary concerns will influence the carrier's decision about the right thing to do for Mr. Ecks. They may offer him the option of continuing his health insurance coverage as an individual, privately paying policyholder. They may also refuse to pay for any rehabilitation services rendered after 2 weeks, the time at which the processing plant will cease to be an active enterprise that accepts responsibility toward its employees.

It could easily be true that the right thing for the insurance carrier to do is to offer Mr. Ecks the option of continuing his insurance as an individual policyholder. If we agree on the rightness of this choice, we would then have to say that it is ethically wrong for the insurance company to cancel Mr. Ecks' coverage altogether in 2 weeks.

A middle ground for the insurance company might be to explore the options with another source of funding for health care such as worker's compensation or shift him to a governmental program designed to provide care for indigent or medically indigent persons. The greatest concern in this case could be continuity of care, assuming that 2 weeks is not enough time to negotiate coverage by any alternative source.

However, the insurance company could say that their obligation to all the policyholders, not just to Mr. Ecks, is the basis on which their decision has to be made. The risk of financial loss from payment for approximately 2 weeks of care or $1,000 may seem a small amount to the outside observer. At the corporate level, this kind of loss could be multiplied a thousand times during the year and therefore result in large-scale financial loss for the company. This kind of logic could easily result in the insurance company deciding that the right action is refusal to pay for Mr. Ecks' rehabilitation beyond the date of the processing plant's official closing, which is 2 weeks from now.

Once again the complexity of ethical dilemmas is elucidated. The difficulty any one participant in the situation faces is compounded by the fact that there are always multiple actors, multiple points of view, and numerous ethical positions to be reckoned with. The need for conflict resolution and tolerance is apparent every step of the way when any one of us is involved in an ethical decision-making process; and process it is! All these kinds of situations are difficult, trying, and time consuming but also challenging and rewarding despite the dissonance and diversity that attend the process.

By consciously facing the ethical dilemmas that confront all of us in everyday practice, we are forced to become increasingly self-reflective and self-critical; we are forced also to become mindful of the diversity of points of view, the value of learning to participate effectively in the project that Veatch (1989) characterized as an "enterprise." Our hope, and our belief, is that active involvement in the fullness of the enterprise helps us cultivate virtues that honor the highest ideals of our professions and of personal maturity.

Assuming that we have undertaken the challenge of becoming virtuous persons, how then would we react to Mr. Ecks' situation? Virtue theorists tell us first that we will be concerned with ourselves as virtuous therapists when we respond to the question Mr. Ecks put to us. Our actions will be "right if they express virtue, wrong if they express vice" (Veatch, 1989, p. 31). Virtuous therapists will therefore be able to know, perhaps intuitively, what the right action is regardless of rules or principles. Furthermore, virtuous therapists wish to do the right thing and avoid doing the wrong thing (Veatch, 1989,

p. 44). How they do things is as important as what they do.

What then will the virtuous physical or occupational therapist do? How does the virtuous person know what is right? What happens when two virtuous people judge the same situation according to different virtues? What does it mean to be virtuous? Is one person's virtue another's vice?

There seems to be tacit agreement among many medical ethicists that virtues are ideals that define and structure our behavior. Service is often thought of as a virtue; honesty is another. Charity as well as selflessness and compassion are qualities that may be described as virtues. Becoming a virtuous person can be a lifelong project. Ethical dilemmas provide us with good opportunities to both cultivate and express virtues.

In the case of Mr. Ecks, a virtuous therapist is less likely to be concerned about the issue of payment of his or her services and more likely to be interested in Mr. Ecks, the sick person, his dignity and autonomy.

Furthermore, the virtuous therapist is quite likely to have a strong commitment to working collegially with other health-care providers, Mr. Ecks and his family, the spokesperson for the processing plant where he worked, and the insurance carrier. The virtuous therapist is concerned about his or her interactions with all the people in the situation, with honoring the humanity of all the participants, including the therapist, and with how to balance often conflicting ideals such as autonomy, beneficence, and fairness with professional competence and integrity. One of the reasons the virtuous therapist cultivates and nurtures networks with all these people is to honor the dignity of Mr. Ecks and all other clients. Being a virtuous health professional can be an awesome responsibility and an arduous task.

Virtue is easiest in close and long-lasting relationships, such as that of Mr. Ecks and the rehabilitation team who have been working with him for several months. In situations of short-term treatment or when the client is not cognitively competent to participate in his or her welfare (e.g., a comatose patient), virtue as an ethical premise for structuring a therapeutic relationship is hardly a viable choice. In those cases, one must rely on principles or rules such as primacy of professional judgment or professional autonomy and doing good while avoiding harm.

RELATIONSHIPS WITH CLIENTS AND COLLEAGUES

Implicit throughout the previous discussion and application of ethical theories in health care is the matter of therapeutic relationships. Especially during the exploration of how a virtuous therapist would behave in Mr. Ecks' situation, it became apparent that we cannot discuss the enterprise of health-care ethics without considerable attention to the relationships between therapist and client and therapist and other members of the health-care team.

Since the 1970s, an impressive literature on therapeutic relationships has been compiled by medical ethicists and physicians. As the allied health professions grow in stature within the health-care arena, we are well advised to focus more attention on the ethical bases of our therapeutic relationships and our relationships with colleagues. There are some valid reasons why we should do more than attempt to extrapolate from the literature about client-physician relationships those concepts and concerns that may be pertinent also for allied health professionals.

One basic difference between allied health professionals and physicians is professional autonomy. Another difference is the lack of scientific validity for many of the treatments and techniques used by allied health professionals. It is beyond the scope of this chapter or this book to explore these differences in depth. However, we can begin to ask pertinent questions and to search for answers that can help elucidate the differing ethical imperatives for allied health professionals and physicians. This search can also be useful in helping us structure our profession's ethical traditions, test the premises on which we are presently making our ethical judgments, and contribute to the evaluation of newer medical specialties such as sports medicine and ergonomics. The broader projects of prevention and rehabilitation of injuries can also be enhanced by our efforts to clarify, refine, and validate our ethical choices and participation in this postmodern world.

A publication by Davis (1989) can be immensely helpful to allied health professionals who wish to participate in this project of structuring ethical therapeutic and collegial relation-

ships among those of us who are engaged in the prevention and rehabilitation of injuries. Davis (1989) provided many helpful questions and exercises designed to guide allied health practitioners in their quest for growth as healing professionals. Her methods are focused on individual maturity through enhancement of self-awareness, values clarification, and refinement of assertiveness and communication skills.

In a chapter on ethical dilemmas, Davis emphasized many of the same issues raised by Veatch and other ethicists in Veatch's *Medical Ethics*. Davis is a physical therapist and an allied health educator. The fact that both medical ethicists and allied health ethicists sometimes raise the same issues and ask the same questions in trying to resolve ethical dilemmas points to the universality of ethical principles and moral imperatives such as truth telling, confidentiality, and client and therapist autonomy. Major differences between medical ethicists and allied health ethicists like Davis in their approaches to ethical concepts are their process and methodology.

Medical ethicists tend to concentrate on explication and application of ethical theories through case studies or casuistry. Allied health ethicists, on the other hand, tend to concentrate on methods of individual professional growth and the process by which individual health professionals seek answers to moral dilemmas and how one participates in ethical decision making. Medical ethicists may be said to focus more often on the situation, whereas allied health ethicists focus on how to become a mature and responsible moral agent. Having said that, however, we are reminded that medical ethicists who profess to honor virtue theories share with the allied health professionals a primary concern for the individual decision maker. The development of a virtuous health professional can be, therefore, a value shared by medical and allied health ethicists.

Davis advocated the use of contextualism in helping individual therapists resolve ethical dilemmas (Davis, 1989, pp. 123, 126). Contextualism, according to Davis, is a method of resolving ethical dilemmas in which "the context of the situation provides the key information in deciding the right thing to do *in that situation*" (Davis, 1989, p. 126). She relied heavily on the work of development psychologists Lawrence Kohlberg, Jean Piaget, and Carol Gilligan to help her structure exercises designed to help therapists clarify their values in preparation for ethical decision making.

What Davis called contextualism, medical ethicists would call act deontology. Although casuistry is a method commonly used by both medical and allied health ethicists, the latter concentrate more heavily on the values clarification, the sophistication of moral reasoning, and communication skills of the individual health professional. In other words, allied health professionals may be said to emphasize more strongly how they make decisions than physicians and medical ethicists.

If that is a true and fair distinction to make, does it mean that physical and occupational therapists are more likely to be virtuous health professionals than physicians? This is not necessarily the case. However, this preference for individual virtue over rules or consequences may reflect the fact that historically and politically the traditions of allied health professions have been shaped by women.

Allied health professionals can learn to become responsible, mature moral agents as we work to prevent and rehabilitate athletic, vehicular, or industrial injuries. Physical and occupational therapy literature offers rich collections for consultation on psychosocial issues and values in the practice of our professions. Undertaking a project of individual professional maturity through pragmatic self-reflection, values clarification, and refinement of communication skills can produce many rewards. First, it can help us become more virtuous people and practitioners. That achievement then can manifest itself every day in our relationships with clients and colleagues alike.

Virtues carry with them responsibilities, such as the willingness to make difficult choices and to tolerate differences of opinion or advocacy of moral imperatives and the will to work hard and long to develop and refine our personal integrity and professional competence.

SUMMARY AND CONCLUSIONS

This chapter has studied ethical considerations for allied health professionals who work to prevent and rehabilitate injuries. An overview of ethical theories commonly invoked to solve dilemmas in medical and health-care situations has focused on discussion of deontologic and virtue theories. Application of rule- and act-deontologic and virtue theories to a clinical situation involving rehabilitation of an injured worker elucidated the complexity and difficulty of resolving ethical dilemmas or making ethical choices.

Preference was expressed for virtue theory as the framework for ethical decision making in allied health practice and for fostering maturity and integrity in individual practitioners. However, rights and responsibilities, rules and situations, as well as virtuous practitioners must also be taken into account. Tolerance of the diversity of theoretic frameworks, individual moral preferences, and choices interacting in any specific situation or dilemma has been urged. Finally, the process of becoming a virtuous health professional through lifelong growth and study as advocated by Davis was supported.

Professional codes of ethics need to be discussed. Both the American Occupational Therapy Association and the American Physical Therapy Association publish and periodically revise codes of ethics for their members as do medical, nursing, and other professional organizations. Ethicists acknowledge these codes but usually speak in reserved tones when discussing them as frameworks or guidelines for clinical ethical decision making among health professionals.

If one applies rigorously the ethical framework outlined in this chapter, we find limited expressions of deontologic, utilitarian, or virtue concepts in the occupational therapy code of ethics (American Occupational Therapy Association, 1988) and in the American Physical Therapy Association (1987) code of ethics for physical therapists who are members of the association. Both of these codes mention concepts such as confidentiality, honesty, justice, and clients' rights. However, neither code offers us much help as we participate in ethical decision making for Mr. Ecks or for most of the real-life client-care situations faced daily by occupational and physical therapists. Furthermore, all health-care professionals, whether or not they are members of a professional organization, are faced with these situations and the necessity for making choices and taking responsibility for their actions.

All of us who are clinicians, educators, or researchers practice in a world that confronts us daily with choices, conflict, and diversity of opinions and ethical premises. To function maturely in this world, we need to remind ourselves of the wisdom expressed in the introduction to this chapter: Ethics is an *enterprise* (Veatch, 1989, p. 2) that requires the active participation of all of us who are involved in the prevention and rehabilitation of injuries. The admonition to embrace that enterprise, along with our commitment to therapeutic competence and efficacy, requires us to raise ethical questions within and among ourselves. We are furthermore challenged to question and refine our choices and responses to those questions and to be tolerant of the multitude of possible choices and decisions.

References

American Heritage Dictionary, 2nd college ed. Boston, Houghton Mifflin, 1985.

American Occupational Therapy Association: Occupational therapy code of ethics. Am J Occup Ther 42(12):795–796, 1988.

American Physical Therapy Association: Guide for Professional Conduct and Code of Ethics. Alexandria, VA, American Physical Therapy Association, 1987.

Aristotle: Ethica nicomanchea. In McKeon R (ed): Introduction to Aristotle. New York, Random House, 1947.

Brody H: The physician/patient relationship. In Veatch RM (ed): Medical Ethics. Boston, Jones & Bartlett, 1989.

Davis CM: Patient Practitioner Interaction: An Experimental Manual for Developing the Art of Health Care. Thorofare, NJ, Slack, 1989.

Frankena WK: Ethics, 2nd ed. Englewood Cliffs, NJ, Prentice-Hall, 1973.

Grover K (ed): Fitness in American Culture: Images of Health, Sport and the Body, 1830–1940. Amherst, University of Massachusetts Press, 1989.

Veatch RM (ed): Medical Ethics. Boston, Jones & Bartlett, 1989.

Bibliography

Bartlett EE: Patient education can lower costs, improve quality. Hospitals 63(21):88, 1989.

Burgess M: Ethical and economic aspects of noncompliance and overtreatment. Can Med Assoc J 141(8):777–780, 1989.

Canquilhem G: The Normal and the Pathological. (Fawcett CR and Cohen RS [trans]). New York, Zone Books, 1989.

Coy JA: Autonomy-based informed consent: Ethical implications for patient noncompliance. Phys Ther 69(10):826–833, 1989.

Doak CC, Doak LG, and Root JH: Teaching Patients with Low Literacy Skills. Philadelphia, JB Lippincott, 1985.

Faden RR and Beauchanys TL: A History and Theory of Informed Consent. New York, Oxford University Press, 1986.

May WF: Code and covenant or philanthropy and contract. Hastings Cent Rep 5(6):29–38, 1975.

Peck CL and King NJ: Compliance and the doctor-patient relationship. Drugs 30:78–84, 1985.

Veatch RM: Models for ethical medicine in a revolutionary age. Hastings Cent Rep 2(3):5–7, 1972.

C H A P T E R
27
Jeffrey Rothman

Problem-Solving Approach to Health and Wellness: An Educational Model

The purpose of this chapter is to describe a curriculum approach that prepares therapists and health professionals to plan and implement programs of health promotion and disease prevention.

Healthy People 2000 (U.S. Department of Health and Human Services, Office of Disease Prevention and Health Promotion [USDHHS-ODPHP], 1990) set new objectives to promote health and prevent disease for the nation over the next decade. The successful attainment of these goals by the year 2000 will depend on the training of health professionals to implement these objectives. The National Council for the Education of Health Professions in Health Promotion, when testifying before the Committee on Health Objectives for the Year 2000, suggested that:

> Students of medicine, nursing, dentistry, and the allied health professions be adequately prepared to intervene effectively with those patients at risk and to organize health promotion/disease prevention services. Therefore, those responsible for the education, training, and certification of health professions must develop goals and objectives to assure that health promotion and disease prevention become an integral part of the repertoire of skills of those charged with the responsibility of providing health care. (USDHHS-ODPHP, 1990, p. 78)

Only recently have medical and allied health curricula begun to incorporate the concepts of health promotion and disease prevention into their educational programs and prepare students to play a role in this area. This process has been delayed because of several factors:

1. The strong influence of the medical model and the disease orientation of health care
2. The popularity of lecture-based teaching compared with problem solving, which is more effective in learning concepts of health promotion and disease prevention
3. The lack of curriculum models on preparing health professionals in health promotion and disease prevention
4. The paucity of research on the effectiveness of teaching health promotion and injury and disease prevention
5. Health insurance plans that have been slow to include reimbursement for health promotion and disease prevention programs
6. Health promotion and disease prevention require individuals to assume responsibility for their own health

Only in the last 10 years has there been a shift away from the biomedical model toward a health-promotion and disease-prevention approach to health care. The pressures for cost containment and society's changing attitude are some of the major reasons for this change in health-care delivery. The objectives contained in *Healthy People 2000* will help to accelerate the acceptance of health promotion and disease prevention programs as did the first *Healthy People: The Surgeon General's Report on Health Promotion and Disease Prevention* (U.S. Department of Health, Education and Welfare, 1979).

Health promotion and disease prevention continue to evolve and expand within the practice of occupational and physical therapy. Therapists are playing a more active role in a variety of settings that offer these services, but the programs are still in the infancy stages of development. The entry-level educational curriculum for physical and occupational therapy must meet accreditation requirements that specifically address health-promotion and disease-prevention concepts and the role of graduates in this area (American Occupational Therapy Association, 1983; American Physical Therapy Association Commission on Accreditation in Physical Therapy Education, effective 1992).

Bezold and colleagues (1985) predicted that a host of new health-care technologies, both diagnostic and therapeutic, will be put to use over the next 25 years. Twenty-first century medicine will also see an equally strong soft technologies component, which is consistent with self-care practices; wellness programs; therapeutic, nutritional, and fitness regimes; and other alternative healing practices.

The chapters in this book exemplify to a degree the type of health promotion, disease prevention, and activities programs in which therapists are participating. Wolfe (1986), when commenting on emerging trends in physical therapy, wrote:

> Given the escalating costs of all medical services, physical therapists must consider branching their skills and interests beyond reparation of injury. Promotion of wellness and prevention of movement limitations are emerging concerns that require the attention and intervention of many health professionals, including physical therapists. It is not unreasonable to suggest that significant financial reimbursement will emerge from pre-morbid interventions because they will be cost-effective. Therefore, the winds of change dictate expansion of patient services beyond the "repair" phase. (Wolfe, 1986, p. 383)

Examining the role of occupational therapy in disease prevention and health promotion, Jaffee (1986) wrote:

> There is now a unique opportunity for occupational therapists to be among those determining significant changes in the outlook on health care. Health, considered in terms of individual and societal fulfillment and accompanied by feelings of purpose and worth, has long been the goal of occupational therapy. As health professionals, occupational therapists must remember the philosophical orientation of the profession and use their many skills to develop techniques and programs that enhance health, prevention disease, and improve the social climate that fosters and promotes a healthy society. (Jaffee, 1986, p. 752)

Although occupational and physical therapists are quickly moving in the direction of health promotion and disease prevention, educators and clinicians need to take a leadership role and prepare therapists with the skills and knowledge necessary to participate effectively in health-promotion and disease-prevention programs. This participation requires a different training from that currently being offered in traditional education programs. According to Grossman (1991), convincing arguments have been made for the role of occupational therapy in health promotion and disease prevention and for the need to move practices into the community. Further support comes from the increasing number of empiric studies and prevention program descriptions in the literature. Despite these examples, according to Grossman, models of practice for prevention research and service provisions are lacking.

PROBLEM SOLVING IN HEALTH AND WELLNESS

The model described in this chapter is based on a problem-solving approach to health and wellness. This model recognizes, first and foremost, the importance of dealing with clients in terms of their totality (i.e., physical, mental, emotional, and environmental dimensions) (Fig. 27–1). Second, this model recognizes the personal power one has to influence one's own state of health.

The problem-solving approach to health and wellness (Fig. 27–2) is based on six premises:

1. The most effective way to incorporate health promotion and injury prevention within health-care curriculum is through a problem-solving learning approach.

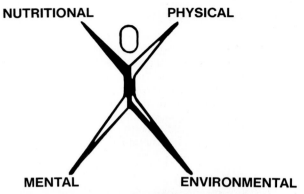

Figure 27–1. The multidimensionality of health.

2. To best understand the importance of dealing with the clients in terms of their totality, students and practitioners should assess their own health status and generate strategies for personal health.
3. The clinical experience for students and therapists should include exposure to health-promotion and disease-prevention programs.

4. Community-based health-promotion and disease-prevention projects provide students with practical experience in preparation for the challenges and benefits of designing and implementing health-promotion and disease-prevention programs.
5. Research is necessary to demonstrate and document the efficacy of health-promotion and disease-prevention programs.
6. Faculty members should serve as role models for students in health-promotion and disease-prevention programs.

Problem solving, individualized experiential learning of one's own health status, faculty role models, clinical experience, community-based practical experience, and research provide an educational climate that helps to develop the future practitioner's ability to develop and implement effective programs in health promotion and disease prevention. Each of these premises is discussed in terms of activities and learning strat-

PROBLEM SOLVING PEDAGOGY

Figure 27–2. Problem solving in health and wellness.

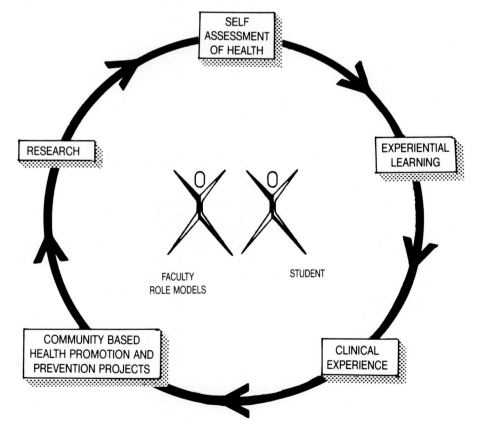

egies that can be incorporated by the educator and clinician.

Premise 1: The Most Effective Way to Incorporate Health Promotion and Prevention Within Health-Care Curricula Is Through a Problem-Solving Learning Approach

Training health-care practitioners to be effective problem solvers is one of the most important goals of education. Strategies of learning should facilitate inquiry, which promotes critical thinking, intellectual curiosity, decision making, and personal growth. The use of a problem-based teaching method gives students a chance to implement the theoretic knowledge they are learning rather than waiting until after graduation to practice what they have learned (Barrows, 1983).

Problem-based learning and clinical decision making have received a great deal of attention in the literature (Barrows, 1983; Olsen, 1983; Schmidt, 1983; Shepard, 1977). Wolfe (1986) provided an excellent reference on decision-analysis methodology for educators, clinicians, and researchers. Readers are referred to these references for a more detailed discussion on the various approaches and systems used to facilitate problem solving and critical decision-making skills.

Health-care professionals must be competent problem solvers to play an effective role in health-promotion and disease-prevention programs. The problem solving approach to health and wellness model emphasizes clinical problem solving applied to health promotion and disease prevention. A problem-centered curriculum is attractive to this model because it provides students and practitioners with the opportunity to conceptualize, analyze, deal with uncertainty and ambiguity, experience new modes of therapy, locate limited resources, and assess the results of one's efforts and intervention. Problem solving in health and wellness helps to foster and develop a high level of critical thinking and decision making; this application will aid in preparing practitioners for this new and continually involving area of practice.

The educational methodology and strategies that can be used to develop the student's ability to problem solve in health and wellness are as follows:

1. Units of instruction are organized around problems that require the integration of clinical skills with concepts of health promotion and disease prevention.
2. The problems emphasize the need to consider the interrelatedness of the physical, environ-

mental, psychologic, and social factors that contribute to the overall quality of a person's life.
3. The objectives and learning experiences aid students in resolving the problems and are used to evaluate the student's performance.
4. The problems integrate subject matter previously learned as well as act as a means of introducing new information.
5. The problems are organized from the simple to the complex. As the program progresses, subject matter and problems increase in difficulty.
6. Group-directed activity is encouraged in all learning activities.
7. Closure will follow each learning unit. Students analyze and synthesize what has been learned and discovered and apply this information to future problems. Suggestions for alternative learning experiences are also discussed. Closure integrates learned information with its relevance to health promotion and disease prevention.

The problems presented to the students are based on clinical case studies that are similar to the typical clinical situations often used in problem-based educational curricula. Laboratory and clinical experiences serve as vehicles to develop students' ability to approach a problem systematically and apply critical decision-making skills. The process of problem solving is emphasized so that students approach problems logically and with confidence. The expected outcome is therapists who are problem solvers in the delivery of health care.

The problems also encourage the importance of the team approach. The need to consult, seek advice, and refer clients to other health professionals is an important strategy used to resolve the problem effectively.

Within the model discussed here, as students develop a resolution to the clinical problem, they must also consider the environmental, lifestyle, psychologic, and physical factors that may be responsible for causing the problem. Three questions are frequently asked throughout the curriculum:

1. How could this problem be prevented?
2. What health-promotion strategies could be implemented to ensure that this problem does not recur?
3. As a therapist, how can I best use my skills and knowledge to develop an effective pro-

gram of health promotion and disease prevention for this population?

Consider the following clinical problem and then ask the three questions.

Mrs. Jones, an 85-year-old woman, fell in her home and suffered a fracture of the right hip. She lives in a senior citizens' home. Her medical history is unremarkable. She was in good condition before the fall. Her rehabilitation program was successful. She is independent in ambulation and activities of daily living. Her strength and general endurance are good.

Question 1: How could this problem be prevented?

To respond to this question, therapists need to work with the client and the other health professionals involved first to determine the cause of the fall. The precipitating factors are used to develop a health-promotion and disease-prevention program. Areas that need to be assessed include environmental, social, psychosocial, and lifestyle factors.

First, the home environment should be evaluated for structures that could have caused the fall. The following questions should be asked: What was the client doing at the time of the fall? What was the client thinking about at the time of the fall? Was the fall a direct result of the environment or improper care of the environment? How can the environment be modified to lessen the chance for recurrent falls?

Second, social and community factors may need to be assessed to develop an effective health-promotion and disease-prevention program. One should ask: Are there community and recreational programs that meet the health-care needs for the elderly?

Third, how does the individual deal with stress? Are psychologic and emotional support systems available if one needs them? Does the individual know where to go for assistance? Psychologic factors may expose an individual to medical illness and injury.

Fourth, aspects of lifestyle that should be assessed include nutritional practices, exercise patterns, self-care, and self-responsibility to maintain an optimum healthy lifestyle.

The key point of this exercise is for the students to recognize and appreciate the importance of the interrelatedness of the physical, psychologic, emotional, social, and environmental factors that may contribute to one's health status.

Question 2: What health-promotion strategies could be implemented to ensure that this problem does not recur?

Based on the health assessment, appropriate interventions of health promotion and disease prevention can be recommended. In the case study just presented, strategies to prevent the recurrence of falls include the following:

Structured exercise and physical fitness program
Changing eating habits after nutritional counseling
Stress-management program
Modification of the environment (i.e., removal of scatter rugs, installing grab bars in bathroom)

Question 3: As a therapist, how can I best use my skills and knowledge to develop an effective program of health promotion and disease prevention for this population?

An important goal of the curriculum is for graduates to function effectively as a contributing member of the health-care team and to identify potential health hazards, formulate remedies and therapy, and promote a healthy community.

To achieve this goal, as students apply critical decisions to resolve case problems and situations, they also develop activities, strategies, and interventions that may best use the skills of a therapist to develop health-promotion and disease-prevention programs.

Programs of interventions for the case study presented include the following:

1. Therapists make a presentation to the senior citizen community on the prevention of falls.
2. Therapists offer individual and group consultation on physical activities and exercises.
3. Working with other health-care professionals, therapists develop a stress-management and nutritional guidance program.
4. Therapists consult with the architect and building management to ensure a barrier-free home environment.

Premise 2: To Best Understand the Importance of Dealing with Clients in Terms of Their Totality, Students and Practitioners Should Assess Their Own Health Status and Generate Strategies for Personal Health

An important aspect of the problem-solving approach to health and wellness model is students' assessment of their own health status and lifestyle behaviors and the formulation of strategies for personal health promotion. The experience of developing and following through on activities that are designed to maximize one's health is emphasized throughout the curriculum. The active participation in evaluating and modifying one's behavioral lifestyle patterns will help to provide a foundation for a lifelong commitment to a high level of wellness. The adage "practice what you preach" exemplifies the need to be a model for good health. This activity helps the therapists when they develop health-promotion strategies with and for clients.

The assessment of one's own health is adapted from the model proposed by Dennison (1984), which focuses on the active participation in personal health assessment, awareness of health values in decision making, and the assumption of personal health responsibility for health and self-care. This approach consists of three phases:

Experiential phase. Students engage in self-assessment, including measurement and recording of indicators of personal health status.

Awareness phase. Students assess positive and negative influences on personal health and evaluate their susceptibility to various illnesses.

Responsibility phase. Students clarify their personal health values, determine actual and ideal health behaviors, identify barriers to establishing ideal behavior, establish personal behavioral goals, and develop a self-management program of illness prevention and health promotion.

The curriculum activities and teaching strategies used to facilitate the students' active participation in their own health include the following:

1. The course "Health and Wellness" introduces students at an early stage of their education to concepts of health promotion and disease prevention. An important aspect of the course is for students to examine and assess their health status and, based on the findings, to develop health-promotion strategies.
2. As part of the course requirements for "Health and Wellness," students complete a health-assessment survey instrument, which provides information that can be used to assist individuals in setting personal goals for health promotion and disease prevention. Various forms are available. The health-survey instrument proposed by Edlin and Golanty (1989) was used most frequently. Students are also encouraged to devise their own form.

3. On the basis of information obtained from the health survey, students formulate a contract with themselves to make appropriate changes in the areas needing improvement. Students are required to keep a health journal in which to record their health-promotion strategies and their progress toward health goals.
4. For the duration of the program, students, working in small groups with faculty guidance, form a health-promotion support group. Peer counseling and group support help to encourage continued participation and fulfillment of health goals.
5. Before completion of the program, students review their progress toward a healthier lifestyle and how they plan to maintain an optimum level of health on a personal and professional manner.

The primary purpose of these activities is to provide students with the means necessary to assess their health status and actively participate in developing strategies to promote a healthy lifestyle. This experience helps to contribute to the students' professional career and augment their decision-making ability to develop health-promotion strategies with and for their clients.

Premise 3: The Clinical Experience for Students and Therapists Should Include Exposure to Health-Promotion and Disease-Prevention Programs

As therapists continue to establish a niche within the health-promotion and disease-prevention areas, it is important that students are prepared to function in nontraditional settings that offer these services. During clinical education experiences, students are sent to traditional sites such as hospitals, rehabilitation centers, and private practice facilities. In these areas, students treat clients who have sustained an injury or disability and, thus, they may not participate in disease prevention or health-promotion activities. Traditional settings are important and provide an invaluable educational experience that is necessary for training practitioners at entry-level practice. However, it is also important that students participate in clinical settings that provide health-promotion and health-protection activities.

According to Huhn and Volski (1985), for physical therapists to use prevention techniques effectively, they must have experience with the problems they are attempting to prevent. As we broaden our practice base, we should also provide students with clinical experiences in nontraditional settings such as worksite health promotion; prevention and employee safety programs; wellness clinics; fitness and exercise clubs; public departments of health and social welfare; preseason sports clinics; mental health clinics; health-maintenance organizations; school-based health-promotion clinics; and senior centers. These are just some of the areas in which health-promotion and disease-prevention activities exist.

Premise 4: Community-Based Health-Promotion and Disease-Prevention Strategies Provide a Practical Experience that Prepares Students for the Challenges and Benefits of Designing and Implementing Health-Promotion and Disease-Prevention Programs

Healthy People 2000 (USDHHS-ODPHP, 1990) emphasized the importance of health professionals collaborating with the community to achieve the health objectives set forth for the nation. To achieve that goal, health professionals need to work with the community and health agencies to develop outreach health-promotion and disease-prevention programs for the population in greatest need.

As part of the curriculum requirements, students are required to design and implement a community-based health-promotion project. They are asked to identify a potential health hazard and establish an intervention program. Students use their own initiative to identify a subject area that would respond to a therapeutic intervention. The subject matter and proposed activities must first be approved by a faculty advisor. The proposal must be short term and not a large-scale project. Occupational therapy students and physical therapy students work in groups of four. The final products of this experience are a written project and an oral report. Because this requirement is due at the end of the educational program, students are able to best use and maximize the clinical and problem-solving skills obtained throughout the curriculum to perform this project.

Feedback after the community projects has been excellent from both the students' and the community's point of view. The students provided a service that contributed to the betterment of the community and helped to promote the image of physical therapy and occupational therapy as playing important roles in health promotion and disease prevention. Joffee and Farrant

(1989) reported similar results when medical students established community health-promotion projects as part of their community medicine course. According to the authors, the gains from this experience were substantial. Educationally, projects enabled students to pursue a particular topic in some depth and to gain insight into the challenge of health promotion in a socially deprived locality. The enjoyable and stimulating experience of the projects also appeared to have a beneficial effect on students' response to other parts of the community medicine course, as reported by the authors.

The health-promotion projects reflected a diversity of areas and specialties. Examples include:

Designed a brochure on prevention of falls for the elderly at a senior citizens facility. This program included a presentation to the residents.
Performed preseason screening of high school athletes and designed an off-season stretching and exercise program.
Designed a cardiac prevention program for a local corporation followed by a presentation on how to exercise properly.
Presented a program, along with a nutritionist, to junior high school students on the importance of exercise and eating the right foods.
Developed a slide presentation on preventing low back problems for a local Elks Club meeting.
Organized a Health Awareness Fair at a local shopping mall.
Prepared posters on proper exercise techniques for local sports and fitness clubs.

The community projects enabled students to develop and implement a community-based program of health promotion and disease prevention. This experience helps prepare graduates to assume an active leadership role in health-promotion efforts for the community at large.

Premise 5: Research is Necessary To Document the Efficacy of Health-Promotion and Disease-Prevention Programs

In an era of cost accountability and because of the need to support the efficacy of clinical practice, research is of paramount importance to all health professions (Rothman and Badyrka, 1991). With the increasing number of health-promotion and disease-prevention programs, the cost effectiveness and validity of these programs in particular are closely being monitored. According to Elias and Murphy (1986), occupational therapists are confronted with many of the same health problems that health-promotion professions are facing, including the need to justify the cost of these programs. Such circumstances, claimed the authors, will increasingly require occupational therapists (and other health professionals) to demonstrate the functional relationship between intervention parameters such as type, length, and intensity of treatment on the one hand and functional change in the client on the other. The economic impact of prevention and health-promotion programs must be assessed if we are to compete successfully with treatment-oriented programs for health-care dollars (i.e., assess whether these programs will decrease health-care costs or only add to current health expenditures) (Pender, 1987).

Health professionals must evaluate the effectiveness of health-promotion and disease-prevention programs to document their disciplines' contributions toward these activities. Successful intervention programs will help to support insurance coverage for these services and encourage federal and state grant allocations. The Committee on Trauma Research and the Institute of Medicine (1985) recommended that training health professionals in injury research is crucial if we are to develop and apply knowledge about the prevention of injury.

The model described in this chapter emphasizes the importance of applying problem-solving skills to practice especially as related to the need to develop a scientific basis for health promotion and disease prevention. Students encounter concepts of health promotion and critically assess the impact of these approaches on themselves and their clients.

Throughout the curriculum, students evaluate the strengths and weaknesses of health-promotion and disease-prevention applications using an objective, analytic approach. They do not accept the intervention on face value. They learn to ask pertinent questions and to seek out potential answers as they discover more information before they incorporate it as part of their treatment regime. What is the purpose of the health-promotion (or prevention) program? Has there been any published research in this area? If so, on what type of sample? What did the investigation show? Are there any side effects or precautions we should be aware of? These are some

of the questions students ponder and attempt to resolve as they evaluate the efficacy of health-promotion and disease-prevention strategies.

When designing the community-based health-promotion project, students propose and implement a pilot study on the effect of the health-promotion intervention on a sample population. Because of the time limitations of an entry-level program, students are confined to the pilot study. However, upon graduation they are encouraged to continue this investigation especially if they pursue graduate study.

The key point in this discussion is not to train entry-level students to be researchers but to teach them to apply problem-solving skills in a confident manner and to recognize the need to investigate new treatment approaches cautiously but receptively.

Premise 6: Faculty Members Should Serve as Role Models for Students in Health Promotion and Disease Prevention

The success of the problem solving in health and wellness model is contingent on how well the faculty is able to model and to reflect the ideals, attitudes, and behaviors that it hopes to develop and foster in students. Jonas (1988), when commenting on how can health promotion be productively incorporated into medical education, wrote that leadership is essential within the institution that is seeking to change a problem-solving health-promotion-oriented medical education program. Faculty understanding and support are equally important. No change of this magnitude, added Jonas, can take place without them.

On-going faculty development and self-evaluation are crucial factors for the success of this curriculum model. Faculty must first be supportive of this teaching pedagogy, program goals, and expectations. The academic institution should provide a structure for which faculty can develop the skills and knowledge necessary to practice and teach health-promotion and disease-prevention concepts. To prepare faculty as role models, it must be understood that this is a developmental process and cannot be achieved overnight. As students develop an understanding and appreciation for health promotion and disease prevention, so does the faculty. Health-promotion and disease-prevention concepts are new frontiers in occupational and physical therapy practice; new programs and activities are evolving from pre-existing ones. The key point for faculty and students is to be open-minded, receptive, and creative as they approach new programs in health promotion and disease prevention. To assist faculty members in developing as role models in health promotion and disease prevention, it is recommended that they formulate a faculty development plan. In this plan, specific goals are identified that faculty members hope to accomplish in health promotion and disease prevention as they relate to research, clinical practice, teaching, and continuing education. Besides serving as a guide for faculty to facilitate their skills in health promotion and disease prevention, this agenda would also serve as a resource for self-assessment and evaluation.

Additional factors to assist faculty in this process include:

1. Faculty and students must work together to support each other individually and collectively as they strive toward achieving the curriculum goals.
2. Invite and work with faculty, clinicians, and students from other disciplines and enthusiastically support multidisciplinary collaboration in teaching, research, and clinical practice activities.
3. Assist supportive staff and adjunct faculty in promoting healthy habits and lifestyle behaviors.
4. Monitor and modify, if necessary, one's progress toward achieving optimum health through self-assessment and feedback from others.
5. Continually assess the effectiveness of the curriculum and revise accordingly. Students and faculty should collaborate on the assessment process.
6. Work with college administration to acquire the resources necessary for faculty development from within or outside the institution.
7. Establish and maintain a learning environment that is conducive for students and faculty to experience and facilitate a healthy lifestyle and positive atmosphere.

SUMMARY

This chapter describes an educational model that uses a problem-solving approach to health and wellness with the goal of preparing graduates with the skills and knowledge necessary to play an effective role in health promotion and disease prevention. Using a problem-solving approach,

students first experience and analyze the effect of health-promotion concepts on themselves. This experience prepares them as they develop health-promotion and disease-prevention programs with and for their clients. The role of faculty in this process is pivotal to the curriculum's success.

Acknowledgments

The problem solving in health and wellness curriculum was developed and implemented by the Department of Physical Therapy, College of Allied Health Sciences, Thomas Jefferson University, Philadelphia, Pennsylvania. The program graduated its first class in 1985.

As the former chairman of the department, I wish to acknowledge the support, assistance, and camaraderie of the faculty and staff that was exigent and necessary to accomplish this new initiative. I also thank the administration for providing the resources and structure necessary for developing this new approach and especially the students, who allowed us to experience with them these new concepts and practice modalities.

References

American Occupational Therapy Association: Essentials and Guidelines of an Approved Educational Therapy Program for Occupational Therapists. Rockville, MD, American Occupational Therapy Association, 1983.

American Physical Therapy Association Commission on Accreditation in Physical Therapy Education: Evaluation Criteria for Accreditation of Educational Programs for the Preparation of Physical Therapists. Alexandria, VA, American Physical Therapy Association, effective 1992.

Barrows HS: Problem-based self-directed learning. JAMA 250:3077–3080, 1983.

Bezold C, Carlson R, and Peck J: The Future of Work and Health. Weston, CT, Greenwood Publishing, 1985.

Committee on Trauma Research and the Institute of Medicine: Injury in America: A Continuing Public Health Problem. Washington, DC, National Academy Press, 1985.

Dennison D: Activated health education: The development and refinement of an intervention model. Health Values: Achieving High-Level Wellness 8(2):18–24, 1984.

Edlin G and Golanty E: Health and Wellness: A Holistic Approach. Boston, Jones and Bartlett, 1989.

Elias W and Murphy R: The case for health promotion programs containing health care costs: A review of the literature. Am J Occup Ther 40(11):759–763, 1986.

Grossman J: A prevention model for occupational therapy. Am J Occup Ther 45(1):33–41, 1991.

Huhn RR and Volski RV: Primary prevention programs for business and industry. Phys Ther 65(12):1840–1844, 1985.

Jaffee E: The role of occupational therapy in disease prevention and health promotion. Am J Occup Ther 40:749–752, 1986.

Joffee M and Farrant W: Medical student projects in practical health promotion. Community Med 11(1):759–763, 1989.

Jonas S: Health promotion in medical education. Am J Health Promotion 3(1):37–42, 1988.

May BJ: An integrated problem-solving curriculum design for physical therapy education. Phys Ther 57:807–813, 1977.

Olsen S: Teaching treatment planning: A problem solving model. Phys Ther 63:526–529, 1983.

Pender N: Health Promotion in Nursing Practice. Norwalk, CT, Appleton and Lange, 1987.

Rothman J and Badyrka R: Utilizing resources to promote research in an entry level program. Clin Management Phys Ther 11(1):38–41, 1991.

Schmidt HG: Problem based learning: Rationale and description. Med Educ 17:11–16, 1983.

Shepard KF: Considerations for curriculum design. Phys Ther 57:1389–1393, 1977.

U.S. Department of Health, Education and Welfare: Healthy People: The Surgeon General's Report on Health Promotion and Disease Prevention, DHEW Publication No. (PHS) 79-55071. Washington, DC, U.S. Government Printing Office, 1979.

U.S. Department of Health and Human Services, Office of Disease Prevention and Health Promotion: Healthy People 2000, Publication No. 017-001-00474-0. Washington, DC, National Academy Press, 1990.

Wolfe S: Summation: Identification of principles underlying clinical decisions. In Wolfe S (ed): Clinical Decision Making in Physical Therapy. Philadelphia, FA Davis, 1986.

Phil Dunphy

Assessment of Exercise and Fitness Equipment

As we enter the last decade of the 20th century, exercise is no longer considered a passing fad: It has become an integral part of our lives. Scientific studies showed that exercise, integrated with nutritional modification and cessation of smoking, will help improve quality of life.

The importance of exercise has never been more evident than in the fields of physical and occupational therapy. Exercise therapy is becoming the dominant modality in clinics and hospitals throughout the country and is replacing the more standard passive approaches to rehabilitation. Exercise therapy is seen as the perfect adjunct to the therapist's unique skills in musculoskeletal evaluation and hands-on care. Clients are demanding a more active role in the rehabilitative process, and exercise gives back to clients some of the independence that may have been lost during the initial acute phase of rehabilitation. Exercise allows clients to reclaim control over their bodies.

As professionals who deal with individuals on a one-to-one basis, we have the opportunity and the responsibility to "physically" educate our clients as well as the public at large. This does not require any fancy or expensive equipment, simply a dedication to the concept of encouraging people to take control of their bodies.

Many people in the United States are still under the impression that performing hundreds of sit-ups per day will slim down their waistlines.

Unfortunately, as we know, this is not true. In fact, the public actually knows very little about exercise and overall fitness. Consider the fact that over 80% of the public will have a back problem in their lifetime (Deyo and Loeser, 1990). The public needs to be educated not only on the importance of exercise but also on how to rehabilitate themselves through the judicious application of exercise therapy.

Over the past decade, hospitals have been seeking ways to better serve their local communities and increase their revenue base. One example of their results is Wellness Centers. These outpatient facilities provide exercise and physical therapy units as well as weight loss, smoking cessation, stress reduction, and other educational programs. These programs have met with varied success. One reason for their lukewarm reception is that the hospitals have not incorporated exercise therapy within their own existing rehabilitation departments.

Health clubs have been in existence for many years. Before the 1970s, these clubs were mostly free-weight gyms. In the 1970s, weight machines were introduced to the public and, with the advent of jogging, the fitness craze had its inception. The problem with the majority of health clubs was the emphasis on membership and not "usership." Many individuals joined health clubs but came away with a negative attitude toward exercise and its possible benefits because of their lack of participation. As we enter the 1990s, this attitude is beginning to change. The public is demanding better educated health club staff, functioning equipment and, ultimately, results from their exercise programs for which they paid. People are becoming better educated about their bodies and the importance of exercise and nutrition. Unfortunately, not enough of this information is coming from the medical community. Less than 10% of the total population participates in a regular exercise program 3 times per week. Children and teenagers of today have a higher body fat percentage and higher total cholesteral (lower high-density lipoproteins) and have blood pressure significantly higher than their parents did as children. As professionals, we have a responsibility not only to our clients but to ourselves to rehabilitate clients with an active, exercise-oriented approach.

The purpose of this chapter is to provide therapists with an overall view of current therapy and fitness testing and exercise equipment. It is hoped that, armed with this information, therapists will move toward a more active approach in the treatment of their clients.

USE OF EXERCISE IN REHABILITATION

The key to a successful exercise therapy program is to make sure the clients understand what is expected of them. It may be necessary to make a verbal "contract" with clients to ensure their compliance to the program (Edwards, 1986). They must realize that the program will be successful only if they actively participate. This means not only regular attendance but an understanding of what they are doing in relation to what they should be doing. This is the element of monitoring.

Motivation is the next key element to any successful exercise program. Incentives can be given to the individual for reaching certain goals or for improving performance. Motivation also must become self-directed. Clients must feel that the time spent exercising will produce the desired result. This is no different than the individuals who work out in a health club to lose weight, tone up, or gain strength; they also are in need of physical rehabilitation and require motivation.

Measurement of clients' progress is another key element to a successful exercise program.

Therapists have always been concerned with many measurements such as joint range of motion (ROM), muscle strength, muscle tone, and so on. How many of us have measured resting and exercise heart rate and blood pressure? Do we use training heart rate zones in our exercise programs? Have we realized the importance of body fat percentage or lean body mass? Have we considered the importance of strength levels beyond just normal or a rating of 5 on the manual muscle test? These are just some of the additional elements we should consider in measuring clients' progress. We must go beyond the basic ROM measurements and even the more sophisticated isokinetic testing so popular in the 1980s. We must involve clients' total body and not just the affected limb. If we do not exercise the total body in our treatment program, we are no different than the lay persons who think they will lose inches from their waistline by doing only sit-ups!

The last and arguably the most important element of a successful exercise program is modification of the intensity, duration, frequency, and mode of exercise by therapists. The exercise program must be continually modified to provide the cardiovascular and neuromuscular systems with the needed stimulus for maximal adaptation. Progression of an exercise therapy program is the basis for maintaining clients' motivation level. Modification of clients' program is the key function of the treating therapist. By using their specialized knowledge of pathomechanics, musculoskeletal evaluation, and exercise therapy, therapists are best able to guide clients to the ultimate goal of increased independence.

A problem that arises in rehabilitation today is what happens to clients when formal therapy is ended and all of the treatment goals have not been realized. Whether the reason for this discharge is the referral source, the insurance carrier, or another agency, clients are left with few alternatives. If clients have been introduced to a total body exercise program during the formal therapy sessions, the process of assimilating into a outside exercise program is improved. If clients are not given a specific and comprehensive training program, full recovery will not be realized. This leaves clients with a greater risk of reinjury and further need for rehabilitation (Immes, 1980; Immes et al, 1977). The key to assisting clients is to educate them not only to their specific injury but to the total body involvement during the rehabilitative process.

BASIC EXERCISE PRIMER

Before specifically assessing exercise equipment, it is important to review the types of muscle contractions, different training methods, and resistance and cardiovascular exercise.

Different types of muscle contractions exist. *Concentric contraction* is the shortening of the muscle. It is sometimes referred to as a positive contraction. *Eccentric contraction* is the lengthening of the muscle. It is sometimes referred to as a negative contraction. *Isometric* or *static contraction* refers to the limb remaining in a fixed position.

Five types of training methods are discussed here (Table 28–1). *Isometric training* involves zero limb velocity and zero limb movement. *Isotonic training* deals with variable velocity and variable resistance. It is sometimes referred to as dynamic training and uses weight machines and free-weights. *Isokinetic training* involves near-constant velocity and accommodating resistance. *Plyometric training* deals primarily with eccentric muscular contractions using the stretch-shortening cycle. *Manual training* involves resistance applied in two different ways: (1) An individual applies resistance with one limb against another using isometric muscle contractions; (2) one individual applies resistance to another's limb using either isometric, concentric, or eccentric muscle contractions. It is beyond the scope of this chapter to discuss the various problems with the precise definitions of these training methods and muscle contractions (Atha, 1981).

Resistance exercise involves high-intensity, short-duration movements using smaller muscle groups. It improves both muscular strength and muscular endurance. Little or no cardiovascular effect is derived from resistance training. Resistance exercise does, however, increase the body's ability to burn calories and prepares the muscles to serve as shock absorbers during cardiovascular exercise. Resistance exercise is the foundation on which we build clients' exercise programs.

Cardiovascular exercise involves total body movement patterns, maintaining the exercise intensity within a training heart rate zone for a minimum of 20 minutes. There is no need to prescribe a 60 to 85% intensity level for clients who have been injured for a long while or who are confined to bed rest. These individuals may have to begin at an intensity level as low as 40 to 60% to receive the cardiovascular benefit. Cardiovascular exercise increases the body's ability to use fat as the primary energy source as well as to retard the loss of lean body tissue. This type of exercise is not the most efficient or effective means of increasing muscle mass.

Exercise has been further delineated into open- and closed-chain exercise (Table 28–2). In *open kinetic chain exercise*, the foot (end segment) is free while the body remains relatively still. An example of this type of exercise is that performed on a leg-extension weight machine or a treadmill.

In *closed kinetic chain exercise*, the foot (end segment) is fixed in a relatively stationary position while the parts proximal to the end segment are free to move. Examples of this type of exercise are a leg-press machine and a cross-country ski simulator.

TYPES OF EXERCISE EQUIPMENT

Resistance equipment comes in various forms such as weight machines; free-weights; combination weight machines and free-weights; machines using pneumatics, hydraulics, and electromagnetics; and those using body weight and elastic type material. Cardiovascular equipment includes treadmills, stationary bicycle ergometers, row ergometers, cross-country ski simulators, upper body ergometers, stair climbers, and vertical treadmills. Testing and evaluation equipment assesses muscular strength and endurance, cardiorespiratory endurance, functional capacity, body fat content, and flexibility. Self-monitoring devices measure heart rate and muscular function. Balance and proprioception exercise devices allow users to improve their neuromuscular rehabilitation.

Resistance Exercise Equipment

Resistance exercise machines are used primarily to develop muscular strength and endurance but not the cardiovascular system. Exercise machines are single-station or multistation units. Because this equipment has been designed primarily for the fitness market, unilateral movement patterns can be difficult.

Weight stacks are selectorized for safe and efficient weight changes. They are also available with plate-loaded resistance, which is more economical. Various types of weight-transport systems are available, including chain, cable, belt, elastic-type material, hydraulics, leverage systems, and the newer electromagnetics.

Table 28–1. Training Methods

Method	Velocity	Limb Motion	Force	Type Contraction
Isometric	Zero	Zero	Variable	Isometric
Isotonic	Variable	Variable	Variable/constant	Concentric/eccentric
Isokinetic	Constant/near	Variable	Variable	Isometric concentric/eccentric
Plyometric	Variable	Variable	Variable	Primarily eccentric
Manual	Variable/controlled	Zero/variable	Variable/constant	Isometric concentric/eccentric

ROM-limiting devices are very beneficial to protect the joint structures from exceeding the desired anatomic limits especially in the knee, shoulder, and trunk. ROM-limiting devices ideally are located away from the weight stack and should limit ROM in both directions. All adjustments to the ROM device for seat height and other body positions should be marked and conveniently displayed for clients to see and record. This is important for repeating the same ROM or for progression to increase or decrease clients' motion. Smaller weight increments are being used at the top of the stack to make progress safer and easier. Side-mounted weight stacks are used to minimize the space requirements for both the single-unit and multiunit stations. These weight stacks also allow for easier weight change without getting out of the seat. Plastic cover guards shield the weight stacks moving assembly and protect clients from any potential hand and finger injuries.

An important consideration in selecting any piece of equipment is the position of clients' neck and lower back (Fig. 28–1). Some companies provide adjustable neck and back supports (Fig. 28–2). The angle of the seat usually determines the position of the head. If the angle is too acute, the neck and head are forced into extension. This creates a strain and potentially aggravates an existing condition. This position could also create a neck and shoulder problem. The material used to upholster the seats, backs, and so on should

be able to withstand sweat and germs so as not to crack and harden prematurely. In certain areas where the upholstery does wear out and cracks prematurely (headrests, elbows pads, and so on), removable outer pad coverings are available. These can be changed easily and are more economical than reupholstering the entire pad. You should always wipe down the upholstery daily no matter what the manufacturer's recommendations indicate. This ensures cleanliness of the material and extends the lifetime of the upholstery.

The smoothness of the equipment is one of the most important things to check before considering a purchase. The machine should glide through the movement evenly.

All of the machine manufacturers will tell you that they have designed the most accurate strength curve into their equipment. The best way to determine the accuracy of the curve is to try the equipment yourself. As therapists, you have sufficient knowledge of biomechanics and kinesiology to make an intelligent decision as to design accuracy. You must also realize that at present no one company makes the best exercise station for each joint movement. One company may design an excellent station for the legs but not for the shoulders. I am not suggesting that you purchase equipment for different body parts from different companies; however, all therapists should be aware of this problem.

Finally, make sure the machine has easy acces-

Table 28–2. Kinetic Chain Exercise

Open	Closed
Foot (end segment) is free	Foot (end segment) is fixed
Proximal parts relatively stationary or can move	Proximal parts free to move
Increased compressive forces	Decreased compressive forces
Treadmill (weight bearing)	Nordic Ski Track
StairMaster 6000, Gauntlet	StairMaster 4000
Leg extension (nonweight bearing)	Leg press, Total Gym squat
Multihip exercising leg	Multihip supporting leg

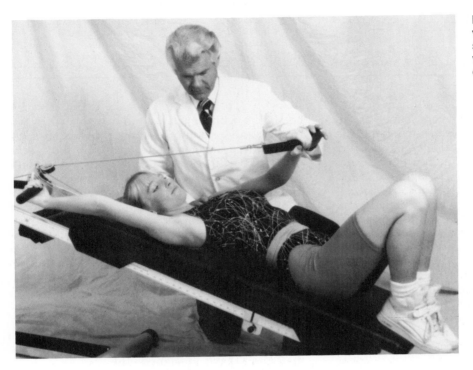

Figure 28–1. Total gym provides the patient with excellent support of the entire spine while allowing for resistance of the upper and lower body.

Figure 28–2. Bodymaster leg extension provides an adjustable lower back support that can be moved easily into position.

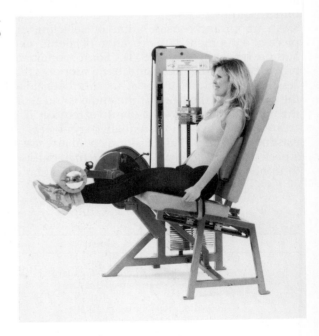

sibility for all of your clients. These machines have been designed for the fitness market and not for therapy clients. Manufacturers need your input to make changes that will better accommodate your and your clients' needs.

Because there are so many different movement patterns within the body, the resistance equipment is evaluated according to joint movement pattern and the pertaining diagnoses.

Ankle

Dorsiflexion. It is difficult to find exercise equipment that allows ankle dorsiflexion. You should be able to perform this exercise while sitting and in supine and prone positions. Zel-X weight equipment allows for seated unilateral motion. Wikco uses hydraulics in their system, which allows for seated, unilateral movement (no eccentric muscle contractions).

Plantar Flexion. One should be able to perform ankle plantar flexion in the seated, prone, supine, and standing positions. The difficulty with the standing position is the pressure placed on the shoulders. Some clients have difficulty with unilateral movement in the standing position. Besides the difficulty with pressure on the shoulders, the standing units create a problem for the lower back. The flexion required to get in or out from under the shoulder pads and lift the weight can create increased compression on the lower back. It is also important to maintain an erect position during the exercise. The height of the shoulder pads must be adjustable. The seated position does not allow for strength development of 'the entire triceps surae group. Nautilus, BodyMaster, and Cybex all have standing calf machines. Nautilus' Multi-Exerciser allows this motion in the standing position, but no pressure is placed on the shoulders. A belt placed around the client's waist is connected to the weight stack. Nautilus and Zel-X have a seated calf-exercise unit (Fig. 28–3). Wikco has a seated calf-exercise device that uses hydraulics. This allows for unilateral movement but not eccentric muscle contraction. Polaris weight-stack equipment has a standing, seated, and supine calf machine. Total Gym, which uses body weight as resistance (concentric and eccentric), allow plantar flexion in the supine position, either bilateral or unilateral (Fig. 28–4). There are many seated and standing plate-loaded (nonselectorized) devices available. Donkey calf machines, which are highly advocated by the body building community, place unnecessary stress on the lower back. The risks outweigh the benefits for the normal client population.

Knee

Extension. Knee-extension machines are the most popular and are available from all manufacturers. Very few companies have unilateral versions of this machine (Kinesi-Arc). Look for adjustable seat backs and an extra pad for the low back. Seat belts are a must. Ideally, the machines should allow for supine positioning, but this option is not available at present. The leg pad should be cushioned enough to prevent undue pressure on the lower leg. The back pad should extend high enough to support the neck and head. Handgrips should be available, but their use should be discouraged to maintain isolation and intensity. N.K. Products produces a unit that allows for unilateral motion and is plate-loaded. Keiser makes a unit that uses pneumatics as the source of resistance. Unilateral and eccentric muscle contractions are possible. Nautilus makes one of the finest machines despite its being bilateral. The rounded leg pad allows for easy unilateral adjustment. A ROM-limiting device is necessary for treatment of anterior cruciate ligament and patellofemoral problems.

Flexion. Flexion machines are designed for various positions; the most common is the prone position with a slight degree of hip flexion. Other positions available are side lying (Nautilus), seated (David equipment—it is important to have a lower back support in this position and the back pad high enough to support the head and neck), and standing (Polaris and BodyMaster—exercise is unilateral and excellent for isolation of this muscle; it should have an adjustable chest pad to assist in maintaining a more vertical position) (Fig. 28–5).

Each company has a different degree of hip flexion built into the unit. Look for an adjustable hip flexion angle. Variable handgrip positions is also a nice feature (Fig. 28–6). Except for the standing unit and those manufactured by Kinesi-Arc and NK Products, the rest are bilateral. The units with the proper leg cushion can be more easily adapted to unilateral motion. Total Gym provides supine knee flexion using body weight as resistance. Knee-flexion exercise is critical in the rehabilitation of certain knee pathologies, as are ROM-limiting devices, and is important for total limb strengthening. If you find yourself with a flat bench-type machine, having the client rest on their elbows may provide better isolation and decreased lower back discomfort.

Hip

Flexion. This motion is found on the multihip

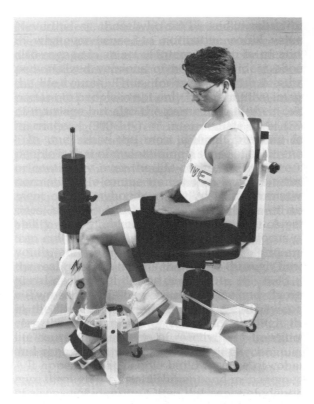

Figure 28–3. Zel-X provides this seated, unilateral calf machine. Concentric and eccentric muscle contractions are available.

Figure 28–4. Total gym demonstrating supine, bilateral, or unilateral plantar flexion.

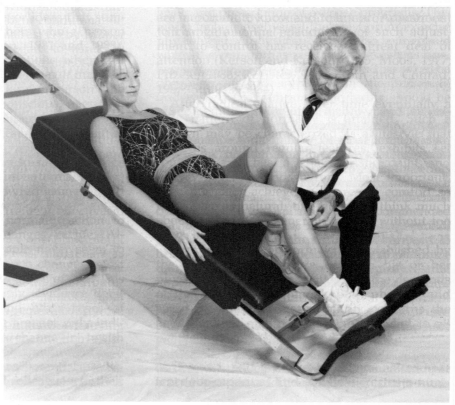

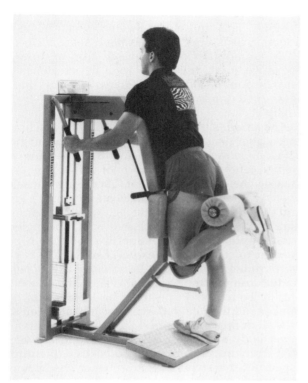

Figure 28–5. Bodymaster standing leg curl with chest supported.

exercise unit now made by most of the companies. BodyMasters and Cybex make this unit, which is excellent for unilateral closed-chain (supporting limb) and open-chain (exercising

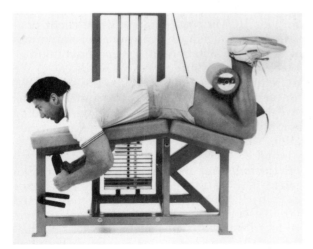

Figure 28–6. Bodymaster prone leg curl with hip flexion. Two different hand grips are available.

limb) exercise (Fig. 28–7). Hydra-Gym's Runner provides unilateral, bilateral, and reciprocal hip flexion and hip extension. Resistance is provided through hydraulic pistons, and no eccentric muscle contractions are available.

Extension. Hip extension is an important motion to strengthen for all lower extremity injuries. Like hip flexion, hip extension can be performed with the multihip exercise unit. Nautilus previously made a unit that strengthened the hip and back extensors unilaterally. This is sometimes a difficult machine for clients to master. A hack squat is designed by most free-weight equipment companies, but this places increased compression on the shoulders. BodyMaster also makes an inverted leg press, which decreases the pressure on the lower back (Fig. 28–8). Leg-press machines that strengthen the knee extensors also place pressure on the shoulders. Examine the shoulder cushion to determine how comfortable the pad is. Leg-press machines have different

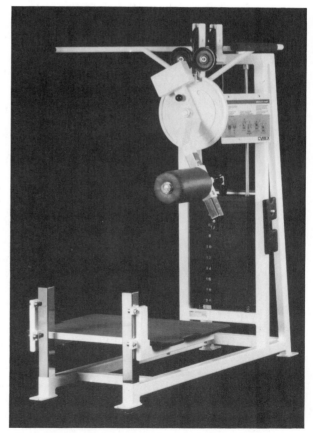

Figure 28–7. Cybex Multihip unit for hip flexion exercises.

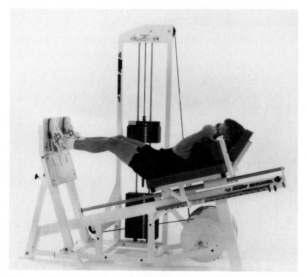

Figure 28–8. Bodymaster "Super Leg Press" provides different foot positions.

back angles from 90 degrees (seated) to approximately 15 degrees (reclined). Markings on the foot plate should be clearly identified for similar foot placement and to afford new positions when change is required. With Total Gym's unit, the exercise can be performed in a supine position with the head, neck, and back supported. Wynmor makes a multileg press that adjusts from 90 degrees to approximately 45 degrees. The classic barbell squat is a very effective exercise for lower body strengthening. Unfortunately, the compression of the bar on the neck and shoulder area and proper technique makes this exercise prohibitive for some clients. Padded bars with counterbalancing to help maintain a more upright position can partly alleviate this problem. A Smith-type machine allows clients to move the bar safely along a guided rail. This permits clients to stop the motion at any point and unload the weighted bar off the shoulders. BodyMaster and Cybex both make excellent units that also have a counterbalancing feature.

A small company in Tennessee makes a unit called Safety Squat, which has several advantages. First, the weight is not on the shoulders. A belt is fastened around the client's waist (several sizes are available) and slipped through a bar attached to the weight (plate loaded only). This keeps the weight below the client's center of gravity. Second, the client holds on to side rails and is better able to maintain a more vertical

position. This unit is not pretty but can be very effective. It is imperative to have some form of ROM-limiting device or soft end stop to protect the knee joint, especially into hyperextension and flexion beyond 90 degrees. Clients must wear an abdominal support.

Hip

Abduction. Once again the multihip machine provides resistance for this important movement. The one difficulty with using this machine is clients' tendency to display poor form. This decreases the intensity on the exercising muscle and creates unnecessary forces on the lower back and the opposite supporting leg. Most companies manufacture a seated version with an angled back support. This back support should be high enough to control the head and neck. The back support angle should not be so acute as to place undue strain on the neck. ROM should be closely monitored to avoid unwanted back extension. A lumbar roll may be necessary with some clients. This is an important muscle to strengthen for all lower body and lower back injuries (seated version with lumbar roll). Total body strengthening, especially the stabilizing muscles of the hip, is important to include in the treatment protocol. This ensures the client's return to independent functional activities and improves his or her understanding of how the total body interacts during movement.

Adduction. The same caveat mentioned previously when using the multihip machine and the seated version applies. However, the advantage of using the multihip machine for this movement is the client's ability to go beyond neutral. A ROM-limiting device is necessary because there are wide ROMs possible among the client population. Once again, this movement is important for total rehabilitation of lower body injuries. Lower back dysfunction responds well to strengthening this muscle group. The seated version appears to be better for treatment of the lower back (lumbar roll) because the standing multihip unit does not provide enough stabilization.

Trunk

Extension. As mentioned earlier, approximately 80% of the population will experience lower back problems in their lifetime. Armed with these statistics, equipment manufacturers produced various types of back-extension machines. All of the weight-loading machines place the client in a seated position. The following features *must* be available on this type of machine to provide safe, effective exercise: (1) ROM-limiting device, which controls the motion into both flexion and extension (in most of these machines clients do not even reach neutral); (2) seat and foot-plate adjustments must be present and clearly identified; (3) proper form must be adhered to in order to maximize the benefits from this exercise; (4) seat belts must be worn, and an adjustable back pad is preferable; (5) position of the head and neck during the exercise is important to avoid undue discomfort. Nautilus has a new moving axis of rotation design to simulate the motion of the lumbar spine better. Lido introduced its lower inertia equipment, which emphasizes the quality of each repetition. This is especially critical with trunk extension (Fig. 28–9).

Flexion. Ever since the exercise became popular, everyone has attempted to discover the perfect exercise machine for the abdominals. In the early 1980s Arthur Jones, founder of Nautilus, developed the first commercially successful abdominal machine. Since then, all of the equipment manufacturers have basically followed the same design. Posterior pelvic tilts, partial sit-ups, and sit-backs are still as or more effective than any machine on the market. As in the trunk-

extension machine, a ROM-limiting device is important. Adjustable seat and back support with restraining belt is necessary. Proper form is imperative, and clients must be kept from hooking their feet (with lower weight this will not be necessary). Neck discomfort is a common side effect from using these machines. Cybex, David, BodyMaster, and Polaris manufacture this type of unit. Check the firmness of the chest pad because one that is too soft can cause undue discomfort. Nautilus used the same moving axis of rotation technology in their abdominal unit.

Rotation. Of all of the machines that have been developed, this torso rotation unit is the machine most frequently misused. Clients enjoy using this machine to assist in ridding themselves of their "love handles!" As therapists, you are aware of the problems created with flexion and rotation of the lumbar spine. There are basically two types of units. In the first, the arms are locked behind two pads. In the second unit the hands are in front of the body gripping two handles. The most important consideration is how comfortable clients feel on the unit. When using the units described previously, clients tend to "twist" their bodies around their stationary head. As in most proper movement patterns, the

Figure 28–9. Cybex 45-degree back extension exercise unit.

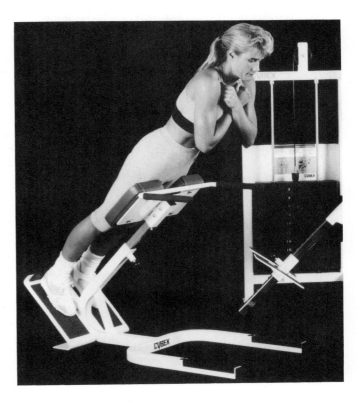

head should move *with* the body. As in all of these trunk movements, proper form may be more important than the type of unit itself. Systems 2000's Rotary Torso-Flex uses a rotary actuator as the source of resistance. Cybex, Nautilus, and BodyMaster offer this type of unit with concentric and eccentric muscle contractions available (Fig. 28–10).

Elbow

Flexion with Shoulder Flexion. For clients to be able to perform these exercises safely, they must have 90 degrees of shoulder external rotation. The padding on the machine where the elbow is placed must be comfortable. The seat must be adjustable to place the shoulder in the desired position. In all upper body exercises, the neck should be kept in axial extension to avoid injury to the structures of the neck. Cybex and Nautilus,

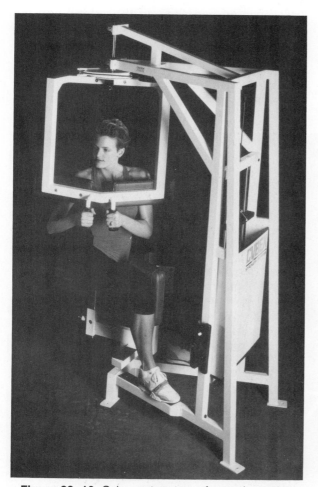

Figure 28–10. Cybex rotary torso for trunk rotation.

which allow for unilateral movement and BodyMaster and Polaris, which allow 45-degree shoulder flexion, provide units with this movement pattern. Dumbbells or a straight bar on a Scott-type bench are also very effective.

Flexion with Shoulder Extension. This motion can be performed in either the seated or standing position. The David unit, Total Gym seated, and free-weights in a standing position with a straight bar or dumbbells can be used. In the standing position, it is important to maintain an erect posture. The David unit allows for unilateral motion.

Extension with Shoulder Flexion. As in elbow flexion, 90 degrees of shoulder external rotation are necessary. Examine the comfort of the padding for the elbow to prevent irritation of the soft tissue. It is necessary to have an adjustable seat and elbow pad that allows for proper alignment of elbows. (Cybex and Nautilus provide this type of unit.) It is important to keep the elbows in at the sides to maintain the intensity and isolation on the muscle groups. Cable pulley machines allow standing 45-degree shoulder flexion elbow extension. As in all standing free-weight exercises, maintaining posture is important for maximal results. Supine shoulder flexion and elbow extension are possible on a tricep bench using free-weights.

Extension with Shoulder Extension. This is the classic "dip" position and is available in the seated position on a David unit (unilateral possible), BodyMaster, Polaris, and Total Gym in the supine position. StairMaster's Gravitron assists clients if they cannot lift their entire body weight. This is ideal for low-level strength clients and back clients who require spine extension (Fig. 28–11). Pacific Fitness manufactures the Imperial, which is a weight-assisted upper body unit. Instead of standing, as in the Gravitron, clients kneel. Units that allow shoulder extension beyond neutral should have a ROM-limiting device. An adjustable seat is important to assist in the alignment of the joint axis during this motion. Maintaining axial extension is extremely important when this movement is performed in a seated position. Dumbbells can be used to perform this motion with an exercise called "kickbacks." It is important to support the chest when performing this exercise to decrease the stress on the back.

Shoulder

Scapular Protraction in Shoulder Abduction. This is the position for strength training the

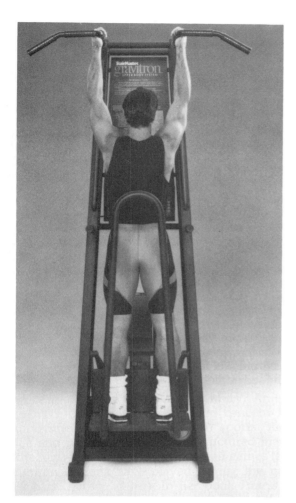

Figure 28–11. Stairmaster developed the gravitron, which allows for standing chins, dips, and wide-grip pull-ups. Ideal for patients who require spinal extension.

soft tissue structures in an unsuitable position (Fig. 28–12). David, BodyMaster, Polaris, and Cybex offer this type of unit. Nautilus offers a unique unit that places users in a supine position with the neck and lower back supported. The users place their elbows around two round rollers to perform the movement. The shoulder is essentially in a neutral rotation position. Two different units are available: One has the bench at a 10-degree angle, and the bench of the other is at a 50-degree angle. With Total Gym, this exercise can be performed in a supine position using body weight as the resistance. Vertical chest-press units are available from Polaris, Cybex, David, BodyMaster, and Hammer Strength. The units must have adjustable seats high enough to support the head and neck. A ROM-limiting device or a foot-driven lifting device should be available. As in all upper body exercises, proper head and neck position is critical. Hand position should be adjustable to allow for shoulder ab-

pectoral musculature. All of the equipment manufacturers make units for this type of exercise. The classic "pec deck" also places the shoulder in complete external rotation. This type of unit, in which clients are in a seated position, must have either a ROM-limiting device or a foot-plate control. The pad for the arms should be long enough to support the hand to the elbow. Otherwise, the elbow moves outward and places the shoulder into internal rotation. This places the shoulder in a compromised position and decreases the total ROM. This significantly decreases the work and power performed by the chest musculature. Clients tend to bring their neck into either a forward head posture or cervical extension placing the neck and shoulder

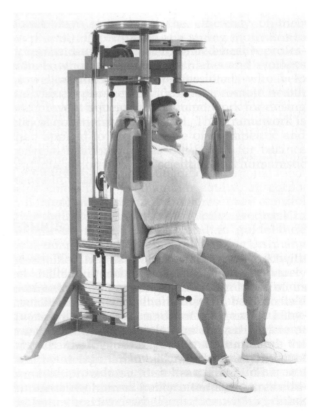

Figure 28–12. Bodymaster's vertical "Pec Deck" provides ROM-limiting device, low back support, and a long pad from the wrist to the elbow.

duction or adduction. Hammer Strength makes a unit that is plate loaded and allows for unilateral motion. The classic bench press is another example of this motion. Most clients, especially those over the age of 30, should avoid this particular exercise because of the technique required and stress placed on the shoulder, back, and elbow. If the bench press is a must, use dumbbells on a flat or inclined bench. On all of these exercises, it is important for clients to keep their shoulders in abduction and avoid full elbow extension.

Scapular Retraction in Shoulder Adduction. This is an extremely important movement pattern in the rehabilitation of all upper body injuries and for clients with cervical, thoracic, and lumbar dysfunction. This unit is referred to as a vertical row or rowing machine. Adjustable seat and chest pads are necessary. Examine the chest pad for angle, comfort, and cushioning. It is critical in this exercise for clients to maintain a position of axial extension. Variable hand position to allow the therapist to place the client in either shoulder adduction or abduction is desirable. Cybex, BodyMaster, Nautilus, Hammer Strength, and Total Gym have this type of unit available. Hammer Strength offers this unit as a plate-loading device with unilateral function possible. The difficulty with performing this exercise in a unilateral manner is that the contralateral limb should be placed into elbow extension. This prevents twisting of the upper body on a stabilized hip. These muscle groups can also be exercised using a pair of dumbbells and a flat or inclined bench. Reminding clients to keep their elbows at their side will facilitate safer and better results.

Abduction. The lateral raise is an ideal component of any shoulder-rehabilitation program. The key is to make sure clients avoid abduction with internal rotation. It is important that the pad for the upper arm extend from the elbow to the wrist. This encourages the clients to avoid dropping the hands into shoulder internal rotation. The second key is to keep clients from exceeding 90 degrees of shoulder abduction. This motion can cause an impingement syndrome or irritate existing tendinitis. David's Rotary Deltoid unit places the shoulder into abduction beyond 90 degrees (actually shoulder adduction) and, because of the pad placement, creates a tendency toward moving into internal rotation. The angle of the seat makes it difficult for clients to maintain axial extension. With the BodyMaster unit,

clients face the unit instead of facing out. This enables the clients to maintain proper position of their neck more easily. Nautilus provides users with both an arm pad and grip handles. Dumbbells are an excellent and safe way to provide strength training to this muscle group. Theraband and Sport Cord use elastic-type material to provide resistance. This allows clients to place themselves in a pain-free position. Shoulder abduction beyond 90 degrees is termed an overhead press. Units for this movement are available from BodyMaster, Total Gym, Cybex, Nautilus, and Zel-X. A key feature to look for on this type of unit is multiple hand positions. Clients will have difficulty with shoulder external rotation and abduction above 90 degrees. The alternative grip position allows clients to place their shoulder in less horizontal abduction. This exercise is done with less difficulty using dumbbells on an upright or inclined bench.

Internal and External Rotation. The lack of this type of exercise unit (plus hip rotation and so on) until the late 1980s demonstrates why therapists must provide direction for equipment manufacturers. The equipment designers must have a clearer understanding of what movement patterns are necessary to better serve the client population. Internal and external shoulder rotation is one of the more important movements in the rehabilitation of rotary cuff injuries and, in fact, of all shoulder dysfunctions. Zel-X provides a unit that allows for seated and standing motion with adjustable degrees of shoulder abduction (Fig. 28–13). The use of Theraband and Sport Cord is a very effective means of strength training this muscle while keeping the shoulder joint in a pain-free ROM. Dumbbells in the supine, prone, side-lying, standing, and sitting positions are also safe and effective and allow for eccentric muscle contractions. As new units are developed, it is important to look for those that stabilize the upper torso, provide adjustable seat and arm attachments, and have various degrees of abduction positioning.

Extension. The latissimus dorsi is one of the larger muscle groups in the body and is certainly important in the rehabilitation of back problems. The pull-over, pull-down, wide-grip pull-up all strengthen this muscle group. The pull-over machine is available from BodyMaster, David, Total Gym, Nautilus, and Polaris. An adjustable seat, a ROM-limiting device, a safety foot plate, a back pad high enough for the head, a seat belt, and a properly angled back pad are necessary to pro-

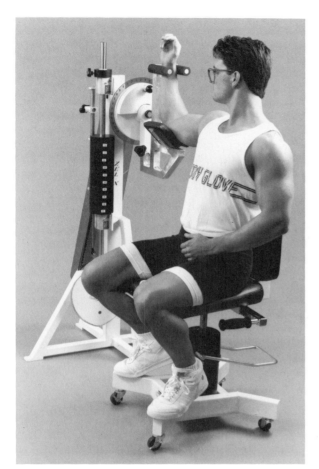

Figure 28–13. Zel-X provides a versatile unit for shoulder external rotation. Varying degrees of shoulder abduction are available. Exercise is performed unilaterally with concentric and eccentric muscle constraints.

Wrist, Hand, and Forearm: All Motions. This is another movement pattern for which most equipment manufacturers have not designed equipment. Nautilus recently demonstrated a unit providing resistance for wrist flexion, extension, grip, forearm supination, and forearm pronation. These exercises are performed in a seated position with excellent stabilization and can be done unilaterally. In the early 1980s, Hydra-Gym designed a unit using hydraulics to resist wrist and forearm motions.

It is impossible to include all of the body's movement patterns in this chapter. It is hoped that as therapists become more oriented to active treatment protocols they will demand better and safer products for their clients and for the public.

Cardiovascular Exercise Equipment

Cross-Country Ski Simulators. Cross-country ski simulators are the most efficient type of exercise device because they incorporate both upper and lower body exercise in a standing position. This closed kinetic chain exercise allows for a gliding motion of the lower extremities. This gliding motion decreases the compressive forces on the lower extremity joints and the lower back area. It is clearly more effective as a cardiovascular conditioner and as a fat-burning exercise device than the stationary bicycle found in most facilities. This device is easy for most clients to master and is ideal for postoperative lower extremity problems and cervical and lumbar dysfunction. The standing posture makes this unit the perfect antidote for a society that spends most of its time sitting. Resistance is provided for both the upper and lower extremities. Elevation is available, which increases the work load considerably and activates the hip flexor as well as hip extensor musculature. It is important to instruct clients in maintaining an erect posture while exercising to avoid undue fatigue of the lower back musculature. Lower level clients can begin by using only their legs, whereas high-level clients can simulate running in preparation for sports activities. NordicTrack makes units to accommodate most budgets. They are the unquestioned leaders in the field (Fig. 28–15).

Stair Climber. The key features to look for in this unit are independent step action and durability. The original unit had escalator-type stairs. Users had to raise each foot while the revolving stairs kept moving. This was an open kinetic

mote proper neck alignment. Clients who have limited motion in the shoulder must be careful not to increase the shoulder ROM by hyperextending the lower back. Clients should maintain a posterior pelvic tilt to avoid this problem. Total Gym's unit places clients in a supine position with the head, neck, and lower back supported. The clients' body weight is the resistance and can be adjusted by changing the angle of the cushioned board (Fig. 28–14). Dumbbells can be used in a similar motion on a flat bench. StairMaster's Gravitron allows for pull-ups, chinups, and wide-grip pull-ups. This unit provides lift assistance to allow clients who cannot lift their full body weight to perform these exercises. Exercising in the standing position is ideal for clients with certain types of back problems.

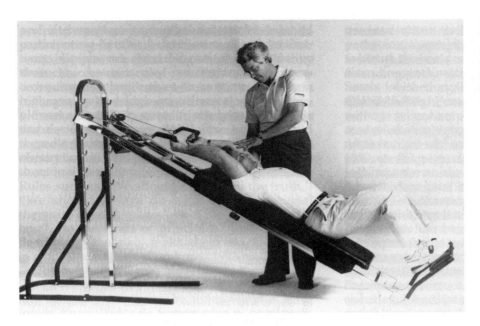

Figure 28–14. Total gym "Pullover" with neck and back support and resistance that is changed easily by moving height of bed. This machine can be used as a portable or wall-mounted unit.

chain exercise. It was excellent for cardiovascular conditioning and weight loss but, because of the compressive forces on the lower extremities and rotation of the hips and spine, not ideal for early rehabilitation. The later model solves some of these problems by keeping the feet stationary on pedals, while each step is independent of the other. This unit becomes a closed kinetic chain exercise device. There is a decrease in anterior shear forces at the knee and a decrease in the compressive forces to the spine. Knee and back dysfunction clients can easily control the step

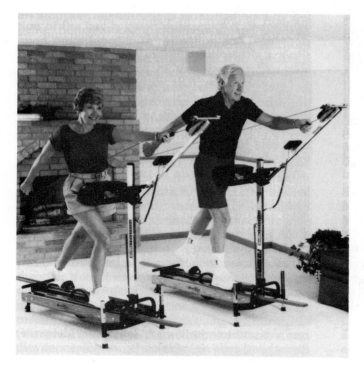

Figure 28–15. NordicTrack displaying "aerobic extension" type exercise. Ideal closed kinetic chain exercise with adjustable hip pad. Separate resistance settings for the upper and lower body.

ROM into knee flexion and extension. Unfortunately, there is no way for therapists to monitor the ROM for clients, and it is therefore difficult to progress objectively. Clients have a tendency to hold onto the side rails and lean forward. This significantly reduces the amount of work produced and places unwanted stress on the spine. Prolonged holding of the side rails, which should be used only for balance, causes increased potential for wrist and elbow injury. Long bouts of exercise can cause the feet to become numb because of lack of movement on the pedal. The only unit on the market to have independent step action is the StairMaster 4000. StairMaster has the most experience with this type of unit and has excellent service facilities. Their stair climbers are state of the art, having both open (Gauntlet) and closed kinetic chain models (4000), and are the safest for clients (Figs. 28–16 and 28–17).

Treadmills. Many decisions need to be made

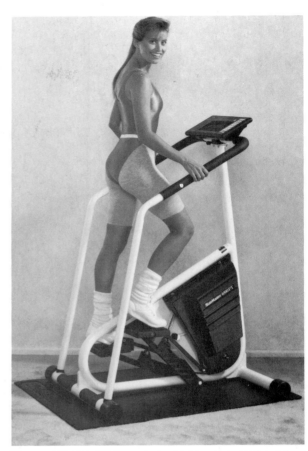

Figure 28–17. Stairmaster's highly successful 4,000 Model provides the patient with a safe, effective closed kinetic chain exercise. Independent step action with improved electronics.

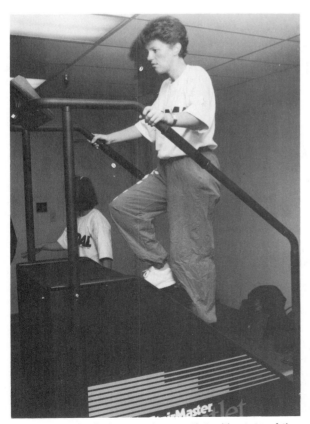

Figure 28–16. Stairmaster's gauntlet with state-of-the-art electronics is an example of an open kinetic chain-type exercise.

concerning treadmills. First, you must decide if an open kinetic chain exercise device will suit your client population. The advantage of a treadmill versus stair climbers is that even the individual at the lowest level of fitness can ambulate on a treadmill if the speed setting is slow enough. Although there are increased forces involved with an open-chain exercise device, the treadmill can be a perfect adjunct to your closed kinetic chain devices. First, you must decide between an AC- and DC-type motor. The AC-type motor runs at a constant speed, which allows for more speed control of the belt because it is completely electronic. The DC motor does not compensate quickly enough to the load created by the client's foot strike. This causes a momentary lag in the belt, which is even further exaggerated if the client is heavy. AC-drive treadmills have a history of high-speed starts. If one client does not manually lower the speed before stopping the unit, the next client might start the unit at a potentially dangerous speed. Make sure the manufacturer has safely resolved this problem. Maintenance is the most important consideration in your decision. Although the AC drive appears to be better, because of its intricate drive system the maintenance may be costlier. The length of the bed, the width of the bed, and the belt–bed interface are other factors to consider when deciding which treadmill to purchase. Elevation and speed controls are normally electronic and extremely accurate. Depending on the client population, you may require side rails. Treadmills are ideal for walking forward and backward (stimulates increased hamstring activity) and for advanced activities such as jogging and side-stepping. Make sure clients wear good footwear and maintain an erect posture. Place a television in front of the treadmill to deter boredom. A cheap, effective method of analyzing gait involves placing a video camcorder 8 to 12 feet behind the treadmill and connecting this to the television in front of the treadmill. Your clients can observe any gait deviations as if they were looking at themselves from behind. You can further analyze the gait pattern on recorded videotape. Quiton, Universal, TrackMaster, and Precor are but a few of the leading treadmill manufacturers.

Vertical Treadmill. This is the newest type of closed kinetic chain exercise device. The vertical treadmill simulates mountain climbing using both arms and legs in a reciprocal manner at an angle of approximately 70 degrees. This exercise is not for the low-level clients, but recent adaptations allow pedaling in a seated position and alternating arm action in a seated position. The vertical treadmill provides excellent ROM for the upper and lower body, and the motion approximates functional human movement. Heart Rate's Versa Climber has a variety of models and all of these adaptations (Fig. 28–18).

Bicycle Ergometers. This piece of exercise equipment is standard in most facilities. It is a closed kinetic chain exercise that involves sitting and in many cases forward trunk flexion. The ROM into knee flexion and the compressive forces on the patella-femoral area preclude the use of this device for most knee clients. Because sitting can increase the lumbar disc compressive forces, this device should be carefully prescribed for neck and back clients. Any bicycle ergometer

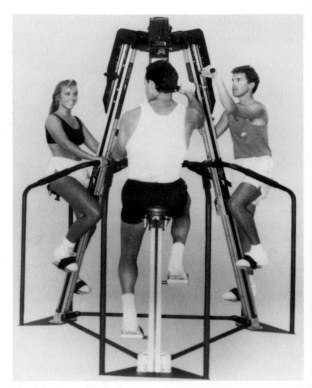

Figure 28–18. Heart Rate's Versaclimber showing full climbing with arms and legs, pedaling (on seat), and lower body only. Ideal closed kinetic chain exercise with reciprocal action.

should have adjustable handlebars and seat. Bicycles are available that have sprockets that limit the ROM into knee flexion to less than 90 degrees. Semirecumbent bicycles place clients in a better anatomic position. This type of bicycle will make clients work harder, requiring more muscles to contract (increase hamstring and gluteal activity), and will keep the back in a better posture. It is ideal for improving lower extremity ROM by changing the seat setting. The recumbent position creates less compressive force on the spine. More than 20 different bicycle manufacturers make units that have hydraulic resistance, wind resistance, mechanical brake resistance, and sophisticated electronics that even monitor workout by measuring heart rate. Some companies introduced units that simultaneously exercise the upper body. The bottom line is that clients are still exercising in a sitting position, and in this day of modern technology we may be better off prescribing activities that require standing. If you feel your clients need a bicycle, look at one of the recumbent models.

Row Ergometer. The days of manual rowers are outdated. Flywheel, hydraulic, and electronic types are more effective. Flywheel types are approximately 8 feet long, which can create a problem, but more closely simulate outdoor rowing. Electronic rowers may be too expensive and more than you need. Look for comfortable seat and pedal design. Adjustable straps should be available for the feet. Rowers are excellent for using both upper and lower body if properly utilized. Clients must maintain their back in an upright position. Clients with low back and cervical problems probably are not good candidates for this device. Rowers are an excellent method of dynamic stretching of the knee into flexion. Improper form, however, can place the knee into unwanted hyperextension. Clients with ankle problems respond well with this device because ROM is improved and strength of the triceps surae group is increased. Clients with upper extremity dysfunction adapt well to this exercise device because all the major muscle groups are involved. Concept II's flywheel-type unit is most like outdoor rowing. StairMaster offers the WindRacer Rower, which is an electronic version with many desirable features. NordicTrack has designed the Nordic Row TBX, which provides a unique seat design to support the lower back.

Upper Body Ergometer. This excellent device provides upper body strength and muscular endurance. The seat should be adjustable, and clients should be able to stand. Variable grip handles allow forward and reverse movement. Cybex offers the UBE, which is an isokinetic-type unit. EDC's UpperCycle unit features electronic speed control and displays power, time elapsed, and speed. Upper back and neck problems respond well with this device. All upper extremity injuries, including hand and wrist fractures, heal more rapidly using this active approach.

Testing and Evaluation Equipment

Muscle Testing. In the late 1960s, muscle dynamometry became more sophisticated with the advent of isokinetic muscle testing. Cybex, with the patented isokinetic muscle-testing device (James Perrine, inventor), introduced the medical community to a more objective method of assessing muscle strength and endurance than had previously been available. The Cybex unit has undergone many changes but still offers isokinetic and isometric testing and exercise units.

In 1981 Chattecx released the Kinetic Communicator (Kin Com), which afforded the medical and athletic communities the first exercise and testing device with eccentric muscle contractions. This was truly an eccentric contraction in which the external force actively lengthens the muscle at a constant velocity or a constant force. This unit also offered constant force isotonics, which allowed clients to vary the velocity (acceleration and deceleration) while maintaining a near-constant force. With the advent of the Kin Com, a new level of accuracy and validity was available to clinicians to determine muscular deficiencies. The Kin Com has become smaller in size and more computer friendly over the years. It has also improved on the accuracy of the isotonic and isometric modes.

In the mid-1980s, Biodex offered a unit that provided isokinetic and isometric training modes. The isokinetic mode functioned with both concentric and eccentric muscle contractions. Both an exercise and testing unit, the Biodex offered adaptors to allow for multijoint exercise and testing.

Loredan's Lido, invented by Dr. Malcolm Barnes, provided isokinetic concentric and eccentric muscle contractions. The Lido is an exercise and testing unit that introduced a new level of computer software and precision in evaluating strength and endurance deficits. This unit also provides isometric exercise and a form of isotonic exercise. A wide variety of joint applications are available with its unique sliding-cuff design. Many different computer programs are available including client-treatment protocols.

In 1989, Med-Ex of Canada introduced the Dynatrac, based on the work of James MacArthur. MacArthur was the inventor of the previously mentioned Kin Com. Dynatrac provides clinicians with the first true constant-force isotonics. Concentric, eccentric, and isometric muscle contractions are available. It also provides clinicians with a method of storing client data on a magnetic card. This is ideal for setting the clients' exercise parameters more easily at each treatment.

MedX of the United States, with founder Arthur Jones, demonstrated a line of testing and exercise units. They are unique in that the testing is performed in the isometric mode. The back and neck are the primary joints tested in this system, but units for other joints are becoming available.

As the 1980s drew to a close, there was a

sudden emphasis on the evaluation of the strength and endurance of the back musculature. Biodex, Kin Com, and Dynatrac introduced add-on back-testing units. Cybex, MedX, Iso-Technologies, and Lido have made available separate testing and exercise units for the back.

It is not the object of this chapter to make recommendations on equipment. Considering the $25,000 plus price tag on these testing units, careful, judicious decision making should precede a purchase of this magnitude.

Functional Capacity

A graded exercise test yields valuable information regarding how a client responds to various levels of exercise. It is important to determine the initial exercise level of each client. This information allows the therapist to monitor the exercise program in a safe, effective manner. By establishing these baseline levels, the client's progress can be more objectively documented. This can be performed by (1) symptom-limited graded exercise stress test and (2) submaximal exercise stress test. The most important evaluation is the electrocardiogram (ECG), which is used to evaluate the action of the heart during exercise. The ECG looks for signs of latent coronary artery disease. The client's resting and maximal heart rate and blood pressure achieved during exercise are measured. The training heart rate zone can be determined with this information. The symptom-limited exercise stress test is performed by a physician and therapist or exercise physiologist. The main function of this test is diagnostic. However, if the client is connected to a gas analyzer during the test, the VO_2 max and RQ range values are assessed, which assists in the determination of clients' functional capacity. VO_2max is the volume of oxygen consumed in millimeters per kilogram of body weight per minute. It is a measure of the client's maximal aerobic work capacity. RQ range, the respiratory exchange ratio, is an important value that monitors what food sources are being used to perform the work. A value of .72 is interpreted to mean that 93% of the energy source is derived from fats. A value of .98 means that 93% of the energy source is derived from carbohydrates.

A submaximal exercise stress test can be performed on a stationary bicycle, treadmill, and even a stair climber. This test primarily screens a client's heart rate and blood pressure response to a graded exercise program. The VO_2max and maximum heart rate can be predicted from the results of this test according to the specific protocol used. This value can be improved as can the exercise intensity within the client's target heart rate zone. This affords the therapist another objective means of measuring the client's progress.

Body composition is probably one of the best means therapists have to measure the client's response to exercise therapy. As we know, the scale only tells the client their total body weight. This is a relatively meaningless number without knowing how much of that total weight is lean body weight (muscle) and how much is fat weight. These figures are expressed as percentages (i.e., percentage of body fat and percentage of muscle). An effective resistance exercise program increases the lean body weight, and an effective cardiovascular program decreases the percentage of body fat. The combination of resistance and cardiovascular programs will help clients achieve the best results. There are several ways to measure body composition:

1. Hydrostatic weighing. This is the gold standard and requires the client to be dunked into a specially designed tank of water. This method measures the body's volume. It is a form of "volumeter." The volume must be converted to density using several standard values for fat and lean body tissue, including the measurement of the client's residual lung volume. Density is then converted to body fat percentage by one of several formulas.
2. Electrical impedance. A small hand-held device estimates the percentage of body fat by measuring the electrical resistance in the skin. The results are affected by the amount of water in the system.
3. Skin-fold test. A pair of specially designed calipers are used to "measure" your skin at several sites on your body. The Lange and Halpender skin-fold calipers are the most accurate type. The accuracy of the tester is extremely important to ensure reliability. The actual formulas used to convert the measurements to body fat are population specific, so be sure to select carefully the most appropriate formula for your clients.

Self-Monitoring Devices

Heart Rate. One of the advantages of incorporating exercise therapy into your program is the importance of your clients' heart rate response to exercise. As therapists, we are constantly trying to find more objective means of evaluating our clients' response to a particular treatment protocol. By knowing clients' heart rate response to cardiovascular exercise, the therapist has the necessary information to modify their exercise protocol. The first step is to instruct clients in counting their own pulse at the wrist or at the neck. In addition, heart rate monitoring devices have been available since the late 1970s. They have attempted to measure exercising heart rate by clipping a sensor on the index finger or ear lobe, or by having the client grip a sensor. Some of these devices have varying rates of accuracy at rest but are not reliable during moderate to intense exercise. Polar USA uses wireless transmission via an unencumbered heart transmitter worn around the chest (over clothes) and a watch-like monitor. They offer a variety of models all with ECG-type accuracy.

Muscular Function. When observing your clients exercising on resistance-type equipment, you will quickly realize how difficult proper form can be. You can prescribe the perfect exercise therapy protocol, but if your clients are unable to perform the activity in a controlled manner, the results may be unsatisfactory. Clients are unaware of how they are performing the exercise. They are lacking the necessary feedback to improve their performance while they are exercising. In fact, clients may not be aware that they are performing the exercise incorrectly. They must be shown a template of the exercise pattern to imitate while they are exercising. ATP Exercise Systems developed a device, Right Weigh, that gives clients visual feedback of the correct movement while they are exercising (real-time visual feedback). The Right Weigh is adaptable to all types of resistance exercises and actually gives clients a performance score based on how well they were able to track the computerized template.

Balance and Proprioception

Balance activities have always been an integral part of therapy programs. The alignment of the body's center of gravity and base of support is critical during all phases of rehabilitation. It is important to train the proprioception system during treatment in order for the client to regain full independence in functional activities. All clients

(orthopedic, neurologic, pediatric, geriatric, industrial, and so on) benefit from exercises that facilitate improved balance and better proprioception. Neurocom Systems and Chattecx's Balance System provide computerized analysis of the clients' equilibrium. These sophisticated systems allow for both quantification of clients' balance and a training system using real-time visual feedback as the ultimate motivator. Codoc Balance Platform, produced by Euroscand, Inc., is an inexpensive method of rehabilitating lower extremity injuries and improving clients' balance and proprioception. Fitter International, Inc.'s Pro-Fitter, a resistive-type balance board, allows side-to-side sliding, which stimulates improved balance, muscular strengthening and endurance, and increased kinesthetic awareness. Euroglide, by Improve Human Performance, allows unrestricted side-to-side motion on a specially designed board. Originally used by speed skaters, this unit has excellent applications in rehabilitation for a wide variety of clients. Interestingly, advocates of free-weights have always stated that one of the benefits of this equipment is the beneficial effect on an individual's balance. Whereas training on weight machines appears to emphasize isolation of the muscle groups, free-weight exercises allow clients greater freedom of movement. This in turn requires a greater need for stabilization and balance.

BASIC RECOMMENDATIONS FOR A TOTAL PROGRAM

As professionals, we realize the key to a successful therapy program is the one-on-one relationship between therapist and client. The following recommendations are designed to enhance this relationship and to provide the client with a program that involves the total body. This is done by using exercise therapy as an adjunct to the therapist's hands-on skills.

Medical History

A client's medical history should include the following:

1. Specific questions relating to coronary risk factors (modifiable and nonmodifiable) for the client and immediate family
2. Client's history of participation in a super-

vised exercise program; specific questions relating to their attitude toward the body should be included such as "What muscles of your body respond best and least to exercise?," "What home exercises do you perform?," "How much time do you plan to devote to your exercise therapy program?," and "What can we do to help you stick with your exercise therapy program?"

3. A series of questions concerning client's involvement in fad diets and their understanding of nutrition
4. Assessment of the primary body positions that their job involves (e.g., sitting, standing, walking, climbing, lifting)
5. Record of client's resting blood pressure and heart rate to screen for any elevated or abnormal values
6. A determination of any medical problems apart from the primary diagnosis that could prevent client's participation in an exercise therapy program. This allows the therapist a better understanding of the client's overall attitude toward movement, exercise, and nutrition.

Goals

As therapists, we are familiar with the importance of setting short-term and long-term goals; however, we should also include in this initial evaluation the client's goals and their referral source, if any. We can then coordinate our goals with those of the client and physician or referral source for a more effective treatment program.

Initial Evaluation

The initial evaluation should include a musculoskeletal and postural evaluation and an assessment of muscle imbalances, flexibility and joint laxity, and postural changes (forward head, rounded shoulders, increased or decreased lordosis, supination or pronation of the foot, and so on). This should be an evaluation of the whole body and not just the joint or body part involved. Movement and exercise should involve the entire body. Training heart rate zone should be determined. The American College of Sports Medicine (ACSM) and the American Heart Association recommend a symptom-limited graded exercise stress test from a physician for an individual with

any coronary risk factors. If this is not feasible, a release from the referring physician is appropriate. Instruct your clients in how to count their own pulse rate during rest and exercise. Finally, the evaluation should also include a functional exercise assessment to determine client's present exercise level.

Prescribing an Exercise Program

The basis of a successful exercise therapy program is the involvement of the clients' total body. Back clients need leg strength and flexibility as well as trunk stability and mobilization. Neck clients need shoulder, upper back, and upper extremity strengthening and flexibility as well as proper neck mechanics. Knee injuries require balance and proprioception activities as well as strengthening and endurance training to the ankle, thigh, and hip musculature. Hand clients require upper extremity strengthening. Paraplegics require more extensive muscular strengthening and endurance with cardiovascular endurance in a normal fitness environment to increase their level of independence. All clients require cardiovascular exercise to maintain proper body fat levels and retard the loss of lean body tissue.

Applying the basic fitness principles of intensity, frequency, duration, and mode of activity assist in establishing a safe, effective program. ACSM guidelines recommend a program involving both cardiovascular and strength training for optimum fitness (ACSM, 1990).

A general outline for establishing an exercise therapy program for various lower extremity diagnoses is as follows:

Step 1. Involuntary muscle contraction (electrical muscle stimulation using various frequencies)
Step 2. Isometric muscle contractions (Cybex, Biodex, Dynatrac)
Step 3. Mat core exercises using body weight (Theraband and Total Gym)
Step 4. Low velocity, limited-ROM isokinetics (Lido, Kin Com, Phoenix)
Step 5. Velocity and ROM-controlled, open-chain non-weight-bearing isotonic training (Right Weigh, Dynatrac, pool therapy); bilateral concentric muscle contractions and unilateral (uninvolved limb) eccentric muscle contractions (lift two up, lower one down [uninvolved

limb]); and unilateral concentric muscle contractions (involved limb) and bilateral eccentric muscle contractions (lift one up [involved limb], lower two down).

Step 6. Closed-chain weight-bearing cardiovascular exercise (NordicTrack and StairMaster 4000)

Step 7. Closed-chain non-weight-bearing isotonic training (Total Gym and Leg Press). Use same progression as in Step 5 plus unilateral concentric muscle contractions (involved limb) and unilateral eccentric muscle contractions (involved limb) (Lift one up [involved limb], lower one down [involved limb]); bilateral concentric muscle contractions and unilateral eccentric muscle contractions (involved limb). (Lift two up, lower one down [involved limb]); and bilateral concentric muscle contractions and bilateral eccentric muscle contractions (lift two up, lower two down).

Step 8. Open-chain weight-bearing cardiovascular exercise (treadmill)

Step 9. Variable velocity isotonic training (Right Weigh Exercise Guidance System or Dynatrac)

Step 10. Variable-velocity isokinetic training (Cybex, Biodex, Kin Com, Lido, Merac, Phoenix)

Step 11. Interval closed- and open-chain weight-bearing training, using NordicTrack, StairMaster (4000, 6000, or Gauntlet), treadmill, recumbent bicycle, rower, upper body ergometer, or VersaClimber)

Step 12. Balance and proprioception activities using CODOC balance board and the Pro-Fitter

The program should also include exercise of the uninvolved limb and other body segments for muscular endurance training. This should begin as soon as clients' symptoms allow. An exercise program for the trunk varies in that unilateral exercise is not available. In this case, Step 5 would be replaced by limited-ROM eccentric trunk flexion or extension (depending on the symptoms) and assistive concentric trunk flexion or extension. Step 7 would be replaced by limited-ROM concentric trunk flexion or extension and assistive eccentric trunk flexion or extension. This would be followed by symptom-free ROM concentric and eccentric trunk flexion or extension and Step 9 with variable velocity concentric and eccentric training.

Flexibility exercises should be introduced into the program as early as possible. This includes stretching for the entire body, emphasizing increased body awareness. Much like body builders who during contests pose off, displaying remarkable control of individual muscle groups, it is important that your clients are able to contract and relax their muscles before initiating their isokinetic or isotonic training program to control these movements better. Appropriate abdominal exercises should also be taught as early in the program as clients' diagnoses permit. Abdominal and stretching exercises are excellent activities for clients to continue for their home program.

All clients benefit from a proper flexibility and abdominal program. This information also serves as a good introduction to their understanding of the importance of lifelong fitness. It also gives your clients increased independence and better control of their bodies.

THE FUTURE

As the medical community, specifically therapists, use a more active approach in their treatment modules, their needs for equipment and exercise protocols will become more sophisticated.

Movement patterns that are more unilateral, rotational, and diagonal will be required. Exercises will be performed in positions of less trunk flexion. Physically challenged clients' needs for more accessibility to exercise equipment will increase. Equipment for younger children and mature adults will become necessary to accommodate the growing numbers of individuals in these age categories.

Possibly the most important improvements in exercise equipment and techniques are the following:

1. More emphasis will be placed on the quality of the exercise and less on the quantity. Physicians, therapists, and clients will place more importance on how well the exercise therapy program is performed versus how much is accomplished. Form will be redefined, and exercise equipment will reflect this new emphasis.
2. Feedback will become an important means of

integrating clients with the exercise equipment. Real-time biofeedback will replace the currently used feedback terminology. The term *feedback* as it is presently used for exercise equipment today is merely a recording of various parameters accomplished during the exercise. This information is normally displayed at the end of the exercise session. It does not allow clients to (1) realize that their movement pattern is being performed incorrectly and (2) correct any deviations of the movement during the exercise. Real-time visual biofeedback enhances the clients' motivation while linking clients' perception of their own motion to the actual predesigned movement pattern. As clients internalize the movement pattern better, further research can be performed to determine which exercise protocols are more advantageous for a safer and more expedient recovery. Occupational therapists can design functional activities that mirror the movement patterns of various exercise equipment. These functional activities will afford more clients the benefits of active therapy protocols.

Pool therapy will become more recognizable as the most effective form of exercise therapy. Pool therapy has all the advantages of open- and closed-chain exercise without the disadvantages. Water offers 10 times the resistance of air, allowing for resistance to occur in all directions. Clients are able to begin ambulation sooner because of the buoyancy effects of water. Clients metabolize approximately 4 times the number of calories walking in 3 to 4 feet of water compared with walking on an open-chain device such as a treadmill. Exercise equipment is being developed that will be placed in the water to further enhance training effects of water.

The future of therapy appears to lie in movement, exercise, and active treatment protocols. The knowledge of therapy, pathomechanics, biomechanics, exercise, and client care will enable therapists to become the experts in exercise therapy.

As we enter the last decade of the 20th century, we must keep our minds open to all the fact and fiction concerning movement, exercise, and exercise equipment. By doing so, we will better serve our clients and become even more respected among the public and our own medical community.

References

American College of Sports Medicine: Position stand on the recommended quantity and quality of exercise for developing and maintaining cardio-respiratory and muscular fitness in healthy adults. Med Sci Sports Exerc 22:265–274, 1990.

Atha J: Strengthening muscle. *In* Miller DI (ed): Exercise and Sport Science Reviews, Vol 9. Philadelphia, The Franklin Institute Press, 1981.

Deyo RA, Loeser JD, and Bigos SJ: Low back pain and the herniated disc. Ann Intern Med 112:598, 1990.

Edwards RHT: Muscle fatigue and pain. Acta Med Scand 711(Suppl):179–188, 1986.

Immes FJ: The use of physiological techniques for monitoring of progress during rehabilitation following fractures of the lower limb. Int J Rehabil Med 2:181–188, 1980.

Immes FJ, Hackett AJ, Prestidge SP, et al: Voluntary isometric strength of patients undergoing rehabilitation following fractures of the lower limb. Rheumatol Rehabil 16:162–171, 1977.

Bibliography

Astrand PO and Rodahl K: Textbook of Work Physiology. New York, McGraw-Hill, 1977.

Burke EJ and Humphreys JHL: Fit to Exercise. London, Pelham Books, 1982.

Downiniguez RH and Gajda R: Total Body Training. New York, Scribner's, 1982.

Falls HB, Wallis EL, and Logan GA: Foundations of Conditioning. New York, Academic Press, 1970.

Garrick JG and Radetsky P: Personal Trainer. New York, Crown Publishers, 1989.

Gutin B and Kessler G: The High-Energy Factor. New York, Random House, 1983.

Kapandji IA: The Physiology of the Joints, Vols. 1–3. New York, Churchill Livingstone, 1970.

McArdle WD, Katch FI, and Katch VL: Exercise Physiology. Philadelphia, Lea & Febiger, 1986.

Miller DI (ed): Exercise and Sport Sciences Reviews, Vol 9. Philadelphia, The Franklin Institute Press, 1981.

Milvy P (ed): The Long Distance Runner. New York, Urizen Books, 1977.

O'Shea JP: Scientific Principles and Methods of Strength Fitness. Reading, MA, Addison-Wesley, 1976.

Pearl B: Keys to the Inner Universe. Pasadena, CA, Physical Fitness Architects, 1979.

Sweigard LE: Human Movement Potential. New York, Harper & Row, 1974.

Westcott WL: Strength Fitness. New York, Allyn & Bacon, 1987.

APPENDIX I: EQUIPMENT MANUFACTURERS

Resistance Training

BodyMaster
P.O. Box 259
Rayne, LA 70578
(800) 325-8964

Cybex
P.O. Box 9003
2100 Smithtown Ave
Ronkonkoma, NY 11779-0903
(800) 645-5392

David Fitness Systems
A Division of Kinetic Resources, Inc.
3725 Cockrell
Fort Worth, TX 76110
(800) 933-2600

Equidyne Physical-Therapy Products
Norsk Sequence Training Equipment
6836 Rovalwood Way
San Jose, CA 95120

First Choice
Heartline
P.O. Box 2982
Setauket, NY 11733
(516) 751-8489

Hammer Strength
P.O. Box 19040
Cincinnati, OH 45219
(800) 543-1123

Hydra-Fitness Industries
Hydra-Gym
P.O. Box 599
2121 Industrial Park Rd
Belton, TX 76513-0599
(800) 433-3111

Keiser
411 S West Ave
Fresno, CA 93706-9952
(800) 888-7009

Kinesi-Arc
Round Valley Industrial Park
P.O. Box 118
Lebanon, NJ 08833
(800) 262-2770

Loredan
Lido Strength Training Systems
P.O. Box 1154
1632 Da Vinci Court
Davis, CA 95617
(800) SAY-LIDO

Nautilus
P.O. Box 708-709
PowerHouse Rd
Independence, VA 24348
(800) 874-8941

N.K. Products Company, Inc.
2500 Rosedale Ave
Soquel, CA 95073
(408) 462-6509

Pacific Fitness
12349 E Telegraph Rd
Santa Fe Springs, CA 90670
(800) 722-3482

Polaris
P.O. Box 1478
Spring Valley, CA 92077
(800) 858-0300

Randal Sports Medical Products
Gravitron
12421 Willows Rd NE
Suite 100
Kirkland, WA 98034
(800) 635-2936

Sport Cord
6 Shimmering Oak Court
Suite 230
Chico, CA 95926
(916) 895-1951

Strive Enterprises, Inc.
P.O. Box 22
Washington, PA 15301
(800) 368-6448

Systems 2000
Rotary Torso-Flex
1899 Sangamon Ave
Springfield, IL 62702
(800) 727-1756

The Hygenic Corp.
Thera Band
1245 Home Ave
Akron, OH 44310

T.K. Star
210 South Second Ave
Mount Vernon, NY 10550
(914) 667-5959

Total Gym
9225 Dowdy Dr
Suite 220
San Diego, CA 92126
(619) 566-8810

Wikco
Route 2 Box 154
Broken Bow, NE 68822
(308) 872-5327

Wynmor Products Ltd.
309 Williamson Ave
Opelika, AL 36803
(205) 749-6516

Zel-X
11 Dorn Place
Centereach, NY 11720
(516) 732-5859

Cardiovascular Training

Combi/Mitsu & Co
Combi System 5RH
200 Public Square
Suite 29-5500
Cleveland, OH 44114
(216) 696-8710

Concept II, Inc.
Lamoille Industrial Park
RR 1 Box 1100
Morrisville, VT 05661-9727
(802) 888-7971

Cybex
Upper Body Ergometer, Fitron
P.O. Box 9003
2100 Smithtown Ave
Ronkonkoma, NY 11779-0903
(800) 645-5392

Engineering Dynamics Corp.
Upper Cycle
120 Stedman St
Lowell, MA 01851
(508) 458-1456

Heart Rate, Inc.
VersaClimber
3188-E Airway Ave
Costa Mesa, CA 92626-6601
(800) 237-2271

NordicTrack
NordicTrack, Nordic TrackRower TBX
141 Jonathan Blvd
North Chaska, MN 55318
(612) 448-6987

Patex
TrackMaster
P.O. Box 12445
Pensacola, FL 32582
(800) 225-2655

Precor
P.O. Box 3004
20001 North Creek Parkway
Bothell, WA 98041-3004
(206) 486-9292

Pro-Tec Sports
2321 Gilberto
Rancho Santa Margarita, CA 92688
(800) 800-5890

Quiton Instrument Company
2121 Terry Ave
Seattle, WA 98121-2791
(800) 426-0347

Randal Sports Medical Products
StairMaster, Windracer, Windracer Rower
12421 Willows Rd NE
Suite 100
Kirkland, WA 98034
(800) 635-2936

Unisen, Inc.
StarTrac
14352 Chambers Rd
Tustin, CA 92680
(800) 228-6635

Universal
Tredex
P.O. Box 1270
930 27th Ave SW
Cedar Rapids, IA 52406
(319) 365-7561

Testing and Evaluation Equipment

Biodex
P.O. Box S
49 Natcon Dr
Shirley, NY 11967
(516) 924-9300

Chattecx
Kin Com
P.O. Box 4287
Chattanooga, TN 37405
(800) 322-7343

Cybex
P.O. Box 9003
2100 Smithtown Ave
Ronkonkoma, NY 11779-0903
(800) 645-5392

Dynatronics
Dynatron 2000 & 3000
470 Lawndale Dr, Bldg D
Salt Lake City, UT 84115
(800) 874-6251

Loredan
Lido
P.O. Box 1154
1632 Da Vinci Court
Davis, CA 95617
(800) SAY-LIDO

IsoTechnologies
P.O. Box 1239
Elizabeth Brady Rd
Hillsborough, NC 27278
(919) 732-2100

Med-Ex
Dynatrac/Phoenix
BTE
7455 L New Ridge Rd
Hanover, MD 21076
(800) 331-8845

MedX
1155 NE 77th St
Ocala, FL 32670
(904) 622-2112

Universal
Merac
P.O. Box 1270
930 27th Ave SW
Cedar Rapids, IA 52406
(800) 553-7901

Functional Capacity

Cambridge Scientific Industries, Inc.
Lange Skinfold Caliper
Cambridge, MD

Self-Monitoring Devices

ATP Exercise Systems, Inc.
Right Weigh Exercise Guidance System
P.O. Box 11246
Chattanooga, TN 37401-2246
(800) The-Weigh

Chattecx
The Balance System
P.O. Box 489
4717 Adams Rd
Hixson, TN 37343-0489
(615) 870-2281

Euroscand, Inc.
CODOC Balance Platform
14040 Leaning Pine Dr
Miami Lakes, FL 33014
(305) 556-1085

Fitter International, Inc.
Pro-Fitter
4515 1st St SE
Calgary, Alberta Canada T2G 212
(800) 661-9458

Improve Human Performance, Inc.
EuroGlide
1143-D Charles View Way
Towson, MD 21204
(301) 321-1540

Neurocom International, Inc.
Neurocom-Equitest
9570 SE Lawnfield Rd
Clackamas, OR 97015
(503) 653-2144

Polar USA, Inc.
470 West Ave
Stamford, CT 06902
(203) 359-1966

CHAPTER
29

Elizabeth DePoy

Program Evaluation

Current trends in health care require practitioners to show that their programs are cost effective and beneficial to patients. Conducting a program evaluation meets that requirement. Program evaluation is a systematic process of determining how to establish the best program to meet an identified need and how to demonstrate that the program's process and outcome have met the need. This chapter introduces basic principles of program evaluation and offers examples of how to implement evaluation strategies in programs aimed at preventing and treating injuries.

DESCRIPTION AND HISTORY OF PROGRAM EVALUATION

Program evaluation can be defined as the application of systematic investigation to the development and assessment of a program. In the past, program evaluation was narrowly conceptualized only as the assessment of outcome of a programmatic effort, including the benefit to client and the cost versus outcome ratio. Simply put, evaluation sought to answer two primary questions about health-care programs:

1. Did the programs solve the health problems that they were initiated to address?
2. Was the program worth its output in health restoration in monetary terms?

While evaluation of health and social programs existed before World War II, it was not until after the war that program evaluation took hold. According to Rossi and Freeman (1989), the proliferation of large social programs such as urban development, preventive health, and community development created expenses for which the program developers and directors would be held responsible. In other words, people wanted "proof" that their money was being spent for a worthy purpose and that the programs were doing what they promised to do. By the 1960s, and with the backdrop of the War on Poverty, evaluation grew and was the rule rather than the exception in grant proposals, human service projects, and health-care programs. The reciprocal relationship between method and need for evaluation developed as program evaluation became a field of inquiry unto its own. By the late 1970s, textbooks and journals exclusively devoted to the evaluation process and method were common in professional libraries and collections. In the 1970s and early 1980s, the methodologic preference in evaluation seemed to be quantitative; that is, the outcomes were expressed in numeric terms. However, an interesting shift, which is still taking place, emerged in the early 1980s. With more value being recognized in qualitative method, evaluators began incorporating field study and qualitative analysis, or narrative explanation of findings, into evaluation designs (Patton, 1987). Regardless of method, the acceptance of program evaluation as the test of the value of a program rendered it essential that clinicians and administrators come to consider program evaluation as a necessary task in their daily routines.

Contemporary program evaluation has taken on several analogous terms, including, among many, development research, needs assessment, quality assurance inquiry, and evaluation research. Each of these terms, in part, describes the purposes of evaluation. Thus, within the past 2 decades, program evaluation has expanded and emerged not only as a process or outcome assessment but also as a method to establish need and set policy for the expenditure of financial, intellectual, and human resource effort.

Different from research, program evaluation does not have the goal of testing theory. However, the extent to which theory forms the basis for program evaluation differs according to the evaluation effort. In earlier years, program evaluation was viewed as totally atheoretical and primarily political in nature. Evaluators were seen as the harbingers of survival or demise of social programs, in that they determined whether the program was worthy of funding. However, current evaluation research, although political, seeks to answer the broader questions presented in Table 29–1.

In summary, within the past 6 decades, program evaluation has grown and has evolved into a specialized field. It is methodologically diverse and accomplishes multiple purposes (Table 29–2). Clinicians and administrators in injury prevention and treatment must begin to see evaluation as a necessary professional activity in

Table 29–1. Issues Addressed by Program Evaluation

1. What are the most urgent health problems that need to be addressed?
2. What is the nature of these problems?
3. Who is affected by the problems?
4. What is the extent of the problems experienced by the identified group?
5. What type of intervention seems most appropriate to the problem within the constraints of the resources available to address the problem?
6. What programmatic goals are priorities?
7. How should the goals be operationalized?
8. What is the program process?
9. What are the program outcomes?
10. What are the program costs?
11. Are the costs justified by the outcomes?
12. To what extent did the outcomes address the problem and the scope of the problem?
13. What changes need to be implemented to strengthen the program?

Table 29–2. Purposes of Program Evaluation

1. Development of an understanding of a problem and a clearly articulated problem statement to which a program speaks
2. Delineation of priorities for program development
3. Understanding of need and resources
4. Development of a program to respond to articulated priorities
5. Assessment of the process of program development and implementation
6. Assessment of outcome
7. Determining areas for improvement in the process and the product
8. Determining survival status of a program

order to demonstrate the value of their interventions, to receive continued financial support, and to improve the effectiveness of existing programs in preventing injury and treating it when it occurs.

METHODS TO DEVELOP AND EVALUATE HEALTH CARE PROGRAMS

Two basic categories of program evaluation are common in the evaluation literature: *summative* and *formative* evaluation (Herman et al, 1987). Although not mutually exclusive, these two sides of the evaluation continuum emerge from different schools of thought about the purpose and function of program evaluation (Fig. 29–1; Table 29–3).

Further on in this chapter, an evaluation model that synthesizes both formative and summative evaluation is presented and analyzed. The model has been anchored on evaluation strategies suggested by numerous authors and seems to be most useful to practitioners who are beginning to engage in evaluation of their practices and programs. (For more specialized and complex evaluation planning, refer to additional resources listed in the bibliography.)

Summative evaluation is defined as the systematic assessment of (1) program outcome, and (2) program impact on the problem to which the program is aimed at solving (Rossi and Freeman, 1989). This type of evaluation is most frequently done when program survival is questioned. In other words, summative evaluation occurs when the purpose of the evaluation is to determine whether to continue, expand, or modify a program. The summative evaluator produces a sum-

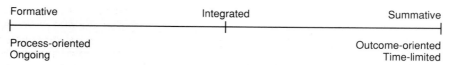

Figure 29–1. Continuum of program evaluation.

mary document of the program, including a description of its mission, activities, and impact. Theoretically, the summative evaluator should not work with or become involved with the program staff beyond the collection of data to avoid conflict of interest. Ideally, summative evaluation represents the interest of the funding agency or the sanctioning body for the program (Herman et al, 1987).

The primary methodologic tools for summative evaluation include systematic observations, standardized measurements, and interview data. In a summative process, the evaluator determines what data need to be obtained. Then, the evaluator obtains and analyzes the data set and draws conclusions about the program impact. These conclusions are used for various purposes, but most commonly to inform funding and policy decisions.

Although the term "summative evaluation" most frequently refers only to the evaluation element of program development and assessment, the summative style can be used throughout the development-evaluation sequence. In this style, an expert or experts usually define the problem, develop the goals, implement the program, and use summative strategies to have it evaluated.

Formative Evaluation

Formative evaluation is a broader and more longitudinal process than summative evaluation. The

purposes of formative evaluation are manifold and include the development of a full understanding of a problem, implementation of a program, monitoring the process of decision making and implementation, and improving the program based on information derived from many different sources. Thus, formative evaluation is an ongoing process that is intended to improve program effectiveness in achieving its goals (Patton, 1987). The formative evaluator most often represents the interests of program staff, and while outcome assessment is conducted, its purpose is to enhance understanding and is not to determine survival.

In formative evaluation, a full spectrum of data collection and analysis strategies are employed. The choice of method is determined by purpose. Although formative evaluation may include summation, the summary of program data is used to improve and assist staff to further develop the program, rather than to address whether or not a program will be funded in the future. Formative evaluation is therefore an ongoing process, which essentially systematizes and formalizes administrative and evaluative activities that are informally and perhaps routinely performed by health-care providers.

Who Conducts Program Evaluation?

The purpose and nature of the evaluation largely determine who structures and conducts the evaluation. Professional evaluators are frequently used for summative evaluation because of their technical expertise and "outsider status." According to Rossi and Freeman (1989), a summative evaluation should be performed by an individual or group who holds no "stake" in the program. The summative evaluator must be capable of posing evaluation research questions relevant to the evaluation purpose, of designing an evaluation research plan, of completing the research, and of reporting the findings in a manner that best accomplishes the purpose of the evaluation.

In formative evaluation, a coordinator may be

Table 29–3. Formative Versus Summative Evaluation

	Formative	Summative
Purpose	Improve	Determine survival
Length of time	Ongoing	One shot
Techniques	Qualitative and quantitative	Quantitative
Domain	Process	Outcome
Who does it	Insiders and consultants	Outsiders
In whose interest	Program staff	Funding source

ultimately responsible for organizing the evaluation activities. However, staff input and participation are essential in order for formative evaluation to be meaningful to program improvement. The formative evaluator therefore needs organization and communication skills, project design skills, and managerial skills to oversee all phases of the formative process.

Can the practitioner structure and conduct an evaluation of his or her own program? Ideally, summative evaluation should be performed by an outsider to avoid conflict of interest. Therefore, a practitioner may want to select someone other than himself or herself to conduct an evaluation that falls into the summative category. However, the resource and time limitations in the health-care industry may preclude the employment of an external evaluator to conduct a program evaluation. In such a scenario, the practitioner may be asked to evaluate the outcome and value of his or her own program. The practitioner therefore must be careful to ensure that the evaluation design is appropriate to the evaluation questions and is acceptable to the funding source. Consultation with a skilled evaluation researcher can help a practitioner to prepare an evaluation plan that serves the needs of the funding agency and of the practitioner.

In the case of a formative evaluation, the practitioner does not face the issue created by being a "stakeholder" in the program, because the evaluation efforts are directed at improving the program rather than judging its merit. However, in this category, the time-consuming nature of the evaluation may create problems for the practitioner. When a practitioner has multiple duties in his or her job, other staff and consultants can be useful in planning and implementing the evaluation at any point in the process. However, if informal evaluation is being routinely conducted, a formative evaluation may be accomplished by systematizing the efforts that are already in place—a seemingly easy task for the practitioner who is already evaluating.

At this point, the practitioner may be questioning his or her skill and ability to conduct a program evaluation. Table 29–4 demonstrates the skill requisites for program evaluation and the relationship of these skills to those already exercised by practitioners in daily professional activity. It may come as somewhat of a surprise to the reader that the practitioner already possesses and uses the foundation skills to conduct an evaluation. The key to translating these practice

Table 29–4. Comparison of Practice and Evaluation Skills

Practice Skill	Evaluation Skill
Assess the client	Develop a problem statement
Validate assessment findings	Assess needs
Plan treatment	Set goals
Conduct treatment intervention	Implement the program
Assess the client's progress	Assess the process and outcome
Modify intervention as necessary	Modify the program or change the program survival status

skills into evaluation skills is to systematize, formalize, and articulate them in the evaluation domain. Although program evaluation is usually applied to total programs, an excellent way to begin to develop confidence as an evaluator is to practice evaluation skills on individual clients.

A MODEL OF PROGRAM EVALUATION FOR HEALTH-CARE PRACTITIONERS

In this chapter, program evaluation is defined broadly as a process that begins with problem identification, proceeds with goal setting and program implementation, and then ends with a determination of the extent to which the problem has been addressed by the intervention. In the case of formative evaluation, the evaluation efforts continue as an ongoing process. However, from the summative perspective, evaluation occurs at the termination of an agreed-upon time frame and determines the continuation status of a program.

Ideally, the sequence of program evaluation suggested in this chapter remains consistent regardless of purpose. Don't forget, however, that the practitioner may not be able to conduct all evaluation activities in this sequence, but he or she should attempt to formally identify the problem, needs, and goals that preceded implementation of the program (even if the program is already in existence). For example, if the practitioner is hired to work in an adolescent drug abuse unit in which drug abuse prevention programs have already been established, the evaluation does not begin with a problem statement. However, in order to determine whether the program is ameliorating the problem to which it is aimed, the nature of the problem must be known. Because so many health-care programs

Problem statement ◄─── Need ◄─── Goals ◄─── Implementation ◄─── Assessment

Figure 29-2. Model sequence of program evaluation.

are not preceded by systematic problem identification, it is therefore not uncommon to create an ex-post facto problem statement, one that is formulated after the program is already operational, and to then subsequently recreate the steps that should have preceded the implementation of the program. In the drug abuse unit discussed earlier, the practitioner, attempting to clarify the problem that the program addresses, may seek information from program staff, patients, and literature to develop a problem statement. If the problem seems to be that adolescents abuse drugs as a function of peer pressure, but the prevention is intended to teach adolescents about the consequences of drug abuse, the practitioner may suggest alternative programs to respond to the problem.

Thus, a sound program evaluation, without regard to where the practitioner enters the program implementation process, begins with a clear and carefully articulated problem statement. All subsequent evaluation activities refer back to the problem statement. In other words, the problem statement is the foundation on which each subsequent step in program development and evaluation is anchored. Following the problem statement, four steps then take place: need statement, goal setting, program planning and implementation, and assessment (Fig. 29-2).

Before delving into the sequence and skills involved in implementing an evaluation, three case examples illustrating different styles of program evaluation that use the aforementioned sequence of evaluation activity are discussed.

BACK INJURY PREVENTION PROGRAM

A local manufacturing plant has contacted a rehabilitation team to design a back injury prevention program for employees. The manager of the plant has observed that workers seem to incur a disproportionate amount of injury during the summer.

Case 1: Rehabilitation team 1 was contracted to develop and implement an injury prevention program. As experts in "back school" provision, the rehabilitation team entered the manufacturing plant and observed the manufacturing per-

sonnel performing their work tasks. They observed that, although the workers performed their tasks in a speedy manner, the majority were using poor body mechanics and conservation techniques. They also interviewed management, who believed that many of the workers malingered in order to have paid vacation in the summer. Thus, their data analysis revealed that:

1. The workers did not use correct body mechanics in their jobs.
2. Increase in injury in the summer was a result of malingering.

Based on these data, the rehabilitation team suggested that the problem was two-fold. The workers did not know proper body mechanics, and they did not have sufficient time off work in the summer. A back school program was needed as well as a modification of vacation schedule. The program goals that they suggested were:

1. To teach proper body mechanics to the manufacturing personnel, and
2. To provide more vacation in the summer in order to reduce malingering.

The rehabilitation team therefore implemented a prevention program in which workers were tested for proper body mechanics, were educated about proper body mechanics and conservation techniques, and were then retested in their work environments to ensure that they knew how to use these techniques effectively. In addition, the rehabilitation team suggested that management examine the vacation policy and offer summer vacation to the cohort of workers who tended to exhibit disproportionate injury during the summer. Summative assessment was then accomplished to ascertain the workers' level of knowledge and use of proper body mechanics and the incidence of injury in June, July, and August following the implementation of the program. Data were collected by the management of the manufacturing firm. Each worker was observed in a task, before and after the educational component of the program, and was scored on his or her demonstration of proper body mechanics. Additional data were collected from personnel records about the incidence of injury. Final data analysis was done to determine if there was a relationship between injury and retest score on the body mechanics test. Analysis revealed no significant change in scores on the retest, no change in incidence of back injury during the summer, and no significant relationship between retest scores and incidence of injury. In addition, the management found that summer vacations decreased and that summer earnings for employees increased. The program was considered a failure, and the rehabilitation team was fired.

Case 2: The manufacturing firm then hired rehabilitation team 2 to implement a back injury program. The first step in their evaluation was the development of a clear understanding of the problem. The team selected three data collection methods: systematic observation; formal, scheduled interview; and document review to answer the following questions:

1. What is the nature of the problem?
2. Why is it occurring?
3. How is it occurring?

In order to answer these questions, the rehabilitation team conducted systematic observations of the work area during the month of May, randomly selected and interviewed a sample of informants representing all levels of employment and management, and reviewed health and personnel records. Their data analysis revealed that:

1. Employees worked in an environment in which using proper body mechanics during lifting tasks would slow the work.
2. Most employees were aware of how to use proper body mechanics because they had either had training or prior experience.
3. During the summer, overtime pay was available to manufacturing employees.
4. Most employees who sustained low back injuries attempted to return to their jobs as soon as possible.
5. Management staff believed that manufacturing employees injured themselves in order to have the summer off work.

These findings led to a problem definition that targeted the area of need at the management level.

Just take a moment and think about the essential nature of being comprehensive in this first step, particularly in light of the failure of the program initiated by team 1. The traditional back injury prevention program, implemented by the first rehabilitation team, did not work because the problem did not lie with the workers. If the first team had conducted a broader and more complete problem assessment, they might not have established the program goals and the subsequent program.

As a result of the problem statement, the second rehabilitation team set the following programmatic goals:

1. Engage management in observing their employees on the job as a basis to improve management understanding of the problem
2. Review the environmental barriers, including human and nonhuman barriers to using proper body mechanics
3. Structure the environment so that the use of proper body mechanics is rewarded.

The program implemented by rehabilitation team 2 began with videotaping the workers on the job. They were also interviewed on videotape about the reasons why they accomplished their tasks in the way that they did. The second step in the program was a series of meetings with management to modify the reward system and the environment so that speed could be maintained with proper body mechanics. By the end of the program, the environment was altered so that proper body mechanics had to be used. For example, heavy loads were placed at different heights and the position of loading platforms was changed to facilitate proper handling of heavy weights. Second, the reward system was modified to reinforce speed and proper motion. An employee of the week who exhibited exemplary safety behavior was selected by a foreman. This employee was chosen from the group who performed above a chosen speed threshold. However, the fastest individual speed was not a consideration. Thus, rewards encouraged safe speed for the entire work group, not competition for the fastest individual at any cost.

The final assessment of the project was directed at ascertaining whether or not the environmental and reinforcement changes allowed for the use of proper body mechanics with speed, whether body mechanics improved while speed was more uniformly maintained, and whether the incidence of back injury significantly decreased in the summer after the implementation of the program. Data collection on the first variable was accomplished by random observation and rating of the work environment to describe the behaviors and speed of the workers. Speed of task completion was charted by a foreman for 3 weeks. The incidence of injury was obtained from personnel records and was reviewed by the management team. The results of the outcome evaluation were positive on all variables. Rehabilitation team 2 was maintained for consultation and periodic re-evaluation of body mechanics, environmental barriers, and prevention in other potential injury areas.

In this scenario, the difference between positive outcome and negative outcome was embedded in the problem definition. Both groups followed a reasonable sequence of program development and evaluation research strategies. However, the foundation of success in evaluation lies in an accurate and complete understanding of the problem. In situations in which programs are already in existence, the luxury of problem clarification is not always an option. However, if outcome findings are unfavorable, then the culprit may not be poor program implementation but may instead be a misunderstanding of the problem to which a program speaks. Rehabilitation team 2 demonstrated a mixture of formative and summative strategies. The team still held the expertise and assessed the outcome of their intervention as a mechanism to determine program survival. However, the assessment of a program by its own developers is more characteristic of the formative approach. In case 3, a formative evaluation example is presented.

Case 3: Using the same manufacturing company, rehabilitation team 3 has been retained to develop and assess the prevention program. Different from teams 1 and 2, team 3 selected a formative evaluation structure. They began with observation of and informal meetings with all levels of employees and management in the manufacturing firm as two methods to define the problem. However, in addition, team 3 asked each employee to render an opinion on what strategies would be most effective in reducing injuries during the summer. Data revealed that:

1. Employees would like to have the opportunity for overtime placed more uniformly throughout the year, because summer incentives come at a time when many employees are also performing heavy lifting around their homes
2. Employees suggested modifications to the work environment that would promote proper body mechanics
3. Middle management suggested that the each work group be assessed for speed as a group rather than as individuals, so that they would regulate themselves as a group and use group pressure to maintain speed and safety
4. The foremen suggested that they should be educated in body mechanics and conservation techniques so that they could train and retrain employees when observing improper body mechanics.

As a result of the formative evaluation model, more worker participation in the process and outcome of the prevention program was elicited and determined as a need. The rehabilitation team was then retained to assist with environmental modification and to do periodic body

mechanics and conservation training with the foremen. Periodic assessment of process, safety behavior, and worker satisfaction by the rehabilitation team occurred frequently and both formally and informally. Findings were used to identify areas for further improvement, not to ascertain whether the rehabilitation team would still have a job.

COMPARISON OF THE THREE PROGRAM EVALUATION STYLES

A comparison of the three styles of program evaluation suggests several important principles. First, the importance of careful and thorough problem definition is critical when planning a program. The example presented in the first scenario clearly demonstrates the pitfalls of assuming which intervention will work without ascertaining the nature and scope of the problem. Unfortunately, the strategy used by rehabilitation team 1 is not unusual, and summative evaluations of programs that are developed in similar manners are often negative. Second, the difference in summative and formative evaluation are demonstrated. Summative evaluation is a cross-sectional rather than a longitudinal view of a program. In other words, summative evaluation is used most effectively when the questions about program effectiveness are time limited. In the third scenario, a formative evaluation was used as a mechanism to change the program to meet the evolving identified problem, not to determine goal accomplishment at one point in time. Furthermore, summative evaluation requires fewer resources. Summative evaluation can therefore take place even with the limited resources that many programs seem to have in the contemporary health-care arena. However, formative evaluation, even though it is lengthy, speaks to the dynamic nature of the relationship between problems and programs. Finally, summative evaluation is aimed at observable outcomes, whereas formative evaluation encompasses a broad spectrum of need and programmatic assessments.

EVALUATION OF EXISTING PROGRAMS

The reader may now be asking questions about evaluating programs that have already been established. Too frequently, rehabilitation professionals do not have the luxury of ascertaining the nature of the problem before developing a program. Although it is always most desirable to begin with problem definition, the program evaluation process can be initiated at any point in the sequence. For example, rehabilitation team 1 could have instituted body mechanics training without obtaining data to define the need. Team 3 could have entered the process after a program was initiated and base the necessary changes on the process and outcome findings in the formative evaluation.

Now that the reader has become familiar with basic distinctions between formative and summative evaluation and with the comparative value, purpose, and application of each, the next section of the chapter should provide a basic foundation for thinking about evaluating prevention and rehabilitation programs.

SEQUENCE OF PROGRAM EVALUATION

Many different models of program evaluation are advanced in the numerous texts and journals that are devoted to the subject. However, there are elements and sequences that are basic to most if not all models. The following model suggests a sequence of evaluation that guides the rehabilitation professional through an ideal evaluation (see Fig. 29–2). Always keep in mind that even though the ideal may not be possible, every effort to systematically develop and assess programs should still be made, no matter where one begins the process. This model works well for both formative and summative evaluative processes.

Problem Statement

The first step in the sequence of program evaluation begins with problem definition. As presented in the aforementioned three vignettes, even when professionals think that they are experts in a particular area, the choice of intervention will be more likely to have a positive outcome if a complete and accurate view of a problem can be advanced. There are many strategies to define problems. *Keep in mind that ultimately, the problem statement itself is the foundation against which program success will be assessed.*

The most common approach to defining problems is to synthesize information from multiple sources into a coherent problem statement. Evaluators use many methods for data collection. First, evaluators often use literature to ascertain the perspectives of others who have been faced

with similar situations. If professionals are relying on theory to frame their programs and evaluations, contemporary literature about the nature, scope, and causes of problems may be included in the problem statement. Data can be obtained from interviews of persons who are directly and indirectly affected by the problem, of those who intervene with the problem, and of those who hold expertise in some aspect of the problem. For example, in the earlier discussion of injury prevention, rehabilitation team 1 sought interview information from management, whereas teams 2 and 3 interviewed the workers and management.

Information can also be obtained through observation and document review. A summative process may rely heavily on observation and interview data that are obtained through standardized measurement. These data form the basis for subsequent evaluation measures. For example, in a head injury prevention program, the baseline incidence of head injury may be the standard against which prevention program success is measured. The desired outcome of a significant reduction in head injury will therefore be measured by the same procedure that was used to establish the baseline in the problem identification.

The formative evaluator may use both qualitative and quantitative strategies to collect data. Rehabilitation team 2 used systematic sampling and observation as well as quantitative review of health and personnel documents to formulate their problem statement and to form the foundation against which to determine program progress. In the example of rehabilitation team 3, the strategies not only involved interview and observation but also included all employees in meetings and suggestions for intervention. The data in their problem statement not only included a view of the problem but also implied that part of the problem may be the "silence" of workers who may have valuable opinions that are not included in the management perspective.

The way in which a problem is stated is very important in the development and evaluation of programs. For example, referring back to the examples, if rehabilitation team 1 had indicated that the problem was the "lack of opportunity to learn body mechanics" rather than "poor body mechanics," they could have evaluated their program on the provision of the opportunity to learn body mechanics rather than the use of good body mechanics in work tasks. Their evaluation would have supported the success of their intervention if the criterion was the provision of the back school for employees. This important concept requires further example. Assume that you are developing a head injury prevention program. From your extensive data collection efforts, you learn that wearing seatbelts in an automobile is one of the most effective means of preventing head injury in an automobile accident. You also learn that teenage boys are most likely to sustain head injuries in automobile accidents. Therefore, your problem statement might look something like:

> Teenage boys, as a result of careless habits such as not wearing seatbelts while driving or riding in a car, sustain a disproportionate amount of head injury as compared to the driving public.

This problem statement implies that intervention should be aimed at encouraging seatbelt use and that evaluation of such an intervention would look only at the numbers of boys who sustain head injuries following the intervention. However, the professionals who are conducting the intervention may have not influenced any change in the incidence of head injury but might have made some change in the boys' awareness of prevention. If success of the program is measured only in terms of head injury reduction, as implied in the problem statement, the valuable intermediate accomplishment of increasing awareness of prevention will not be reflected in success criteria. Furthermore, many variables outside of the control of the program staff could influence the incidence of head injury in a group of teenage boys even if the program impact was positive. Perhaps injury occurred as a result of another driver who did not participate in the intervention and who increased the incidence rates such that no improvement on the outcome measure of reduction of head injury incidence is illustrated. If a summative approach is used to evaluate the extent to which the problem stated earlier is remediated, the narrow definition and subsequent limited evaluation will not be adequate to determine the positive influence of prevention on the targeted population.

A more realistic problem statement, based on the same data set that was used to formulate the first problem statement, which would lend itself to more reasonable evaluation, might be stated as follows:

> Teenage boys who drive or ride in cars are at high risk for head injury.

This type of problem statement creates a broader scope for the problem. For example, an intervention may aim at uncovering the driving habits of teenagers as a basis for education and prevention. The evaluation of such an intervention is not limited to reduction in trauma incidence, which may not be a realistic target for intervention at the time of problem definition.

In summary, the problem statement forms the foundation for any evaluation effort, regardless of where the evaluation begins. The key element in conducting a sound program evaluation is to define a problem in such a manner that realistic goals can be set, accomplished, and demonstrated. Stating a problem so that the goals derived from it are beyond the reach of any intervention program is a common fault of novice evaluators and should be avoided.

The Need

The need statement frames the rationale for the program. Although problem statement and need statement are frequently used interchangeably, it is not advisable. Look what can happen if one defines a problem in terms of a need. One experience that almost everyone has had is the "battle of the bulge." If the problem is defined as "I need to lose weight," only one intervention option is possible—weight loss. The evaluation criterion can only be weight loss with the traditional outcome measure being the scale. We are very disappointed if we do not lose weight. The intervention has failed, and frequently it is abandoned. Think instead of defining the problem not in terms of need but rather something like, "I don't like my weight." The need statement deriving from such a problem could be varied. For example, an individual might need to develop acceptance of his or her body. Another possibility is that the individual needs to exercise. A third need is to diet. This example demonstrates the distinction between the need and the problem as well as the relationship between the two. In health maintenance and prevention, the same principles apply. Return to the example of the head injury prevention effort. If the problem is defined as boys who ride in cars are at high risk for head injury, many needs can be developed. The key to developing an accurate and reasonable need statement is to use literature and data to determine the nature of need based on the initial problem. As in the head injury prevention example, a staff planning a prevention program needs to establish the reason why boys do not wear seatbelts as a basis for implementation of meaningful prevention efforts. In other words, the need for a clinician, administrator, or consultant to conduct evaluation research is the first step in prevention.

The collection and analysis of data to define need is called *needs assessment*. In the needs assessment phase of program evaluation, research skills should be used to determine what questions are asked and how these questions are answered. For example, in the manufacturing plant examples, each team had a different plan for determining need. Rehabilitation team 1 used observation and management staff interviews to determine what type of program was needed, whereas rehabilitation teams 2 and 3 used more inclusive strategies by involving the workers in needs assessment. Rehabilitation team 1 determined that a back school approach was needed, whereas rehabilitation team 2 ascertained that a management-oriented approach was needed. Don't forget that one problem statement may give rise to varied needs statements. It is essential that the need should be clearly related to the problem statement and that it remains realistic. The need statement is the basis from which programmatic goals are extracted.

Goals

Goals form the conceptual guidelines for the program. Based on the need statement, programmatic goals state what the program will accomplish in order to improve the problem by addressing the need. Goals do not state "how" the program will meet the need. Rather, specific objective statements related to each goal delineate program operation. Goals constrain the scope of a program. For example, the goal statement generated by rehabilitation team 3 in the aforementioned example identified worker participation as the need. Goal statements then delineated what types of worker participation would be elicited. In the example of head injury prevention, the need statement led to the goals of conducting a research effort to determine the patterns of seatbelt use in boys who were at risk. From the goal statements, clear objectives can be detailed that guide the implementation of programs. Thus, each step of a program evaluation has been developmental and relies on careful and accurate execution of the previous step.

Implementation

Implementation, as all other steps, is anchored on previous developmental efforts. For each program goal presented in the previous step, objectives that specify how goals will be achieved are stated. (Refer to the other chapters in this book for detailed preventive implementation strategies.) The basic steps of implementation include planning all phases of a program (including cost) through specifying objectives and then operationalizing the objectives. In formative evaluation, program implementation is a process that is consistently monitored. Data collected in the formative process inform future implementation and operation. In the implementation phase, the following six questions are answered:

Who, what, how, where, when, and how much?

Answers to "who" state which personnel will carry out the program. Answers to "what" indicate what personnel will do, including a discussion of who will be served and what the program will include. How the program will be carried out is commonly known as operations and procedures. "Where" specifies not only location but also the design of the environment in which the program will be implemented. "When" delimits time and includes a proposed daily schedule and timeline for objective accomplishment. Finally, "how much" details costs and expected cost/benefit ratio. (A discussion of cost/benefit analysis is beyond the scope of this chapter. Refer to Rossi and Freeman [1989] for a complete discussion of cost setting and assessment.)

A brief example will serve as an illustration. Rehabilitation team 3 operationalized the goal of employee participation through involving foremen in safety promotion. The team determined that they would ask for volunteer foremen who were willing to participate rather than selecting persons without their consent. The team trained the foremen and then, with management, observed the interaction between the foremen and the workers. The goal of employee participation therefore gave rise to the following objectives, among many others:

1. Recruit volunteer foremen—"the who"
2. Train foremen in safety promotion and body mechanics—"the how"
3. Ask foremen to carry out training and safety promotion in the workplace during the daily

routine—"the what, the when, and the where"
4. Request that rehabilitation team and management observe interaction among the foremen and workers as an evaluative measure—"the who, what, and where"
5. Retrain foremen or continue with the current program, depending on the performance of the foremen—"the how much"

Thus, the implementation phase not only specifies how the program will be implemented but is also the phase during which the program is conducted. This phase can be time limited or indefinite, depending on the nature of the program and the purpose and findings of the evaluation.

Assessment

The assessment phase is the determination of program process or outcome. In this phase, systematic inquiry skills are essential to ask evaluative questions and to answer them. The first step in assessment is defining the extent and limit of the assessment. For example, in some cases, only cost analysis is conducted whereas in others, a full assessment of program process and specified outcomes occurs.

The guideline for what and how to assess lies in goal and objective statements. Quantitative strategies primarily measure objective attainment, whereas qualitative investigation more frequently addresses program description and the influence of the program on the problem. Because all elements of a program are based on the problem statement, all assessment either directly or indirectly investigates the extent to which a program addressed the problem.

In general, the sequence of program assessment begins with specific evaluation research questions. These questions address either program outcome or program process. For example, rehabilitation team 3 posed the following assessment questions:

1. To what extent are workers participating in the prevention program?
2. What environmental changes are being made?
3. What periodic body mechanics and conservation activities are foremen conducting with workers?
4. What safety behaviors are being demonstrated by the workers as a result of the prevention program?

5. What level of worker satisfaction is expressed by participants in the prevention program?
6. What changes need to be made to improve the prevention program?

Questions 1 to 3 and 6 are formative questions, and questions 4 and 5 are summative. Thus, questions 1 to 3 and 6 inquire about process and program change, whereas questions 4 and 5 investigate specific outcomes related to the problem statement, needs assessment, and goals.

The next step in assessment is data collection. In order to answer questions 1 to 4, rehabilitation team 3 selected systematic scheduled interview and periodic observation of the workplace as data collection methods. Data collection for questions 5 and 6 occurred through an anonymous closed-ended questionnaire of participating employees for their opinions.

Data analysis follows data collection, which was descriptive for questions 1 to 4. The occurrence of specific tasks was described by the frequency with which each task occurred each day. For questions 5 and 6, responses to the written questionnaire were analyzed by frequencies (the number of times that the same answer was given) and by percentages of responses (the percentage of total answers of each response item) to closed-ended questions.

The final step of assessment is reporting. In the example of team 3, all results were reported in writing to the managers of the manufacturing firm.

In summary, in the assessment phase research techniques are used to obtain and analyze data on program outcome and process. The techniques and scope of assessment are determined by the purpose of program evaluation and by the resources available.

CONCLUSION

This chapter has presented introductory information and examples of program evaluation. In the current health-care arena, program evaluation is becoming more of a necessity than a luxury, both for obtaining and maintaining financial support and for assessing the process and outcome of prevention efforts. Readers are urged to explore program evaluation in more depth as a vehicle for establishing meaningful interventions, improving prevention programs, and demonstrating the value of existing programs.

References

Herman JL, Morris LL, and Fitz-Gibbon CT: Evaluator's Handbook. Newbury Park, CA, Sage, 1987.

Patton MQ: Creative Evaluation, 2nd ed. Newbury Park, CA, Sage, 1987.

Rossi PH and Freeman HE: Evaluation: A Systematic Approach, 4th ed. Newburg Park, CA, 1989.

Bibliography

Alters C and Evens W: Evaluating Your Practice: A Guide to Self-Assessment. New York, Springer, 1990.

Bloom M and Fischer J: Evaluating Practice: Guidelines for the Accountable Professional. Englewood Cliffs, Prentice-Hall, 1982.

Currier DP: Elements of Research in Physical Therapy. Baltimore, Williams & Wilkins, 1984.

Fitz-Gibbon CT and Morris LL: How to Design a Program Evaluation. Newbury Park, CA, Sage, 1987.

Fuhrer MJ: Rehabilitation Outcomes: Analysis and Measurement. Baltimore, Brookes, 1987.

Herman PH and Freeman HE: Evaluation: A systematic approach. Newbury Park, CA, Sage, 1989.

Isaac S and Michael WB: Handbook in Research and Evaluation, 2nd ed. San Diego, EDITS, 1981.

King JA, Morris LL, and Fitz-Gibbon CT: How to Assess Program Implementation. Newbury Park, CA, Sage, 1987.

Ostrow, PC, Williamson JW, and Joe BE: Quality Assurance Primer. Silver Springs, MD, AOTA, 1984.

Ottenbacher KJ: Evaluating Clinical Change: Strategies for Occupational and Physical Therapists. Baltimore, Williams & Wilkins, 1986.

Pilcher DM: Data Analysis for the Helping Professions: A Practical Guide. Newbury Park, CA, Sage, 1990.

Schaefer M: Designing and Implementing Procedures for Health and Human Services. Newbury Park, CA, Sage, 1985.

Trochim WM: Research Design for Program Evaluation: The Regression-Discontinuity Approach. Newbury Park, CA, Sage, 1984.

CHAPTER

30

Ernest A. Burch, Jr.
Quinten M. Davis

Marketing, Health Promotion, and Injury Prevention Programs

As people use health care more and more each year, its total cost increases dramatically. In analyzing these escalating costs, people discovered that prevention was much more effective than rehabilitation. Historically, prevention was tied to community health. The most obvious example of early prevention activities was the institution of inoculation programs to stop the spread of diseases and ultimately to prevent them.

Society has applied the concepts learned in these disease prevention programs to the prevention of acute injury and trauma in the workplace. In disease, prevention practitioners looked for the etiologic factors of the disease and then worked to eliminate them. This is basically the same tactic that is applied to trauma in injury prevention; the initial step taken in industrial injury prevention initially focused on jobs that required brute strength and had a high incidence of injury.

Today practitioners are also analyzing jobs that consist of repetitive tasks which are causing injury and trauma. In addition, prevention programs have sought to modify behaviors that led to disease (e.g., smoking, excessive eating). Agencies have developed smoke cessation, weight loss, and fitness programs. In the same manner, industrial prevention programs also seek to modify the worker's behavior that may have contributed to the industrial injury.

In light of the evolution of health care programs designed to promote health and prevent injury, marketing tactics must be modified. This chapter provides an overview of general marketing concepts, aspects of the prevention industry that have an impact on marketing and respective marketing programs effective for each component of the prevention industry. At the conclusion of this chapter, readers should be able to objectively analyze their current marketing strategies and potential prevention population, and to modify their marketing plans to successfully reach this emerging and expanding population.

THE NEED FOR PREVENTION PROGRAMS

Health care reimbursement programs have been challenged by the high cost of technology, increasing numbers of surviving trauma and congenital dysfunction cases, and a growing elderly population. Federal health programs are being overwhelmed today by an aging population as evidenced by the fiscal problems of the Medicare and Medicaid programs. State Workman's Com-

488

pensation programs are taxed today by the increasing numbers of injured workers who expect treatment.

The need for preventive programs is obvious, especially in the workplace. Keckley, a noted health care/market research and analysis expert, stated: "Each year approximately 0.5% of employed persons receive injury or illness that will keep them off the job for at least five months." He also stated that only 48% of severely disabled workers ever return to work (Keckley, 1987). While all companies suffer when employees are injured, the self-insured in particular feel the loss of every dollar spent to treat an injury. As Oldner, U.S. Area Safety Director for self-insured Dow Chemical Corporation said: "Safety must be monitored every day. It is not something that can be done sporadically and then forgotten for awhile. With the average cost of employee injury approaching $30,000, and I think that this is probably underestimated, it is obviously important from both human and financial standpoints to be certain that the work is safe." Oldner's corporation considers injury prevention so vital that his department does not have a budget. They do not keep track of their expenditures. They just do whatever it takes to get the job done safely. Oldner goes on to say, "Rehabilitation personnel must now become educators rather than just the treatment specialists that they have traditionally been in the past" (Keyes, 1990). Thus, OTs and PTs must seize this opportunity to expand their services to individuals in need.

HEALTH CARE PROVIDERS AND MARKETING

To institute a prevention program, someone must be convinced in the executive level that prevention is worth the expense on a long-term basis. The process of convincing is actually a selling or marketing activity.

Marketing, as a selling or convincing process, has been with us since the beginning of time. Various components of the process occur whenever an individual or group of individuals possesses something that someone else needs or wants. New health programs, professions, and competition have brought an increased awareness of marketing to all health care providers. Increased awareness among the general public and increased competition for a given patient in

light of cost-containment efforts by insurance carriers have all made medical practitioners more likely to apply marketing techniques to create a stable patient population.

Often, health-care providers are hesitant to admit that marketing is a vital and worthwhile component of today's practice. Perhaps this is due to a misunderstanding of the term "marketing" or perhaps it is marketing's negative connotation.

An operational definition of marketing is that it is the process of identifying the needs and wants of a given individual or populations and designing and implementing a mechanism to meet those needs. It is the most basic function of any business; in the words of management expert Peter Drucker, "Marketing is so basic that it cannot be considered a separate function. It is the whole business as seen from the standpoint of its final result, that is, from the customer's point of view" (Drucker, 1973).

THE "FOUR P'S" OF MARKETING

Most marketing theory is based on a marketing mix or a set of controllable variables to influence consumer behavior. One of the most popular means of classifying these variables is called the "Four P's," specifically: product, place, promotion, and price (McCarthy, 1971).

With regard to educating in disease and injury prevention, there are several possibilities of how those "Four P's" can be applied.

Product

The product as stated is the service of educating clients in disease and injury prevention. However, there are various methods by which this product could be designed:

1. Is this education meant to be a "one-shot deal" or is it meant to be given over a series of sessions?
2. Do you include written materials with this education program?
3. Is the material presented in the form of a lecture, film, or slides?
4. Is a guarantee going to be offered to the user regarding the benefits of this program as exemplified by a decrease in worker's compensation claims made or money spent?
5. What kind of follow-up service will be given?

Place

This variable speaks to the process through which the product will be delivered to the consumer. A few pertinent questions would be:

1. Will these services be marketed directly to the client or to some "middleman" who will in turn encourage the worker to participate? In other words, would a person be taught to return to work in an industry preventative program?
2. Will these services be at a medical office or some other location?
3. Geographically, how large a territory will the program cover?

Price

Pricing a product determines the product's profit-generating feature and its attractiveness to the consumer. Price should be demand-oriented and consumer-sensitive rather than cost-sensitive and competitor-sensitive (reactive pricing to meet or undercut competitor pricing). The price of a prevention program should be based on the following items:

1. Pricing objectives—is the program being sold to generate income, to market the corporation, or to break even as a goodwill effort?
2. Price influences—the program should consider the consumer, competitor, legal constraints (Worker's Compensation regulations), and the general economy as environmental factors. Cost of program development and implementation and corporate policies and strategic plans are internal factors of price influence.
3. Pricing strategy—developed based on price objective and influences.
4. Price levels—cost, competition, and demand analysis determine price level of the program and is modified in response to consumer reactions. Even after the price of the prevention program is set, based on the aforementioned components, the physical therapist must be willing to adjust the price in accordance with changes in the price objectives or price influences over time. However, the therapist should only modify the price in response to factors within predetermined limits. These limits may be determined by the cost of pro-

gram delivery, staff availability, or shifting environmental and economic factors.

Promotion

This component of marketing is the process by which potential customers will be made aware of the health prevention service. Generally, promotion consists of four separate components: personal selling, sales promotion, advertising, and publicity. Personal selling is imparted when, one on one, an individual directly attempts to inform another individual of the health prevention program. Sales promotion is informing a large population about your product. Advertising is a paid presentation of your product, which uses a visual or audio media. The key to effective advertising is to gear the promotion toward your target population. For example, a physical therapist may advertise his or her services only to primary care providers who offer wellness programs to the employers, the insurance carriers, unions or organized employee groups, or the employees themselves. The cost of these components of the promotion vary, depending on the mode of communication selected and on the extent of the population.

In contrast, publicity is the process of informing the potential customer at no cost. The advantage of publicity is that your target market often accepts this information more readily owing to the mode of communication (i.e., television or the newspaper). Because by definition this exposure is at no expense, it is often perceived as information that is being reported by the source rather than intentionally placed or distributed by the subject of the promotion. Since it does not cost the marketer, one can target a larger population than is usually identified in a market process, which could be very expensive.

A therapist who offers an injury prevention program could speak with a local newspaper about writing an article on him or her for the health section of that newspaper. This article will be read by potential consumers who will perceive it as a news report rather than as self promotion. Publicity is a form of promotion that is vastly underutilized by small medical practices today.

MARKETING PLAN: CONSIDERING THE TARGET POPULATION

To effectively market a health prevention program, the practitioner must begin with a marketing plan. When attempting to develop a marketing plan, one must begin with a basic philosophy of marketing. This process is necessary irrespective of the product that is being offered. The marketing philosophy involves initially identifying the needs of the available consumer group and then developing mechanisms to meet those needs as they apply to the specific product offered. The importance of this philosophy cannot be overstated. It is vital that the therapist first consider the consumer:

1. Who is the consumer—the user, the end-user, or a middleman?
2. How would the consumer utilize this service?
3. How does the consumer want this service to be delivered?
4. Where does the consumer prefer to utilize this service?
5. Who makes the purchase decision?
6. Does the consumer understand the product, or is education necessary?

We can refer to this approach as "defining the target population."

One example of a target population is recently injured workers in the hospital. With this population, the practitioner is primarily dealing with the etiologic factors of the injury, the hows and whys, and the mode of the injury. Compliance usually comes quite easily to the inpatient population, because the trauma is recent and the symptoms are acute. Treatment and general activity are maximally controlled by the care giver. Multiple instructional prevention approaches can be focused on inpatients who are essentially a captive audience. Techniques that may be used on inpatients include video instructions, group sessions, or private consultations. There is also perhaps the intervention of the family who, also, are at their peak motivational level in their desire to get the family member out of the hospital and back home.

The prevention focus for an outpatient target population is more on the practical modification of the lifestyle and activities of daily living as physical capabilities return. The outpatient is likely to be less focused than the inpatient because of home distractions, but he or she probably still wants to return to work. Properly designed group therapy sessions are usually very effective with this type of client, because the clients motivate each other.

Long-term client is the most difficult to instruct in prevention, primarily because the worker has the tendency to fall back on his or her old patterns of behavior. The worker must be given the motivation to alter work habits and daily activities. Work site evaluations are extremely valuable at this point to ensure restructuring the job and environment. Job safety evaluation and specific task analysis are critical components in prevention of re-injury. Client cooperation in this phase is also important, but the long-term program of effectiveness really depends on compliance in the inpatient and outpatient phases of the prevention programming.

Another target population to consider is the employer-consumer. An effective approach to this target population is to emphasize the potential cost savings to the employer who would adopt an injury prevention program.

Understanding marketing philosophy guides the therapist toward successfully addressing each component of marketing. These components determine how readily your service will be purchased and utilized by the targeted consumer.

Another approach to marketing would be to address the product itself, the prevention program. *Product concept* assumes that if a product is of good quality and reasonably priced, consumers will respond favorably. This approach assumes that consumers understand the product well enough to make decisions based on quality. More important, this approach does not consider if the product solves a particular problem or fulfills a particular need. Therefore, one should decide if the product designed is appropriate to fulfill the consumer's need. If this is accomplished, the consumer can then effectively appraise the product's quality.

All marketing must begin with the consumer rather than with the service that is to be offered. By taking a consumer-oriented approach, the marketing program is matched to the specific characteristics and tends to be more efficient and has a greater opportunity to be effective, whereas a program oriented to the product could more easily fail and not communicate well with the consumer.

Another commonly utilized approach is *the selling philosophy*, which assumes that consumers will purchase a particular product or service if the appropriate amount of selling and promotional efforts are used. This assumes that consumers can be persuaded to make a purchase through various selling or promotional techniques. The obvious flaw in this philosophy is that the needs of the consumer are not taken into consideration. It assumes that the role of the service provider is to simply sell the product rather than to fill a particular need. It also assumes that consumer choice is directly proportional to the cost and effort of the marketing activity. Even if this approach did work in the short term, few repeat sales would be generated because the product has not been designed to meet a particular consumer need.

One cannot overemphasize the importance of therapists buying into the marketing philosophy as he or she attempts to provide education in disease and injury prevention programs. A logical and systematic approach to market the provisions of these services will result in a very successful practice. The days of medical providers simply hanging out a shingle and waiting for the patients to herd into their office are long gone.

MARKETING TECHNIQUES

In-Patient Marketing. For the inpatient, you would market directly to the hospital or their specialty clinic. The marketing is done with two potential options. One option is to sell the whole package so that the hospital or clinic staff can do it or to sell yourself or your program so that you will get the contract to provide all of the services.

When selling the whole package, you will be expected to educate the staff that is assigned to the hospital. In order for the package to be effective, you must plan to have an ongoing instruction program for the staffing changes plus a constant updating of the subject matter being taught. If this policy is not adhered to, the program will inevitably and absolutely fail. The failure could occur by no more than being watered down by slight errors that compound themselves over time, especially if the hospital staff proceeds to instruct new staff members assigned to the program. The other more obvious cause of failure would be neglecting program modifications essential to meet the needs of a changing patient population (i.e., from a lifting [back injury] clientele to a high materials handling [carpal tunnel] industry).

Two ideas come to mind regarding marketing to hospitals that may be valuable for obtaining a contract. One idea is to have slides, videos, brochures, handouts, and so forth for the population that the hospital would be most likely to

see. Second, you perhaps would want to do your own program on an injury entity on which you can do the very best job of selling yourself. In short, impress them! A portion of this presentation should be a video of you or your staff actually interacting with patients. The diverse audience that you will be addressing, such as the hospital administrator or his or her assistant, nurses, doctors, the comptroller, the rehabilitative staff, and so forth, can all assess your ability as a possible value to their program. They must be made to perceive the cost effectiveness of your program.

Outpatient Marketing. The outpatient tends to identify with his or her own environment. You must be able to specifically focus on the injured worker's job as it relates to the injury. You are selling to the employer now and also to the worker, perhaps on an equal basis. The worker has motivation. He or she wants to get better and stronger. The employer has motivation. His thrust is, "Don't let him, the worker, back until he is 100% cured."

Long-Term Marketing. You are now selling worksite and job analysis. You are selling prevention of injury to the employer. The employer has the cost containment of the market place to contend with also. The job site evaluation and analysis must not only help to prevent injuries but must also be acceptable to work on a production line, or your ideas may not be embraced. You cannot, generally, sell just an injury prevention program. The workers may not even be interested in just injury prevention if they are working on a production line with their paychecks calculated on a payment for a piecework type of job. If your program causes them to have a reduction in pay (even though they are potentially safer and will not have as great a probability of being hurt), they will most likely not be compliant.

Prevention Marketing. The individual must be marketed all the way through the program to ensure that he or she understands the importance of compliance. You may be able to elicit compliance by eliminating the stigma of the previous injury and by enabling the client to demonstrate the ability to function now in a full capacity. You cannot omit prevention if you expect to demonstrate lower cost to the employer.

Marketing Pre-Employment Screening. It is very important to convince the union that pre-employment screening is not a job-eliminating process. You must demonstrate that you are finding jobs that are safe for potential employees, not that you are eliminating any jobs. You must convince the employers that it works and that you are saving them money. You must convince the individual that it is for his or her own good. The pre-employment screening workers must be tested, not only for strength but also for endurance, agility, and dexterity.

STEP-BY-STEP MARKETING STRATEGY

The therapist's prevention marketing strategy is a step-by-step approach to market analysis, goal setting and action planning. This approach is presented schematically in Figure 30–1 (Cottler, 1976).

The first step in this process is for the physical and. occupational therapist to identify market opportunities. In the area of education program and injury prevention, the sources of these market opportunities are varied: employees, medical practitioners, insurance carriers, local health clubs, local schools, or even senior citizen organizations. The therapist should ask himself or herself, what groups of people are interested in maintaining their health. This may even expand the market opportunities beyond traditional sources.

Once the opportunities are analyzed and selected, the therapist should develop his or her set of objectives. These objectives will vary depending on the specific identified market and should be stated in objective, measurable terms. His or her objectives should be quantitative and realistic. They must be compatible and should not be mutually exclusive. Once the objectives have been identified, the therapist will be better

able to move to the next phrase, which is developing marketing strategy.

Marketing strategy is the process by which the therapist will define the prevention product, the market, and the means by which this product will be delivered to potential consumers.

Market Segmentation. The first step in developing marketing strategy is the marketing segmentation. This is the process of segregating the various components of the entire market according to specific characteristics. Because different marketing techniques could be utilized for different segments of the market, the technique of separating the entire market into smaller groups is the logical effective means of developing and implementing this strategy.

Markets can be segmented according to many demographic characteristics: geography, age of the consumer, sex, socioeconomic status, and so forth. In attempting to segment the market, the provider should use his or her imagination and expertise and professional network in the area to identify the groups of significant size to which he or she has access.

Separate marketing strategies can be used to market prevention programs to younger individuals in organizations such as health clubs, sports teams, and local schools. On the other hand, an entirely different program could be developed to market these services to members of senior citizen's groups and to residents in retirement communities.

The end-user strategy calls for identifying different individuals or groups who will utilize the product in different manners, or at different levels (direct and indirect). Basically, by this approach we could market these services through "middlemen." Insurance carriers might be a very logical choice. These programs can be marketed through group health insurance carriers, work-

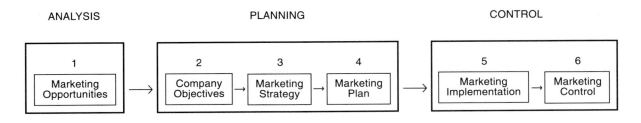

STRATEGIC MARKETING PROCESS

Figure 30–1. Strategic marketing process. (Adapted from Drucker PF: Management: Tasks, Responsibilities, Practices. New York, Harper & Row, 1973.)

ers' compensation, insurance carriers, and even HMOs. All those groups have a vested interest in keeping their members healthy and in avoiding and preventing medical problems.

One other group that might fall into this category could be the primary care physician. Although different from the groups mentioned earlier, they do share similar interests in keeping their patients healthy. In this situation, the services would not necessarily be marketed to the patient who would actually participate in the program but to the physician or to someone on his or her staff, who would in turn sell the idea to the patient along with its benefits.

Creative and imaginative methods of segmenting the market can actually help to identify new characteristics to subdivide the target group to even smaller segments of the population. This enables the practitioner to apply very specific marketing techniques that consider the subgroup's unique characteristics and increase the successful potential of the marketing plan.

No idea should be dismissed without careful consideration and thought. Creative market segmentation has led to certain products being offered in new and different ways. For example, pharmaceutical manufacturing companies now advertise directly to the patient through the media. Ten years ago, this practice was unheard of. By segmenting the market among physicians who prescribe the medication and among the patients who use it, an entirely new marketing strategy has been developed. The keys to this component of the marketing strategy are imagination and creativity.

Once the market has been segmented, a decision must be made with regard to whether the therapist intends to provide services for one segment of the market or to many different segments. This decision must be based on the available resources.

Incorporating the "Ps." The next phase of marketing involves the "Four Ps" of marketing: product, place, promotion, and price. These variables are manipulated as part of the organization's "marketing mix." The various combinations depend on the market segment that you wish to capture.

Because segmentation by age requires a program designed differently for younger individuals than for older individuals, the place or the manner in which services are distributed will also be affected. Promotion activities and adjustments in price may also be required. The key in

utilizing the "Four Ps" is to adjust them specifically by addressing the market characteristics that you are targeting.

Client Compliance. In addition to marketing strategy, the practitioner must consider the compliance of the patient or program participant to ensure program success. Hebert, a physical therapist, lists five items that successful (back school) prevention programs must contain. These five factors can be adapted to fit into any program to develop patient compliance. The five factors as listed by Hebert are:

1. Address *all* risk factors (not just materials-handling risks) emphasis—mine.
2. Be taught by a valid expert (in the eyes of the workers).
3. Teach current injury avoidance techniques.
4. Include actual practice of techniques.
5. Choose a program specifically designed to fit the needs of workers.

Summary. Keeping these factors in mind, the rehabilitation program is not only a means of treatment, but it is also a preventative program which should be embraced by the employer because it can potentially eliminate the significant expenses associated with employee re-injury.

SALES AND MARKET TARGETS

There are many sophisticated mechanisms for developing sales goals, quotas, or market targets. A great deal of information can be found in any business school library in various marketing tests. A unique approach for therapists marketing prevention programs is to look beyond focusing on specific sales goals. The therapist should determine the most efficient sales approach to sell the prevention program. The approach in turn will determine the individuals in the potential market population who should be contacted. The practitioner can set a goal for the number of "quality contacts" to be made in a particular period of time. The ratio of "new sales" to "quality contacts" is developed through experience (i.e., how many contacts must be made to sign a potential client or facility). Because most practitioners do not market on a full-time basis, the therapist must project the number of contacts to be made over a longer time span. It is probably that the therapist would realize the necessity to employ a full-time marketing person simply because of the marketing requirement and the cost effectiveness. If personal selling is found to be the most effective means, effort should go into developing quality sales, staff person(s), and presentation. Once this has been done, analyze the amount of new sales desired and then translate this information into the number of sales contacts necessary to achieve the desired results. This can ultimately be translated into the amount of time necessary to perform the designed amount of sales calls to achieve the desired results.

Product Life Cycle

Once the population target has been identified and targeted, the product and its life cycle must be addressed. The product life cycle, a basic marketing concept, is illustrated in Figure 30–2 (Cox, 1967).

Introduction is a period of relatively slow growth—the time when the product has just been introduced into the market. Profits are usually very low during this period, generally attributable to the high start of costs. During the growth phase, the product becomes more acceptable in the marketplace, which results in the substantial improvements in profit. The third phase, maturity, is one in which growth starts to slow and in which the market becomes saturated. Profits reach a maximum level during this phase, which is also characterized by increased costs. Competition, a byproduct of any success, is also now occurring. Lastly, the decline is one in which sales and profits begin to decrease.

The provision of programs for educating in disease and injury prevention are still in the introduction phases of the life cycle. This is characterized by an unwillingness on the part of the employer or the employees as well as the insurance carriers to accept the benefits of these programs. However, it is probably shifting to the end of the introduction stage due to an increased awareness of the general public on health issues in general and the physical fitness boom that the United States experienced in the late 1980s. This means that the market should be ripe for injury prevention and rehabilitation programs. Typically, when a new product appears, it first has to overcome resistance to the current purchasing patterns. This is certainly the case with regard to these programs. Consumers, especially the insurers, are not used to paying for prevention.

Therefore, the strategy utilized should be to stimulate interest and awareness. This requires a high-profile promotion strategy, which can be costly. Many marketers believe that during the introductory phase, a particular group of consumers should be targeted. These individuals are considered to be leaders of innovators who are not afraid to try new and different ideas and products. Although rehabilitation is an accepted entity, injury prevention is probably only at the latter of the introductory phase.

Nevertheless, promotional programs to get industry to try this idea could be effective at this stage. The market is very price-sensitive at this stage despite limited competition. Marketing strategy that sells the benefit to your marketing group should be effective. Remember, the eco-

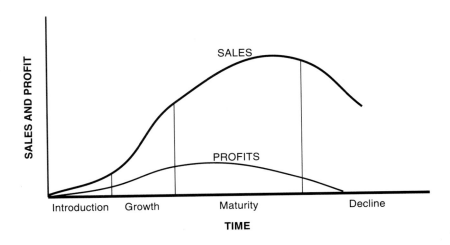

Figure 30–2. A graph of the product life cycle. (From Kotler P: Marketing Management: Analysis, Planning, Implementation and Control. Englewood Cliffs, NJ, Prentice-Hall, 1976, p. 350.)

nomic benefit must be demonstrated to the group to whom you are marketing rather than to the patient participating in the program. For example, if these services are being marketed to an HMO, the benefits of utilizing the program that the HMO would experience through lower utilization, therefore, higher profits must be highlighted. This is very different from marketing the health benefits that the patient will receive.

As long as prevention programs are in the late introduction stage, providers should concentrate on three areas. First, the targeted segments must be educated about this relatively unknown product and the benefits. Second, various techniques should be used to induce potential customers to try this product. The providers of the service must diligently work to secure a unique and loyal distribution mechanism(s). This is important, because as the product grows in acceptance, so will the competition. The more securely any particular provider is linked to the distributor of the prevention program, the better he or she will be to fend off potential competitors and to maintain a successful market position in health-care prevention programming.

SUMMARY

To contain costs, the health-care industry continues to attempt to reduce utilization of health services and at the same time reduce the costs of these services. Programs of health promotion and injury prevention address the first cost containment approach; while work hardening and return to work rehabilitation programs address the latter by specifically reconditioning workers in short-term individual therapeutic programs. Despite the obvious advantages of these two approaches, providers of these services must actively market to inform the employer and the worker to utilize these programs. It is difficult to convince an employer that it is prudent to spend money on health promotion or injury prevention programs to save money at a time when they are cutting back on actual health care expenses. It is equally difficult to convince an injured worker that "a bad back is not always a bad back" and that they can safely return to work in a reasonable time period following physical conditioning and minor job or task modification. Therefore, to be a successful provider of health promotion and industry prevention programs, the practitioner must be a comprehensive investigator and analyzer of the product, the environment, and consumer; a powerful salesperson to make the consumers aware of the product and willing to use the product; and, last but certainly not least, an effective practitioner to implement the service as promised.

References

Kotler P: Marketing Management: Analysis, Planning, Implementation and Control. Englewood Cliffs, NJ, Prentice-Hall, 1976.

Drucker P: Management: Tasks, Responsibilities, Practices. New York, Harper & Row, 1973.

Hebert LA: A change of place. Clin Management 8(6):6, 1988.

Keckley P: Health care market research. October 26, 1987.

Keyes K: Reducing liability costs. Rehab Management May 1990.

McCarthy EJ: Basic Marketing: A Managerial Approach. Homewood, IL, Irwin, Inc, 1971.

Bibliography

Anderson GBJ: Epidemiologic aspects on low-back in industry. Spine Vol. 6, No 1. January-February, 1981.

Assael H: Marketing Management. Boston, Kent Publishing Co, 1985.

Isernhagen SJ: Work Injury. Rockville, MD, Aspen Publishers, Inc, 1988.

Key GL: Industrial PT: An Introduction: Orthopaedic and Sports PT, 2nd ed. CV Mosby, 1990.

Leiter P and Jacobson S: Sound marketing. Rehab Management 3(7):37–40, 1990.

MacStravic RES: Managing Health Care: Marketing Communications. Rockville, MD, Aspen Systems Corporation, 1986.

Reibstein DJ: Marketing Concepts: Strategies and Decisions. Englewood Cliffs, NJ, Prentice-Hall, 1985.

Washington Business Group: An employer's guide to obtaining physical therapy services. Healthcare Management and PT, March 1988.

INDEX

Note: Page numbers in italics refer to illustrations; page numbers followed by t refer to tables.

497